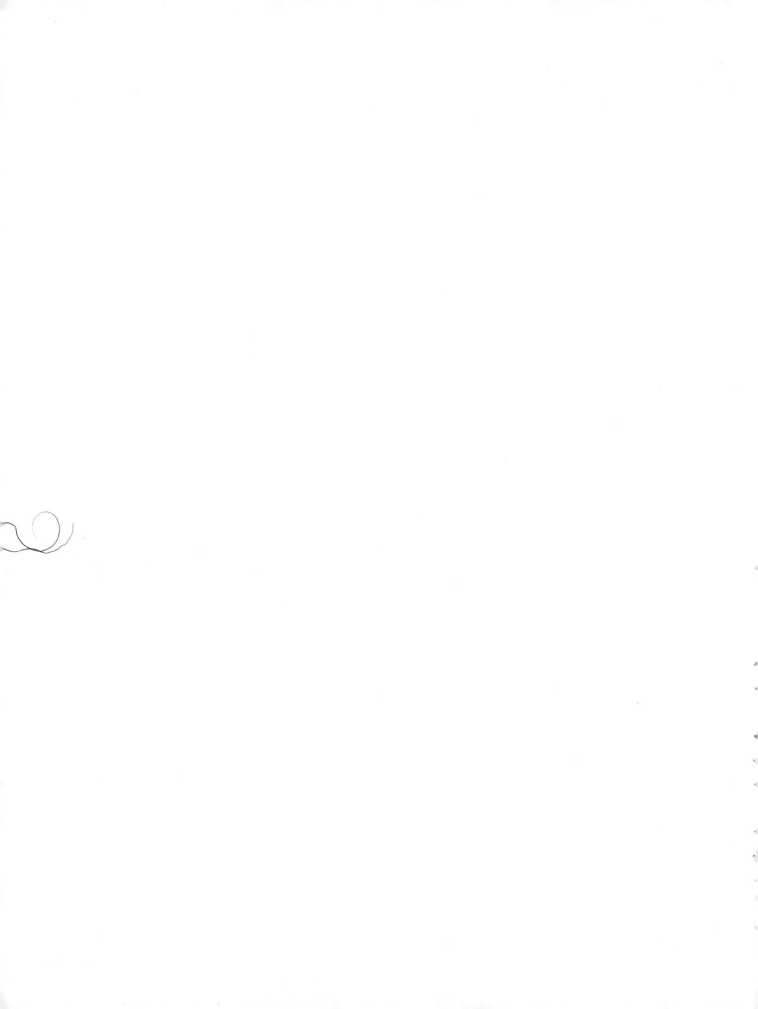

The Food and Nutrition Board of the National Academy of Sciences determines recommended nutrient intakes that apply to healthy individuals. Beginning in 1997, the Food and Nutrition Board (with the involvement of Health Canada) began releasing updated recommendations under a new framework called the Dietary Reference Intakes (DRI). In these revisions, target intake levels for healthy individuals in the U.S. and Canada are listed as either Adequate Intake (AI) levels or Recommended Dietary Allowances (RDA). Also, the DRI values include a set of Tolerable Upper Intake Levels (UL) which are levels of nutrient intake that should not be exceeded due to the potential for adverse effects from excessive consumption.

Dietary Reference Intakes (DRI)

Life stage group	Vitamin A (μg/d)[1]	Vitamin D (μg/d)[2]	Vitamin E (mg/d)[3]	Vitamin K (μg/d)	Thiamin (mg/d)	Riboflavin (mg/d)	Niacin (mg/d)[4]	Pantothenic Acid (mg/d)	Biotin (μg/d)	Vitamin B$_6$ (mg/d)	Folate (μg/d)[5]	Vitamin B$_{12}$ (μg/d)	Vitamin C (mg/d)	Choline (mg/d)	Sodium (g/d)
Infants															
0-6 mo	400*	15	4*	2.0*	0.2*	0.3*	2*	1.7*	5*	0.1*	65*	0.4*	40*	125*	0.12*
7-12 mo	500*	15	5*	2.5*	0.3*	0.4*	4*	1.8*	6*	0.3*	80*	0.5*	50*	150*	0.37*
Children															
1-3 y	300	15	6	30*	0.5	0.5	6'	2*	8*	0.5	150	0.9	15	200*	1.0*
4-8 y	400	15	7	55*	0.6	0.6	8	3*	12*	0.6	200	1.2	25	250*	1.2*
Males															
9-13 y	600	15	11	60*	0.9	0.9	12	4*	20*	1.0	300	1.8	45	375*	1.5*
14-18 y	900	15	15	75*	1.2	1.3	16	5*	25*	1.3	400	2.4	75	550*	1.5*
19-30 y	900	15	15	120*	1.2	1.3	16	5*	30*	1.3	400	2.4	90	550*	1.5*
31-50 y	900	15	15	120*	1.2	1.3	16	5*	30*	1.3	400	2.4	90	550*	1.5*
51-70 y	900	15	15	120*	1.2	1.3	16	5*	30*	1.7	400	2.4[7]	90	550*	1.3*
>70 y	900	20	15	120*	1.2	1.3	16	5*	30*	1.7	400	2.4[7]	90	550*	1.2*
Females															
9-13 y	600	15	11	60*	0.9	0.9	12	4*	20*	1.0	300	1.8	45	375*	1.5*
14-18 y	700	15	15	75*	1.0	1.0	14	5*	25*	1.2	400[6]	2.4	65	400*	1.5*
19-30 y	700	15	15	90*	1.1	1.1	14	5*	30*	1.3	400[6]	2.4	75	425*	1.5*
31-50 y	700	15	15	90*	1.1	1.1	14	5*	30*	1.3	400[6]	2.4	75	425*	1.5*
51-70 y	700	15	15	90*	1.1	1.1	14	5*	30*	1.5	400	2.4[7]	75	425*	1.3*
>70 y	700	20	15	90*	1.1	1.1	14	5*	30*	1.5	400	2.4[7]	75	425*	1.2*
Pregnancy															
≤18 y	750	15	15	75*	1.4	1.4	18	6*	30*	1.9	600	2.6	80	450*	1.5*
19-30 y	770	15	15	90*	1.4	1.4	18	6*	30*	1.9	600	2.6	85	450*	1.5*
31-50 y	770	15	15	90*	1.4	1.4	18	6*	30*	1.9	600	2.6	85	450*	1.5*
Lactation															
≤18 y	1,200	15	19	75*	1.4	1.6	17	7*	35*	2.0	500	2.8	115	550*	1.5*
19-30 y	1,300	15	19	90*	1.4	1.6	17	7*	35*	2.0	500	2.8	120	550*	1.5*
31-50 y	1,300	15	19	90*	1.4	1.6	17	7*	35*	2.0	500	2.8	120	550*	1.5*

This table presents Recommended Dietary Allowances (RDA) and Adequate Intakes (AI). An asterisk (*) indicates AI. RDAs and AIs may both be used as goals for individual intake.

[1]As retinol activity equivalents (RAE).

[2]As cholecalciferol.

[3]As α-tocopherol.

[4]As niacin equivalents (NE).

[5]As dietary folate equivalents (DFE).

[6]In view of evidence linking folate intake with neural-tube defects in the fetus, it is recommended that all women capable of becoming pregnant consume 400 μg of folic acid from supplements or fortified foods in addition to intake of food folate from a varied diet.

[7]Because 10 to 30% of older people may malabsorb food-bound vitamin B$_{12}$, it is advisable for those older than 50 years to meet their RDA mainly by consuming foods fortified with vitamin B$_{12}$ or a supplement containing vitamin B$_{12}$.

Life stage group	Potassium (g/d)	Chloride (g/d)	Calcium (mg/d)	Phosphorus (mg/d)	Magnesium (mg/d)	Iron (mg/d)	Zinc (mg/d)	Selenium (µg/d)	Iodine (µg/d)	Copper (µg/d)	Manganese (mg/d)	Fluoride (mg/d)	Chromium (µg/d)	Molybdenum (µg/d)	Water (L/d)[8]
Infants															
0-6 mo	0.4*	0.18*	200	100*	30*	0.27*	2*	15*	110*	200*	0.003*	0.01*	0.2*	2*	0.7*
7-12 mo	0.7*	0.57*	260	275*	75*	11	3*	20*	130*	220*	0.6*	0.5*	5.5*	3*	0.8*
Children															
1-3 y	3.0*	1.5*	700	460	80	7	3	20	90	340	1.2*	0.7*	11*	17	1.3*
4-8 y	3.8*	1.9*	1000	500	130	10	5	30	90	440	1.5*	1*	15*	22	1.7*
Males															
9-13 y	4.5*	2.3*	1,300	1,250	240	8	8	40	120	700	1.9*	2*	25*	34	2.4*
14-18 y	4.7*	2.3*	1,300	1,250	410	11	11	55	150	890	2.2*	3*	35*	43	3.3*
19-30 y	4.7*	2.3*	1,000	700	400	8	11	55	150	900	2.3*	4*	35*	45	3.7*
31-50 y	4.7*	2.3*	1,000	700	420	8	11	55	150	900	2.3*	4*	35*	45	3.7*
51-70 y	4.7*	2.0*	1,200	700	420	8	11	55	150	900	2.3*	4*	30*	45	3.7*
>70 y	4.7*	1.8*	1,200	700	420	8	11	55	150	900	2.3*	4*	30*	45	3.7*
Females															
9-13 y	4.5*	2.3*	1,300	1,250	240	8	8	40	120	700	1.6*	2*	21*	34	2.1*
14-18 y	4.7*	2.3*	1,300	1,250	360	15	9	55	150	890	1.6*	3*	24*	43	2.3*
19-30 y	4.7*	2.3*	1,000	700	310	18	8	55	150	900	1.8*	3*	25*	45	2.7*
31-50 y	4.7*	2.3*	1,000	700	320	18	8	55	150	900	1.8*	3*	25*	45	2.7*
51-70 y	4.7*	2.0*	1,200	700	320	8	8	55	150	900	1.8*	3*	20*	45	2.7*
>70 y	4.7*	1.8*	1,200	700	320	8	8	55	150	900	1.8*	3*	20*	45	2.7*
Pregnancy															
≤18 y	4.7*	2.3*	1,300	1,250	400	27	12	60	220	1,000	2.0*	3*	29*	50	3.0*
19-30 y	4.7*	2.3*	1,000	700	350	27	11	60	220	1,000	2.0*	3*	30*	50	3.0*
31-50 y	4.7*	2.3*	1,000	700	360	27	11	60	220	1,000	2.0*	3*	30*	50	3.0*
Lactation															
≤18 y	5.1*	2.3	1,300	1,250	360	10	13	70	290	1,300	2.6*	3*	44*	50	3.8*
19-30 y	5.1*	2.3	1,000	700	310	9	12	70	290	1,300	2.6*	3*	45*	50	3.8*
31-50 y	5.1*	2.3	1,000	700	320	9	12	70	290	1,300	2.6*	3*	45*	50	3.8*

[8]The AI for water represents total water from drinking water, beverages, and moisture from food.

Sources: Data compiled from *Dietary Reference Intakes for Calcium, Phosphorus, Magnesium, Vitamin D, and Fluoride.* Washington, DC: National Academies Press; 1997. *Dietary Reference Intakes for Thiamin, Riboflavin, Niacin, Vitamin B₆, Folate, Vitamin B₁₂, Pantothenic Acid, Biotin, and Choline.* Washington, DC: National Academies Press; 1998. *Dietary Reference Intakes for Vitamin C, Vitamin E, Selenium, and Carotenoids.* Washington, DC: National Academies Press; 2000. *Dietary Reference Intakes for Vitamin A, Vitamin K, Arsenic, Boron, Chromium, Copper, Iron, Manganese, Molybdenum, Nickel, Silicon, Vanadium, and Zinc.* Washington, DC: National Academies Press; 2000. *Dietary Reference Intakes for Water, Potassium, Sodium Chloride, and Sulfate.* Food and Nutrition Board. Washington, DC: National Academies Press; 2005. *Dietary Reference Intakes for Calcium and Vitamin D.* Washington, DC: National Academies Press; 2011. These reports may be accessed via http://nap.edu.

Practical Applications in

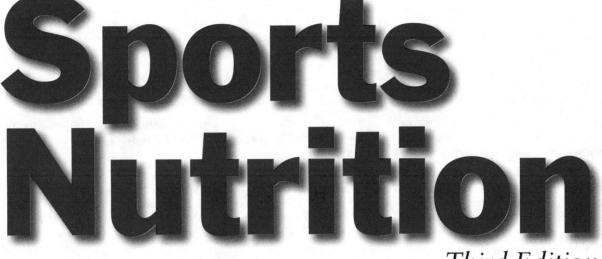

Sports Nutrition

Third Edition

Heather Hedrick Fink, MS, RD, CSSD
Assistant Director of Educational Services
National Institute for Fitness and Sport
Indianapolis, Indiana

Alan E. Mikesky, PhD, FACSM
Professor
School of Physical Education and Tourism Management
Indiana University–Purdue University Indianapolis
Indianapolis, Indiana

Lisa A. Burgoon, MS, RD, CSSD, LDN
Visiting Teaching Associate
College of Agricultural, Consumer and Environmental Sciences
University of Illinois
Urbana–Champaign, Illinois

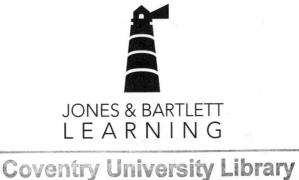

JONES & BARTLETT
LEARNING

World Headquarters

Jones & Bartlett Learning
5 Wall Street
Burlington, MA 01803
978-443-5000
info@jblearning.com
www.jblearning.com

Jones & Bartlett Learning
Canada
6339 Ormindale Way
Mississauga, Ontario L5V 1J2
Canada

Jones & Bartlett Learning
International
Barb House, Barb Mews
London W6 7PA
United Kingdom

Jones & Bartlett Learning books and products are available through most bookstores and online booksellers. To contact Jones & Bartlett Learning directly, call 800-832-0034, fax 978-443-8000, or visit our website, www. jblearning.com.

Substantial discounts on bulk quantities of Jones & Bartlett Learning publications are available to corporations, professional associations, and other qualified organizations. For details and specific discount information, contact the special sales department at Jones & Bartlett Learning via the above contact information or send an email to specialsales@jblearning.com.

The authors, editor, and publisher have made every effort to provide accurate information. However, they are not responsible for errors, omissions, or for any outcomes related to the use of the contents of this book and take no responsibility for the use of the products and procedures described. Treatments and side effects described in this book may not be applicable to all people; likewise, some people may require a dose or experience a side effect that is not described herein. Drugs and medical devices are discussed that may have limited availability controlled by the Food and Drug Administration (FDA) for use only in a research study or clinical trial. Research, clinical practice, and government regulations often change the accepted standard in this field. When consideration is being given to use of any drug in the clinical setting, the health care provider or reader is responsible for determining FDA status of the drug, reading the package insert, and reviewing prescribing information for the most up-to-date recommendations on dose, precautions, and contraindications, and determining the appropriate usage for the product. This is especially important in the case of drugs that are new or seldom used.

Production Credits

Publisher, Higher Education: Cathleen Sether
Senior Acquisitions Editor: Shoshanna Goldberg
Senior Associate Editor: Amy Bloom
Editorial Assistant: Prima Bartlett
Production Manager: Julie Champagne Bolduc
Senior Production Editor: Renée Sekerak
Production Editor: Jessica Steele Newfell
Production Assistant: Sean Coombs
Associate Marketing Manager: Jody Sullivan

V.P., Manufacturing and Inventory Control: Therese Connell
Photo Researcher: Sarah Cebulski
Composition: Publishers' Design and Production Services, Inc.
Cover Design: Kate Ternullo
Cover Image: © Ron Kloberdanz/ShutterStock, Inc.
Printing and Binding: Malloy, Inc.
Cover Printing: Malloy, Inc.

To order this product, use ISBN: 978-1-4496-4643-1

Library of Congress Cataloging-in-Publication Data
Fink, Heather Hedrick.
  Practical applications in sports nutrition / Heather Fink, Alan Earl Mikesky, Lisa Burgoon. — 3rd ed.
      p. cm.
  Includes bibliographical references and index.
  ISBN 978-1-4496-0208-6 (pbk.)
  1. Athletes—Nutrition. 2. Exercise—Physiological aspects. I. Mikesky, Alan E. II. Burgoon, Lisa A.
III. Title.
  TX361.A8F56 2012
  613.2024796—dc22
                                                                                          2011012887
6048

Printed in the United States of America
15 14 13 12 11   10 9 8 7 6 5 4 3 2 1

Brief Contents

Contents

CHAPTER 4   **Fats.. 98**

CHAPTER 5   **Proteins 128**

CHAPTER 6   **Vitamins...154**

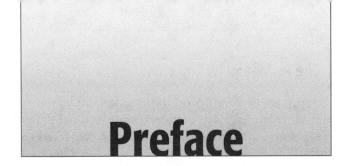

Preface

Sports nutrition is an exciting field that combines the sciences of nutrition and exercise physiology. The generally accepted notion that proper nutrition can positively impact athletic performance has created the need for exercise and nutrition professionals to acquire knowledge that goes beyond the basics of general nutrition.

In addition, emerging career opportunities in sports nutrition require that academic programs preparing registered dietitians expand the application of nutrition beyond the clinical population. Strength coaches and personal trainers also need to go beyond the nutrition basics to help their athletes achieve optimal performance. The growing research base supporting the importance of sports nutrition and the inherent interest of athletes seeking a nutritional edge has created an increased demand for sports nutrition courses in dietetic and exercise science programs.

In order to obtain a job in the sports nutrition field, readers need to understand current nutrition guidelines, be aware of the results of emerging research, and be able to practically apply sports nutrition knowledge to athletes of all ages, sports, and abilities. This text has been developed to meet these needs, providing readers with an opportunity to learn the most up-to-date information related to diet and athletic performance while also addressing consultation skills and giving readers the tools they need to educate others properly. The focus on research, current guidelines, and practical application of information makes this sports nutrition textbook unique among other texts currently on the market.

Undergraduate and graduate students as well as professionals from several different backgrounds will benefit from this textbook. Students in dietetics, exercise science, and athletic training programs will enhance their education with an understanding of the relationship among essential nutrients, energy metabolism, and optimal sports performance. Dietetics students seeking the registered dietitian (RD) credential will appreciate the thorough explanations and many helpful tips on how to guide an athlete through nutrition consultations. Exercise science and athletic training students will learn how to educate athletes regarding public domain sports nutrition guidelines as well as how to work together as a team with a registered dietitian and physician. Current professionals in the field of sports nutrition will benefit from adding this text to their reference library due to the straightforward and complete presentation of current sports nutrition recommendations as well as examples of practical applications for athletes participating in endurance, strength/power, and team sports.

Third Edition Enhancements

The *Third Edition* of *Practical Applications in Sports Nutrition* is divided into two sections. Chapters 1–9 provide an introduction to sports nutrition, including definitions of sports nutrition and general nutrition concepts; a review of digestion and energy metabolism; a thorough explanation of macronutrients, micronutrients, and water and their relation to athletic performance; and finally an overview of nutritional ergogenics. New features within Chapters 1–9 in this *Third Edition* include the new 2010 Dietary Guidelines, MyPlate initiative, and World Anti-Doping Association Prohibited Substances List; updated calcium and vitamin D recommendations; new sports beverage comparison chart; revised health and nutrient content claims; additional meal planning and snack ideas; nutrition analyses for all recipes in the book; and updated information and references, particularly for hot topics such as artificial sweeteners, carbohydrate loading, and carbohydrate intake immediately prior to exercise.

Several of this textbook's unique features appear in the second half of the text, within the practical and applied section. Chapter 10 focuses on how to educate, communicate with, and empower athletes to make behavior changes through nutrition consultations. Chapter 11 covers enhancing athletic performance through nutrition while also focusing on weight management, including weight loss, weight gain, and eating disorders. Highlights of this *Third Edition* include an expanded section on weight gain, example meal plans for athletes aiming to gain weight in a healthy way, and updated references regarding weight management and eating disorders.

In Chapters 12–14, sports are divided into three categories—endurance, strength/power, and team—and each is covered separately. Each chapter reviews the most current research as it relates to the energy systems and specific nutrition needs of athletes in these various categories of sports. Chapters 12–14 are examples of one of the main objectives of this book—to empower individuals to excel in the sports nutrition field by teaching sports nutrition guidelines and showing how to apply the concepts to athletes in various sports. These chapters demonstrate how to give advice that is practical and easy to follow. Chapters 12–14 have been the favorites of many reviewers; therefore, only a few changes were made in this *Third Edition* such as research updates and recommendation clarifications.

Due to the increased occurrence of athletes with special medical or nutritional considerations, including those who are pregnant, vegetarian, masters athletes, or have chronic diseases, Chapter 15 targets the unique nutrition requirements of these special populations. The text concludes with a chapter dedicated to helping readers discover and understand the pathway to becoming a sports dietitian through education and experience. *Third Edition* enhancements to Chapters 15 and 16 include updated references, resources, and Web sites.

The Pedagogy

The pedagogy developed for this text includes many special features. Each chapter begins with the **Key Questions Addressed**; these questions are asked to introduce the student to information that will be covered, stimulate his or her curiosity, and help focus the student's attention before he or she begins reading. In other words, the Key Questions Addressed encourage purposeful reading.

You Are the Nutrition Coach is a case study presented at the beginning of each chapter that requires the application of specific information from the chapter in a real-life scenario. Thoughtful consideration and/or discussion of the case study prior to reading the chapter will engage the readers and help students identify preconceived misconceptions or shortcomings in their current level of nutritional knowledge. After reading the chapter, the case study should be reconsidered and answers compared to the solutions provided in Appendix A.

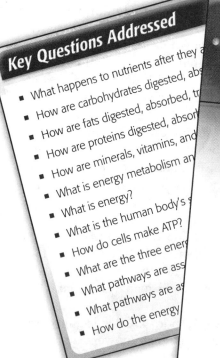

Key Questions Addressed

- What happens to nutrients after they a
- How are carbohydrates digested, abs
- How are fats digested, absorbed, t
- How are proteins digested, absor
- How are minerals, vitamins, and
- What is energy metabolism an
- What is energy?
- What is the human body's
- How do cells make ATP?
- How do the three ener
- What pathways are ass
- What pathways are a
- How do the energy

You Are the Nutrition Coach

Meggan is a 15-year-old soccer player. She is very athletic, plays midfielder, and is noted for her speed and endurance. She has been trying to lose a few pounds to achieve a more comfortable playing weight, and therefore has decreased her carbohydrate intake from 65% of her total daily caloric intake to 40%. Lately she has been feeling fatigued in the middle of her 2- to 3-hour practices and weekend games, which is affecting her performance. Meggan's coach has suggested that she bring a water bottle filled with a sport drink to their next practice. However, Meggan dislikes the taste of sports drinks and decides to find an alternative. She enjoys juices of any kind; therefore, the following Saturday she fills her water bottle with orange juice and drinks diligently throughout practice. Halfway through practice, instead of feeling tired, she is feeling nauseous and has intestinal cramping.

Questions

- What are the possible causes of Meggan's earlier-than-usual fatigue?
- What dietary suggestions might you give to Meggan to get her back to peak sport performance?

Key Terms within each chapter are bolded within the text and defined in a sidebar.

Gaining the Performance Edge statements throughout each chapter highlight important information or special tips on how to apply sports nutrition knowledge when working with individual athletes or entire sporting teams.

gaining the performance edge

Dietary carbohydrates can be obtained from a variety of foods throughout the MyPlate food guidance system. Each food group provides a unique blend of carbohydrates and other nutrients. Athletes should focus on the most nutrient-dense carbohydrate sources including whole grains, fruits, vegetables, low-fat dairy/alternatives, beans/legumes, and nuts.

more flavorful and enjoyable. Sweets and sodas do not need to be permanently excluded from the diet but should be used sparingly. Diet sodas, desserts, and snacks replace sugar with artificial sweeteners, thus providing minimal or no carbohydrates. Diet foods can be incorporated into a healthy diet, but should also be used sparingly to make room for carbohydrate-rich and nutrient-dense foods.

What happens to the fats once they are absorbed?

Once absorbed, the water-soluble glycerol and short- and medium-chain fatty acids pass through the intestinal cells and diffuse into capillaries, thus entering directly into the bloodstream (see Figure 2.13). The monoglycerides and long-chain fatty acids that are absorbed are reassembled into triglycerides within the intestinal cells. The resynthesized triglycerides are then combined with protein carriers to form **lipoproteins**. These lipoproteins with their fatty cargo then pass through the intestinal cells. Once they leave the intestinal cells they are called **chylomicrons**. Chylomicrons do not enter directly into the bloodstream, but instead enter into the lymphatic system (see Figure 2.13). The lymphatic system then delivers the chylomicrons to the large veins of the neck via the thoracic duct. The fats then empty into the blood and are distributed throughout the body.

lipoproteins Substances that transport lipids in the lymph and blood. These substances consist of a central core of triglycerides surrounded by a shell composed of proteins, phospholipids, and cholesterol. Various types of lipoproteins exist in the body and differ based on size, composition, and density.

chylomicron A droplet made of resynthesized triglycerides that is wrapped in lipoproteins that is produced inside the intestinal cells. Chylomicrons are released from the intestinal cells and then pass into the lymphatic system.

Fortifying
Your Nutrition Knowledge

The National Cholesterol Education Program's Therapeutic Lifestyle Recommendations

In May 2001, the National Cholesterol Education Program (NCEP) released the Third Report of the Expert Panel on Detection, Evaluation, and Treatment of High Blood Cholesterol in Adults (Adult Treatment Panel III). The series of seven steps posted in the report provides a framework for detecting risk for heart disease and treating those who have heart disease or who present significant risk factors for developing heart disease. Also included in the report are therapeutic lifestyle changes that can be implemented to lower LDL cholesterol levels in the blood.

The therapeutic lifestyle changes suggested are as follows:

- *Consume a diet with <7% of total calories from saturated fat*: Saturated fat comes mainly from animal products such as meats and full-fat dairy. The only vegetable oils containing a significant amount of saturated fat are coconut, palm, and palm kernel oils.
- *Keep dietary cholesterol intake to <200 mg per day*: Cholesterol is found only in animal products such as meats and higher-fat dairy products.
- *Increase soluble fiber to 10–25 grams per day*: Soluble fiber is found only in plant products such as oats, oat bran, legumes, and some fruits and vegetables.
- *Consider consuming plant stanols/sterols (2 grams per day) to help lower cholesterol*: Derived from plant foods, plant stanols/sterols can be found in commercial products such as Take Control or Benecol margarines and have been shown to actively aid in lowering blood cholesterol.
- *Maintain a healthy body weight*: Balance calorie intake (diet) with calorie expenditure (exercise, training, competition, and daily movement) on a daily basis.
- *Increase physical activity*: Achieve at least 30 minutes, preferably 60 minutes, of physical activity every day of the week.

For more information on the Third Report of the Expert Panel on Detection, Evaluation and Treatment of High Blood Cholesterol in Adults, visit www.nhlbi.nih.gov/guidelines/cholesterol/atglance. htm. In 2004, the NCEP updated the report based on the results from new clinical trials. The updates applied to moderately high and high-risk patients only and thus will not be discussed. However, to get the updated information, go to www.nhlbi.nih.gov/guidelines/cholesterol/atp3upd04.htm.

The in-depth coverage of timely topics related to sports nutrition in the **Fortifying Your Nutrition Knowledge** segments will enhance students' learning and overall nutrition knowledge.

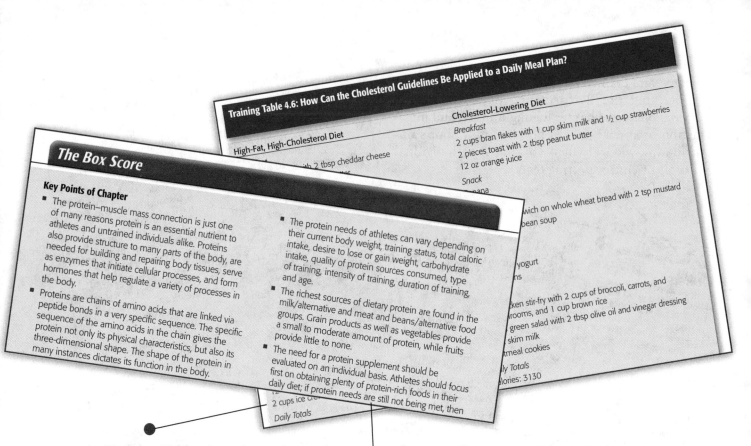

Training Table 4.6: How Can the Cholesterol Guidelines Be Applied to a Daily Meal Plan?

Cholesterol-Lowering Diet

Breakfast
2 cups bran flakes with 1 cup skim milk and ½ cup strawberries
2 pieces toast with 2 tbsp peanut butter
12 oz orange juice

Snack

High-Fat, High-Cholesterol Diet

...with 2 tbsp cheddar cheese

...wich on whole wheat bread with 2 tsp mustard

...bean soup

...yogurt

...ken stir-fry with 2 cups of broccoli, carrots, and
...rooms, and 1 cup brown rice
...green salad with 2 tbsp olive oil and vinegar dressing
...skim milk
...tmeal cookies

...ly Totals
...lories: 3130

The Box Score

Key Points of Chapter

- The protein–muscle mass connection is just one of many reasons protein is an essential nutrient to athletes and untrained individuals alike. Proteins also provide structure to many parts of the body, are needed for building and repairing body tissues, serve as enzymes that initiate cellular processes, and form hormones that help regulate a variety of processes in the body.

- Proteins are chains of amino acids that are linked via peptide bonds in a very specific sequence. The specific sequence of the amino acids in the chain gives the protein not only its physical characteristics, but also its three-dimensional shape. The shape of the protein in many instances dictates its function in the body.

- The protein needs of athletes can vary depending on their current body weight, training status, total caloric intake, desire to lose or gain weight, carbohydrate intake, quality of protein sources consumed, type of training, intensity of training, duration of training, and age.

- The richest sources of dietary protein are found in the milk/alternative and meat and beans/alternative food groups. Grain products as well as vegetables provide a small to moderate amount of protein, while fruits provide little to none.

- The need for a protein supplement should be evaluated on an individual basis. Athletes should focus first on obtaining plenty of protein-rich foods in their daily diet; if protein needs are still not being met, then

2 cups ice cr...

Daily Totals

The **Training Tables** demonstrate how to translate sports nutrition knowledge into actual meal planning ideas, recipes, or individual food selections.

At the conclusion of each chapter, the **Key Points** provide a summary of the topics presented and the important key messages.

The **Study Questions** posed after the Key Points will continue to engage students in thoughtful review and application of chapter topics, while also aiding in the preparation for course examinations.

Throughout the text the primary, secondary, and tertiary section headings are phrased as questions. We formatted the section headings as questions to help readers focus their attention and to foster interest in the topic before they begin to read. In other words, they are "directed" to read about topics with the specific purpose of obtaining an answer to a question.

This is an effective way of reading and borrows from the work of Francis Robinson, who developed the widely used "preview-question-read-recite-review" (PQ3R) reading technique. The goal is to prevent "hollow reading," in which a person reads the words on the pages but without a specific understanding or perspective of why he or she is reading.

Our mission is for readers to become engrossed in their reading with the hope that they will be inspired to learn more about the relatively new and growing field of sports nutrition. After all, regardless of where a reader's academic and career paths may lead, knowledge of good nutrition is universally applicable to one's personal health and well-being, to enjoyment of recreational and sports activities, and in the case of dietitians and fitness professionals, to career success.

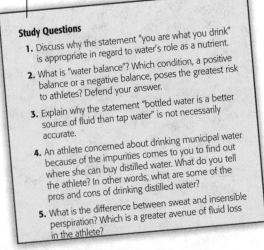

Study Questions

1. Discuss why the statement "you are what you drink" is appropriate in regard to water's role as a nutrient.

2. What is "water balance"? Which condition, a positive balance or a negative balance, poses the greatest risk to athletes? Defend your answer.

3. Explain why the statement "bottled water is a better source of fluid than tap water" is not necessarily accurate.

4. An athlete concerned about drinking municipal water because of the impurities comes to you to find out where she can buy distilled water. What do you tell the athlete? In other words, what are some of the pros and cons of drinking distilled water?

5. What is the difference between sweat and insensible perspiration? Which is a greater avenue of fluid loss in the athlete?

Integrated Learning and Teaching Package

Integrating the text and ancillaries is crucial to deriving their full benefit. Based on feedback from instructors and students, Jones & Bartlett Learning offers the following supplements.

Diet analysis software is an important component of the behavioral change and personal decision-making focus of a nutrition course. **EatRight Analysis**, developed by ESHA Research, offers dietary software online at http://EatRight.jblearning.com. With this online tool, you and your students can access personal records from any computer with Internet access. Through a variety of reports, students learn to make better choices regarding their diets and activity habits.

Nutrition Science Animations

These scientifically based animations give nutrition students an accurate, accessible explanation of the major scientific concepts and physiological principles presented in *Practical Applications in Sports Nutrition, Third Edition*. More than 30 of the most difficult processes are graphically presented in an interactive, easy-to-understand format. These Nutrition Science Animations, available at http://nutrition.jbpub.com/animations, complement online courses, classroom lectures, and independent studying. Access is free and does not require a password. The Nutrition Science Animations are also available on CD-ROM (ISBN-13: 978-0-7637-4497-7).

The companion **Web site** for *Practical Applications in Sports Nutrition, Third Edition*, http://go.jblearning.com/fink3 offers students and instructors an unprecedented degree of integration between the text and the online world through many useful study tools, activities, and supplementary health information.

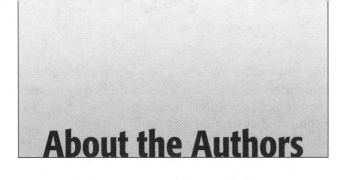
About the Authors

Heather Hedrick Fink, MS, RD, CSSD

Heather Hedrick Fink is the assistant director of the Center for Educational Services within the National Institute for Fitness and Sport. She is a registered dietitian, has her master of science in kinesiology, and is a Board-Certified Specialist in Sports Dietetics. She completed her Bachelor of Science degree in dietetics as well as her Master of Science degree at the University of Illinois, Urbana–Champaign. Heather is certified by the American College of Sports Medicine as a Health/Fitness Specialist®. Heather's interests and extensive experience are in the areas of wellness, weight management, exercise prescription, vegetarian nutrition, and sports nutrition, ranging from the recreational to the ultra-endurance athlete. At the National Institute for Fitness and Sport, she develops educational materials, implements programs, and delivers presentations to various groups on nutrition and fitness topics related to healthy eating, weight control, disease prevention, and improving athletic performance. She routinely appears on local NBC, CBS, and cable television shows and news broadcasts to educate central Indiana residents on the benefits of a healthy lifestyle. She was the dietitian for the first team of four men aged 70-plus to successfully complete Race Across America, the non-stop bicycle race across the United States. Heather is the author of the *Absolute Beginner's Guide to Half-Marathon Training*. She has been interviewed and quoted in *Women's Day*, *Ladies Home Journal*, and *Newsweek*. Heather is also an accomplished triathlete, duathlete, and marathon runner, including qualifying for and competing in the 2003 Hawaii Ironman.

Alan E. Mikesky, PhD, FACSM

Alan Mikesky is a professor at the School of Physical Education and Tourism Management, Indiana University–Purdue University Indianapolis, and Director of the Human Performance and Biomechanics Laboratory. He also has an adjunct appointment with the School of Medicine, Department of Anat-

omy, and serves as research associate at the National Institute for Fitness and Sport in Indianapolis. Dr. Mikesky received his Bachelor of Science in biology from Texas A&M University and his Master of Science in physical education with a specialization in exercise physiology from the University of Michigan. He received his Doctorate in anatomy/cell biology from the University of Texas Southwestern Medical Center at Dallas where he studied the adaptations of skeletal muscle to heavy resistance exercise. He is a Fellow of the American College of Sports Medicine (ACSM), a member of ACSM's national media referral network, and was fitness editor for ACSM's quarterly newsletter, *Fit Society Page*. He has served as a member of the editorial board for the *National Strength and Conditioning Association's Journal of Strength and Conditioning Research* and *Strength and Conditioning Journal*. He is also coauthor of the *Sixth Edition* of *Physical Fitness: A Way of Life*, a textbook published by Cooper Publishing Group. His research focuses on the functional improvements and physiological adaptations to various forms of resistance exercise. He has investigated the impact of strength training on gait, balance, incidence of falls, joint proprioception, functional ability, and chronic diseases such as osteoarthritis. His most recent research interests involve exploring the effects of low-intensity, resistance exercise combined with blood flow restriction. Finally, his teaching responsibilities include both undergraduate and graduate exercise science courses and sports conditioning.

Lisa A. Burgoon, MS, RD, CSSD, LDN

Lisa A. Burgoon is a visiting teaching associate in the College of Agricultural, Consumer and Environmental Sciences at the University of Illinois at Urbana–Champaign. Her primary teaching and research centers around student leadership development, but she also teaches at least one sports nutrition course per year through the Department of Food Science and Human Nutrition. She is a registered and licensed dietitian and is Board Certified as a Specialist in Sports Dietetics. She received her Bachelor of Science degree in dietetics from Michigan State University, her Master of Science degree in sports medicine from Chapman University and her Master of Education in higher education administration from the University of Illinois at Urbana–Champaign. A practicing sports dietitian for more than a decade,

Lisa has worked with Division I athletes and teams, recreational athletes competing in numerous sports, and athletes of all ages. She continues some consulting work with local athletes and provides lectures and practical experiences on sports and wellness nutrition topics for students in kinesiology, community health, athletic training, and other applied health studies majors.

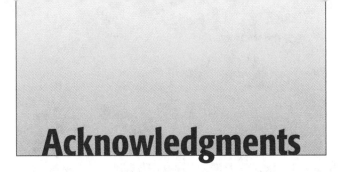

Acknowledgments

We would like to thank Jones & Bartlett Learning's Health Development Team for making this *Third Edition* a reality. Thanks to Shoshanna Goldberg, Amy Bloom, Rachel Isaacs, and Prima Bartlett on the editorial team for their support, encouragement, and direction for the development of this *Third Edition*. Thank you to Julie Bolduc, Renée Sekerak, and Jessica Newfell on the production team for their tireless efforts in the production of the book and ancillary materials. Thanks to Jody Sullivan and the entire Jones & Bartlett marketing and sales teams. Their dedication to our book has helped us to surpass our goals.

We are grateful to the reviewers who obviously spent a large part of their valuable time reviewing the *Third Edition* of our book:

Craig Biwer, MS, ATC/L, CSCS, HFS
University of Wisconsin, Oshkosh

Lorrie Brilla, PhD, FACSM, FACN
Western Washington University

Jamie A. Cooper, PhD
Texas Tech University

Kathleen L. Deegan, PhD, MS, RD
California State University, Sacramento

Samuel A. E. Headley, PhD, FACSM, RCEP, CSCS
Springfield College

Jessica Hodge, PhD
Folsom Lake College

Dennis Hunt, EdD, CSCS
Florida Gulf Coast University

Astrid Mel, PhD, HFS
Methodist University

Elizabeth Nicklay, LAT, CSCS
Luther College

Jennifer Spry-Knutson
Des Moines Area Community College

Amy J. Reckard, MS, LAT, ATC
Nova Southeastern University

Scott C. Swanson, PhD
Ohio Northern University

Their thoughtful, constructive comments provided the feedback necessary to enhance our book with accurate and timely sports nutrition updates.

Finally, we would be remiss not to acknowledge the patience, understanding, and support of our spouses and families. The countless hours spent on this project took away from precious family time and could not have been done without help "picking up the slack" in the other areas of our lives. Without their support, keeping this project on schedule would never have been possible.

1

Introduction to Sports Nutrition

Key Questions Addressed

- What is sports nutrition?
- Why study sports nutrition?
- What are the basic nutrients?
- How does the body produce energy?
- What are the Dietary Reference Intakes?
- What are enriched and fortified foods?
- What are the basic nutrition guidelines?
- How should athletes interpret the information on food labels?
- What are the factors to consider when developing an individualized sports nutrition plan for athletes?
- How can sports nutrition knowledge be converted into practical applications?

Jennifer is a 42-year-old tennis player. She states that recently her energy levels have dropped and she has had a hard time recovering from long tennis matches. She also complains of being "hungry all the time." The constant hunger has been frustrating because she is trying to maintain her current weight and thus attempting to control her total daily intake. She has been "eating well" since she found out two years ago that she has high cholesterol. She counseled with a dietitian at the time of her diagnosis and subsequently made major changes in her diet such as switching to nonfat foods and eliminating dairy. Her goals are to increase her energy levels, decrease recovery time, and create a meal plan that will also be healthy for her husband and three sons.

Question

- What should be considered her top priority—her high cholesterol, struggle to maintain her weight, constant hunger, low energy levels, or long recovery time?

What is sports nutrition?

Sports nutrition is a specialization within the field of nutrition that partners closely with the study of the human body and exercise science. Sports nutrition can be defined as the application of nutrition knowledge to a practical daily eating plan focused on providing the fuel for physical activity, facilitating the repair and rebuilding process following hard physical work, and optimizing athletic performance in competitive events, while also promoting overall health and wellness. The area of sports nutrition is often thought to be reserved only for "athletes," which insinuates the inclusion of only those individuals who are performing at the elite level. In this text, the term *athlete* refers to any individual who is regularly active, ranging from the fitness enthusiast to the competitive amateur or professional. Differences may exist in specific nutrient needs along this designated spectrum of athletes, creating the exciting challenge of individualizing sports nutrition plans.

To fully understand and subsequently apply sports nutrition concepts, professionals instructing athletes on proper eating strategies first need to have a command of general nutrition as well as exercise science. The second step is to gain the knowledge of how nutrition and exercise science are intertwined, understanding that physical training and dietary habits are reliant on each other to produce optimal performance. The final step can be considered one of the most critical—the practical application of sports nutrition knowledge to individual athletes participating in any sport or physical activity.

Sports nutrition professionals must be able to teach athletes by putting "book" knowledge into practice with actual food selection and meal planning, while keeping in mind the challenges presented by busy schedules of exercise, competitions, work, school, and other commitments. It is this third step that many professionals lack after graduating from an undergraduate or graduate program in sports nutrition, dietetics, exercise science, or athletic training. The focus of this book is to review sports nutrition concepts while also translating the information into specific meal plans, recipes, and case study scenarios. Students are encouraged to seek additional opportunities outside the classroom to work with recreational and elite athletes to gain more experience in applying sports nutrition concepts before searching for a job in the "real world."

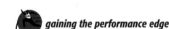

gaining the performance edge

The field of sports nutrition requires a command of general nutrition and exercise science, an understanding of their interrelationship, and the knowledge of how to practically apply sports nutrition concepts. This text provides a review of the current sports nutrition research, established dietary recommendations for athletes, and guidance on how to develop individualized nutrition plans for athletes participating in various sports.

Why study sports nutrition?

Sports nutrition has recently emerged as a recognized specialty area within the field of nutrition. Athletes challenge their bodies on a regular basis through physical training and competitions. To keep up with the demands of their activity or sport, athletes need to fuel their bodies adequately on a daily basis. This fueling process requires a specialized approach; therefore, athletes who want to make dietary changes should seek out professionals who are experts in sports nutrition and experienced in developing individualized plans.

Because of its relative infancy, sports nutrition research is providing new and exciting information on a regular basis. Over the years, this information has been compiled to form dietary guidelines geared specifically for athletes. Professionals who have studied sports nutrition and have experience in the field can help athletes interpret research and determine how, or if, the information relates to their sport and individual needs.

Studying sports nutrition and becoming an expert require years of education and experience. The last chapter of this text outlines the traditional pathway to becoming an expert in this area, which can lead to an exciting and fulfilling career.

gaining the performance edge

The field of sports nutrition is growing, and thus creating a demand for qualified sports nutrition professionals. To be considered an "expert" in sports nutrition, a professional must obtain the appropriate education and certification background as well as hands-on experience working with athletes.

What are the basic nutrients?

Foods and beverages are composed of six nutrients that are vital to the human body for producing energy, contributing to the growth and development of tissues, regulating body processes, and preventing deficiency and degenerative diseases. The six nutrients are carbohydrates, proteins, fats, vitamins, minerals, and water and are classified as **essential** nutrients. The body requires these nutrients to function properly; however, the body is unable to endogenously manufacture them in the quantities needed daily, and therefore these nutrients must be obtained from the diet. Carbohydrates, proteins, and fats are classified as **macronutrients** because they have a caloric value and the body needs a large quantity of them on a daily basis. The **micronutrients** include vitamins and minerals; the prefix *micro* is used because the body's daily requirements for these nutrients are small. Water fits into its own class, and requirements for it vary greatly among individuals. These nutrients will be introduced in this section; individual chapters later in this book will provide a more thorough review of their application to athletics.

essential A nutrition descriptor referring to nutrients that must be obtained from the diet.

macronutrients These include carbohydrates, proteins, and fats and are classified as such because they have caloric value, and the body has a large daily need for them.

micronutrients Vitamins and minerals are classified as micronutrients because the body's daily requirements for these nutrients are small.

What are carbohydrates?

Carbohydrates are compounds constructed of carbon, hydrogen, and oxygen molecules. Carbohydrates are converted into glucose in the body, providing the main source of fuel (4 calories per gram of carbohydrate) for all physical activity. Carbohydrates are found in a wide variety of foods, including grains, fruits, and vegetables, as well as in the milk/alternative (soy, rice, nut, or other nondairy products) group.

What are proteins?

Amino acids are the building blocks of proteins, constructed of carbon, hydrogen, oxygen, and nitrogen molecules. Amino acids can be made within the body (**nonessential**) or obtained from dietary sources. Proteins are involved in the development, growth, and repair of muscle and other bodily tissues and are therefore critical for recovery from intense physical training. Proteins ensure that the body stays healthy and continues working efficiently by aiding in many bodily processes. Protein can also be used for energy, providing 4 calories per gram; however, it is not used efficiently and therefore is not a source of energy preferred by the body. Proteins are found in

nonessential A nutrient descriptor referring to nutrients that can be made within the body.

a variety of foods, including grains and vegetables, but are mainly concentrated in the milk/alternative as well as meat and beans/alternative (soy products, nuts, seeds, beans, and other nonanimal products) group.

What are fats?

Fats, like the other macronutrients, are compounds made up of carbon, hydrogen, and oxygen molecules. Fats are also known as lipids and come from both plant and animal sources in our diet. Triglycerides are the most common type of fat. Other fats include cholesterol and phospholipids. With 9 calories per gram, fats are a concentrated source of energy. Fat is primarily used as a fuel at rest and during low-to-moderate intensity exercise. Fats are also involved in providing structure to cell membranes, aiding in the production of hormones, forming the insulation that wraps nerve cells, and facilitating the absorption of fat-soluble vitamins. Fats are concentrated in butter, margarines, salad dressings, and oils but are also found in meats, dairy products, nuts, seeds, olives, avocados, and some grain products.

What are vitamins?

Vitamins are a large class of nutrients that contain carbon and hydrogen, as well as possibly oxygen, nitrogen, and other elements. There are two main requirements for a substance to be classified as a vitamin. First, the substance must be consumed exogenously because the body cannot produce it or cannot produce it in sufficient quantities to meet its needs. Second, the substance must be essential to at least one vital chemical reaction or process in the human body. Vitamins do not directly provide energy to the body; however, some vitamins aid in the extraction of energy from macronutrients. Vitamins are involved in a wide variety of bodily functions and processes that help to keep the body healthy and disease-free. Vitamins are classified as either water soluble (B vitamins and vitamin C) or fat soluble (vitamins A, D, E, and K), depending on their method of absorption, transport, and storage in the body. Vitamins are found in nearly all foods, including fruits, vegetables, grains, meat and beans/alternative, milk/alternative, and some fats.

What are minerals?

Minerals are also a large group of nutrients. They are composed of a variety of elements; however, they lack carbon. Minerals have a role in the structural development of tissues as well as the regulation of bodily processes. Physical activity places demands on muscles and bones, increases the need for oxygen-carrying compounds in the blood, and increases the loss of sweat and electrolytes from the body, all of which hinge on the adequate intake and replacement of dietary minerals. Minerals are categorized into major minerals (calcium, sodium, potassium, chloride, phosphorus, magnesium, and sulfur) and trace minerals (iron, zinc, copper, selenium, iodine, fluoride, molybdenum, and manganese) based on the total quantity required by the body on a daily basis. Similar to vitamins, minerals are found in a wide variety of foods, but mainly are concentrated in the meat and beans/alternative and milk/alternative groups.

What is water?

Forming a category of its own, water deserves to be highlighted because of its vital roles within the body. The human body can survive for a much greater length of time without any of the macro- or micronutrients than without water. The body is made of 55–60% water, representing a nearly ubiquitous presence in bodily tissues and fluids. In athletics, water is important for temperature regulation, lubrication of joints, and the transport of nutrients to active tissues. In addition to plain water, water can be obtained from juices, milk, coffee, tea, and other beverages, as well as watery foods such as fruits, vegetables, and soups.

How does the body produce energy?

The body derives its energy from foods ingested daily. Carbohydrates, fats, and proteins are known as the **energy nutrients** because they serve as the body's source for energy. These energy nutrients are quite literally chemicals that have energy trapped within the bonds between the atoms of which they are made. The energy trapped within these nutrients is released when

energy nutrients Carbohydrates, proteins, and fats serve as the body's source of energy and are considered the energy nutrients.

metabolic pathways within the cells break down the foods into their constituent parts, carbon dioxide and water. Some of the energy released is conserved or captured and used to make another high-energy chemical called **adenosine triphosphate** (**ATP**). The rest of the energy is lost as heat. ATP is the body's direct source of energy for cellular work. Without a constant source of ATP, muscles would not be able to generate force and thus athletes would not be able to move or perform any physical activity. In Chapter 2, the importance of the energy nutrients, the metabolic pathways that break them down, and their role in energy production during sport are discussed in more detail.

adenosine triphosphate (ATP) The molecule that serves as the body's direct source of energy for cellular work.

What are the Dietary Reference Intakes?

Several different terms are used to classify the recommendations for macronutrients and micronutrients. The **Recommended Dietary Allowances (RDAs)** were developed in 1941 by the U.S. National Academy of Sciences. The RDAs were the primary values health professionals used to assess and plan diets for individuals and groups, and to make judgments about excessive intakes. The RDAs still exist for many nutrients; however, a newer way to quantify nutrient needs and excesses for healthy individuals has been developed and termed the **Dietary Reference Intakes (DRIs)**. The DRIs expand on the RDAs and take into consideration other dietary quantities such as **Estimated Average Requirement (EAR)**, **Adequate Intake (AI)**, and **Tolerable Upper Intake Level (UL)**. DRIs are continually being reviewed, and reports on various groups of nutri-

Recommended Dietary Allowance (RDA) The average daily dietary intake level that is sufficient to meet the nutrient requirements of the overwhelming majority (i.e., 98%) of a healthy population.

Dietary Reference Intakes (DRIs) A newer way to quantify nutrient needs and excesses for healthy individuals. The DRI expands on the older Recommended Dietary Allowance (RDA) and takes into consideration other dietary quantities such as Estimated Average Requirement (EAR), Adequate Intake (AI), and Tolerable Upper Intake Level (UL).

Estimated Average Requirement (EAR) The estimated daily intake level of a vitamin or mineral needed to meet the requirements, as defined by a specified indicator of adequacy, of half of the healthy individuals within a given life stage or gender group.

Adequate Intake (AI) A reference intake for nutrients that is used instead of the Recommended Dietary Allowance. When insufficient scientific evidence is available to calculate an Estimated Average Requirement (EAR), then an AI is used. Similar to the EAR and the Recommended Dietary Allowance (RDA), the AI values are based on intake data of healthy individuals.

Tolerable Upper Intake Level (UL) The highest level of daily nutrient intake that poses no adverse health effects for almost all individuals in the general population.

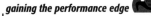

gaining the performance edge

The DRIs encompass the EARs, RDAs, AIs, and ULs for each macronutrient, vitamin, and mineral based on recent research and epidemiological data of healthy populations. As more information and data are discovered, these recommendations will be updated and revised.

ents are published as scientific data are gathered. This comprehensive effort to develop all components of the DRIs is under the auspices of the Standing Committee on the Scientific Evaluation of Dietary Reference Intakes of the Food and Nutrition Board, the Institute of Medicine, and the National Academy of Sciences of the United States, along with Health Canada.[1] The definitions of these values are reviewed in **Table 1.1**.

What are enriched and fortified foods?

In the milling process of grains, the germ and bran are removed. The germ and bran contain a majority of the vitamins and minerals in whole grains, and thus the resulting refined product is less nutritious. Refined grain products include white flours, bread, pasta, rice, crackers, and cereals. To prevent deficiency diseases, the Food and Drug Administration mandated in 1943 that the nutrients lost during the milling process of wheat, rice, and corn be replaced. The nutrients identified and thus added to refined grain products include thiamin, riboflavin,

gaining the performance edge

Enrichment and fortification of foods and beverages are intended to help individuals meet their daily nutrient needs.

niacin, and iron. The addition of vitamins and minerals to refined products is termed **enrichment**.

Fortification is the addition of a vitamin or mineral to a food or beverage in which it was not originally present. The first successful fortification program was the addition of iodine to salt in the 1920s to prevent goiter and other iodine deficiency conditions. In general, fortification is not required by the FDA, with the exception of folic acid in grains and vitamin D in milk. Other fortification programs are designed to enhance the quality of a product, such as the addition of vitamin A to milk and other dairy foods, as well as lysine to specific corn products to enhance protein quality. The food industry has the freedom to add any vitamin or mineral to a product. However, the FDA does require companies to show that a dietary insufficiency exists and therefore requires fortification in otherwise standardized products. Some products contain vitamins or minerals not naturally found in the food or beverage, such as added vitamin D and vitamin B_{12} in soy milk. Other products boost existing vitamin or mineral content, such as extra vitamin C added to orange juice. Sport supplements, such as bars and shakes, are highly fortified with a variety of vitamins and minerals. Athletes should check labels to ensure that total daily consumption of any vitamin or mineral is not in excess of upper dietary limits. For more information about enrichment and fortification, visit

enrichment The addition of vitamins and minerals to refined/processed products to increase their nutritional value.

fortification The process of adding vitamins or minerals to foods or beverages that did not originally contain them.

TABLE 1.1	Review of the DRI Values
DRI Value	**Definition**
Dietary Reference Intake (DRI)	Umbrella term for all nutrient classifications, including RDA, EAR, AI, and UL.
Recommended Dietary Allowance (RDA)	Average daily dietary intake level that is sufficient to meet the nutrient requirements of nearly an entire (i.e., 98%) healthy population. The established RDAs can vary based on life stage, including age, gender, and, if appropriate, pregnancy and lactation.
Estimated Average Requirement (EAR)	Daily intake level of a vitamin or mineral estimated to meet the requirements, as defined by a specified indicator of adequacy, in half of the healthy individuals within a life stage or gender group.
Adequate Intake (AI)	Intake recommendation when insufficient scientific evidence is available to calculate an EAR/RDA. AI values are based on intake data of healthy individuals. However, the results of studies regarding the nutrient in question are not conclusive enough or more study is required before an EAR/RDA can be established.
Tolerable Upper Intake Level (UL)	The highest level of daily nutrient intake that poses no adverse health effects for almost all individuals in the general population. At intakes above the UL, the risk of adverse effects increases.

the Food and Drug Administration's Web site at www.fda.gov.

What are the basic nutrition guidelines?

The keys to healthful eating are to consume a diet that provides adequate nutrients to maintain health, includes a variety of foods, is balanced, and is consumed in moderation. Government agencies have developed several tools that provide general healthful eating guidelines that include balance, variety, and moderation to help the American population maintain or improve health. The Dietary Guidelines for Americans and the MyPlate[3] food guidance system are two such tools that convert scientific evidence into practical applications that Americans can use to eat more healthfully. These general guidelines are applicable to sedentary and athletic individuals alike.

What are the Dietary Guidelines for Americans?

The Dietary Guidelines for Americans, developed jointly by the U.S. Department of Health and Human Services (HHS) and the U.S. Department of Agriculture (USDA), are revised and published every 5 years. The first publication was in 1980. The most recent version of the Dietary Guidelines for Americans was published in 2010.[2] The guidelines provide science-based advice for people 2 years and older on dietary and physical activity habits that can promote health and reduce the risk for chronic illnesses and conditions such as cardiovascular disease, diabetes, and hypertension. A healthful diet that is not excessive in calories, follows the nutrition recommendations contained in the guidelines, and is combined with physical activity should enhance the health of most individuals.

The primary purpose of the Dietary Guidelines is to provide the public with information about nutrients and food components that are known to be beneficial for health and to provide recommendations that can be implemented into an eating and exercise plan. The 2010 Dietary Guidelines cover four interrelated focus areas. When the guidelines are implemented as a whole, they encourage Americans to: a) maintain calorie balance over time to achieve and sustain a healthy weight, b) focus on consuming nutrient-dense foods and beverages.

The four interrelated themes and the key recommendations from the 2010 Dietary Guidelines report are as follows (www.dietaryguidelines.gov):[2]

1. *Balance Calories to Manage Weight*
   - Prevent and/or reduce overweight and obesity through improved eating and physical activity behaviors.
   - Control total calorie intake to manage body weight. For people who are overweight or obese, this means consuming fewer calories from foods and beverages.
   - Increase physical activity (see Figure 1.1) and reduce time spent in sedentary behaviors.
   - Maintain appropriate calorie balance during each stage of life—childhood, adolescence, adulthood, pregnancy and breastfeeding, and older age.

2. *Reduce the Following Foods and Food Components*
   - Reduce daily sodium intake to less than 2300 milligrams (mg) and further reduce intake to 1500 mg among persons who are 51 and older and those of any age who are African American or have hypertension, diabetes, or chronic kidney disease. The 1500 mg recommendation applies to about half of the U.S. population, including children, and the majority of adults.

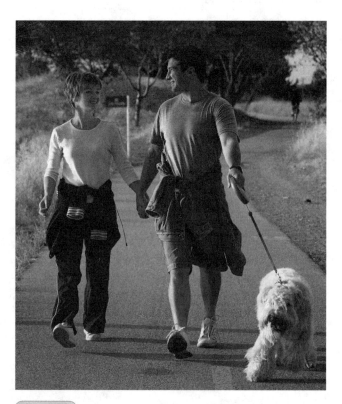

Figure 1.1   Exercising regularly, combined with a diet that does not exceed calorie needs, helps manage weight.

- Consume less than 10% of calories from saturated fatty acids by replacing them with monounsaturated and polyunsaturated fatty acids.
- Consume less than 300 mg per day of dietary cholesterol.
- Keep *trans* fatty acid consumption as low as possible by limiting foods that contain synthetic sources of *trans* fats, such as partially hydrogenated oils, and by limiting other solid fats.
- Reduce the intake of calories from solid fats and added sugars.
- Limit the consumption of foods that contain refined grains, especially refined grain foods that contain solid fats, added sugars, and sodium.
- If alcohol is consumed, it should be consumed in moderation—up to one drink per day for women and two drinks per day for men—and only by adults of legal drinking age.

3. *Increase Intake of the Following Foods and Nutrients*

Individuals should meet the following recommendations as part of a healthy eating pattern while staying within their calorie needs.
- Increase vegetable and fruit intake.
- Eat a variety of vegetables, especially dark green, red, and orange vegetables and beans and peas.
- Consume at least half of all grains as whole grains. Increase whole grain intake by replacing refined grains with whole grains.
- Increase intake of fat-free or low-fat milk and milk products, such as milk, yogurt, cheese, or fortified soy beverages.
- Choose a variety of protein foods, which include seafood, lean meat and poultry, eggs, beans and peas, soy products, and unsalted nuts and seeds.
- Increase the amount and variety of seafood consumed by choosing seafood in place of some meat and poultry.
- Replace protein foods that are higher in solid fats with choices that are lower in solid fats and calories and/or are sources of oils.
- Use oils to replace solid fats where possible.
- Choose foods that provide more potassium, dietary fiber, calcium, and vitamin D, which are nutrients of concern in American diets. These foods include vegetables, fruits, whole grains, and milk and milk products.

Recommendations for specific population groups:
- *Women capable of becoming pregnant*
  a. Choose foods that supply heme iron, (which is more readily absorbed by the body), additional iron sources, and enhancers of iron absorption such as vitamin C–rich foods.
  b. Consume 400 micrograms (mcg) per day of synthetic folic acid (from fortified foods and/or supplements) in addition to food forms of folate from a varied diet.
- *Women who are pregnant or breastfeeding*
  a. Consume 8 to 12 ounces of seafood per week from a variety of seafood types.
  b. Due to its high methyl mercury content, limit white (albacore) tuna to 6 ounces per week and do not eat the following four types of fish: tilefish, shark, swordfish, and king mackerel.
  c. If pregnant, take an iron supplement, as recommended by an obstetrician or other health care provider.
- *Individuals aged 50 years and older*
  a. Consume foods fortified with vitamin B_{12}, such as fortified cereals, or dietary supplements.

4. *Build Healthy Eating Patterns*
- Select an eating pattern that meets nutrient needs over time at an appropriate calorie level.
- Account for all foods and beverages consumed and assess how they fit within a total healthy eating pattern.
- Follow food safety recommendations when preparing and eating foods to reduce the risk of foodborne illnesses.

Although the Dietary Guidelines listed here were developed with the American population's health in mind, athletes can benefit from implementing the guidelines in their daily nutrition planning. By selecting a variety of nutrient-dense foods, as dictated in the guidelines, athletes can meet their energy, macronutrient, and micronutrient needs for a high level of sport performance. The MyPlate food guidance system can be used to further plan an athlete's daily food intake by practically applying the information in the Dietary Guidelines.

What is the MyPlate food guidance system?

The United States Department of Agriculture (USDA) released the MyPlate food guidance system in 2011 (www.ChooseMyPlate.gov). The USDA's Center for

Nutrition Policy and Promotion, established in 1994, developed the MyPlate system to improve the nutrition and well-being of Americans. The MyPlate system (see Figure 1.2) is a revision of the MyPyramid released in 2005. The new icon was developed for two main purposes: (1) to improve the effectiveness in motivating consumers to make healthier food choices and (2) to incorporate the latest nutrition science information into the new system. MyPlate and the Dietary Guidelines for Americans complement each other and can provide basic guidelines and practical applications for healthful eating to improve health and well-being.

On the ChooseMyPlate.gov website, seven selected messages are reviewed in association with the MyPlate icon. The selected messages are intended to help consumers focus on key nutrition behaviors. The selected messages, which correlate with the four interrelated themes and key recommendations of the 2010 Dietary Guidelines, include:

- Enjoy your food, but eat less.
- Avoid oversized portions.
- Make half your plate fruits and vegetables.
- Switch to fat-free or low-fat (1%) milk.
- Make at least half your grains whole grains.
- Compare sodium in foods such as soup, bread, and frozen meals—and choose foods with lower numbers.
- Drink water instead of sugary drinks.

Graphically, the MyPlate food guidance system is a useful and intuitive way for athletes to eat well and improve their health. The MyPlate icon provides a visual representation of a balanced, nutritious meal. The icon is a plate split into four sections, each representing a different type of food (protein, whole grains, fruits, and vegetables). The sections vary in size depending on the recommended portion of each food an athlete should eat. A circle shape next to the plate represents dairy products, especially milk. Each of the food groups are further described in print and electronic format to help consumers make positive nutrition changes. The concepts and main messages in each food category are described briefly in the following paragraphs.

The key message in the grain group of MyPlate is that at least half of the total grains consumed

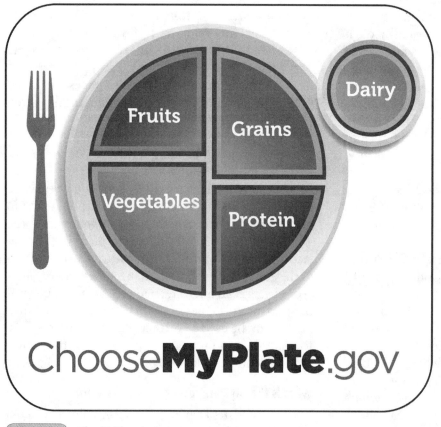

Figure 1.2   The MyPlate icon.

should be from whole grain sources. The goal is to eat three or more ounce-equivalents of whole grain products each day. Individuals that require more calories will need to consume more than this amount daily. Examples of whole grains include brown rice, bulgur, oatmeal, and whole wheat breads, crackers, and pastas. Consumers can check the food label for the words "whole grain" and the ingredient panel for the word "whole" or "whole grain" before the grain ingredient.

In the vegetable category, emphasis is placed not only on consuming enough vegetables daily, but also on choosing different vegetables throughout the week to obtain a greater variety of the nutrients provided from vegetables. The vegetables are listed in five subgroups based on nutrient content: dark green, orange, starchy, dry beans and peas, and other vegetables. The main consumer message with vetetables and fruits, is to "make half of your plate vegetables and fruits."

Similar to the vegetable group, MyPlate encourages not only consuming the recommended amount of fruit each day, but also consuming a wide variety of fruits. Fruits consumed fresh, canned, frozen, dried, or as 100% juice all count toward the fruit recommendation. However, MyPlate recommends focusing on whole fruits versus fruit juices. This recommendation is made because fruit juices tend to be more calorie-dense and contain little fiber compared to whole fruits.

A variety of different foods are part of the oils and empty calories categories of MyPlate. Please note that these categories are not food groups. Americans are encouraged to minimize sources of empty calories, however, there are some essential nutrients provided by oils. The key concept in the oils category is to choose mainly monounsaturated and polyunsaturated fats contained in foods such as fish, nuts, seeds, and vegetable oils. Oils used in liquid form such as canola, corn, olive, and sunflower are considered unsaturated and commonly used in cooking. Other foods that are composed primarily of oils include items such as mayonnaise, salad dressing, and soft margarine. Consumers should review the Nutrition Facts label of these foods to ensure no trans fats are present. Foods and beverages containing solid fats and added sugars are considered empty calories because they provide extra calories with few to no nutrients. While small amounts of these foods can be included daily, most Americans are consuming far more than is healthy, and therefore, should focus on limiting their intake. Examples of empty calories include butter, shortening, desserts, and sodas.

The dairy group of MyPlate contains liquid milk products, yogurt, cheeses, and many foods made from milk. The key concept for the dairy category is to consume three cups of fat-free or low-fat (1%) milk or an equivalent amount of yogurt or cheese per day. Foods made from milk that retain calcium after processing (such as cheese and yogurt) are part of this food group, but foods made from milk that do not contain appreciable calcium (such as cream cheese and butter) are not included in this group. Individuals who do not or cannot consume milk and milk products should consume dairy alternative products (soy, nut or grain milk, yogurt and cheese) and other calcium-rich foods daily.

The protein foods group includes items made from meat, poultry, fish, dry beans or peas, eggs, nuts, and seeds. The key concept for this group is to make choices that are low-fat or lean when selecting meat and poultry. The dry beans and peas, including soy products, are part of this group as well as the vegetable group. Dry beans and peas are naturally low in fat and nutrient-dense. Nuts, seeds, and some fatty fishes contain higher fat content, but these fats are from healthy oils and should be chosen frequently as a substitute for meat or poultry.

Physical activity is not depicted in the MyPlate icon, but is encouraged as part of a healthy lifestyle. The key message is to become less sedentary and to engage in regular physical activity. Physical activity includes movement that uses energy. Adults should engage in at least 2 hours and 30 minutes of aerobic physical activity at a moderate level each week or 1 hour and 15 minutes of aerobic physical activity at a vigorous level each week. For example, moderate or vigorous activities include walking briskly, hiking, gardening/yard work, golf (walking and carrying clubs), weight training, bicycling, swimming, and aerobics. Physical activities that are not intense enough to meet the recommendations might include walking at a casual pace or doing light household chores.

To personalize a plan, individuals can go to www.ChooseMyPlate.gov[3] to get information that is specific to their needs for energy, nutrient composition, and physical activity level. For example, a 32-year-old female recreational runner can enter her age, gender, and average amount of daily physical activity, and the online MyPlate program will calculate the recommended servings in each of the five major food groups and information on the amount of oils, solid fats, and added sugars per day. Figure 1.3 shows the food group recommendations, suggested maximum intake of oils, solid fats, and added sugars, and states what calorie level the pattern is based on for this 32-year-old runner at the moderate activity level. Following the recommendations from this calculation should help this female athlete maintain a healthful weight and meet nutrient requirements. If energy expenditure should increase (for example, if this female runner decided to train for a marathon), she could return to the Web site and enter the new information using the 60 minutes or more physical activity level and a new calorie level, and recommended servings would be calculated. This individualization is helpful because not all individuals at the same age and gender have the same physical activity level and energy needs. Ath-

letes with extremely high exercise levels will need to consume more than the MyPlate plan recommends because these athletes are exercising at daily levels significantly greater than 60 minutes.

The MyPlate food guidance system provides a wealth of information for consumers to apply healthful eating and exercise patterns into their daily lifestyle. Athletes can use this system to learn their personalized nutrient needs. Many athletes who train extensively daily will need a significantly higher number of calories than the average person. These additional calories should be consumed in nutrient-dense foods from the MyPlate food groups. In summary, MyPlate provides detailed guidelines for improving overall health, as well as athletic performance, with adequate daily nutrition and physical activity.

My Daily Food Plan

Based on the information you provided, this is your daily recommended amount for each food group.

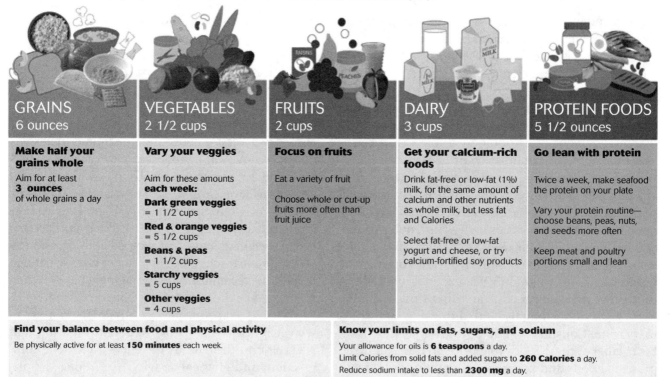

GRAINS 6 ounces	VEGETABLES 2 1/2 cups	FRUITS 2 cups	DAIRY 3 cups	PROTEIN FOODS 5 1/2 ounces
Make half your grains whole Aim for at least **3 ounces** of whole grains a day	**Vary your veggies** Aim for these amounts **each week:** **Dark green veggies** = 1 1/2 cups **Red & orange veggies** = 5 1/2 cups **Beans & peas** = 1 1/2 cups **Starchy veggies** = 5 cups **Other veggies** = 4 cups	**Focus on fruits** Eat a variety of fruit Choose whole or cut-up fruits more often than fruit juice	**Get your calcium-rich foods** Drink fat-free or low-fat (1%) milk, for the same amount of calcium and other nutrients as whole milk, but less fat and Calories Select fat-free or low-fat yogurt and cheese, or try calcium-fortified soy products	**Go lean with protein** Twice a week, make seafood the protein on your plate Vary your protein routine—choose beans, peas, nuts, and seeds more often Keep meat and poultry portions small and lean

Find your balance between food and physical activity	**Know your limits on fats, sugars, and sodium**
Be physically active for at least **150 minutes** each week.	Your allowance for oils is **6 teaspoons** a day. Limit Calories from solid fats and added sugars to **260 Calories** a day. Reduce sodium intake to less than **2300 mg** a day.

Your results are based on a 2000 Calorie pattern.   Name: _____

This Calorie level is only an estimate of your needs. Monitor your body weight to see if you need to adjust your Calorie intake.

Figure 1.3   The MyPlate food guidance system allows individuals to personalize their food plan based on gender, age, and level of physical activity.

How should athletes interpret the information on food labels?

The nutrition guidelines presented in this text are a combination of the current research in sports nutrition and the practical application of that knowledge. A large part of the practical portion is athletes' awareness of how the foods they eat contribute to their total daily needs. The food label (see Figure 1.4) allows athletes to obtain credible and reliable nutrition information about various food and beverage products, ultimately empowering them to make wise food choices on a daily basis. However, some athletes find the food label confusing and difficult to interpret. This section will provide a brief overview of the food label, the components that pertain directly to sports nutrition, and how to apply the label information to individual scenarios. A full report and explanation of the food label and associated regulations can be found at www.fda.gov.

Who created the food label regulations?

Food and Drug Administration (FDA) The governing body responsible for ensuring the safety of foods sold in the United States. This includes oversight of the proper labeling of foods.

The **Food and Drug Administration (FDA)** is the governing body responsible for ensuring the safety of foods sold in the United States, which includes overseeing the proper labeling of foods. In 1990, Congress passed the Nutrition Labeling and Education Act (NLEA) based on the demand for consistent consumer information and labeling of all foods. With the passing (1990) and implementation (1994) of the NLEA, a series of changes was seen on food packages. A nutrition label is now required on most food packages, with a few exceptions such as small, individual food packages (modified label required) and meat products (governed by the USDA, therefore no labeling is required). The nutrition labeling of food products must follow specific FDA guidelines and include the following: (1) statement of identity, (2) net contents, (3) name and address of the manufacturer, packer, or distributor, (4) ingredient list, and (5) Nutrition Facts panel. The statement of identity is prominently displayed on the front of the food label and gives the commonly used name or a descriptive title to the food contained within the package. Also on the front of the food label along the bottom edge, the net contents can be found. The net contents give the quantity of food within the package and are expressed in units of weight, vol-

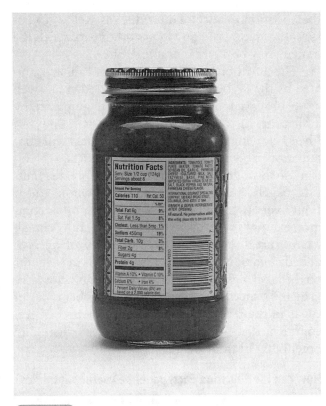

Figure 1.4 Information on food labels. Federal regulations determine what can and cannot appear on food labels.

ume, or numeric count. The name and address of the producer or distributor of the product is usually in the small print found beneath the list of ingredients. Contact information is important in case the athlete has further questions about the product or needs to report problems. The food label may also include FDA-approved **nutrient content claims** or **health claims** that highlight certain characteristics or potential benefits of the food. Finally, the list of ingredients and Nutrition Facts panel must be shown on the label. Each is discussed in the following sections.

nutrient content claims Nutrition-related claims on food labels that highlight certain characteristics of the food.

health claim A description placed on a food label that describes potential health benefits of a food or nutrient.

How can the ingredient list be useful to athletes?

An ingredients list is required on all foods that contain more than one ingredient. The ingredients must be listed in descending order of predominance in the product. The order of predominance is determined by weight, with the ingredient that weighs the most listed first and the one that weighs the least listed last. Athletes can use this nutrition tool to evaluate the nutrition quality of a product as well as to ensure that they avoid any food/additive to which the athlete may be allergic or intolerant.

The nutrition quality of a product can be evaluated by the presence of a specific ingredient as well as the order of listed ingredients. For example, many athletes are instructed to increase their daily intake of fiber. Knowing that whole grain products will contain more fiber than refined flour products, athletes can use the ingredients label to choose breads, muffins, bagels, and pasta that contain "whole wheat flour" versus "enriched white flour." Another common example pertains to choosing a healthy cereal. Many cereals contain a large quantity of refined, added sugars. By studying the order of ingredients on the label and choosing a brand that does not have "sugar," "sucrose," "corn syrup," or other types of sugar in the first 2–3 ingredients, athletes can feel confident that they have chosen a lower-sugar, and potentially healthier, cereal.

How can the Nutrition Facts panel be useful to athletes?

The Nutrition Facts panel informs consumers about the specific nutrient content of foods in quantifiable terms. Manufacturers must use the Nutrition Facts panel within the specified FDA guidelines and must provide accurate information about the nutrient content of the food. An example and description of the Nutrition Facts panel are presented in (Figure 1.5). Foods that are not required to carry a Nutrition Facts panel include delicatessen-style foods, restaurant foods, fresh bakery products, foods that provide no significant nutrition such as instant coffee and most spices, and multiunit packages. Smaller packages may require a modified Nutrition Facts panel, as shown in (Figure 1.6).

Starting just below the Nutrition Facts heading on each food label, the following required components are all applicable to athletes:

- *Serving size and number of servings per container:* Athletes need to understand what counts as one serving. Often, athletes consider one package to be "one serving," when in fact there could be multiple servings included in a container, as stated in the Nutrition Facts panel. Because the nutrition information is presented for one serving, athletes will need to multiply the nutrition information listed on the Nutrition Facts panel

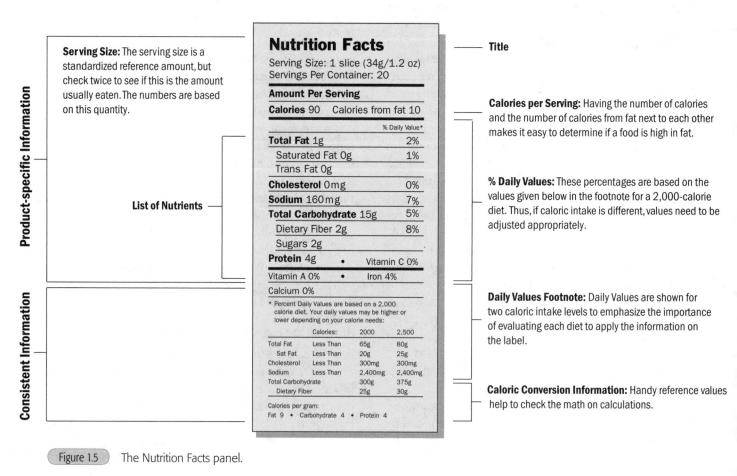

Figure 1.5   The Nutrition Facts panel.

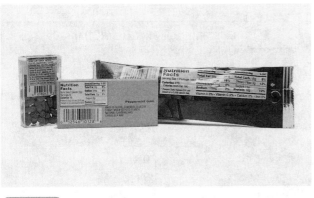

Figure 1.6 Nutrition Facts panel on small packages. Food products that have small packages can use an abbreviated version of the Nutrition Facts panel.

by the number of servings consumed to obtain an accurate estimate of total nutrient intake.

- *Calories and percentage of calories from fat:* Reviewing the calorie content of foods eaten throughout the day will allow athletes to ensure adequate total energy consumption. To obtain the percentage of calories from fat, the "calories from fat" can be divided by the total "calories" and then multiplied by 100. Athletes should aim for a diet that includes no more than 30–35% of total calories from fat, indicating it is low to moderate in fat. Calculating the percentage for each food chosen throughout the day can help athletes make healthy choices. Chapter 4 of this text will discuss in greater detail the importance of fat and how to calculate the percentage of calories from fat in several different ways.

- *Total fat and saturated fat:* Fat is important in an athlete's diet; however, it should be consumed in moderation. Athletes can compare different brands or types of food to find low/moderate fat options. Saturated fat is detrimental to heart health, and therefore athletes should attempt to minimize their saturated fat intake.

- *Cholesterol:* Cholesterol, also discussed in Chapter 4 of this text, is not a required nutrient in the diet. Cholesterol is made in the body and therefore does not need to be consumed daily. If it is consumed, athletes should keep intake to a minimum because dietary cholesterol has been shown to increase blood cholesterol levels, thus increasing the risk for cardiovascular disease.

- *Sodium:* Classified as an electrolyte, sodium is an essential nutrient for athletes because it is lost in sweat. Sodium has also been linked to high blood pressure, and therefore athletes should consume

enough to meet their needs while also avoiding excessive intake. Sodium will be discussed in Chapter 7 of this text.

- *Total carbohydrates, dietary fiber, and sugar:* Carbohydrates are the master fuel for all athletics and should compose a majority of an athlete's diet. Dietary fiber plays a role in weight management and disease prevention, and aids in the maintenance of blood sugar levels that deliver a consistent dose of energy to the body. The "dietary fiber" section on the Nutrition Facts panel represents the total quantity of fiber present in a product but does not distinguish between soluble and insoluble fibers. The "sugar" category is a combination of naturally occurring and refined sugars. Because there is no distinction, an athlete should review the ingredients list for the presence of fruits and fruit juices (naturally occurring sugars often accompanied by many other nutrients) or any refined sugar product (providing calories and carbohydrates but devoid of other nutritional value). There is no Percent Daily Value (%DV, discussed in the following section) for sugars because there are no RDA values or Daily Reference Values (DRV) established specific to sugars. The role of carbohydrates in an athlete's diet and the determination of individual needs are presented in Chapter 3 of this text.

- *Protein:* The total quantity of protein, another indispensable nutrient for athletes, is provided on the Nutrition Facts panel. Chapter 5 of this text reviews the roles and sources of protein in the athlete's diet.

- *Vitamins and minerals:* Only two vitamins (vitamins A and C) and two minerals (calcium and iron) are required on the food label. Of course, all vitamins and minerals are important for athletes; however, these four nutrients are generally consumed in suboptimal quantities in the United States and therefore deserve special attention. Information regarding all of the vitamins and minerals can be found in Chapters 6 and 7 of this text.

- *Daily Values footnote and calorie conversion:* The concept of Daily Values will be discussed in the following section. The calorie conversion information is a handy reference for athletes to allow them to perform their own calculations based on individual needs and goals.

Many food manufacturers provide additional allowable information on their food labels in an effort to educate the public and to sell their products. As consumers become more aware of the health benefits of specific foods and food categories, they become more interested and demanding of food labeling information. As information about the health benefits of nutrients becomes available, allowable nutrients on the Nutrition Facts panel may increase.

How can the Percent Daily Value be useful to athletes?

The Percent Daily Value (%DV) is listed on the food label for a variety of macronutrients, vitamins, and minerals. The %DV can be used to determine how a particular product meets the needs of an athlete as well as to compare the nutrient content of two different products. For example, the DV for cholesterol is less than 300 milligrams. The %DV represents what percentage of the daily total is provided in one serving of a product. If the product provides 100 milligrams of cholesterol, the %DV will be 33% because 100 is one-third of 300. The overall concept is that athletes can tally up the percentages of all foods consumed throughout the day and aim for a grand total of 100%, indicating that all needs have been met. However, the caveat is that the %DV is based on the needs of an individual following a 2000-calorie diet. Many athletes require substantially more than 2000 calories daily, and therefore obtaining 100% of all nutrients may not necessarily be adequate. The Daily Values footnote, listed on most Nutrition Facts panels, presents additional information for those following a 2500-calorie diet; however, even the 2500-calorie goals may not be enough for most athletes. In general, athletes may find it easier to know their individual daily needs and evaluate a product based on their own goals versus the %DV goals. **Table 1.2** and **Table 1.3** summarize the reference

TABLE 1.3	Reference Daily Intakes (RDI) for Athletes Older Than 4 Years
Food Component	**RDI**
Protein	50 g
Vitamin A	1000 RE[a]
Vitamin D	400 IU[b]
Vitamin E	30 IU
Vitamin K	80 µg[c]
Vitamin C	60 mg[d]
Folate	400 µg
Thiamin	1.5 mg
Riboflavin	1.7 mg
Niacin	20 mg
Vitamin B_6	2 mg
Vitamin B_{12}	6 µg
Biotin	300 µg
Pantothenic acid	10 mg
Calcium	1000 mg
Phosphorus	1000 mg
Iodide	150 µg
Iron	18 mg
Magnesium	400 mg
Copper	2 mg
Zinc	15 mg
Chloride	3400 mg
Manganese	2 mg
Selenium	70 µg
Chromium	120 µg
Molybdenum	75 µg

[a]RE = retinal equivalents
[b]IU = international units
[c]µg = micrograms
[d]mg = milligrams

Note: RDI values were developed based on older RDAs and do not reflect new DRI values.

Source: Food and Drug Administration, www.fda.gov.

TABLE 1.2	Daily Reference Values on Food Labels	
	2000 Kcal Intake	**2500 Kcal Intake**
Fat	<65 g	<80 g
Saturated fat	<20 g	<25 g
Protein	50 g	65 g
Cholesterol	<300 mg	<300 mg
Carbohydrates	300 g	375 g
Fiber	25 g	30 g
Sodium	<2400 mg	<2400 mg

Source: Food and Drug Administration, www.fda.gov.

amounts used to develop the %DV for macronutrients and micronutrients.

Whether or not the %DV can be useful for an athlete's individual needs, it can be used to compare the nutrient density of various products. As an example, athletes needing to consume more iron can look at the %DV of several brands of cereal and know that the brand with the highest %DV for iron contains the greatest total quantity of iron, therefore making that brand the best choice. The benefit of this type of comparison is that athletes are not required to memorize how much iron they need in a day; they merely need to look for the product with the highest percentage (highest %DV). See Figure 1.7 for an example of this type of comparison.

How can nutrient content claims be useful to athletes?

The Nutrition Labeling and Education Act (NLEA) of 1990 included guidelines for food manufacturers to place nutrition-related claims on food labels in addition to the Nutrition Facts section. These claims highlight certain characteristics of the food and are called nutrient content claims. Foods can be labeled with claims such as "low fat," "reduced sugar," or "high in fiber" only if they meet certain criteria. The definitions of the approved nutrient content claims are presented in **Fortifying Your Nutrition Knowledge**. These nutrition descriptor statements allow athletes to quickly identify the products that meet their individual needs or dietary goals. For

Nutrition Facts

Serving Size: 1 Cup (28g/1.0 oz.)
Servings Per Container: About 18

Amount Per Serving	Cereal	with 1/2 cup Skim Milk
Calories	100	140
Fat Calories	0	0
	% Daily Value*	
Total Fat 0g*	0%	0%
Saturated Fat 0g	0%	0%
Trans Fat 0g		
Cholesterol 0mg	0%	0%
Sodium 300mg	13%	15%
Potassium 25mg	1%	7%
Total Carbohydrate 24g	8%	10%
Dietary Fiber 1g	4%	4%
Sugars 2g		
Other Carbohydrates 21g		
Protein 2g		
Vitamin A	15%	20%
Vitamin C	25%	25%
Calcium	0%	15%
Iron	45%	45%
Vitamin D	10%	25%
Thiamin	25%	30%
Riboflavin	25%	35%
Niacin	25%	25%
Vitamin B₆	25%	25%
Folate	25%	25%
Vitamin B₁₂	25%	35%

Nutrition Facts

Serving Size: 1 Cup (30g)
Servings Per Container: About 15

Amount Per Serving	Cereal	with 1/2 cup Skim Milk
Calories	60	100
Calories from Fat	10	10
	% Daily Value*	
Total Fat 1g*	2%	2%
Saturated Fat 0g	0%	0%
Trans Fat 0g		
Cholesterol 0mg	0%	1%
Sodium 125mg	5%	8%
Potassium 230mg	7%	12%
Total Carbohydrate 24g	8%	10%
Dietary Fiber 13g	52%	52%
Sugars 0g		
Other Carbohydrates 11g		
Protein 2g		
Vitamin A	0%	4%
Vitamin C	15%	15%
Calcium	6%	20%
Iron	25%	25%
Vitamin D	0%	10%
Thiamin	25%	30%
Riboflavin	25%	35%
Niacin	25%	25%
Vitamin B₆	25%	25%
Folic Acid	25%	25%
Phosphorus	15%	30%
Magnesium	15%	20%
Zinc	8%	10%
Copper	10%	10%

Figure 1.7 Comparing iron content of two cereals. These labels are from two different breakfast cereals: cornflakes on the left and wheat bran on the right. Comparing the iron content of both cereals is easy using the Percent Daily Values of each.

example, if an athlete has high cholesterol levels, a product labeled "cholesterol free" would be easily identifiable.

Currently there are no approved regulations on nutrition descriptors or content claims regarding total carbohydrates. Because of the growing trend of consumers choosing low-carbohydrate foods in hopes of losing weight, food manufacturers are placing terms such as "low carb" and "net carbs" on food labels. The FDA is currently gathering evidence and developing a statement outlining carbohydrate food-labeling guidelines. Guidelines are likely to be similar to those established for such terms as "low fat" or "reduced sugar." In the meantime, athletes should recognize that carbohydrates are the master fuel for athletics, and therefore products touting a lower carbohydrate content may not be an ideal choice.

How can health claims be useful to athletes?

Health claims describe the potential health benefits of a food or nutrient. The FDA strictly regulates allowable health claims on food labels and allows only health claims that have been well supported in the scientific literature. To date, the following health claims have been approved (www.fda.gov):

1. *Calcium and osteoporosis:* Adequate calcium may reduce the risk of osteoporosis.
2. *Sodium and hypertension (high blood pressure):* Low-sodium diets may help lower blood pressure.
3. *Dietary fat and cancer:* Low-fat diets decrease the risk for some types of cancer.
4. *Dietary saturated fat and cholesterol and the risk of coronary heart disease:* Diets low in saturated fat and cholesterol decrease the risk for heart disease.
5. *Fiber-containing grain products, fruits, and vegetables and cancer:* Diets low in fat and rich in high-fiber foods may reduce the risk of certain cancers.
6. *Fruits, vegetables, and grain products that contain fiber, particularly soluble fiber, and the risk of coronary heart disease:* Diets low in fat and rich in soluble fiber sources may reduce the risk of heart disease.
7. *Fruits and vegetables and cancer:* Diets low in fat and rich in fruits and vegetables may reduce the risk of certain cancers.
8. *Folate and neural tube defects:* Adequate folate status prior to and early in pregnancy may

reduce the risk of neural tube defects (a birth defect).

9. *Dietary noncariogenic carbohydrate sweeteners and dental caries (cavities):* Foods sweetened with sugar alcohols, D-tagatose, and sucralose do not promote tooth decay.
10. *Soluble fiber from certain foods and risk of coronary heart disease:* Diets low in fat and rich in these types of fiber can help reduce the risk of heart disease.
11. *Soy protein and risk of coronary heart disease:* Foods rich in soy protein as part of a low-fat diet may help reduce the risk of heart disease.
12. *Plant sterol/stanol esters and risk of coronary heart disease:* Diets low in saturated fat and cholesterol that also contain several daily servings of plant stanols/sterols may reduce the risk of heart disease.
13. *Whole grain foods and risk of heart disease and certain cancers:* Diets high in whole grain foods and other plant foods and low in total fat, saturated fat, and cholesterol may help reduce the risk of heart disease and certain cancers.
14. *Potassium and the risk of high blood pressure and stroke:* Diets that contain good sources of potassium may reduce the risk of high blood pressure and stroke.
15. *Fluoridated water and reduced risk of dental caries:* Drinking fluoridated water may reduce the risk of dental caries or tooth decay.
16. *Saturated fat, cholesterol, and trans fat, and reduced risk of heart disease:* Replacing saturated fat with similar amounts of unsaturated fats may reduce the risk of heart disease. To achieve this benefit, total daily calories should not increase.

New health claims can be approved at any time based on scientific evidence, and, therefore, this list may expand in the future.

What are the factors to consider when developing an individualized sports nutrition plan for athletes?

As mentioned earlier, one of the exciting aspects of the field of sports nutrition is individualizing eating plans for athletes. Each athlete is different—there is not a "one-size-fits-all" type of meal plan, training diet, or competition hydration schedule. Certainly the basic sports nutrition concepts and guidelines can be applied universally; however, each athlete will require a unique approach by tweaking those guidelines to fit individual needs. For example, all athletes should consume a combination of carbohydrates and protein after exercise to initiate the repair and rebuilding process. However, one athlete may enjoy a turkey sandwich with a banana, while another athlete craves an omelet, toast, and orange juice. Both of these meals meet the carbohydrate–protein combination requirement but also take into consideration personal taste preferences. This individualized approach is much more challenging and requires a greater breadth of knowledge than "cookie-cutter" plans. Sports nutrition professionals with this philosophy will succeed because of the recognition that their plans are based on solid research and current guidelines while also being practical, easy to implement, and specific to an athlete's sport and lifestyle.

Several factors must be considered when calculating nutrient needs and developing a meal plan for an athlete, including the individual's health history, the bioenergetics of the athlete's sport, total weekly training and competition time, living arrangements, access to food, and travel schedules.

Why should a sports nutrition plan consider an athlete's health history?

First and foremost, an athlete must be healthy to train and compete to his or her potential. Proper nutrition

gaining the performance edge

The food label can be very helpful to athletes choosing to follow a more healthful diet. Athletes should review all the information on the Nutrition Facts panel as well as the ingredients list to aid in making informed food and beverage choices. Nutrient content claims and health claims identify products that might be appealing to individual athletes based on their nutrition goals and needs; however, these statements should not take the place of reviewing the Nutrition Facts panel and ingredients list.

Fortifying
Your Nutrition Knowledge

Approved Nutrient Content Claims

Free: Food contains no amount (or trivial or "physiologically inconsequential" amounts). May be used with one or more of the following: fat, saturated fat, cholesterol, sodium, sugar, and calorie. Synonyms include without, no, and zero.

   Fat-free: Less than 0.5 g of fat per serving.
   Saturated fat-free: Less than 0.5 g of saturated fat and less than 0.5 g trans fat per serving.
   Cholesterol-free: Less than 2 mg of cholesterol per serving.
   Sodium-free: Less than 5 mg of sodium per serving.
   Sugar-free: Less than 0.5 g of sugar per serving.
   Calorie-free: Fewer than 5 calories per serving.

Low: Food can be eaten frequently without exceeding dietary guidelines for one or more of these components: fat, saturated fat, cholesterol, sodium, and calories. Synonyms include little, few, and low source of.

   Low fat: 3 g or less per serving.
   Low saturated fat: 1 g or less of saturated fat; no more than 15% of calories from saturated fat.
   Low cholesterol: 20 mg or less per serving.
   Low sodium: 140 mg or less per serving.
   Very low sodium: 35 mg or less per serving.
   Low calorie: 40 calories or less per serving.

High, Rich in, Excellent source of: Food contains 20% or more of the Daily Value for a particular nutrient in a serving.

(continued)

Good source, Contains, Provides: Food contains 10–19% of the Daily Value for a particular nutrient in one serving.

Lean and Extra Lean: The fat content of meal and main dish products, seafood, and game meat products.

　Lean: Less than 10 g fat, 4.5 g or less saturated fat, and less than 95 mg of cholesterol per serving and per 100 g.

　Extra Lean: Less than 5 g fat, less than 2 g saturated fat, and less than 95 mg of cholesterol per serving and per 100 g.

Reduced, Less: Nutritionally altered product containing at least 25% less of a nutrient or of calories than the regular or reference product. (Note: A "reduced" claim can't be used if the reference product already meets the requirement for "low.")

Light: This descriptor can have two meanings:

1. A nutritionally altered product contains one-third fewer calories or half the fat of the reference food. If the reference food derives 50% or more of its calories from fat, the reduction must be 50% of the fat.
2. The sodium content of a low-calorie, low-fat food has been reduced by 50%. Also, light in sodium may be used on a food in which the sodium content has been reduced by at least 50%.
   Note: The term *light* can still be used to describe such properties as texture and color as long as the label clearly explains its meaning (e.g., light brown sugar or light and fluffy).

More, Fortified, Enriched, Added, Extra, Plus: A serving of food, whether altered or not, contains a nutrient that is at least 10% of the Daily Value more than the reference food. May only be used for vitamins, minerals, protein, dietary fiber, and potassium.

Healthy: A healthy food must be low in fat and saturated fat and contain limited amounts of cholesterol (≤95 mg) and sodium (<480 mg for individual foods and ≤600 mg for meal-type products). In addition, a single-item food must provide at least 10% or more of one of the following: vitamins A or C, iron, calcium, protein, or fiber. A meal-type product, such as a frozen entrée or dinner, must provide 10% of two or more of these vitamins or minerals, or protein, or fiber, in addition to meeting the other criteria. Additional regulations allow the term *healthy* to be applied to raw, canned, or frozen fruits and vegetables and enriched grains even if the 10% nutrient content rule is not met. However, frozen or canned fruits or vegetables cannot contain ingredients that would change the nutrient profile.

Fresh: Food is raw, has never been frozen or heated, and contains no preservatives. *Fresh frozen*, *frozen fresh*, and *freshly frozen* can be used for foods that are quickly frozen while still fresh. Blanched foods also can be called fresh.

Percent fat free: Food must be a low-fat or a fat-free product. In addition, the claim must reflect accurately the amount of nonfat ingredients in 100 g of food.

Implied claims: Implied claims suggest that a nutrient is absent or present in a certain amount or suggests a food may be useful in maintaining healthy dietary practices. These claims are prohibited when they wrongfully imply that a food contains or does not contain a meaningful level of a nutrient. For example, a product cannot claim to be made with an ingredient known to be a source of fiber (such as "made with oat bran") unless the product contains enough of that ingredient (in this case, oat bran) to meet the definition for "good source" of fiber. As another example, a claim that a product contains "no tropical oils" is allowed, but only on foods that are "low" in saturated fat, because consumers have come to equate tropical oils with high levels of saturated fat.

Source: Food and Drug Administration. Food Labeling and Nutrition: Nutrient Content Claims Definitions and Approved Claims. Available at: http://www.fda.gov/Food/LabelingNutrition/. Accessed January 24, 2011.

plays a vital role in preventing deficiency and degenerative diseases, while also aiding in the treatment of existing medical conditions. An athlete's health history must be the "team captain" in the sports nutrition game plan, with sport-specific planning, training/competition schedules, living arrangements, and personal preferences rounding out the starting lineup.

For example, an athlete with diabetes must carefully balance his or her intake of carbohydrates with daily doses of insulin to prevent hyper- or hypoglycemia. Whereas most athletes would not think twice about drinking a large glass of juice in the morning before a workout, a diabetic athlete consuming only juice (a carbohydrate source without a protein source to stabilize the digestion of food and blood sugar levels) may experience blood sugar swings that can potentially affect performance. In addition to performance in a single workout, long-term poor blood sugar management can lead to a plethora of associated medical conditions later in life.

An athlete's health history must be considered first and then, subsequently, recommendations can intertwine with sport-specific suggestions. Chapter 10 reviews in further detail the health history and health parameters to consider with athletes during a nutrition consultation.

Why should a sports nutrition plan consider a sport's bioenergetics and logistics?

Energy metabolism is the foundation of sports nutrition. Consideration of the cellular machinery and metabolic pathways responsible for making the energy needed to participate in a specific sport is critical for the development of an individualized eating plan. Chapter 2 of this text explains the different energy pathways in detail, and Chapters 12, 13, and 14 provide examples of how various sport activities differ in using energy for exercise. For example, the calorie, macronutrient, and micronutrient needs of a football player (intermittent exertion over the course of several hours) will be different from the needs of a rower (continuous effort for typically less than 10–20 minutes). Even within one sport, such as running, different events (100-meter sprint versus a marathon) will highlight various energy systems (short, intense effort versus sustained moderate effort). In addition to the bioenergetics of a sport, nutrition plans for athletes must also consider the logistics of training sessions and competitions. Some sports are very conducive for drinking and eating during ac-

tivity (biking), whereas other sports make fluid and energy consumption close to impossible (open water swimming). Sports nutrition professionals must devise plans that are specific for the energy systems utilized during training and competition as well as realistic to the nature of an athlete's sport.

Why should a sports nutrition plan consider an athlete's total weekly training and competition time?

Athletes can range from the weekend warrior to the full-time professional. Each athlete will dedicate a period of time each day to training and competition. Obviously, the athletes who are more active will have greater energy and nutrient needs. However, it is not always as simple as telling highly active athletes to "eat more." Many athletes struggle to meet their daily needs because of the time constraints of meal planning and preparation, as well as short periods of time between workouts, work, school, and other life commitments. Sports nutrition professionals need to be creative in helping athletes to determine how to consume adequate amounts of energy and nutrients while making meal planning easy, convenient, and quick.

A sports nutrition plan also includes the development of a fueling and hydration schedule for training and competition. The timing of meals and snacks must be strategically scheduled to provide enough time for food to digest before training sessions, and to prevent too much time from elapsing after training. Fluid requirements vary considerably among athletes. Therefore, the construction of a hydration schedule is individualized for the athlete and specific to the sport. The energy and nutrients consumed before, during, and after exercise are part of an overall daily sports nutrition plan that can literally make or break an athlete's performance. The more time an athlete spends training each week, the more strategic planning needs to occur to create an appropriate, individualized regimen. Chapters 12, 13, and 14 provide practical applications that are sport-specific for planning and implementing sports nutrition and hydration guidelines before, during, and after training or competitive events (see Figure 1.8).

Why should a sports nutrition plan consider an athlete's living arrangements, access to food, and travel schedule?

A perfectly calculated nutrition plan is worthless if the athlete cannot execute the plan because of a lack of control over the foods available to him or

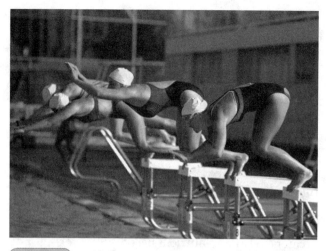

Athletes may travel to events and stay at the competition venue for several hours or all day. Athletes need to plan ahead to fuel and hydrate adequately throughout the event day.

nutrients after exercise is also of great importance. Each athlete will vary in ability to pack a postexercise snack or decipher the most appropriate food/beverage option from a buffet of available items.

Proper nutrition while traveling is a challenge for everyone—athletes and nonathletes alike. Travel forces individuals to change their routine, sometimes wreaking havoc on an athlete's good intentions and typical nutrition habits. Athletes must be educated on how to make healthy choices and appropriate substitutions while on the road. Creative planning, packing nonperishable foods for the trip, and learning to be flexible will help athletes remain optimally fueled while traveling. Chapter 14 provides tips for healthy eating while on the road.

How can sports nutrition knowledge be converted into practical applications?

One of the biggest challenges facing all health promotion professionals is helping people make permanent behavior changes. When working with individuals, possessing "book" knowledge is only one part of the equation; professionals must know how to assess a person's readiness for change, engage in active listening, and then provide the appropriate information or guidance. This process is particularly applicable to counseling athletes on dietary changes to improve performance. Not only should meal plans be based on individual needs, but the construction of the plans also must take into consideration the athlete's preparedness for change. Chapter 10 provides detailed information on the process of counseling athletes, including the use of the Transtheoretical Model,[1] which assesses a person's readiness for change.

The skill of active listening can be a powerful tool for helping athletes initiate change. Athletes want to know that a sports nutrition professional cares about them, their performance, and their capabilities for change. Sports nutrition professionals should refrain from developing a "dictatorship" where athletes simply sit quietly and listen to the dietary changes they "need" to make to improve their performance and/or health. Instead, athletes should be active participants in their meal planning and goal set-

her on a daily basis. For example, a college athlete who lives in a dorm is at the mercy of what is served in the university cafeterias. Therefore, the cafeteria menus should be built into the sports nutrition plan for this athlete. Sports nutrition professionals must fully understand each athlete's living arrangements and access to food before developing an individualized program.

Access to food can also be a factor before, during, or after competitions. Many athletes are required to eat with the team at their training table before a game, thereby limiting their food choices to what is provided by the team. Recreational athletes who are participating in weekend events, such as running or walking road races, often must rely on the products supplied on the course for hydration and fueling. Developing an appropriate race day plan for these athletes involves investigating the foods and beverages available on the course and then planning for the athletes to practice with these specific items throughout training to prevent any surprises on race day. Consuming the optimal blend of

gaining the performance edge

Individualization in nutrition planning for athletes is essential for success as a sports nutrition professional. Standardized plans will contribute to the great success of some athletes, while leaving others on the sidelines. Incorporating factors such as an athlete's health history, the bioenergetics and logistics of the sport, weekly training/competition time, living arrangements, access to food/beverages, and travel schedules into an individualized nutrition program will ultimately lead to the athlete's success and peak performance.

gaining the performance edge

Knowing the current sports nutrition research, established dietary guidelines, and performance-enhancing recommendations is not enough; sports nutrition professionals must be skilled in helping athletes convert the sports nutrition knowledge into practical, daily guidelines for food and beverage intake.

ting. Food selections should be based on an athlete's likes and dislikes versus which foods are "best" for them—if an athlete does not enjoy the foods in the established meal plan, adherence will be poor. Goals should be realistic and manageable to plant the seeds for success and accomplishment that will motivate athletes to continue working on healthy eating behaviors. Listen to athletes—know their goals, questions, and concerns—and then build an individualized plan that is mutually acceptable and productive.

The Box Score

Key Points of Chapter

- Sports nutrition can be defined as the conversion of nutrition knowledge into a practical daily eating plan focused on providing the fuel for physical activity, facilitating the repair and rebuilding process following hard physical work, and optimizing athletic performance in competitive events, while also promoting overall health and wellness.

- In this text, the term athlete refers to any individual who is regularly active, ranging from the fitness enthusiast to the competitive amateur or professional.

- Sports nutrition professionals must have a command of general nutrition and exercise science, understand how nutrition and physical training are intertwined, and practice the practical application of sports nutrition knowledge.

- The area of sports nutrition is a growing field, with many opportunities for a rewarding and exciting career.

- Foods and beverages are composed of six nutrients that are vital to the human body for producing energy, contributing to the growth and development of tissues, regulating body processes, and preventing deficiency and degenerative diseases. The six nutrients are carbohydrates, proteins, fats, vitamins, minerals, and water.

- The body derives its energy from carbohydrates, fats, and proteins, which are collectively known as the energy nutrients. Their breakdown within the cells of the body provides the energy to make ATP, which is the body's direct source of energy for not only sport performance but also all biological work.

- The Dietary Reference Intakes were developed to expand on the Recommended Dietary Allowance values and to set new recommendations for nutrients that did not have an RDA. The DRIs identify the reference amount of a specific nutrient needed for individuals to prevent deficiency conditions in generally healthy individuals. The DRIs include the RDA, EAR, AI, and UL for each vitamin, mineral, and macronutrient.

- Processing of foods often destroys or removes vitamins. Enrichment is a process by which vitamins are restored to foods after processing. Fortification is another way to improve the nutrient value of foods, and involves adding vitamins or minerals to foods in which the vitamins or minerals were not originally present.

- The 2010 Dietary Guidelines for Americans emphasize the fact that nutrition choices and physical activity interact to improve health and prevent chronic conditions. The guidelines focus on making smart choices from all food groups, balancing food intake with physical activity to maintain weight, and choosing nutrient-dense foods.

- MyPlate, along with the 2010 Dietary Guidelines for Americans, encourages individuals to make better food choices. The MyPlate icon provides a visual representation of a balanced, nutritious meal.

- The food label allows athletes to obtain credible and reliable nutrition information about various food and beverage products, ultimately empowering them to make wise food choices on a daily basis.

- Developing an individualized sports nutrition plan for athletes involves considering the individual's health history, the bioenergetics and logistics of the athlete's sport, total weekly training and competition time, living arrangements, access to food, and travel schedules.

- When working with athletes, possessing "book" knowledge is only one part of the equation; professionals must know how to assess a person's readiness for change, engage in active listening, and then provide the appropriate information or guidance.

- Sports nutrition professionals should listen closely to the goals, questions, and concerns of athletes and then build an individualized nutrition plan that is mutually acceptable and productive. Athletes should be active participants in their meal planning and goal setting.

Study Questions

1. What is sports nutrition? Is it applicable only to competitive athletes? Defend your answer.

2. What are the six nutrient categories? Which nutrients are termed the "energy nutrients"?

3. What is the difference between Dietary Reference Intake (DRI) and Recommended Dietary Allowance (RDA)? What do EAR, AI, and UL stand for?

4. What do the terms enriched and fortified mean? How are they different?

5. What information can be learned about a food from its food label?

6. What is the MyPlate food guidance system? In what ways does it apply to sports nutrition?

7. When developing an individualized nutrition plan for an athlete, what factors must be taken into consideration?

References

1. Prochaska JO, Velicer WF. The transtheoretical model of health behavior change. *Am J Health Promotion*. 1997;12(1):38–48.

2. U.S. Department of Health and Human Services, U.S. Department of Agriculture. Dietary Guidelines for Americans 2010: executive summary. Available at: www.dietaryguidelines.gov. Accessed February 2, 2011.

3. United States Department of Agriculture. ChooseMyPlate.gov. Available at: http://www.choosemyplate.gov. Accessed June 7, 2011.

CHAPTER 2

Nutrients: Ingestion to Energy Metabolism

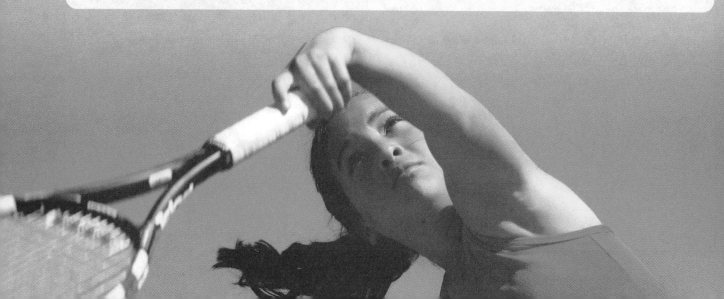

Kay is an aspiring 800-meter track athlete who has read various nutrition books with the hope of finding the ideal diet for her sport. From her reading she has learned that fats yield more calories per gram than carbohydrates. In addition, she knows that dietary proteins are needed to help her muscles recover from training and additionally can be used for energy. She is now convinced that one of the popular high-fat, high-protein, low-carbohydrate diets is her best choice. Her coach disagrees with her decision. She recommends that Kay speak with a sports nutrition professional prior to changing her current diet in which the majority of calories come from carbohydrates.

Questions

- Bioenergetically speaking, is Kay on the right track with her thinking?

- What energy system does an athlete running the 800-meter event rely on for energy?

- Is a diet of energy-dense fats really better for Kay's event?

- How would you explain to her why she should or should not follow this new diet?

What happens to nutrients after they are ingested?

When nutrients are ingested they have not technically entered the body. The digestive tract is merely an internalized conduit that connects the mouth to the anus (see Figure 2.1). Substances in the digestive tract are technically still outside of the body until they are absorbed across the membrane linings of this system. Once absorbed across the membranes of the digestive tract, the nutrients have officially entered the body and can be transported via blood and lymph throughout the body. Because most foods are too large to be absorbed, they first must be broken down into smaller pieces via digestion.

Digestion is the process of breaking down ingested food through mechanical and enzymatic activity so that it can be absorbed into the body. The

remainder of this section will discuss the various parts of the gastrointestinal system and their function in nutrient digestion and absorption.

What are the functions of the various parts of the digestive system?

The anatomical organization and functions of the various parts of the digestive tract are shown in Figure 2.2 . The digestive system extends from the mouth to the anus and is more than 25 feet long in most individuals. The mouth, or **oral cavity**, is the entry point for ingested nutrients. The main digestive process that occurs in the mouth is **mastication**, more commonly known as "chewing." The mechanical process of mastication breaks foods into pieces, thereby increasing the exposed surface area of the food and facilitating enzymatic action. Three pairs of **salivary glands,** namely the parotid, submandibular, and sub-

digestion The process of breaking down ingested foods into their basic units in preparation for absorption by the cells of the gastrointestinal tract.

oral cavity Another name for the mouth, which makes up the first segment of the gastrointestinal tract.

mastication The process of chewing.

salivary glands Glands of the mouth that produce and secrete saliva.

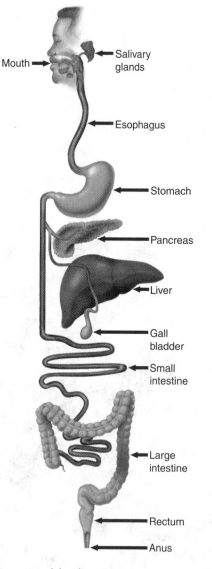

Figure 2.1 Anatomy of the digestive system.

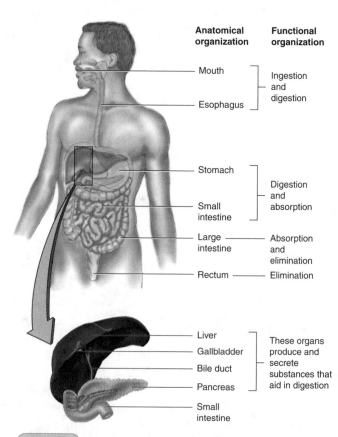

Figure 2.2 Functional organization of the digestive system. Although digestion begins in the mouth, most digestion occurs in the stomach and small intestine. Absorption occurs primarily in the small intestine.

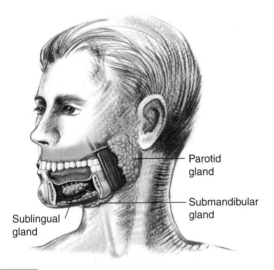

Parotid gland

Submandibular gland

Sublingual gland

Figure 2.3 The salivary glands. The three pairs of salivary glands supply saliva, which moistens and lubricates food. Saliva also contains salivary enzymes that begin the digestion of starch.

lingual glands, secrete saliva into the oral cavity (see **Figure 2.3**). The saliva not only moistens the food particles, but also contains enzymes that initiate the enzymatic breakdown of carbohydrates and fats.

The bolus of food is then swallowed and passes into the **esophagus**, which is a tube leading from the back of the oral cavity to the **stomach**. Food passes so quickly through the esophagus that relatively little digestion occurs there. Once in the stomach, the food is subjected to stomach acids and other enzymes that further the digestive process. The stomach has a muscular wall that churns the food, mixing it with stomach acids and enzymes. This digestive process continues for roughly an hour before food begins to exit the stomach. Although some absorption of nutrients does occur in the stomach, the overwhelming majority occurs in the next portion of the **gastrointestinal tract (GI tract)** known as the **small intestine**.

The small intestine makes up the majority of the length of the GI tract and is approximately 20 feet long. It is divided into three segments: the duodenum, the jejunum, and the ileum (see **Figure 2.4**). As the partially digested food exits the stomach, it enters the duodenum, which is a short segment of the small intestine. Although approxi-

esophagus The segment of the digestive system that connects the oral cavity to the stomach.

stomach The distensible, pouch-like portion of the gastrointestinal system that receives foods from the esophagus. It has muscular walls that mechanically churn food and assist in the digestive process. Ingested foods pass from the stomach into the duodenum.

gastrointestinal tract (GI tract) The regions of the digestive system that include the stomach, small intestine, and large intestine.

small intestine The portion of the gastrointestinal system where the bulk of digestion and absorption occurs. The small intestine is divided into three segments: duodenum, jejunum, and ileum.

mately only a foot in length, the duodenum is where the food from the stomach is barraged with more digestive enzymes from the gall bladder and pancreas. Much of the digestion of foodstuffs is completed in the duodenum, making the food ready for absorption.

In addition to the small intestine being long, the walls inside it are convoluted and lined with **villi**, which are small tubular-shaped projections (see **Figure 2.5**). Each villus has blood and lymphatic supply so that absorbed nutrients can gain easy access into the circulatory systems of the body. The combination of the small intestine's length and the convoluted, villi-lined interior results in a large surface area with which to absorb foodstuffs. In fact, most of the absorption of nutrients occurs in the remaining segments of the small intestine: the jejunum and ileum.

villi Small rod-shaped projections that cover the walls of the small intestine.

large intestine The terminal portion of the gastrointestinal tract, which receives undigested, partially digested, and unabsorbed contents from the small intestine. It is in the large intestine that the formation of feces occurs. The large intestine consists of the colon, rectum, and anal canal.

defecation The physical process of excreting feces from the rectum.

From the small intestine, the remainder of the undigested, partially digested, and unabsorbed contents pass into the **large intestine**. The large intestine includes the colon (ascending, transverse, and descending), the rectum, and the anal canal, which exits the body at the anus (see **Figure 2.6**). Passage of the intestinal contents along the GI tract slows in the large intestine, normally taking 18 to 24 hours to pass through. The intestinal contents are subjected to bacteria that not only continue digesting some of the undigested and unabsorbed foodstuffs, but also produce intestinal gas and certain vitamins. Some of the bacterially produced vitamins are absorbed along with excess water as the remaining contents pass through the colon. Water absorption in the colon helps to solidify the remaining excrement, which by the time it reaches the rectum is 60% solid matter and 40% water. The rectum is basically the storage site for the excrement until elimination or **defecation** occurs. The following sections will provide a more detailed explanation of how and where each nutrient is digested and absorbed.

How are carbohydrates digested, absorbed, transported, and assimilated in the body?

Many different types of carbohydrates are found in foods. The commonality regarding the differ-

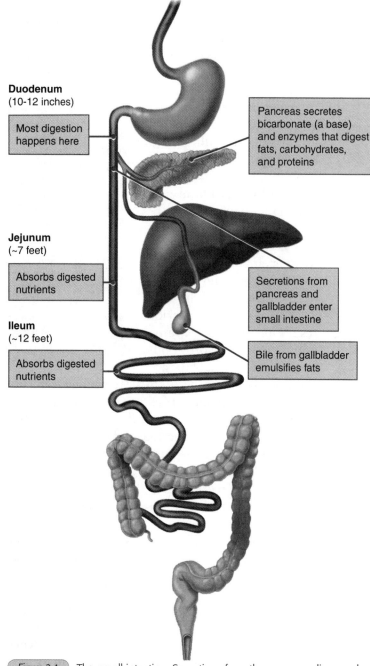

Duodenum
(10–12 inches)

Most digestion happens here

Pancreas secretes bicarbonate (a base) and enzymes that digest fats, carbohydrates, and proteins

Jejunum
(~7 feet)

Absorbs digested nutrients

Secretions from pancreas and gallbladder enter small intestine

Ileum
(~12 feet)

Absorbs digested nutrients

Bile from gallbladder emulsifies fats

Figure 2.4 The small intestine. Secretions from the pancreas, liver, and gallbladder assist in digestion. All along the intestinal walls, nutrients are absorbed into blood and lymph. Undigested materials are passed on to the large intestine.

ent types of carbohydrates is that they are made up of simple sugars, known as **monosaccharides**. Carbohydrates are classified based on the number of simple sugars making up their structure. For example, **disaccharides** are made up of two linked simple sugars. **Oligosaccharides** are carbohydrates composed of 3 to 10 linked sugars, and **polysaccharides** are complex carbohydrates made of 11 or more linked simple sugars. The monosaccharide most important to the human body is glucose. To obtain glucose from ingested foods, the carbohydrates must undergo digestion. The digestive process breaks down the carbohydrates into their constituent sugars so that they can be absorbed, transported, and used by the cells of the body.

What happens to carbohydrates once they are put into the mouth?

The digestive process begins with the mechanical actions of mastication and the activity of an enzyme found in the saliva secreted by the salivary glands. Saliva contains the enzyme **amylase**, which begins the breakdown of starchy foods to individual glucose molecules. **Starch** is the only type of carbohydrate and, besides fats, the only nutrient in which enzymatic breakdown begins in the mouth. Although digestion starts in the mouth, very little of the starch is completely broken down to glucose by the time the food is swallowed and enters the esophagus. In the short transit time through the esophagus to the stomach, amylase continues its breakdown of starch.

Once in the stomach, the food is subjected to hydrochloric acid, which denatures the salivary amylase, thus halting enzymatic digestion of starches in the stomach. However, the mechanical breakdown of food continues through the churning and powerful contractions of the smooth muscle in the stomach walls. The smooth muscle actions help to mix the stomach acid into the food bolus. This process, which prepares the food bolus for movement into the small intestine, usually takes 1 to 4 hours. No absorption of carbohydrates or other nutrients, except for alcohol, occurs in the stomach (see Figure 2.7); these nutrients therefore pass on with the other gastric contents into the small intestine.

monosaccharide A single sugar molecule. Monosaccharides are the building blocks for more complex carbohydrates.

disaccharide A simple carbohydrate that consists of two linked sugar molecules.

oligosaccharide A complex carbohydrate made up of 3 to 10 linked simple sugars.

polysaccharide A complex carbohydrate composed of 11 or more linked simple sugars. Starches and glycogen are examples of polysaccharides.

amylase A digestive enzyme that breaks down carbohydrates into simple sugars.

starch The major plant storage form of carbohydrates. Starch is composed of long chains of linked glucose molecules.

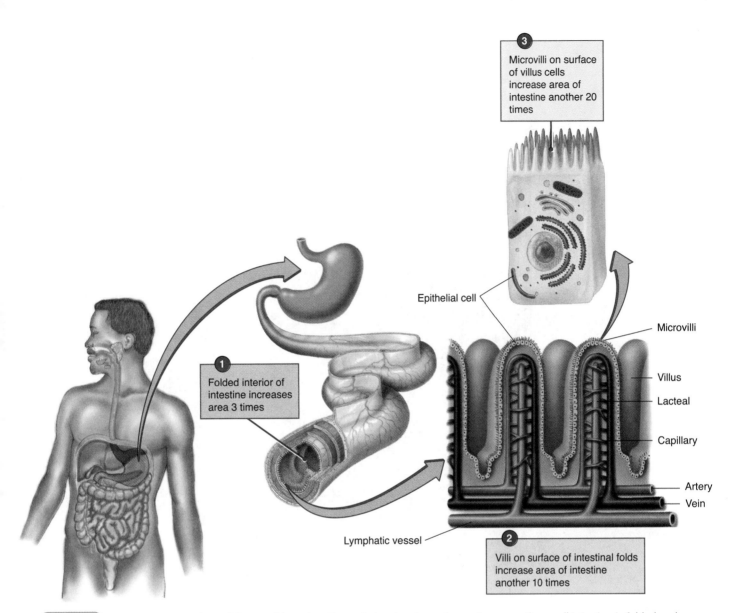

③ Microvilli on surface of villus cells increase area of intestine another 20 times

Epithelial cell

Microvilli

Villus

Lacteal

Capillary

Artery

Vein

① Folded interior of intestine increases area 3 times

Lymphatic vessel

② Villi on surface of intestinal folds increase area of intestine another 10 times

Figure 2.5 The absorptive surface of the small intestine. To maximize the absorptive surface area, the small intestine is folded and lined with villi. You have a surface area the size of a tennis court packed into your gut.

pancreatic amylase An enzyme secreted by the pancreas into the duodenum that assists in the digestion of starches.

brush border disaccharidases Digestive enzymes produced by cells of the intestinal wall that break disaccharides into simple sugars.

The small intestine is where the majority of digestion and absorption of carbohydrates and other nutrients occurs. In the duodenum, the bolus of food is exposed to digestive enzymes from the pancreas, gallbladder, and cells of the small intestine (see Figure 2.4). The pancreas secretes **pancreatic amylase**. This enzyme continues the digestion of starch, breaking it down into the disaccharide maltose. The mucosal cells and microvilli of the intestinal tract contain their own enzymes called the **brush border disaccharidases**. These enzymes go to work on the food as it enters the small intestine

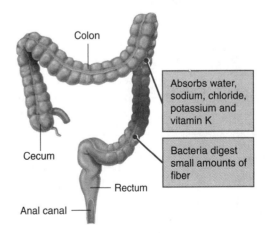

Colon

Absorbs water, sodium, chloride, potassium and vitamin K

Cecum

Bacteria digest small amounts of fiber

Rectum

Anal canal

Figure 2.6 The large intestine. In the large intestine, bacteria break down dietary fiber and other undigested carbohydrates, releasing acids and gas. The large intestine absorbs water and minerals, and forms feces for excretion.

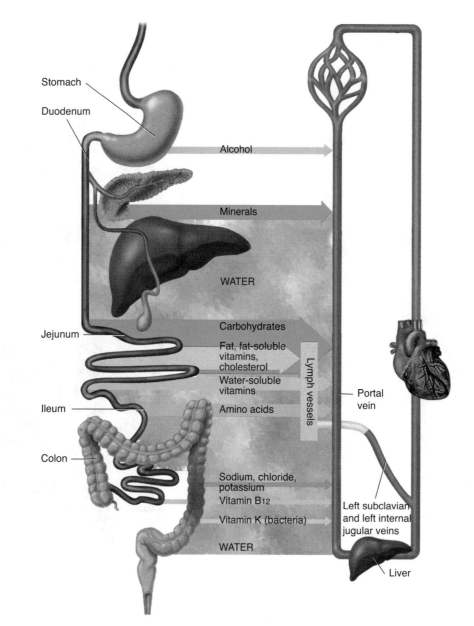

Labels in figure:
Stomach
Duodenum
Alcohol
Minerals
WATER
Jejunum
Carbohydrates
Fat, fat-soluble vitamins, cholesterol
Water-soluble vitamins
Lymph vessels
Amino acids
Ileum
Portal vein
Colon
Sodium, chloride, potassium
Vitamin B12
Left subclavian and left internal jugular veins
Vitamin K (bacteria)
WATER
Liver

Figure 2.7 Absorption of nutrients.

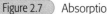

maltase A digestive enzyme that breaks down maltose into two glucose molecules.

sucrase A digestive enzyme that breaks down sucrose into glucose and fructose molecules.

lactase A digestive enzyme that breaks lactose into the simple sugars galactose and glucose.

and break down disaccharides into monosaccharides, which are then ready for absorption. There are a variety of disaccharidases that function to digest specific carbohydrates. For example, **maltase** splits disaccharide maltose into two single glucose molecules. **Sucrase** splits sucrose into glucose and fructose. **Lactase** splits lactose into glucose and galactose. After enzymatic digestion of the carbohydrates, the resulting simple sugars are absorbed through the intestinal wall in the jejunum and upper ileum (see Figure 2.7) and enter the bloodstream.

When individuals have an insufficient supply of the enzyme lactase in their intestinal tract, they are not able to break down the milk sugar lactose. As a result, lactose goes undigested and is passed on to the large intestine, where it is exposed to bacteria. The bacteria ferment lactose in the colon, producing gas and bloating. Consuming dairy products that have added lactase or taking products like Lactaid® prior to consumption of dairy foods can decrease or eliminate these symptoms.

Any unabsorbed and/or undigested polysaccharides, such as fiber, that make it through the small intestine enter into the large intestine, where some bacterial digestion and gas formation can occur. However, no absorption of carbohydrates occurs in the large intestine, and thus any remaining carbohydrates pass through the system and are eliminated as feces. Figure 2.7 provides a graphic summary of nutrient absorption, showing that the majority of carbohydrates are absorbed in the jejunum.

How are the simple sugars absorbed into the intestinal wall?

There are four ways that nutrients can be absorbed into the intestines: passive diffusion, facilitated diffusion, active transport, and endocytosis (see Figure 2.8). The following is a brief overview of how

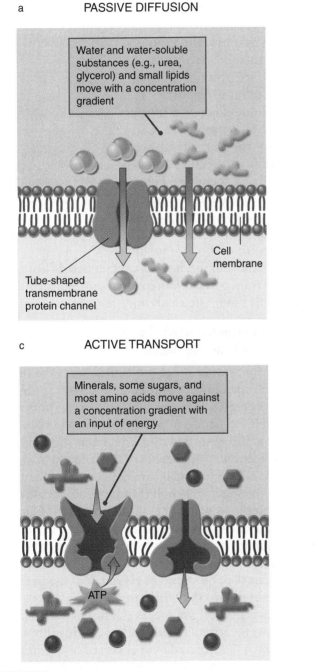

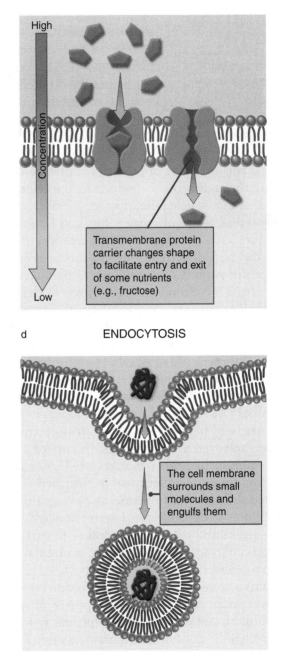

Figure 2.8   Mechanisms for nutrient absorption. (a) Passive diffusion. Using passive diffusion, some substances easily move in and out of cells, either through protein channels or directly through the cell membrane. (b) Facilitated diffusion. Some substances need a little assistance to enter and exit cells. The transmembrane protein helps out by changing shape. (c) Active transport. Some substances need a lot of assistance to enter cells. Similar to swimming upstream, energy is needed for the substance to penetrate against an unfavorable concentration gradient. (d) Endocytosis. Cells can use their cell membranes to engulf a particle and bring it inside the cell. The engulfing portion of the membrane separates from the cell wall and encases the particle in a vesicle.

passive diffusion A means of cellular absorption in which the movement of molecules through permeable cell membranes is driven only by differences in concentration gradient.

facilitated diffusion A means of cellular absorption in which protein carrier molecules are required to move substances across membranes driven only by differences in concentration gradient.

active transport An energy-requiring means of cellular absorption in which substances are carried across membranes by protein molecules. Active transport is not dependent on concentration gradients.

endocytosis A means of cellular absorption in which substances are encircled by the cell membrane and internalized into the cell.

glycogen The storage form of carbohydrates in animal cells. Glycogen consists of intricately branched chains of linked glucose molecules.

insulin A hormone secreted by specialized cells within the pancreas that lowers blood glucose levels after snacking or meals.

beta cells Specialized cells within the pancreas that secrete the hormone insulin.

diabetes A medical disease that is characterized by high blood glucose levels. Diabetes results when either the beta cells of the pancreas do not produce enough insulin or the body's tissues do not respond normally to insulin when it is produced.

these absorptive processes are used for carbohydrates.

Passive diffusion involves the movement of molecules through permeable cell membranes driven only by differences in concentration gradient. Passive diffusion is a non-energy requiring mechanism of absorption, and molecules always move from high concentration to low concentration. The bigger the difference in concentration, the greater the movement of molecules across the membrane. Molecules can enter cells by passively diffusing through the cell membrane or by passing through protein channels in the cell membrane (see Figure 2.8a). Because cell membranes are composed of fatty substances, fats and fat-soluble molecules such as oxygen, carbon dioxide, and alcohol can pass directly through membranes during passive diffusion. Conversely, water passively diffuses across membranes using the protein channels in the cell membranes. Unlike water, the water-soluble nutrients such as carbohydrates, amino acids, minerals, and some vitamins are not absorbed via passive diffusion and must rely on another form of transport, known as facilitated diffusion.

Facilitated diffusion, similar to passive diffusion, does not require energy, and molecules move from areas of high concentration to low concentration; however, molecules must be carried across the membrane by protein carriers (see Figure 2.8b). The monosaccharide fructose is absorbed via facilitated diffusion, but because its passage through membranes is dependent solely on concentration gradients, its absorption is slower than that of other monosaccharides such as glucose and galactose, which are absorbed by active transport.

Active transport is an energy-requiring form of absorption that requires transporter proteins, but unlike facilitated diffusion, nutrient uptake is not dictated by concentration gradients (see Figure 2.8c). As a result, molecules can be actively transported into a cell despite their concentration inside the cell. The monosaccharides glucose and galactose are absorbed across the intestinal lining via active transport. The name of the transporter protein is SGLUT1. For SGLUT1 to transport these simple sug-

ars through the intestinal cell membrane, it must first bind to a sodium ion. Conversely, if no sugars are available, the bound sodium is not transported into the cell either. In other words, SGLUT1 must bind both a sodium ion and sugar for transport into the cell to occur. This is the reason why physiology books refer to this specific active transport process as a glucose-sodium symport.

Endocytosis is a means of cellular uptake that involves the cell membrane encircling molecules and internalizing them (see Figure 2.8d). Although the process of endocytosis does occur in cells lining the GI tract, it is not a process that accounts for carbohydrate uptake.

Of the four mechanisms, facilitated diffusion and active transport explain carbohydrate absorption by the cells lining the small intestine.

What happens to carbohydrates once they make it into the blood?

Once the simple sugar molecules cross the intestinal cell membranes and enter the blood, they are transported to the liver via the hepatic portal system. This system is a network of blood vessels that collects the absorbed nutrients from the small and large intestines and delivers them to the liver (see Figure 2.7). No special carrier proteins are required when the sugars reach the bloodstream because they are soluble in water (i.e., blood plasma). Once the bloodborne simple sugars reach the cells of the liver, those that are not in the form of glucose (e.g., fructose, galactose) are converted to glucose. The glucose can then be stored as **glycogen** in the liver cells or released into the bloodstream.

Rising blood glucose levels after ingestion of carbohydrates stimulates the release of **insulin**, which is a hormone secreted by specialized cells within the pancreas known as **beta cells**. The release of insulin into the bloodstream causes glucose transporter proteins (see next section) within the cell membranes of muscles and other tissues to begin the uptake of glucose, thereby preventing blood glucose levels from rising too high. **Diabetes** results when the beta cells do not produce enough insulin to lower blood glucose levels, or the beta cells produce insulin, to which the body's tissues do not respond normally. The end result is abnormally high blood glucose levels, sometimes in excess of 2 to 4 times the normal level.

What happens to carbohydrates once they make it to the cells of the body?

Once glucose is transported to various bodily tissues, such as skeletal muscle, it must gain access to the inside of tissue cells in order to be used for energy or to be stored. Unlike in intestinal absorption, glucose is carried across the cell membrane by specialized proteins via facilitated diffusion. The specialized membrane carrier proteins are called **glucose transporters (GLUT)** and are present in all cells in the body. Some

glucose transporters (GLUT) Specialized membrane carrier proteins that are responsible for the active transport of glucose into muscle cells.

of these glucose transporters are stimulated by the hormone insulin, which in turn increases the rate of cellular glucose uptake.

Several different types of glucose transporters are present in various tissues throughout the body. In regard to muscle, the transporters are called GLUT1 and GLUT4. At rest or when blood levels of the hormone insulin are low, most glucose enters muscle cells via the GLUT1 transporter. However, when glucose and insulin levels in the blood are high (e.g., after a meal) or when muscle is active (e.g., during exercise), the GLUT4 transporter protein is stimulated and becomes the major transporter of glucose into the muscle cells. Once the glucose has gained entrance into the cell, it basically has one of three fates. It can be stored as glycogen in the muscle, it can be converted into fat and stored as adipose tissue, or it can be used for energy (see Figure 2.9). If it is stored, the glucose molecule can be linked to

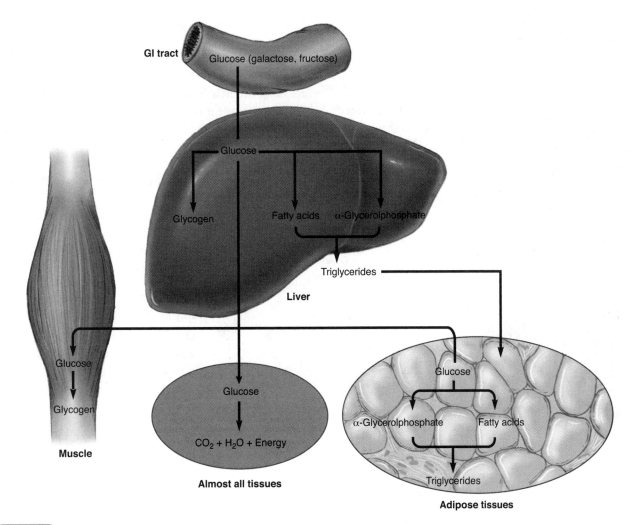

Figure 2.9   Flow chart of glucose and other simple sugars immediately after a meal.
Source: Brooks GA, Fahey TD, Baldwin KM. *Exercise Physiology: Human Bioenergetics and Its Applications.* 4th ed. Boston, MA: McGraw-Hill; 2004:31–42. Reproduced with permission of the McGraw-Hill Companies.

How are carbohydrates digested, absorbed, transported, and assimilated in the body?   **33**

other glucose molecules, forming the complex carbohydrate known as glycogen. Glucose can remain stored as glycogen in the cell until needed for energy, at which point it is cleaved from the glycogen chain and metabolized for energy.

How are fats digested, absorbed, transported, and assimilated in the body?

Although fats are made up of carbon, hydrogen, and oxygen atoms similar to carbohydrates, they have very different chemical structures and physical properties. Fats are molecules that belong to a group of compounds known as **lipids**, which are organic compounds that are insoluble in water and feel greasy to the touch. Sources of dietary lipids are butter, margarines, salad dressings, and oils. Lipids are also found in meats, dairy products, nuts, seeds, olives, avocados, and some grain products. Most dietary lipids exist in the form of **triglycerides**, and as a result, the following discussion will focus on the digestion, absorption, transport, and assimilation of triglycerides (see Figure 2.10).

lipids A class of organic compounds that is insoluble in water and greasy to the touch. Lipids are commonly referred to as fats and exist in the body primarily as triglycerides.

triglyceride A lipid that is composed of a glycerol molecule with three attached fatty acids.

Fatty acids are basically carbon atoms that are linked in a chainlike fashion (see Figure 2.11). These chains of carbon can be of varying lengths and thus fatty acids can be classified as short (4

or fewer carbons), medium (6 to 10 carbons), or long (≥12 carbons). During triglyceride digestion, one fatty acid may be removed, leaving a **diglyceride**, or two fatty acids may be removed, leaving a **monoglyceride**. The fatty acids cleaved off the glycerol backbone become what are known as **free fatty acids**.

Fat digestion, absorption, and transport are more elaborate than that of other macronutrients because of fat's insolubility in water. For example, the majority of enzymes involved in digestion are water soluble, which under normal circumstances would prohibit them from effectively acting on fats. However, the body's digestive system subjects fats to substances known as **emulsifiers**, which work around the insolubility issue and allow enzymes to do their job. Emulsifiers are substances that break lipids into very small globules, which stay suspended in the watery contents of the GI tract and increase the exposed surface area of fats to the actions of digestive enzymes. Without being emulsified, the fats would tend to stick together in large clumps, making it difficult for enzymes to do their jobs. As noted earlier, the following discussion focuses on the digestion of triglycerides.

diglyceride A lipid that is composed of a glycerol molecule with two attached fatty acids.

monoglyceride A lipid composed of a glycerol molecule with one attached fatty acid.

free fatty acid Compounds composed of long hydrogen-carbon chains that have a carboxyl group on one end and a methyl group at the other. Free fatty acids can be formed when a fatty acid is cleaved from a triglyceride molecule.

emulsifier A substance that breaks lipids into very small globules so that they are more manageable in watery fluids.

lingual lipase An enzyme for fat digestion that is secreted by cells located at the base of the tongue.

gastric lipase A fat-digesting enzyme secreted by cells of the stomach.

What happens to fats once they are put into the mouth?

Mastication breaks up fat into smaller pieces, while **lingual lipase** in saliva initiates the enzymatic digestive process. However, because food is in the mouth for a relatively short period of time before being swallowed, very little fat is actually digested in the mouth.

When food is swallowed, the lingual lipase is passed into the stomach, where it continues to break down the fats, at least until it is denatured by stomach acid. **Gastric lipase** is secreted from the

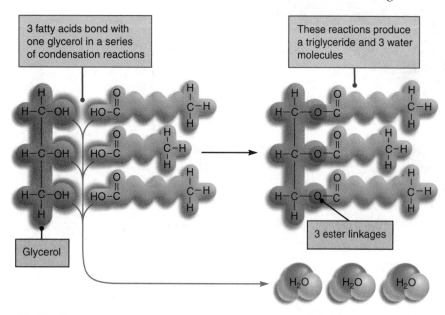

3 fatty acids bond with one glycerol in a series of condensation reactions

These reactions produce a triglyceride and 3 water molecules

Glycerol

3 ester linkages

H₂O   H₂O   H₂O

Figure 2.10   Forming a triglyceride. Concentration reactions attach three fatty acids to a glycerol backbone to form a triglyceride. These reactions release water.

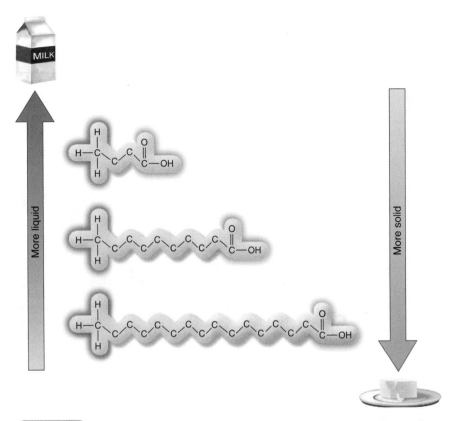

More liquid

More solid

Figure 2.11   Fatty acids vary in length and can be classified as short, medium, or long. The longer the fatty acid, the more solid it is at room temperature.

zymes can continue to do their job. **Secretin**, released from duodenal cells, stimulates the pancreas to release bicarbonate, which neutralizes the acidity of the intestinal contents. Neutralizing the acids prevents denaturation of protein enzymes, such as **pancreatic lipase** and other digestive enzymes, allowing the enzymatic breakdown of foods to progress. The pancreatic lipase is released in large amounts and finishes the digestive process of fats, thereby breaking the remaining triglycerides into glycerol, monoglycerides, and free fatty acids of various lengths. Short- and medium-chain fatty acids, which are water soluble, are absorbed into the intestinal lining via passive diffusion. The monoglycerides and long-chain fatty acids, which are water insoluble, are encircled by bile salts, forming microscopic bubbles known as **micelles**. The micelles transport the long-chain fatty acids and monoglycerides to the cells lining the intestinal walls, at which time they are released from the micelles and passively diffused into the interior of the intestinal cells. Figure 2.12 provides a graphic summary of triglyceride digestion.

Fat digestion and absorption are for the most part completed by the time the food contents reach the large intestine. Minimal amounts of fat are found in the large intestine or passed in fecal matter. However, some disease conditions can cause fat malabsorption, resulting in **steatorrhea** or fatty stools. Radiation therapy for cancer, digestive surgeries requiring a large portion of the small intestine to be removed, Crohn's disease, and cystic fibrosis all can cause fat malabsorption.

cholecystokinin (CCK) A hormone produced by cells of the small intestine that stimulates the release of bile salts and pancreatic enzymes.

stomach lining and continues the enzymatic digestive process in the stomach. The gastric lipase breaks the triglycerides into diglycerides, which help in the digestive process by serving as emulsifiers. Churning and muscular contractions of the muscles in the stomach wall also assist in breaking apart large pieces of food and, in combination with emulsifiers, help keep the fats dispersed and in suspension. After 2 to 4 hours in the stomach, approximately one-third of the dietary triglycerides have been broken down into diglycerides and free fatty acids.[1]

As the food contents reach the small intestine, they stimulate the duodenal cells to release hormones that further assist in digestion. **Cholecystokinin (CCK)** is released and travels to the gallbladder. The CCK stimulates the gallbladder to contract, forcing bile into the bile duct, which empties into the duodenum (see Figure 2.2). Bile is important in the fat digestion process because it contains bile salts and lecithin (a type of lipid), which keep the fats emulsified so that the water-soluble digestive en-

secretin A hormone released from the duodenum that stimulates the release of bicarbonate from the pancreas.

pancreatic lipase A digestive enzyme secreted by the pancreas into the duodenum that breaks down triglycerides.

micelles Tiny bubbles made up of monoglycerides and long-chain fatty acids that are wrapped in bile salts. Micelles help transport digested fats to the intestinal wall for absorption.

steatorrhea An abnormal condition in which large amounts of fat are found in the feces.

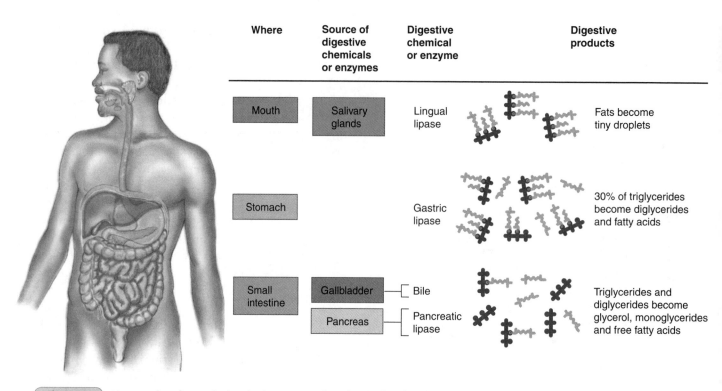

Where	Source of digestive chemicals or enzymes	Digestive chemical or enzyme	Digestive products
Mouth	Salivary glands	Lingual lipase	Fats become tiny droplets
Stomach		Gastric lipase	30% of triglycerides become diglycerides and fatty acids
Small intestine	Gallbladder	Bile	Triglycerides and diglycerides become glycerol, monoglycerides and free fatty acids
	Pancreas	Pancreatic lipase	

Figure 2.12 How are fats digested, absorbed, transported, and assimilated in the body? Triglyceride digestion. Most triglyceride digestion takes place in the small intestine.

What happens to the fats once they are absorbed?

Once absorbed, the water-soluble glycerol and short- and medium-chain fatty acids pass through the intestinal cells and diffuse into capillaries, thus entering directly into the bloodstream (see Figure 2.13). The monoglycerides and long-chain fatty acids that are absorbed are reassembled into triglycerides within the intestinal cells. The resynthesized triglycerides are then combined with protein carriers to form **lipoproteins**. These lipoproteins with their fatty cargo then pass through the intestinal cells. Once they leave the intestinal cells they are called **chylomicrons**. Chylomicrons do not enter directly into the bloodstream, but instead enter into the lymphatic system (see Figure 2.13). The lymphatic system then delivers the chylomicrons to the large veins of the neck via the thoracic duct. The fats then empty into the blood and are distributed throughout the body.

lipoproteins Substances that transport lipids in the lymph and blood. These substances consist of a central core of triglycerides surrounded by a shell composed of proteins, phospholipids, and cholesterol. Various types of lipoproteins exist in the body and differ based on size, composition, and density.

chylomicron A droplet made of resynthesized triglycerides wrapped in lipoproteins that is produced inside the intestinal cells. Chylomicrons are released from the intestinal cells and then pass into the lymphatic system.

What happens to fats once they make it to the cells?

Fats have many functions within the body, and a thorough description of their roles is covered in Chapter 4; however, bioenergetically, depending on the physical state of the body, the type of cell, and the need for energy, once fats reach the cells they can be either used for energy or stored for later use. For example, if energy demands are low and the bloodborne chylomicrons and their fatty payloads enter capillaries within adipose tissue or the liver, the chylomicrons can be acted upon by an enzyme located on the capillary wall called **lipoprotein lipase (LPL)**. LPL breaks the triglycerides inside the chylomicrons into free fatty acids and glycerol. The free fatty acids immediately diffuse into the fat or liver cells, where they are recombined with a new glycerol from inside the cells and once again reformed into triglycerides. These newly formed triglycerides are stored until needed for energy. On the other hand, if the muscles are active and need energy, free fatty acids and chylomicrons in blood flowing through the capillaries of muscles can be used for energy. LPL in the capillaries of muscles acts upon the triglycerides in the chylomicrons, similar to the LPL in adipose tissues. The

lipoprotein lipase A specialized enzyme that breaks down triglycerides into glycerol and free fatty acids.

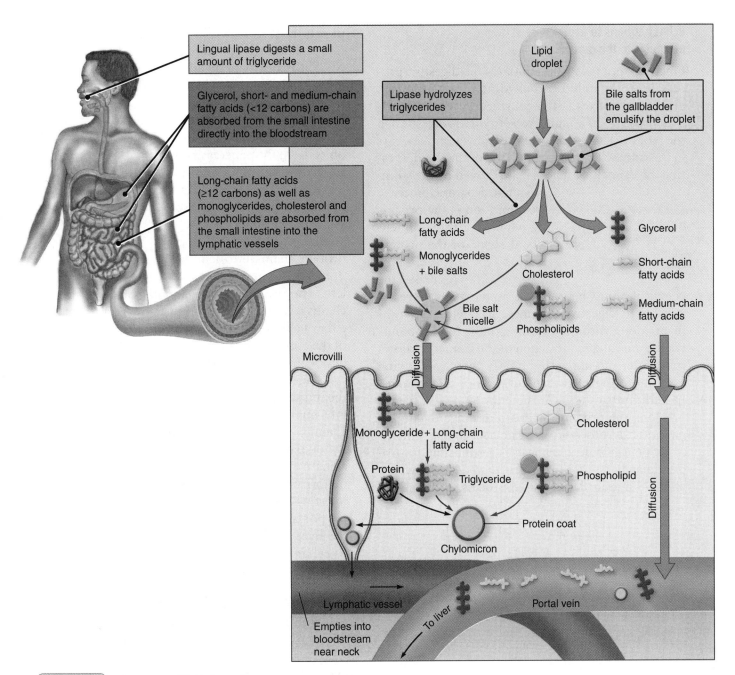

Lingual lipase digests a small amount of triglyceride

Glycerol, short- and medium-chain fatty acids (<12 carbons) are absorbed from the small intestine directly into the bloodstream

Long-chain fatty acids (≥12 carbons) as well as monoglycerides, cholesterol and phospholipids are absorbed from the small intestine into the lymphatic vessels

Lipid droplet

Lipase hydrolyzes triglycerides

Bile salts from the gallbladder emulsify the droplet

Long-chain fatty acids

Glycerol

Monoglycerides + bile salts

Cholesterol

Short-chain fatty acids

Bile salt micelle

Phospholipids

Medium-chain fatty acids

Microvilli

Diffusion

Diffusion

Monoglyceride + Long-chain fatty acid

Cholesterol

Protein

Triglyceride

Phospholipid

Protein coat

Diffusion

Chylomicron

Lymphatic vessel

To liver

Portal vein

Empties into bloodstream near neck

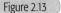 **Figure 2.13**   Summary of lipid absorption.

free fatty acids in the blood, in addition to those released from the chylomicrons, are transported across the muscle cell membrane and into the interior of the cell, where they are used for energy.

How are proteins digested, absorbed, transported, and assimilated in the body?

Of the three macronutrients, proteins are the least used by the body as a source of chemical energy; however, they play the biggest role in providing structure to the body. Proteins also form the enzymes critical to the thousands of chemical reactions required to sustain life.

Proteins are made up of basic building blocks called amino acids. The proteins important to the human body are composed of 20 different amino acids. To make the proteins required, dietary proteins must supply the necessary amino acids. The following sections discuss how dietary proteins are digested and utilized by the body. A more in-depth discussion of the roles of proteins can be found in Chapter 5.

What happens to proteins once they are put into the mouth?

Once again, mastication initiates the digestive process; however, unlike carbohydrates and fats, which are subjected to digestive enzymes present in the saliva, proteins do not undergo enzymatic digestion in the mouth. The majority of protein digestion occurs in the stomach and upper portion of the small intestine. Hydrochloric acid (HCl) secreted by the stomach lining denatures proteins. **Denaturation** is the process by which the three-dimensional shape of the protein begins to unravel (see Figure 2.14). This makes the chemical bonds between the amino acids more accessible to digestive enzymes. The acidic environment, along with the churning of the food contents via the muscular contraction of the stomach, allows for greater mixing with the HCl, thereby allowing for a more thorough denaturation of the proteins. In addition to the HCl, the enzyme pepsin begins breaking the proteins made up of longer chains of amino acids into shorter amino acid chains. The enzyme pepsin in the stomach is responsible for approximately 10–20% of protein digestion.[2] However, at this stage in the digestive process, proteins are mostly broken down into smaller protein chains rather than single amino acids.

denaturation A process by which proteins lose their three-dimensional shape and as a consequence their enzymatic activity.

The majority of digestion of protein takes place in the small intestine, where additional protein-digestive enzymes called **proteases** break down the protein chains into even smaller units. Both the pancreas and small intestine make and release proteases. Cells lining the small intestine also secrete **peptidases**, which continue to break the short protein chains into lengths of only three amino acids or less. The resulting single amino acids and protein chains of two or three amino acids are absorbed by either facilitated diffusion or active transport. Most of the absorption takes place in the cells that line the duodenum and jejunum.

proteases A class of protein-digesting enzymes that break the chemical bonds holding amino acids together.

peptidases A group of protein-digesting enzymes that are released from cells of the small intestine. Peptidases work on breaking the chemical bonds of short-chain proteins (i.e., three or fewer amino acids), thereby yielding single amino acids.

The final stage of protein digestion occurs inside the intestinal cells after absorption. Once inside the intestinal cells, other peptidases break the remaining chemical bonds in the protein chains to produce individual amino acids. Some of the absorbed amino acids are used by the intestinal cells themselves. The majority of amino acids are transported out of the intestinal cells via facilitated diffusion and enter into the portal system of blood vessels that go directly to the liver. Amino acids are then either used by the liver or released into the general circulation. Figure 2.15 provides a graphic summary of protein digestion.

Digestion and absorption of protein are quite efficient in the stomach and small intestine, and as a result, very little protein makes it to the large intestine. Protein that does end up in the large intestine is excreted in the feces. Some medical conditions may cause protein digestion and absorption problems, and it is important for the sports nutrition professional to be aware of these conditions to adapt the dietary plan, particularly when dealing with athletes. For example, celiac disease is a digestive disorder that involves the inability to digest certain plant proteins. Athletes with celiac disease are not able to digest the protein in wheat, rye, oats, and other grains. Because these grains are excellent sources of carbohydrates that athletes need for energy, the sports nutrition professional must work closely with the athlete to find alternative plant protein/energy sources that will not exacerbate the symptoms and/or progression of the disease.

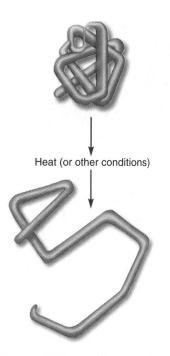

Heat (or other conditions)

Figure 2.14 Denaturation. Exposing a protein to heat, acids, oxidation, and mechanical agitation can destabilize it, causing it to unfold and lose its functional shape.

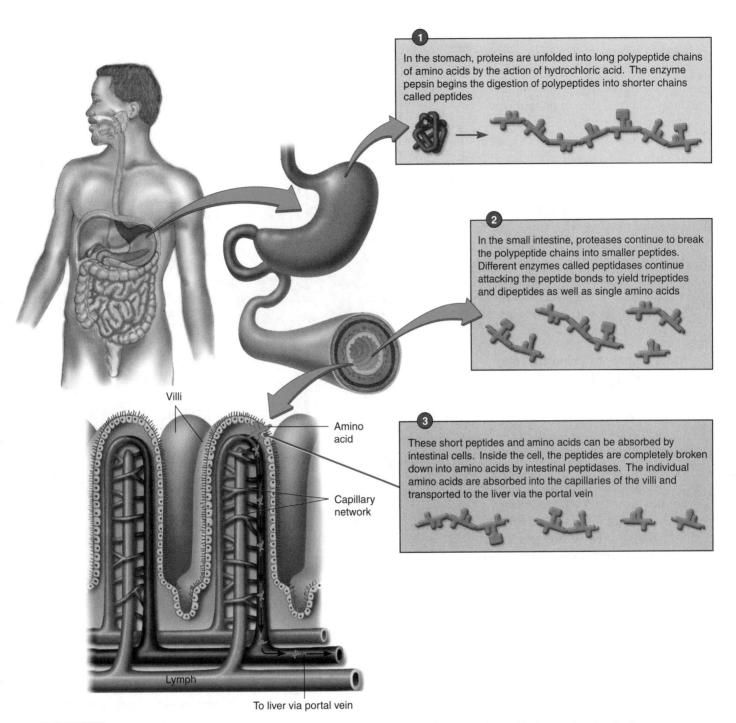

1 In the stomach, proteins are unfolded into long polypeptide chains of amino acids by the action of hydrochloric acid. The enzyme pepsin begins the digestion of polypeptides into shorter chains called peptides

2 In the small intestine, proteases continue to break the polypeptide chains into smaller peptides. Different enzymes called peptidases continue attacking the peptide bonds to yield tripeptides and dipeptides as well as single amino acids

3 These short peptides and amino acids can be absorbed by intestinal cells. Inside the cell, the peptides are completely broken down into amino acids by intestinal peptidases. The individual amino acids are absorbed into the capillaries of the villi and transported to the liver via the portal vein

Villi

Amino acid

Capillary network

Lymph

To liver via portal vein

Figure 2.15 The breakdown of protein in the body. Digestion breaks down protein into amino acids that can be absorbed.

How are proteins absorbed into the intestinal wall?

Amino acid absorption occurs through facilitated diffusion and active transport (see Figures 2.8b and 2.8c). The majority of amino acids require active transport to gain access into the intestinal cells. The active transport process for amino acids is the same as described for glucose earlier in the chapter, although amino acids and glucose use different transport proteins. Similar amino acids share the same active transport systems and carrier proteins. For example, the branched chain amino acids—leucine, isoleucine, and valine—all depend on the same carrier protein for absorption. Proteins consumed in the daily diet usually contain a variety of amino acids needed by the body. Because a variety of amino acids are being moved into cells through a variety of different carrier proteins, competition for the same membrane transporter is minimized, and the amino acids tend to be taken into the cell in proportions representative of the food's composition.

Taking supplements containing large amounts of a single amino acid can affect the absorption of other amino acids if they share the same transport carrier. For example, athletes trying to increase muscle mass may take supplements containing high doses of a specific amino acid or combination of amino acids. This may actually work against them because it could create competition for transport carriers that would result in the overabsorption of one amino acid at the expense of another.

What happens to amino acids once they make it to the bloodstream?

The amino acids that enter the bloodstream after digestion of ingested proteins become part of the body's **amino acid pool**, which consists of not only bloodborne amino acids, but also the amino acids found in other tissues, primarily skeletal muscle and the liver (see Figure 2.16). The blood and its circulating amino acids make up the central part of the body's amino acid pool. Amino acid concentrations in the blood are in equilibrium with the amino acids in the other compartments making up the amino acid pool. However, there are relatively few amino acids circulating in the blood compared to the quantity found in muscle and the liver. If amino acid levels fall in one compartment, amino acids from the other compartments are mobilized to correct the imbalance. This sharing of amino acids between compartments can help ensure that needed amino acids are available when deficits arise.

Amino acids in the pool can be used for a variety of functions depending on needs. They are primarily used to synthesize new structural proteins, enzymes, hormones, or other nitrogen-containing compounds. They

amino acid pool The collection of amino acids found in body fluids and tissues that is available for protein synthesis.

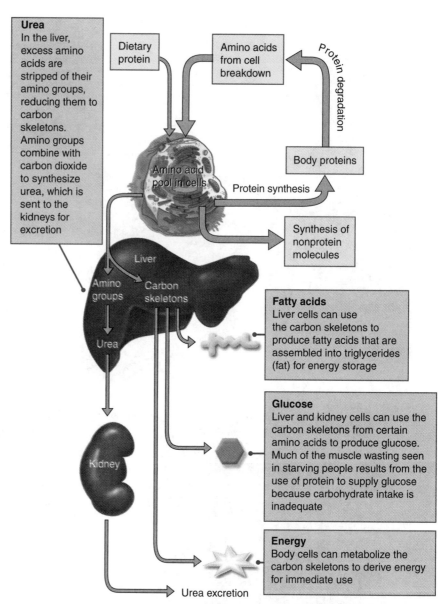

Urea
In the liver, excess amino acids are stripped of their amino groups, reducing them to carbon skeletons. Amino groups combine with carbon dioxide to synthesize urea, which is sent to the kidneys for excretion

Fatty acids
Liver cells can use the carbon skeletons to produce fatty acids that are assembled into triglycerides (fat) for energy storage

Glucose
Liver and kidney cells can use the carbon skeletons from certain amino acids to produce glucose. Much of the muscle wasting seen in starving people results from the use of protein to supply glucose because carbohydrate intake is inadequate

Energy
Body cells can metabolize the carbon skeletons to derive energy for immediate use

Figure 2.16   Amino acid pool turnover. Cells draw upon their amino acid pools to synthesize new proteins. These small pools turn over quickly and must be replenished by amino acids from dietary protein and degradation of body protein. Dietary protein supplies about one-third, and the breakdown of body protein supplies about two-thirds of the roughly 300 grams of body protein synthesized daily. When dietary protein is inadequate, increased degradation of body protein replenishes the amino acid pool. This can lead to the breakdown of essential body tissue.

from the other compartments are mobilized to correct the imbalance. This sharing of amino acids between compartments can help ensure that needed amino acids are available when deficits arise.

Amino acids in the pool can be used for a variety of functions depending on needs. They are primarily used to synthesize new structural proteins, enzymes, hormones, or other nitrogen-containing compounds. They

can be metabolized for energy, particularly when carbohydrate stores of energy are low and demands for energy are high. Alternatively, when amino acid levels are in excess they can be converted to fat and stored for later energy use by the body (see Figure 2.16).

The sharing of amino acids between compartments is

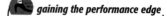
gaining the performance edge

Maintaining adequate protein intake for athletes is essential for the continual replenishment of the amino acid pool.

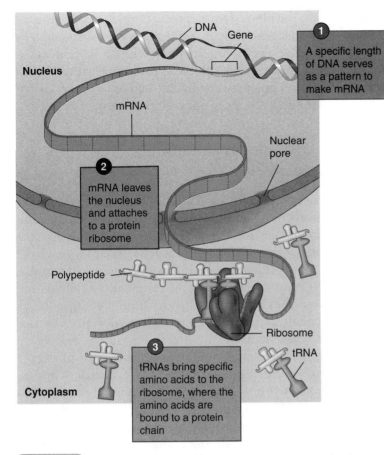

Nucleus

DNA
Gene

1 A specific length of DNA serves as a pattern to make mRNA

mRNA

Nuclear pore

2 mRNA leaves the nucleus and attaches to a protein ribosome

Polypeptide

Ribosome

tRNA

3 tRNAs bring specific amino acids to the ribosome, where the amino acids are bound to a protein chain

Cytoplasm

Figure 2.17 Protein synthesis. Ribosomes are our protein-synthesis factories. First mRNA carries manufacturing instructions from DNA in the cell nucleus to the ribosomes. Then tRNA collects and delivers amino acids in the correct sequence.

as hormones. For example, the hormone testosterone causes muscle cells to increase production of contractile proteins, thus causing the muscle to become bigger and stronger.

The actual instructions for making the specific proteins needed by the cell lie in the strands of **DNA (deoxyribonucleic acid)** found in the nucleus (see Figure 2.17). Segments of DNA that call for specific proteins are called **genes**. When a cell needs a particular protein, the specific gene with the instructions for that protein is copied in a process known as **transcription**. Transcription results in the formation of **messenger ribonucleic acid (mRNA)**, which is a genetic set of instructions on how to make the protein. Upon leaving the cell nucleus, messenger RNA delivers the instructions to the **ribosomes**, which are the cellular organelles located in the cell cytoplasm that build the protein. In a process known as **translation**, the ribosomes read the mRNA segment and begin attaching amino acids together in the sequence called for by the instructions. The amino acids needed by the ribosomes are delivered to the "protein construction site" by **transfer ribonucleic acid (tRNA)**. This process of tRNA delivering the needed amino acids to the ribosomes continues until the protein has been constructed.

If an amino acid is required but not present at the time of protein construction, the protein-building process is stopped. If the required amino acid is a nonessential amino acid, the cell makes the amino acid and tRNA delivers it, continuing the building process. However, if the amino acid needed is an essential amino acid, the building process cannot continue, and the protein requested is

deoxyribonucleic acid (DNA) The molecular compound that makes up the genetic material found within the nuclei of cells.

gene A specific sequence of DNA found within cell nuclei that contains information on how to make enzymes or other proteins.

transcription The process of copying genetic information from a specific DNA sequence through the formation of messenger RNA.

messenger ribonucleic acid (mRNA) A type of nucleic acid that carries the genetic instructions for protein synthesis from the cell nucleus to the ribosomes located in the cell cytoplasm.

ribosomes Cellular organelles that are responsible for protein synthesis.

translation The process in which proteins are produced by ribosomes as they read the genetic instructions found on messenger RNA.

transfer ribonucleic acid (tRNA) A type of ribonucleic acid that is responsible for delivering specific amino acids to the ribosome during production of protein.

dynamic and ongoing. Proteins in the body are constantly turning over, requiring amino acids from the pool on a continual basis. However, this sharing of amino acids between compartments is a short-term fix for providing necessary amino acids. Daily dietary protein intake is essential to maintaining the body's amino acid pool. If protein intake is not adequate, proteins from muscle and other tissues will be cannibalized to provide the necessary amino acids, negatively affecting an athlete's training abilities and competitive performance.

What happens to amino acids once they make it to the cells of the body?

The amino acids circulating in the blood enter the cells of the body by facilitated diffusion. Once inside the cells, the amino acids become the building blocks for specific proteins. The specific protein constructed inside the cell is determined by current needs and/or the influences of outside factors such

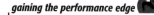
not completed. This is why an athletic diet should include high-quality, complete, or complementary proteins so that all of the essential amino acids are available when needed. One missing essential amino acid can stop the construction of a protein. When this happens, the partially constructed protein is degraded, and its amino acids are used elsewhere or metabolized for energy.

How are minerals, vitamins, and water absorbed and transported in the body?

Minerals, vitamins, and water (unlike carbohydrates, proteins, and fats) do not need to be broken down into smaller units via digestion to be absorbed into the body. As foodstuffs are being digested, the vitamins and minerals within the foods are released into the intestinal contents. The majority of minerals released during digestion are absorbed in the duodenum and jejunum of the small intestine. The exceptions are sodium, potassium, and chloride, which are absorbed in the large intestine.

Vitamins are categorized as being either water soluble or fat soluble. The water-soluble vitamins (i.e., B-complex vitamins and vitamin C) dissolve in the watery mix of food in the GI tract and are absorbed along with the water. The majority of water and all of the water-soluble vitamins (see Figure 2.7) are absorbed in the small intestine. The water-soluble vitamins easily gain access to the blood and move freely throughout the body within the fluids both inside and outside of cells.

The fat-soluble vitamins (i.e., vitamins A, D, E, and K), when released from the digesting foods, dissolve in the fatty portions of the GI contents. As a result, they are transported along with the digested fats in micelles to the intestinal wall where they are absorbed via passive diffusion. Similar to the water-soluble vitamins, the majority of fat-soluble vitamins are absorbed in the small intestine (see Figure 2.7). A small amount of vitamin K is produced by bacteria in the large intestine and is then also absorbed. Once inside the intestinal cells the fat-soluble vitamins are packaged into the chylomicrons and then, along with other fats, transported via the lymph

into the bloodstream. From there they are delivered throughout the body. Some are delivered and used by cells; others are stored along with fat in adipocytes. The fact that fat-soluble vitamins are stored in the body is one reason why taking high dosages of fat-soluble vitamins is not recommended.

What is energy metabolism, and why is it important?

Energy metabolism is a foundational component of sports nutrition. Knowledge of the cellular machinery and metabolic pathways responsible for deriving energy from the macronutrients once they reach the cells is critical to the sports nutrition professional. Without knowledge of the three energy systems and how they work together to supply energy during specific activities, the sports nutrition professional is severely disadvantaged in regard to creating an individualized dietary plan. Knowledge of energy metabolism also enables the sports nutrition professional to objectively assess the potential effectiveness of dietary supplementation. Finally, comprehending energy metabolism enables sports nutrition professionals to educate their athletes about the energy needs of their sport, thus helping to dispel many of the misconceptions that abound in sports nutrition. The remainder of this chapter will define energy, identify which nutrients supply energy, and discuss how cells derive energy during rest and exercise.

What is energy?

Energy is an entity that is better explained or defined than shown because it has no shape, no describable features, and no physical mass. Energy is what enables cells, muscles, and other tissues of the body to perform work, or in layperson's terms, to get things done. The cellular and bodily functions that keep humans alive require energy. Similar to an automobile that relies on the chemical energy of gasoline to run the motor, the cells of the body require chemical energy from foods to power their many different functions. In the case of sport performance, the muscle cells must acquire energy to fuel muscle contraction. In short, energy is what fuels **metabolism**.

Metabolism is the sum total of all the energy required to power cellular processes and activities. The absolute minimal amount of energy required to keep

metabolism The sum total of all the energy required to power cellular processes and activities.

humans alive is called **basal metabolic rate (BMR)**. A slightly higher amount of energy is required for **resting metabolic rate (RMR)**. BMR and RMR are expressed in **kilocalories (kcals)**, which are the commonly used units of measurement for energy. A kilocalorie is the amount of heat energy required to raise the temperature of 1 liter of water 1 degree centigrade, specifically from 14.5° C to 15.5° C. BMR and RMR measurements are obtained in different ways. BMR is measured under very stringent conditions and requires subjects to spend the night in a sleep lab. The subjects must be well rested, thermally neutral (i.e., not hot or cold), and in a transitional state of waking (i.e., not asleep but not fully alert) at the time of actual BMR measurement. RMR measures are much easier to obtain. Subjects must fast for 12 hours but can drive to the laboratory, where they relax for 20 to 30 minutes in a supine/reclined position before their RMR is measured. BMR and RMR are used by sports nutrition professionals to determine an athlete's 24-hour energy expenditure. This total daily energy expenditure can be used both to establish the dietary caloric intake necessary to achieve energy balance and when counseling athletes in weight management (see Chapter 11).

Energy exists in six basic forms: chemical, nuclear, electrical, mechanical, thermal, and radiant. However, the form of energy that humans and animals directly rely upon for survival is **chemical energy**. Chemical energy is energy that is stored within bonds between atoms of molecules. When the bonds between these atoms are broken, energy is released and can be used to perform work. On earth, the primary source of chemical energy for animal life originates from plants. Specifically, the plants use radiant energy from the sun to build high-energy bonds between atoms of carbon, hydrogen, nitrogen, and oxygen. In doing so, plants form molecules of carbohydrates, proteins, and fats, which serve as energy nutrients for the plants themselves, any animals that eat plants, and on up the food chain. Because

animals digest the consumed carbohydrates, fats, and proteins and can convert them into their own forms of each (see Figure 2.18), we can get energy nutrients, also known as macronutrients, from both

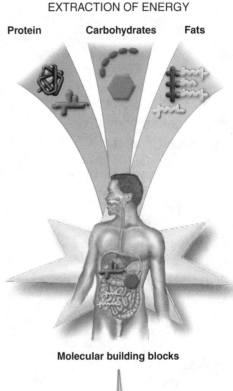

EXTRACTION OF ENERGY

Protein   Carbohydrates   Fats

Molecular building blocks

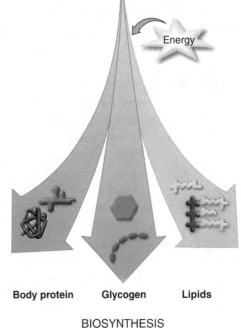

Energy

Body protein   Glycogen   Lipids

BIOSYNTHESIS

Figure 2.18   Metabolism. Cells use metabolic reactions to extract energy from food and to form building blocks for biosynthesis.

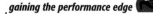
plant and animal sources. When plant and animal foods are eaten, the digestive system breaks the nutrients into their constituent parts so that they can be absorbed and transported to the cells. The cells can then use the blood-borne nutrients as building blocks for biosynthesis, store them for later use, or metabolize them for energy production.

What is the human body's source of chemical energy?

Based on the previous section, it could be concluded that the chemical energy in carbohydrates, fats, and proteins is the direct source of energy for cellular function. However, this is not the case. The direct source of energy for all biological processes comes from a high-energy molecule known as adenosine triphosphate (ATP). In short, the chemical energy from macronutrients is used to make another high-energy chemical known as ATP. The energy stored in the chemical bonds of ATP is released when the bonds are broken and can be used by the cells to perform biological work, as shown in   Figure 2.19 .

ATP is an adenosine molecule with a chain of three phosphate groups attached to it in series (see   Figure 2.20). The energy used by the body is stored in the molecular bonds between the second and third phosphate groups as well as between the first and second groups. When the bonds between the second and third or first and second phosphate groups are broken, energy is released. Some of the released energy is used to perform work, and the remainder is lost as heat energy, which cannot be used by the body. When the bond to the third phosphate group is broken, the resultant products formed are an **adenosine diphosphate (ADP)** and an unattached inorganic phosphate group (P_i) (see Figure 2.20). ADP still has some energy potential for use by the body. If the last phosphate group is cleaved from the ADP, the result is the formation of **adenosine monophosphate (AMP)** and another P_i (see Figure 2.20).

adenosine diphosphate (ADP) A chemical compound that contains two phosphate groups attached to an adenosine molecule. ADP, when phosphorylated, becomes ATP.

adenosine monophosphate (AMP) A chemical compound that contains a single phosphate group attached to an adenosine molecule.

THE ADP–ATP CYCLE

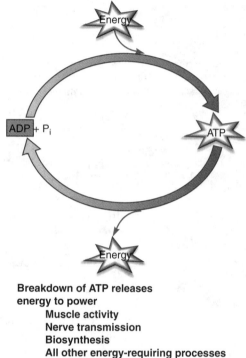

Formation of ATP requires energy from the metabolic breakdown of energy nutrients

Energy

ADP + P_i

ATP

Energy

Breakdown of ATP releases energy to power
   Muscle activity
   Nerve transmission
   Biosynthesis
   All other energy-requiring processes

  Figure 2.19   The ADP–ATP cycle. When extracting energy from nutrients, the formation of ATP from ADP + P captures energy. Breaking a phosphate bond in ATP to form ADP + P releases energy for biosynthesis and work.

Although ATP is the direct source of energy for cellular functioning, it is stored in very small quantities in the cells. For example, in muscle cells, ATP stores are so small they can be depleted in as little as 3 seconds of muscle activity. Despite the fact that ATP is stored in very limited amounts, it is important to note that cells never completely deplete their ATP stores.   Figure 2.21   shows ATP levels during an intense sprint lasting 14 seconds. Note that at the point of exhaustion, roughly 30% of the muscle's ATP still remains. Obviously, athletes perform activities that last longer than 3 seconds every day, so the body must have ways of replenishing ATP once it is used. In fact, every cell, particularly muscle cells, can replenish any ATP that is used to keep the ATP fuel tank somewhat full. If ATP levels fall too low because the activity is so intense that the muscle cells cannot make

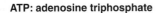

ATP, ADP, AMP, AND HIGH-ENERGY
PHOSPHATE BONDS

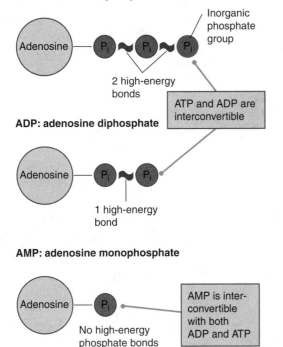

ATP: adenosine triphosphate

Adenosine

Inorganic phosphate group

2 high-energy bonds

ATP and ADP are interconvertible

ADP: adenosine diphosphate

Adenosine

1 high-energy bond

AMP: adenosine monophosphate

Adenosine

No high-energy phosphate bonds

AMP is inter-convertible with both ADP and ATP

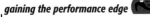
Figure 2.20   ATP, ADP, AMP, and high-energy phosphate bonds. Your body can readily use the energy in high-energy phosphate bonds. During metabolic reactions, phosphate bonds form or break to capture or release energy.

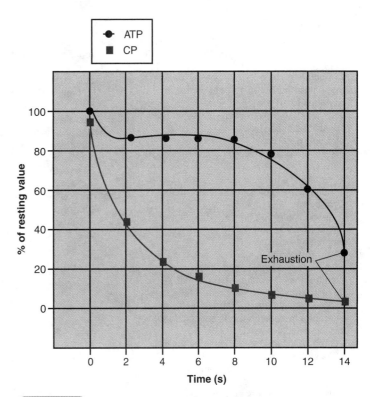

Figure 2.21   Effect of intense activity on ATP levels in muscle. Even when an activity results in exhaustion, ATP levels are not totally depleted.
Reprinted with permission from J.H. Wilmore, D.L. Costill, and W.L. Kenney, 2008, *Physiology of Sport and Exercise*, 4th ed. (Champaign, IL: Human Kinetics), 52.

gaining the performance edge

Poor nutrition can directly affect ATP production and thus decrease sport performance.

ATP fast enough, protective mechanisms kick in that in turn cause **fatigue**. Fatigue is a noted decrease in performance level, which slows down or even stops the activity and thus protects the cell's ATP levels. Poor nutrition can directly affect ATP production and thus decrease sport performance. As a result, there must be a way for cells to make or replenish ATP once it has been used.

How do cells make ATP?

To metabolize the energy nutrients and in the process make ATP, the cells must possess the right metabolic equipment. Although there are many different types of cells that make up the body, they all have similarities.   Figure 2.22   provides the names and functions of many of the parts of typical cells. For example, all cells have a **cell membrane** that encloses the contents of the cell, known as the **cytoplasm**. The cell membrane serves as a barrier that regulates

or prevents the influx of substances into or out of the cytoplasm. The watery component of the cytoplasm that fills much of the interior of the cell is known as the **cytosol**. Dissolved in the cytosol are enzymes, which are proteins responsible for accelerating each step in the metabolic pathways responsible for generating ATP. In addition, within the cytoplasm there are cellular structures known as **organelles** that perform specific functions. The organelle of most importance in regard to the production of ATP is the **mitochondrion**. The mitochondrion is sometimes more descriptively called the "aerobic powerhouse of the cell" because many of the metabolic pathways responsi-

fatigue A physical condition marked by the point in time at which the work output or performance cannot be maintained.

cell membrane The membrane that makes up the outer boundary of a cell and separates the internal contents of the cell from the external substances.

cytoplasm The interior of the cell. It includes the fluid and organelles that are enclosed within the cell membrane.

cytosol The watery or fluid part of the cytoplasm.

organelles Specialized structures found inside cells that perform specific functions. For example, the mitochondria are organelles responsible for the aerobic production of energy for the cell.

mitochondrion A specialized cellular organelle responsible for the aerobic production of ATP within the cell.

Organelles

Endoplasmic reticulum (ER)
- An extensive membrane system extending from the nuclear membrane.
- Rough ER: The outer membrane surface contains ribosomes, the site of protein synthesis.
- Smooth ER: Devoid of ribosomes, the site of lipid synthesis.

Golgi apparatus
- A system of stacked membrane-encased discs.
- The site of extensive modification, sorting, and packaging of compounds for transport.

Lysosome
- Vesicle containing enzymes that digest intracellular materials and recycle the components.

Mitochondrion
- Contains two highly specialized membranes, an outer membrane and a highly folded inner membrane. Membranes separated by narrow intermembrane space. Inner membrane encloses space called mitochondrial matrix.
- Often called the "powerhouse" of the cell. Site where most of the energy from carbohydrate, protein, and fat is captured in ATP (adenosine triphosphate).
- About 2,000 mitochondria in a cell.

Ribosome
- Site of protein synthesis.

Nucleus
- Contains genetic information in the base sequences of the DNA strands of the chromosomes.
- Site of RNA synthesis—RNA needed for protein synthesis.
- Enclosed in a double-layered membrane.

Cytoplasm
- Enclosed in the cell membrane and separated from the nucleus by the nuclear membrane.
- Filled with particles and organelles that are dipersed in a clear fluid called cytosol.

Cytosol
- The fluid inside the cell membrane.
- Site of glycolsis and fatty acid synthesis.

Cell membrane
- A double-layered sheet, made up of lipid and protein, that encases the cell.
- Controls the passage of substances in and out of the cell.
- Contains receptors for hormones and other regulatory compounds.

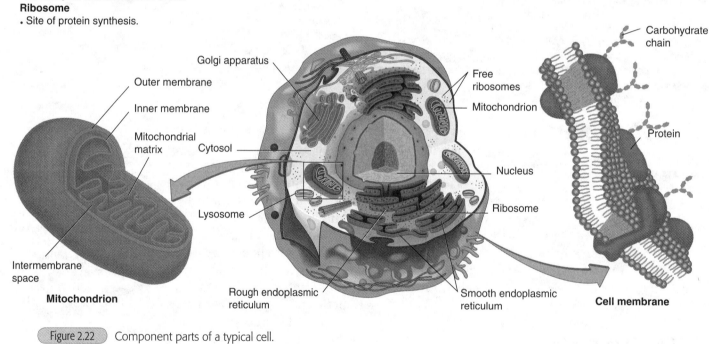

Figure 2.22 Component parts of a typical cell.

ble for the aerobic production of ATP are found inside. Finally, each cell possesses a nucleus that contains the genetic information needed for making the enzymes and cellular structures required for ATP production.

To further explain ATP formation, a basic understanding of **bioenergetics** is necessary. Bioenergetics is the study of how energy is captured, transferred, and/or utilized within biological systems. Because this book deals with sports, the specific biologic system we will discuss in this chapter is muscle. To rebuild ATP, unattached phosphates must be reattached to AMP or ADP to reform ATP. The process of resynthesizing ATP requires energy in and

> **bioenergetics** The study of energy transfer within a biological system.

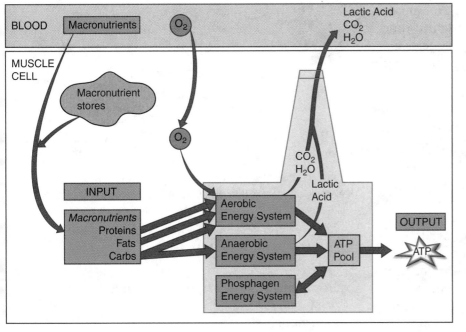

BLOOD

MUSCLE CELL

Macronutrients

O_2

Lactic Acid
CO_2
H_2O

Macronutrient stores

O_2

CO_2
H_2O
Lactic Acid

INPUT

Aerobic Energy System

OUTPUT

Macronutrients
Proteins
Fats
Carbs

Anaerobic Energy System

ATP Pool

ATP

Phosphagen Energy System

Figure 2.23 Metabolic factory analogy of energy metabolism.

metabolic factory The cellular enzymes, organelles, and metabolic pathways responsible for the production of energy within the cells.

ATP pool The muscle cell's inventory of readily available ATP.

of itself, and this is where the energy trapped in the bonds of foods (i.e., macronutrients) comes into play. Using the analogy of a real-life factory, each of the muscle cells in the human body possesses what can be called a **metabolic factory**. These metabolic factories are responsible for manufacturing the cells' ultimate energy source, ATP (see  Figure 2.23).

Continuing with the metabolic factory analogy, inside the factory is an **ATP pool** (i.e., the cell's inventory of readily available ATP). However, the inventory of ATP is very small and must be maintained during exercise and at rest via three different energy systems (see Figure 2.23). One energy system, known as the phosphagen system, is simply

the readily available stores of high-energy phosphates. In other words, the metabolic factory has a small inventory of energy ready for immediate use. To protect the cells from running out of the small inventory of high-energy phosphates, there are two other systems capable of making more ATP when the demand increases (i.e., during exercise). These two systems involve the enzymatic breakdown of macronutrients. One of the systems (i.e., the aerobic energy system) requires oxygen to break down the macronutrients, and the other does not (i.e., the anaerobic energy system). The following section discusses each energy system in greater detail.

What are the three energy systems?

The three energy systems that function within the metabolic factories of muscle cells are the **phosphagen system**, the **anaerobic system**, and the **aerobic system** (see Figure 2.23). These three energy systems have different properties when it comes to the speed with which they can supply ATP (i.e., rate of production) and their capacity to generate ATP (i.e., production capacity) (see **Table 2.1**). The important point to remember is that all three of these energy systems are working together to make sure the

phosphagen system The energy system composed of the high-energy phosphates ATP and creatine phosphate. It is also known as the immediate energy system. Of the three energy systems, it is capable of producing ATP at the fastest rate.

anaerobic system (anaerobic glycolysis) The energy system that has the capability to generate ATP in the absence of oxygen. The anaerobic system results in the formation of ATP and lactic acid.

aerobic system The energy system that relies upon the presence of oxygen to make ATP. Of the three energy systems, it is the slowest at producing ATP but has an almost unending capacity to make ATP.

TABLE 2.1	Comparison of Characteristics of the Three Energy Systems			
Energy System	Energy System Complexity	Maximal Rate of ATP Production	Capacity to Make ATP	Lag Time to Increased ATP Production
Phosphagen	Low; one-step process	Very fast	Very limited	None; instantaneous
Anaerobic	Moderate; 12-step process	Fast; runs a close second	Limited	Seconds
Aerobic	Very high; many processes and steps	Very slow; distant third	Unlimited	Minutes

output of the metabolic factory is meeting the muscle cell's demand for ATP at any given point in time. By working together, the three energy systems can maintain the ATP pool for various activities, ranging from rest to a fast, explosive movement (e.g., a jump or sprint) and everything in between.

What are the characteristics of the phosphagen system?

The phosphagen system is the simplest of the three energy systems. It is also known as the **immediate energy system** because it serves the immediate energy needs of the muscle cells. For example, when athletes burst from the starting blocks in a race, there must be an immediate source of energy available to enable them to go from no movement to maximum speed in fractions of a second. If ATP was not readily available at the start of the race, then the muscles of the athlete could work only as fast as the metabolic pathways could produce energy. Because the pathways are lengthy, there would be a lag period before the increased production of ATP would be available. Using the metabolic factory example, the phosphagen system is the inventory of high-energy product that is stored on-site and readily available for immediate use. The inventory of high-energy phosphates serves as a buffer, thus allowing the other energy systems time to ramp up ATP production without a lag in energy availability. Specifically, the high-energy products are the cell's stores of ATP (i.e., the ATP pool) and another high-energy molecule, called **creatine phosphate (CP)** or alternatively **phosphocreatine**.

CP is a high-energy phosphate that in a one-step metabolic reaction can give its phosphate group to ADP to rebuild another ATP (see Figure 2.24). This metabolic reaction is accelerated by the enzyme **creatine kinase**.[3] The ATP pool and the one-step creatine kinase reaction that comprise the phosphagen energy system give it the highest rate of production of ATP of the three energy systems and enable it to provide instantaneous energy to the cells. Its high rate of ATP production makes the phosphagen energy system most relied upon when energy is needed

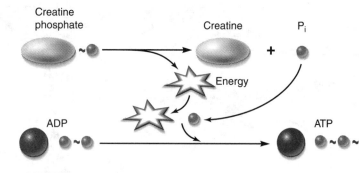

Figure 2.24 The ATP–CP energy system. To maintain relatively constant ATP levels during the first few seconds of a high-intensity activity, creatine phosphate releases energy and its phosphate (P_i) to regenerate ATP from ADP.

quickly during very fast, powerful muscle contractions (see Figure 2.25).

Although the phosphagen system can supply ATP at very high rates, it has a limited capacity to generate ATP. Specifically, if the other two energy systems were not available to help in the production of ATP, the phosphagen system would only be able to provide energy for 5 to 15 seconds, depending on the intensity of the activity.[4] The phosphagen system serves as an energy buffer, which fills the immediate need for ATP until the other two energy systems with higher capacities for generating ATP can ramp up their production of ATP.

What are the characteristics of the anaerobic and aerobic energy systems?

As mentioned earlier, unlike the phosphagen system, which is basically an inventory of readily available high-energy phosphates within cells, the anaerobic and aerobic energy systems must generate ATP via more complex cellular processing (see Table 2.1). As a result, there is a slight lapse in time before the aerobic and anaerobic systems can ramp up and begin contributing ATP when an activity begins or changes in intensity. The cellular processing required to make ATP anaerobically or aerobically occurs via **metabolic pathways**. Metabolic pathways can be **anabolic pathways**, which require energy and result in the formation of more complex molecules, or **catabolic pathways**, which release energy and result in

immediate energy system The energy system composed of the high-energy phosphates ATP and creatine phosphate; as a result it is also known as the phosphagen system. Of the three energy systems, it is capable of producing ATP at the fastest rate.

creatine phosphate (CP) A high-energy phosphate stored inside muscle cells.

phosphocreatine A high-energy phosphate stored inside muscle cells. It is also known as creatine phosphate.

creatine kinase The enzyme that catalyzes the reaction transferring phosphate from creatine phosphate to adenosine diphosphate to make ATP.

metabolic pathways Sequentially organized metabolic reactions that are catalyzed by enzymes and result in the formation or breakdown of chemicals within the body.

anabolic pathway A metabolic pathway that requires energy and results in the formation of more complex molecules.

catabolic pathway A metabolic pathway that degrades complex compounds into simpler ones and in the process gives off energy.

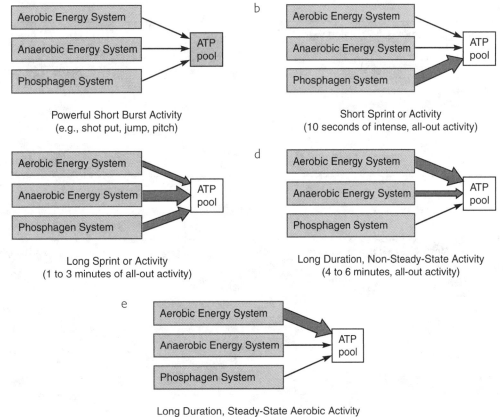

a
Aerobic Energy System
Anaerobic Energy System
Phosphagen System
→ ATP pool

Powerful Short Burst Activity
(e.g., shot put, jump, pitch)

b
Aerobic Energy System
Anaerobic Energy System
Phosphagen System
→ ATP pool

Short Sprint or Activity
(10 seconds of intense, all-out activity)

c
Aerobic Energy System
Anaerobic Energy System
Phosphagen System
→ ATP pool

Long Sprint or Activity
(1 to 3 minutes of all-out activity)

d
Aerobic Energy System
Anaerobic Energy System
Phosphagen System
→ ATP pool

Long Duration, Non-Steady-State Activity
(4 to 6 minutes, all-out activity)

e
Aerobic Energy System
Anaerobic Energy System
Phosphagen System
→ ATP pool

Long Duration, Steady-State Aerobic Activity
(30 minutes of continuous activity)

Figure 2.25   The three energy systems work together to meet the energy demands of any level of physical activity. Width of arrow denotes degree of energy contribution.

the breakdown of molecules (see Figure 2.26). The anaerobic and aerobic metabolic pathways are catabolic. In short, anaerobic and aerobic metabolic pathways are sequential steps in which the energy in foods (i.e., carbohydrates, fats, and proteins) is broken down (see **Table 2.2** and **Table 2.3**). In other words, these metabolic pathways are assembly lines in reverse (i.e., disassembly lines). Instead of building something in a stepwise systematic fashion, metabolic pathways slowly break apart food molecules in an organized stepwise order. This helps the cells to capture as much energy as possible from foods to make ATP. Although there is some commonality in the metabolic pathways required to break down carbohydrates, fats, and proteins, there are a couple pathways that are unique depending on the energy nutrient being processed and/or the availability of oxygen.

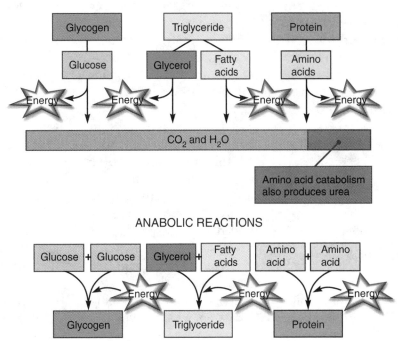

CATABOLIC REACTIONS

Glycogen → Glucose → Energy
Triglyceride → Glycerol → Energy, Fatty acids → Energy
Protein → Amino acids → Energy
CO_2 and H_2O
Amino acid catabolism also produces urea

ANABOLIC REACTIONS

Glucose + Glucose → Glycogen (Energy)
Glycerol + Fatty acids → Triglyceride (Energy)
Amino acid + Amino acid → Protein (Energy)

Figure 2.26   Catabolism and anabolism. Catabolic reactions break down molecules and release energy and other products. Anabolic reactions consume energy as they assemble complex molecules.

TABLE 2.2	Metabolic Pathways Associated with the Three Energy Systems		
	Phosphagen	Anaerobic	Aerobic
Metabolic pathways	None	Glycolysis	Beta-oxidation
			Glycolysis
			Deamination
			Citric acid cycle
			Electron transport chain

TABLE 2.3	Energy Nutrients and the Sequence of the Aerobic Metabolic Pathways That Metabolize Them for Energy		
	Carbohydrates	Fats	Proteins
Glycolysis	1		
Beta-oxidation		1	
Deamination			1
Citric acid cycle	2	2	2
Electron transport chain	3	3	3

What metabolic pathway is involved with the anaerobic energy system?

The second energy system is the anaerobic energy system (see Figure 2.27), which involves one metabolic pathway called anaerobic glycolysis. The only macronutrient that can be broken down via glycolysis is carbohydrates. Energy from fats and proteins is derived from the metabolic pathways involved with the aerobic energy system.

Glycolysis is unique in that it can be part of both the anaerobic and aerobic energy systems. When adequate amounts of oxygen are not available and energy is needed, the end product of glycolysis (i.e., pyruvate) is converted to lactic acid (see Figure 2.27). This last step or reaction enables glycolysis to continue producing ATP without the need for oxygen, which is why it is called the anaerobic energy system. **Anaerobic** means without oxygen. Alternatively, if oxygen is present, then pyruvate is not converted to lactic acid. Instead,

glycolysis A metabolic pathway that is responsible for the breakdown of glucose. It is unique in that it can function with or without the presence of oxygen.

anaerobic A term used to describe a condition in which oxygen is not present.

it is metabolized in other metabolic pathways that are associated with the aerobic energy systems discussed in the following section.

Unlike the phosphagen system, which at its longest is one step, the anaerobic system involves a metabolic pathway (i.e., glycolysis) of 12 steps. Because it is lengthier and more complex than the phosphagen system, it is a little slower to adapt to changes in activity level. However, it is much faster to adapt than the aerobic energy system, which is the slowest of the three systems. The anaerobic energy system is a major contributor to intense (i.e., maximal effort) activities that last from 1 to 3 minutes (see Figure 2.25c). During these activities, oxygen availability is limited because of the intense muscle contractions that close off blood vessels and limit delivery of oxygen, at least in large enough quantities to completely meet the energy demands of the activity.

Although the anaerobic system's rate of production of ATP is fairly high, its capacity for making ATP is limited (see Table 2.1). The resulting product of anaerobic glycolysis is lactic acid. When lactic acid is produced quickly it accumulates in the muscle, and when levels get high enough, fatigue

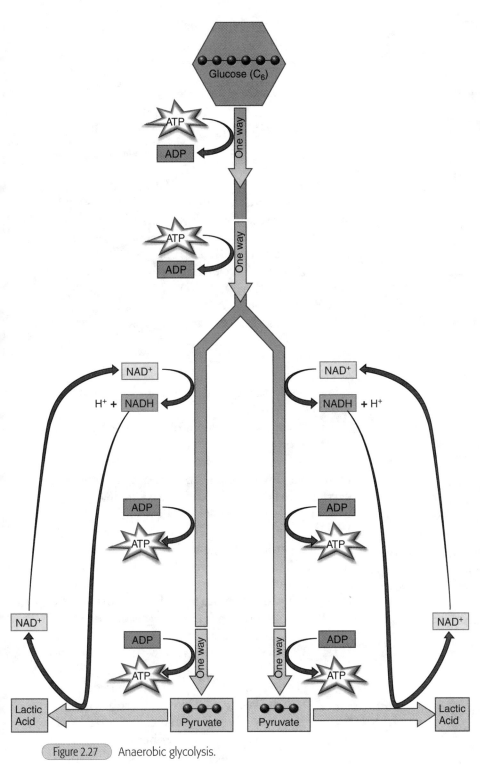

Compared to the other energy systems, the aerobic system is the slowest at producing ATP, but it has an unlimited ability to make ATP. The aerobic system provides the fuel for resting metabolic needs. It also is the energy system most relied upon for longer duration, continuous activities that can be performed for minutes to hours. The aerobic energy system is also the longest and most complex of the three energy systems (see Table 2.1). It involves five different metabolic pathways (see Table 2.2). The metabolic pathways involved depend on the chemical structure of the food molecule being broken down (see Table 2.3 and Figure 2.28). The end products of the aerobic energy system are ATP, carbon dioxide, and water. It should be noted that carbon dioxide and water are the very same molecules used by plants to make carbohydrates, along with fats and proteins. In short, plants use carbon dioxide from the air, water from the soil, and light energy from the sun to make the energy nutrients. During aerobic metabolism our cells break the foods back down to their constituent parts of carbon dioxide and water, thus releasing the chemical energy in the foods (see Figure 2.26) and using it to make ATP. The carbon dioxide and water released from the body can then be reused by plants to make more energy nutrients, thus completing the ongoing energy cycle.

Figure 2.27   Anaerobic glycolysis.

ensues. To experience the fatigue caused by lactic acid buildup, one only needs to run around an outdoor track as fast as possible. The burning feeling experienced in the muscles is caused by lactic acid buildup.

What pathways are associated with the aerobic breakdown of carbohydrates?

The first metabolic pathway carbohydrates must pass through is the glycolytic pathway (see Figure

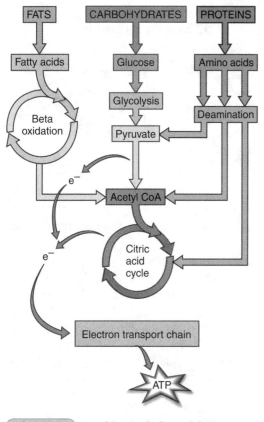

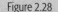

Figure 2.28   Aerobic metabolism of the macronutrients.

pyruvate The end product of glycolysis.

2.27). When sufficient oxygen is present, **pyruvate**, which is the end product of glycolysis, is converted to acetyl coenzyme A (acetyl CoA) (see Figure 2.29) rather than converted to lactic acid as during anaerobic metabolism. The acetyl

CoA then enters into the **citric acid cycle** (see Figure 2.30), which is a series of reactions that occur inside of the mitochondria of the cell. The primary purpose of the citric acid cycle is to strip hydrogens from the molecules as they pass through. The stripped hydrogens are picked up by special carrier molecules known as **nicotinamide adenine dinucleotide (NAD)** and **flavin adenine dinucleotide (FAD)**. NAD and FAD combine with the stripped hydrogens to form NADH and FADH, respectively. The attached hydrogens are transported to the final aerobic pathway, the **electron transport chain (ETC)** (see Figure 2.31).

The hydrogen transfer molecules associated with the electron transport chain are located on the inner membrane of the mitochondria. The transfer of hydrogens down the ETC begins once the hydrogen carriers NADH and FADH release their hydrogens to the ETC (see Figure 2.31). The resulting NAD and FAD are available to cycle back to the citric acid cycle to pick up more hydrogens. The hydrogens dumped into the ETC are transferred from one transfer molecule to another. In the process of hydrogen transfer, energy is given off and captured in the form of ATP.

The final acceptor molecule for the hydrogens being passed down the ETC is oxygen, which results in the formation of water (see Figure 2.31). The ETC is the metabolic pathway that generates the most ATP during aerobic metabolism. The problem is that the ETC is the final pathway in aerobic metabolism and as a result it takes time for ATP formation to increase in response to exercise or activity.

The citric acid cycle and the electron transport chain are aerobic pathways that are common to all three energy nutrients. As already noted, both of these metabolic pathways are found in the mitochondria of the cells. For this reason, mitochondria are called "aerobic

citric acid cycle One of the major metabolic pathways of the aerobic energy system. It is also known as the Krebs cycle or the tricarboxylic acid cycle. Its main role is to strip hydrogens from compounds passing through it.

nicotinamide adenine dinucleotide (NAD) One of two electron carriers that is responsible for shuttling hydrogens from one metabolic step or pathway to another.

flavin adenine dinucleotide (FAD) One of two electron carriers that is responsible for shuttling hydrogens from one metabolic step or pathway to another.

electron transport chain (ETC) The final metabolic pathway of the aerobic energy system. It is responsible for transferring hydrogens from one chemical to another and in the process making ATP and water.

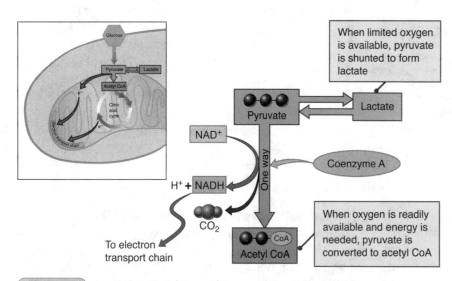

Figure 2.29   Pyruvate to acetyl CoA. When oxygen is readily available, each pyruvate formed from glucose yields one acetyl CoA and one NADH.

beta-oxidation The first metabolic pathway of fat metabolism, which cleaves off two carbon molecules each time a fatty acid chain cycles through it.

deamination The metabolic pathway that is responsible for removing the nitrogen or amine group from the carbon structure of amino acids.

powerhouses" of the cells. Endurance-type training challenges these metabolic pathways to produce energy more rapidly. The cells adapt to endurance training by increasing the size and number of mitochondria, allowing for greater production of ATP aerobically.[5] This is one of the reasons why endurance athletes can perform at higher intensities for a longer duration than untrained persons.

What pathways are associated with the aerobic breakdown of fats and proteins?

Fats and proteins cannot be metabolized via glycolysis and therefore must pass through other pathways before entering into the citric acid cycle and ETC (see Figure 2.28). Fats must first be metabolized via **beta-oxidation**, which is a cyclical pathway that is found within the confines of the mitochondria. Each pass of a fatty acid through beta-oxidation cleaves off two carbon fragments from the end of the fatty acids. Each pass also results in the formation of an NADH and an FADH. The two carbon fragments are converted to acetyl CoA, which then enters the citric acid cycle and ultimately the ETC. The NADH and FADH transfer their hydrogens to the ETC for use in ATP production.

Proteins contain nitrogen components in their molecular structure. These nitrogen-containing components cannot be used by the body and thus must first be cleaved from the protein before it can be metabolized for energy. The process in which the nitrogen group is cleaved from proteins is called **deamination** (see Figure 2.32). Once the nitrogen is removed, the remaining carbon molecule can pass through the citric acid cycle and then the ETC to produce ATP (see Figure 2.28). However, it should be noted that proteins are not normally a major source of energy (they provide less than 10% of energy for exercise) unless energy expenditure is high and/or carbohydrate intake is low.[6]

How does carbohydrate intake affect protein metabolism?

When diets are low in carbohydrates or when an athlete is in-

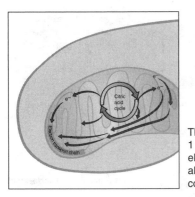

The citric acid cycle produces 3 NADH and 1 FADH$_2$ which carry pairs of high-energy electrons to the electron transport chain. It also forms one GTP which is readily converted to 1 ATP.

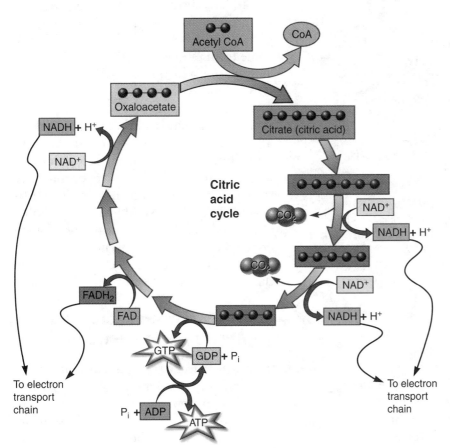

Figure 2.30 The citric acid cycle. This circular pathway conserves carbons as it accepts one acetyl CoA and yields two CO$_2$, three NADH, one FADH$_2$, and one guanosine triphosphate (GTP), a high-energy compound that can be readily converted to ATP.

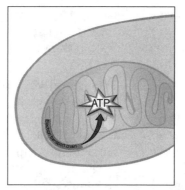

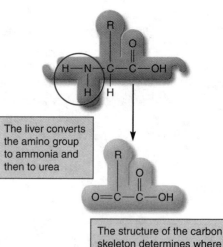

The liver converts the amino group to ammonia and then to urea

The structure of the carbon skeleton determines where it can enter the energy producing pathways.

Figure 2.32 Deamination. A deamination reaction strips the amino group from an amino acid.

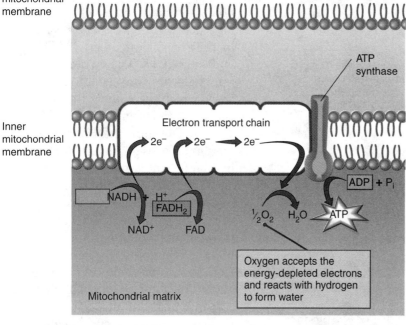

Cytosol

Outer mitochondrial membrane

Inner mitochondrial membrane

ATP synthase

Electron transport chain

$2e^-$ $2e^-$ $2e^-$

NADH + H$^+$
FADH$_2$
NAD$^+$
FAD
$\frac{1}{2}O_2$ H$_2$O ATP
ADP + P$_i$

Oxygen accepts the energy-depleted electrons and reacts with hydrogen to form water

Mitochondrial matrix

Figure 2.31 Electron transport chain. This pathway produces most of the ATP available from glucose, as well as fats and amino acids. Mitochondrial NADH delivers pairs of high-energy electrons to the beginning of the chain. Each of these NADH molecules ultimately produces 2.5 ATP. The pairs of high-energy electrons from FADH$_2$ enter this pathway farther along, so one FADH$_2$ produces 1.5 ATP.

volved in training that depletes carbohydrate stores, the body must get its carbohydrates from somewhere else. It does so by converting proteins in the body to carbohydrates in a process known as **gluconeogenesis** (see Figure 2.33). During gluconeogenesis, proteins are broken down into amino acids, transported to the liver, and converted to the carbohydrate glucose, which can then be used for energy by the body tissues.

gluconeogenesis The formation of glucose from noncarbohydrate sources such as proteins.

Unfortunately for the athlete, most of the proteins used in gluconeogenesis come from muscle.[7] This is one reason why carbohydrate intake is so important to the athlete. If carbohydrate intake is adequate to meet energy demands and carbohydrate stores are replenished after training, then proteins do not need to be converted to carbohydrates, and muscle protein is spared. The relationship between carbohydrate intake and protein breakdown for energy is a critical concept to understand. Put in other words, adequate carbohydrates in the diet spare muscle protein.

gaining the performance edge

Carbohydrates spare muscle protein by decreasing the body's reliance on gluconeogenesis to make its own carbohydrates.

How do the energy systems work together to supply ATP during sport performance?

During sports, the energy requirement of muscle is related to the intensity and duration of the activity. In other words, slow movements do not require ATP to be supplied as rapidly as more powerful, fast movements. As discussed earlier, the existing ATP pool in muscle cells is very small. Therefore it is imperative that the three energy systems work together to maintain ATP levels. Remember, muscle cells never

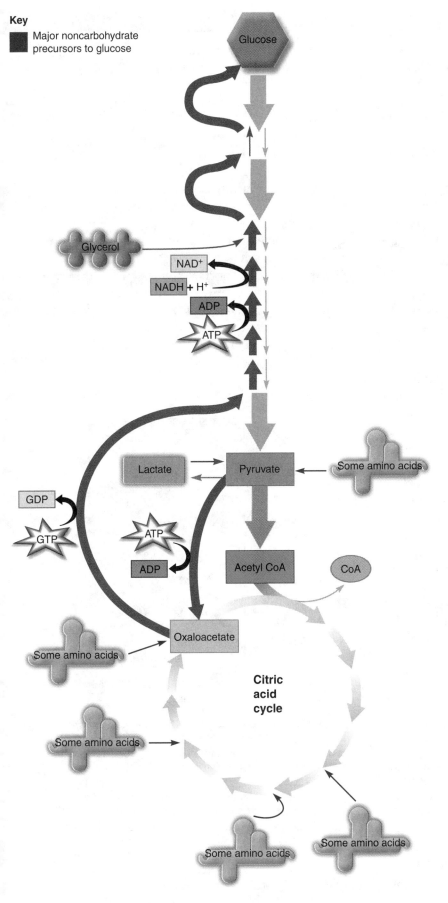

Key

■ Major noncarbohydrate precursors to glucose

Glucose

Glycerol

NAD⁺

NADH + H⁺

ADP

ATP

Lactate → Pyruvate ← Some amino acids

GDP

GTP

ATP

ADP

Acetyl CoA

CoA

Oxaloacetate

Some amino acids

Citric acid cycle

Some amino acids

Some amino acids

Some amino acids

run out of ATP. Thus, if an activity is so intense and burns ATP so quickly that the three energy systems cannot supply ATP fast enough to prevent ATP depletion, fatigue ensues (Figure 2.21). Fatigue causes a decrease in the level of activity, resulting in a lower energy demand, thereby giving the energy systems a chance to begin replenishing the level of ATP.

To prevent fatigue and maintain ATP levels above the threshold for fatigue, the energy systems must work together, taking advantage of their unique characteristics to meet the metabolic demands for ATP. Of the three energy systems, the muscle cells rely predominantly on the aerobic system because of its unending ability to make ATP. If the energy requirements of an activity are low enough for the aerobic energy system to meet the energy demands, exercise can be continued for a long duration. This results in a condition called **steady state exercise**, where the energy demands are being met primarily by the aerobic system (see Figure 2.25e). The more

> **steady state exercise** Any level or intensity of physical activity in which the energy demand for ATP is met by the aerobic production of ATP.

highly trained the aerobic energy system, the faster a person can move while remaining in a steady state.

Endurance athletes train every day to challenge and improve the aerobic systems of their muscle cells. Their muscles respond to the daily demands by increasing the cellular organelles where aerobic production of ATP occurs: the mitochondria. As mentioned earlier, increasing the number and size of mitochondria enables the cell to greatly increase the speed with which it makes ATP. Because ATP can be

Figure 2.33 Gluconeogenesis. Liver and kidney cells make glucose from pyruvate by way of oxaloacetate. Gluconeogenesis is not the reverse of glycolysis. Although these pathways share many reactions, albeit in the reverse direction, gluconeogenesis must detour around the irreversible steps in glycolysis.

supplied much more rapidly, the speed of the activity can be performed more quickly while the athlete remains in a steady state. This is why highly trained marathoners can run 26.2 miles at speeds that untrained persons could not run for even 1 mile without fatiguing.

When the energy needs of the muscle cannot be met by the aerobic system, the other two systems are needed to supplement the deficiency in ATP. If the activity is just slightly above the ability of the aerobic system to supply ATP, then the amount supplemented by the other two systems is low, and the activity can be continued for quite a while before fatigue sets in (see Figure 2.25d). As the intensity of the activity increases, the ability to produce energy through the aerobic pathways decreases, and therefore the reliance on the other two systems increases, causing fatigue to ensue more quickly. For example, if a marathoner decided to increase her running speed to something faster than her normal race pace, the demand for ATP production would go up. If the increase in speed was slightly above the aerobic system's ability to supply ATP, then the phosphagen and anaerobic systems would have to help fill the slight energy deficit. However, the energetic demand placed on the phosphagen and anaerobic systems would be relatively low, and the runner could maintain this increased pace for approximately a mile or two before fatigue sets in. On the other hand, if the marathoner decided to sprint as fast as possible, then the all-out sprint would require ATP to be supplied at rates well above the aerobic system's ability to supply it. In this scenario the muscles would have to rely much more heavily on the other two energy systems, and exhaustion would set in much more quickly. If the marathoner timed the final sprint just right, sprint speed could be maintained for approximately 200 meters before the muscles' ATP stores fell to critically low levels. Recall that, when ATP levels get low, exhaustion sets in (see Figure 2.21). Sprinting places a huge demand on the phosphagen and anaerobic energy systems, and as a result, regular sprint training causes muscles to adapt. The muscles increase their stores of ATP and CP. In addition, the muscle cells make more enzymes such as creatine kinase and others associated with anaerobic metabolism. The end result is a sprint athlete who can maintain his or her maximum running speed for fractions of a second longer than the competition and thus perhaps win the race. **Creatine monohydrate** (see Chapter 9) is a dietary supplement that increases the levels of CP in the muscle, and thus is a popular

item with sprint and power athletes.[8] Creatine monohydrate bolsters the immediate energy system's ability to supply ATP, thus delaying fatigue in high-intensity activities.[9,10]

Athletes with energy needs somewhere between those of the sprinter and those of the marathoner rely on the three energy systems working together. The reliance on each of the systems depends on the nature of the sport. In other words, there exists an **energy continuum** (see Figure 2.34). The energy required for various sports activities falls at different points along this energy continuum. For example, an athlete who runs the mile moves at speeds somewhere between those of the sprinter and those of the marathoner (see Figure 2.25d). The intensity of the

> **creatine monohydrate** A dietary supplement that can help improve an athlete's anaerobic strength and power by increasing levels of creatine phosphate in muscles.
>
> **energy continuum** A continuum of activity levels spanning from lowest to maximum, with all points in between requiring slightly increasing rates of energy production.

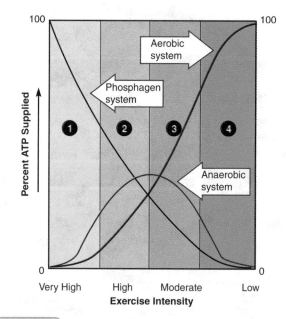

Figure 2.34   ATP contribution of the three energy systems to maximally sustained activities of very short, high-intensity exercise, such as the shot put (i.e., left margin of graph), to low-intensity maximally sustained exercise lasting longer than 3 minutes, such as running a marathon (i.e., right margin). Note: The longer the duration of "maximally sustained activity," the lower the exercise intensity. Area 1 spans from fractions of a second to 30 seconds, area 2 spans from 30 seconds to 1.5 minutes, area 3 spans from 1.5 minutes to 3 minutes, and area 4 is for time longer than 3 minutes.
Source: Bower RW, Fox EL. *Sport Physiology*, 3rd ed. Dubuque, IA: William C Brown Publishers; 1992. Reprinted with permission of the McGraw-Hill Companies.

miler's run is higher than that which can be provided by the aerobic system but not so intense that it puts a huge demand on the phosphagen system. In this case the anaerobic system plays a larger role in working with the aerobic system to provide the needed ATP. The bottom line is that any activity relies on the optimal blending of energy production by the three energy systems (see Figure 2.34).

Key Points of Chapter

- The digestive system is basically a long, internalized tube that passes through the body. Foods enter via the mouth and exit from the anus. Substances in the digestive system have not entered the body until they are absorbed across the intestinal wall.

- The anatomy of the digestive system includes the mouth, esophagus, stomach, small intestine, and large intestine. Associated structures including the salivary glands, pancreas, liver, and gallbladder secrete enzymes and bile salts that help in the digestive process.

- Digestion of carbohydrates begins in the mouth as a result of the mechanical process of mastication and the enzymatic actions of salivary amylase. However, the majority of digestion occurs in the small intestine, where the foodstuffs are subjected to the actions of various pancreatic and intestinal enzymes.

- During digestion, carbohydrates are broken down into their component parts, monosaccharides (i.e., simple sugars).

- Absorption of monosaccharides occurs in the small intestine via facilitated diffusion or active transport, depending on the type of sugar.

- Once the bloodborne simple sugars reach the cells of the liver, those that are not in the form of glucose (e.g., fructose) are converted to glucose. The glucose can then be stored as glycogen in the liver cells or released back into the bloodstream to be used for energy or stored by other cells of the body.

- Digestion of dietary fats begins in the mouth via mastication and the enzymatic actions of salivary lipase. The digestive process continues in the stomach through muscle actions of the stomach wall and the enzymatic actions of gastric lipase. However, the majority of fat digestion occurs in the small intestine, where various lipases act on the dietary fats (i.e., triglycerides), breaking them into free fatty acids and monoglycerides.

- Absorption of fats also occurs in the small intestine. The short- and medium-chain fatty acids are absorbed via passive diffusion and enter directly into the bloodstream. Long-chain fatty acids and monoglycerides are wrapped by bile salts to form micelles and carried to the intestinal wall, where the fats are released from the micelles and absorbed via passive diffusion. The absorbed fats from the micelles are resynthesized into triglycerides and packaged into chylomicrons. The chylomicrons are released from the cells and enter into the circulatory system via the lymph.

- Lipoprotein lipase, which is located on capillary walls and inside adipocytes, is the enzyme responsible for the entrance and exit of fats from the adipocytes.

- Fatty acids in the blood are transported into muscle cells via facilitated diffusion while triglycerides in bloodborne chylomicrons are acted upon by lipoprotein lipase in the capillaries found in muscle. Lipoprotein lipase breaks down the triglycerides into fatty acids, which are then transported across the muscle cell membrane. Once inside the muscle cells, the fats can be stored or used for energy.

- During digestion, dietary proteins are broken into their basic building blocks, known as amino acids.

- Digestion of proteins begins in the mouth via mastication and continues in the stomach where they are denatured by hydrochloric acid. Once they leave the stomach, protease enzymes in the small intestine continue to break the proteins into single amino acids or small chains of two or three amino acids.

- The small digested protein remnants are absorbed via facilitated diffusion or active transport in the small intestine. Once inside the intestinal cells, any existing chains of amino acids are broken up into single amino acids and then released into the bloodstream.

- When ingested amino acids make it into the bloodstream, they become part of the body's amino acid pool. The amino acid pool also includes amino acids found in other tissues, primarily skeletal muscle and the liver. The blood, with its circulating levels of amino acids, makes up the central part of the amino acid pool, which remains in equilibrium with the other compartments. This helps to maintain the blood's levels of amino acids, thereby serving as a constant and readily available source of amino acids for the body.

■ Amino acid absorption from the bloodstream into the cells of the body tissues occurs through facilitated diffusion. Once inside, the amino acids can be used to make needed proteins through the processes of transcription and translation. Genes in the nucleus are transcribed to form mRNA. The mRNA leaves the nucleus and is translated by ribosomes, which attach the amino acids together to form the specific protein required.

■ Minerals, vitamins, and water do not need to be broken down into smaller units via digestion to be absorbed into the body.

■ Digestion of food releases minerals and vitamins, thereby making them available for absorption. Most vitamins and minerals are absorbed in the small intestine. The exceptions are sodium, potassium, chloride, and some vitamin K, which are all absorbed in the large intestine.

■ Without knowledge of the three energy systems and how they work together to supply energy during specific sports activities, the sports nutrition professional is severely disadvantaged with regard to creating an individualized dietary plan.

■ Energy is an entity that is better explained or defined than shown because it has no shape, no describable features, and no physical mass. Energy enables athletes to perform physical work and is measured in kilocalories (kcals). All cellular and bodily functions require energy. The sum total of all the energy (i.e., total daily calories) required by the body to power cellular processes and activities is known as metabolism.

■ Energy exists in six basic forms: chemical, nuclear, electrical, mechanical, thermal, and radiant. However, the form of energy that humans and animals directly rely upon for survival is chemical energy.

■ The macronutrients—carbohydrates, fats, and proteins— are also known as the energy nutrients. The energy trapped in the bonds of macronutrients is used to make a high-energy compound known as adenosine triphosphate (ATP). ATP is the body's direct source of energy for all biological work. The role of the cellular metabolic factory is to release the chemical energy stored in the macronutrients and use it to make ATP.

■ Energy metabolism or bioenergetics is the study of how energy is captured, transferred, and/or utilized within biological systems. The three energy systems responsible for production of ATP are the phosphagen, anaerobic, and aerobic systems. Each of these systems has unique characteristics, but they work together to supply the specific ATP needs of the athlete.

■ To metabolize the energy nutrients and in the process make ATP, the cells must possess enzymes that sequentially break down the energy nutrients and in the process capture energy in the form of ATP. The enzymes for the phosphagen and anaerobic systems lie within the cytoplasm of the cell. The majority of enzymes and molecular compounds important to the aerobic system are found within specialized organelles known as mitochondria. As a result, mitochondria are sometimes referred to as the "aerobic powerhouses" of cells.

■ Carbohydrates can be metabolized for energy both aerobically and anaerobically. In fact, carbohydrates are the only macronutrient that can be metabolized for energy via the anaerobic system. Fats and proteins can be metabolized only via the aerobic system. This is just one reason why carbohydrates are so important to athletes.

■ The aerobic energy system is composed of five metabolic pathways, three of which are unique to each energy nutrient. Carbohydrates are metabolized via glycolysis, then the citric acid cycle, followed by the electron transport chain. Fats must go through beta-oxidation, then the citric acid cycle, and finally the electron transport chain. Proteins, which are not usually a major energy source, are first deaminated and then metabolized via the citric acid cycle and the electron transport chain.

■ The three energy systems are constantly working together to maintain the small ATP pools that exist in cells. Anywhere along the energy continuum, from rest to maximal physical movements, the three energy systems work together to maintain the ATP levels. ATP levels are never depleted in cells; if the energy systems cannot keep up with energy demand, fatigue occurs. The decrease in performance caused by fatigue lowers energy demand and enables the energy systems to prevent ATP depletion.

Study Questions

1. What are the various anatomical components of the digestive system?

2. What are some of the similarities in the digestive processing of carbohydrates, fats, and proteins? How does digestion differ among them?

3. What are the four processes of cellular absorption?

4. Digestion breaks the macronutrients into their constituent parts so that they can be absorbed. What are the constituent parts of each macronutrient?

5. What is the difference between a micelle and a chylomicron?

6. What are the possible fates of the sugars, fats, and amino acids released into the bloodstream during the digestion of foods?

7. How do cells make proteins? Where are the instructions for protein synthesis found, and what processes are involved in making proteins?

8. What is energy? What are the various forms of energy? Which form is most important to human physiology?

9. What are the macronutrients? What role do they play with regard to supplying the body with energy?

10. What are the three energy systems? What are their characteristics with regard to rate of production and capacity to make energy?

11. What cellular organelles are called the "aerobic powerhouses" of the cell? Explain why.

12. An elite marathoner is at mile 17 in the race and bioenergetically in steady state. What energy systems are contributing to the energy needs of the athlete? Which energy system is the major contributor?

13. What energy system is the major contributor of ATP during a discus throw?

14. An athlete is running an 800-meter race in a track meet. What energy systems are contributing to the energy needs of the athlete? Which energy system is the major contributor of ATP?

15. What metabolic pathways are required to aerobically metabolize fats? Can fats be metabolized anaerobically?

16. Which energy system is also called the "immediate energy system"? What high-energy compounds make up this system?

17. Which compounds are known as hydrogen carriers and play a big role in transferring hydrogen ions to the electron transport chain?

References

1. Jones PJH. Lipids, sterols and their metabolites. In: Shils ME, Olson JA, Shike M, Ross AC, eds. *Modern Nutrition in Health and Disease*. 9th ed. Philadelphia, PA: Lippincott Williams and Wilkins; 1999:67–94.

2. Guyton A. *Textbook of Medical Physiology*. 9th ed. Philadelphia, PA: WB Saunders; 1996.

3. Brooks GA, Fahey TD, Baldwin KM. *Exercise Physiology: Human Bioenergetics and Its Applications*. 4th ed. Boston, MA: McGraw-Hill; 2005:31–42.

4. McArdle WD, Katch FI, Katch VL. *Exercise Physiology: Nutrition, Energy, and Human Performance*. 7th ed. Philadelphia, PA: Lippincott Williams and Wilkins; 2001:134–161.

5. Bizeau ME, Willis WT, Hazel JR. Differential responses to endurance training in subsarcolemmal and intermyo-fibrillar mitochrondria. *J Applied Physiol*. 1988;85(4):1279–1284.

6. White TP, Brooks GA. [U-^{14}C] glucose, alanine, and leucine oxidation in rats at rest and two intensities of running. *Am J Physiol*. 1981;240:E155–E165.

7. Paul GL, Gautsch TA, Layman DK. Amino acid and protein metabolism during exercise and recovery. In: Wolinsky I, ed. *Nutrition in Exercise and Sport*. Boca Raton, FL: CRC Press; 1998.

8. Harris RC, Soderlund K, Hultman E. Elevation of creatine in resting and exercised muscle of normal subjects by creatine supplementation. *Clin Science*. 1992;83(3):367–374.

9. Earnest CP, Beckham S, Whyte BO, Almada AL. Effect of acute creatine ingestion on anaerobic performance. *Med Sci Sports Exerc*. 1998;30(suppl):141.

10. Casey A, Constantin-Teodosiu D, Howell S, Hultman E, Greenhaff PL. Creatine ingestion favorably affects performance and muscle metabolism during maximal exercise in humans. *Am J Physiol*. 1996;271(1 Pt 1): E31–E37.

CHAPTER 3

Carbohydrates

Key Questions Addressed

- What's the big deal about carbohydrates?
- What are carbohydrates?
- How are carbohydrates classified?
- What functions do carbohydrates serve in the body?
- How can carbohydrates affect overall health?
- How much carbohydrates should be consumed daily?
- What are the various sources of dietary carbohydrates?
- What are the "glycemic index" and "glycemic load" and how can they be used in sports nutrition?
- How are carbohydrates utilized during exercise?
- What type, how much, and when should carbohydrates be consumed before exercise?
- What type, how much, and when should carbohydrates be consumed during exercise?
- What type, how much, and when should carbohydrates be consumed after exercise?

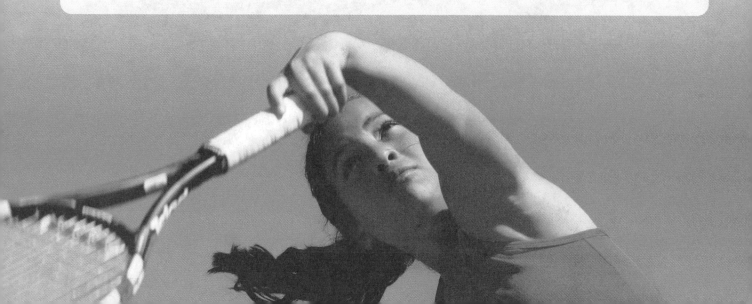

You Are the Nutrition Coach

Meggan is a 15-year-old soccer player. She is very athletic, plays midfielder, and is noted for her speed and endurance. She has been trying to lose a few pounds to achieve a more comfortable playing weight, and therefore has decreased her carbohydrate intake from 65% of her total daily caloric intake to 40%. Lately she has been feeling fatigued in the middle of her 2- to 3-hour practices and weekend games, which is affecting her performance. Meggan's coach has suggested that she bring a water bottle filled with a sport drink to their next practice. However, Meggan dislikes the taste of sports drinks and decides to find an alternative. She enjoys juices of any kind; therefore, the following Saturday she fills her water bottle with orange juice and drinks diligently throughout practice. Halfway through practice, instead of feeling tired, she is feeling nauseous and has intestinal cramping.

Questions

- What are the possible causes of Meggan's earlier-than-usual fatigue?

- What dietary suggestions might you give to Meggan to get her back to peak sport performance?

What's the big deal about carbohydrates?

Extensive research on the importance of carbohydrates in the diet has been conducted since the 1970s. There is little doubt that this macronutrient is critical to a healthy diet and crucial for optimal athletic performance. The popularity of distance sports such as triathlons, marathons, and distance cycling has sparked even more interest in carbohydrates within the scientific community and dietary supplement industry. The challenge for athletes is to consume the best sources and establish ideal practices for carbohydrate intake to improve sport performance. Athletes and active individuals are becoming increasingly exposed to both facts and misconceptions regarding the role of carbohydrates; thus sports nutrition professionals need to have a clear understanding of carbohydrates and their dietary and performance-related roles. Most individuals know that dietary carbohydrates are an energy source for the body, but they do not understand how important a role carbohydrates actually play, particularly for sports and exercise activities. Furthermore, many athletes do not have an appreciation for the fact that adequate intake of carbohydrates is also crucial for recovery from exercise and maintenance of carbohydrate stores in the body. Finally, many people do not understand the impact of the various types of carbohydrate foods and the timing of their intake in regard to exercise and sport performance. The purpose of this chapter is to clarify the understanding of this "master fuel."

What are carbohydrates?

Carbohydrates are a class of organic molecules consisting of a carbon (C) backbone with attached oxygen (O) and hydrogen (H) atoms. "Carbo" means carbon and "hydrate" means water or H_2O, thus giving a hint as to how these molecules are formed.[1] The simplest of carbohydrates in terms of molecular structure, the **simple sugars**, exist in arrangements of one or two molecules.

The arrangement and number of carbon molecules dictate the type of simple sugar. The chemical formula for these simple sugars is $C_nH_{2n}O_n$, where *n* equals a number from three to seven. For example, the most important simple sugar for the human body is glucose. It has six carbons in its chemical structure, and thus its formula is $C_6H_{12}O_6$. In addition to glucose, there are literally hundreds of other simple sugars that exist in nature. However, glucose and a few other simple sugars are the most important to the human body because they can be digested, absorbed, and utilized for energy.

Glucose and most of the other types of carbohydrates that exist in nature are synthesized by plants in a process known as **photosynthesis** (see Figure 3.1). The energy required to construct a carbohydrate comes from the sun. The sun's light energy is captured by plants and used to combine carbon dioxide (CO_2) from the air and water (H_2O) from the soil to create simple sugars. The simple sugars are linked together to make **complex carbohydrates**, such as starch and glycogen. Starch (found in plant cells) and glycogen (found in animal cells) are complex carbohydrates that are stored inside cells and used for energy when needed. Starch and glycogen are nothing more than glucose molecules linked together in chains of various lengths and configurations (see Figure 3.2).

How are carbohydrates classified?

There are several types of carbohydrates that can be classified in different ways. The most common way to classify carbohydrates is using the terms *simple* and *complex*. The different simple and complex carbohydrates are listed in **Table 3.1**. The **simple carbohydrates** are made up of only one or two sugar molecules linked together, whereas complex carbohydrates are composed of longer and more complex chains of sugars.

What are simple sugars?

Simple sugars are a classification of carbohydrates that includes monosaccharides and disaccharides. A monosaccharide is nothing more than a single molecule of sugar. Many different types of monosaccharides exist in nature; however, the three simple sugars that serve as nutrients to humans are glucose, fructose, and galactose.

Glucose is the most abundant simple carbohydrate found in nature (see Figure 3.3). It rarely exists as a monosaccharide in food

simple sugars Another name for simple carbohydrates. These are sugars that exist as single sugar molecules (i.e., monosaccharides) or two linked simple sugar molecules (i.e., disaccharides).

photosynthesis An energy-requiring process in which plants capture light energy from the sun and use the energy to combine carbon dioxide and water to form carbohydrates.

complex carbohydrate A carbohydrate composed of three or more linked simple sugar molecules.

simple carbohydrate A form of carbohydrate that exists as a monosaccharide or disaccharide.

glucose One of the most commonly occurring simple sugars in nature. It is the carbohydrate that humans rely upon for cellular energy.

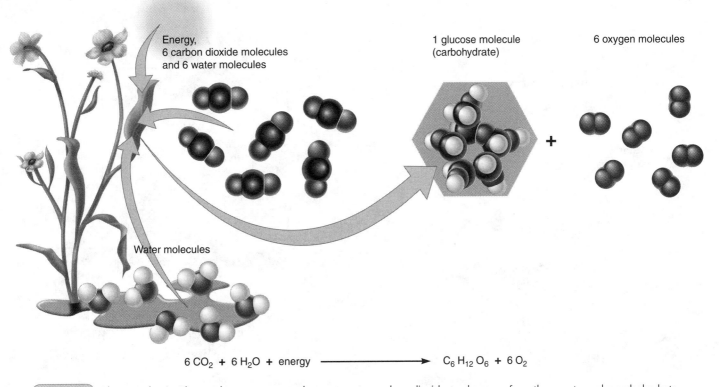

Energy,
6 carbon dioxide molecules
and 6 water molecules

1 glucose molecule
(carbohydrate)

6 oxygen molecules

Water molecules

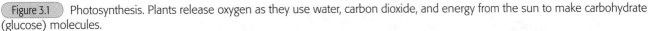

$$6\ CO_2\ +\ 6\ H_2O\ +\ energy\ \longrightarrow\ C_6\ H_{12}\ O_6\ +\ 6\ O_2$$

Figure 3.1   Photosynthesis. Plants release oxygen as they use water, carbon dioxide, and energy from the sun to make carbohydrate (glucose) molecules.

but is joined with other sugars to form disaccharides and other complex carbohydrates. In the body, glucose supplies energy to cells. The blood glucose level in the body is closely regulated to ensure that adequate energy is available to vital cells and organs at all times. The brain uses glucose exclusively except in times of starvation, when glucose is scarce. **Galactose** (see Figure 3.3) is rarely found alone in nature or in foods. It is most commonly linked with glucose, forming the disaccharide lactose, or milk sugar.

Fructose (see Figure 3.3) has the sweetest taste of the monosaccharides. It occurs naturally in fruits and some vegetables and provides the sweet taste. Honey is approximately half fructose and half glucose. A common sweetener containing fructose is high fructose corn syrup, which is added to sweeten many soft drinks, candies, jellies, and desserts.

Disaccharides, also considered to be simple carbohydrates, are made of two simple sugars ("di" means two) that are linked (see Figure 3.4). Examples of disaccharides are sucrose (fructose + glucose), lactose (glucose + galactose), and maltose (glucose + glucose).

galactose A simple sugar found in milk.

fructose A simple sugar known for its sweet taste that is commonly found in fruits.

Sucrose is commonly referred to as table sugar and is composed of one glucose and one fructose molecule. Sucrose is manufactured using extraction processes from sugar beets and sugar cane to produce granulated sugar and powdered sugar. When a food label lists sugar as the first ingredient, the term refers to sucrose. Sucrose and other common nutritive sweeteners that can be found on food labels are listed in **Table 3.2**. Lactose is commonly known as milk sugar and is composed of one molecule of glucose and one molecule of galactose. Lactose gives milk and other dairy products their sweet taste. Some individuals are intolerant to lactose. As a result, milk and other dairy products cause gastric upset because these people lack or have reduced levels of the enzyme necessary to digest and absorb the lactose sugars. Another disaccharide, **maltose** is composed of two glucose molecules. It seldom occurs naturally in foods, but forms whenever long molecules of starch are broken down. In the human body, digestive

sucrose A commonly consumed disaccharide also known as table sugar. It is composed of linked glucose and fructose molecules.

lactose The disaccharide found in milk that is composed of the simple sugars glucose and galactose.

maltose A disaccharide made up of two linked molecules of glucose.

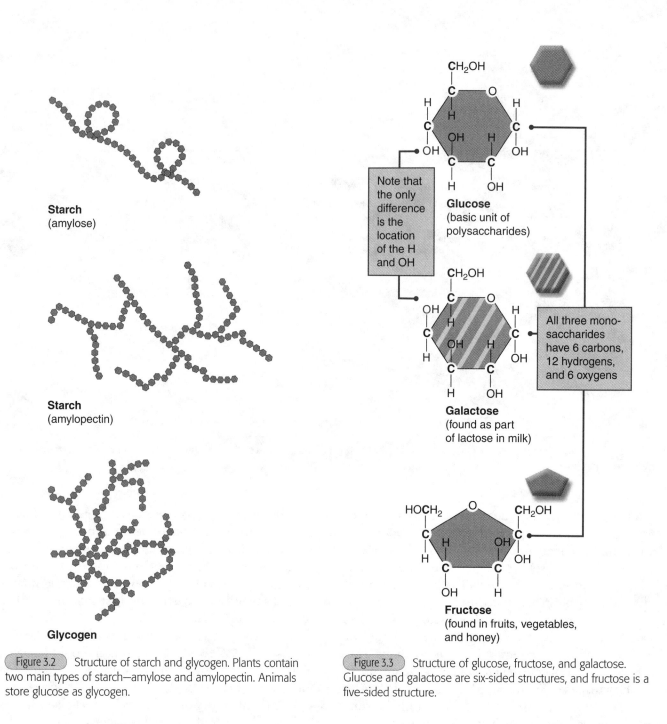

Starch
(amylose)

Starch
(amylopectin)

Glycogen

Note that the only difference is the location of the H and OH

CH₂OH

Glucose
(basic unit of
polysaccharides)

All three mono-saccharides have 6 carbons, 12 hydrogens, and 6 oxygens

CH₂OH

Galactose
(found as part
of lactose in milk)

HOCH₂   CH₂OH

Fructose
(found in fruits, vegetables,
and honey)

Figure 3.2   Structure of starch and glycogen. Plants contain two main types of starch—amylose and amylopectin. Animals store glucose as glycogen.

Figure 3.3   Structure of glucose, fructose, and galactose. Glucose and galactose are six-sided structures, and fructose is a five-sided structure.

TABLE 3.1	Carbohydrate Classifications and Common Examples		
Simple Carbohydrates		**Complex Carbohydrates**	
Monosaccharides	*Disaccharides*	*Oligosaccharides*	*Polysaccharides*
Glucose	Sucrose	Maltodextrin	Fiber
Fructose	Lactose	High fructose corn syrup	Starch
Galactose	Maltose	Corn syrup	

DISACCHARIDES

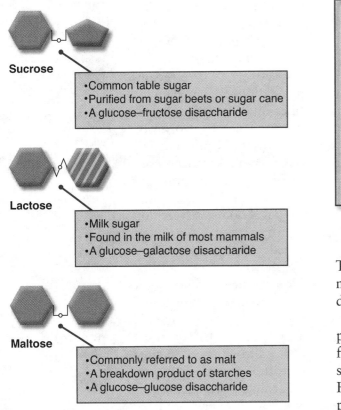

Sucrose

- Common table sugar
- Purified from sugar beets or sugar cane
- A glucose–fructose disaccharide

Lactose

- Milk sugar
- Found in the milk of most mammals
- A glucose–galactose disaccharide

Maltose

- Commonly referred to as malt
- A breakdown product of starches
- A glucose–glucose disaccharide

Figure 3.4 Structure of disaccharides. The three monosaccharides pair up in different combinations to form the three disaccharides.

enzymes begin to break starch down into maltose in the mouth. Although a sugar, maltose is very bland tasting.

What are complex carbohydrates?

The complex carbohydrates found in foods are starches and fiber. Glycogen is the storage form of carbohydrates in the body and is considered a complex carbohydrate because of its similarity in structure to starch (see Figure 3.2). Complex carbohydrates are composed of many sugar molecules linked in often very long and complicated carbon chains. Carbohydrates that are composed of short chains of 3 to 10 linked sugars are known as oligosaccharides. Examples of oligosaccharides are the maltodextrins, corn syrup, and high fructose corn syrup. Polysaccharides are complex carbohydrates composed of even longer chains of 11 or more sugars. Polysaccharides can be straight chains of linked sugars or can be highly branched (see Figure 3.2).

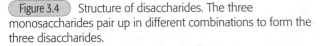

TABLE 3.2	Common Nutritive Sweeteners in Foods
Sucrose	**Corn syrup**
Corn sweetener	Dextrin
High fructose corn syrup	Concentrated fruit juice
Molasses	Maple syrup
Malt	Cane sugar
Honey	Maltose
Dextrose	Fructose
Sugar	Confectioner's sugar
Brown sugar	Turbinado sugar

The molecular structure of a polysaccharide determines how soluble it is in water, how easy it is to digest, and how it behaves when heated.

Complex carbohydrates are found stored in plant cells in the form of starch and in animals in the form of glycogen. Starches are polysaccharides and serve as a major source of carbohydrates in our diet. Food sources rich in starch include grains, legumes, potatoes, and yams (see Figure 3.5). Starches give foods some of their sticky or moist properties. Glycogen, also called animal starch, is the storage form of carbohydrate in animals.[2] Glycogen is not found in plants. It is composed of long, highly branched chains of glucose molecules (see Figure 3.2). Stored glycogen in humans can be rapidly broken down into single glucose molecules for use by cells for energy.

Dietary fiber, yet another complex carbohydrate, is found in plant cell walls and inside plant cells. All plant foods contain some fiber of varying types. Most fiber is indigestible by the body, and therefore

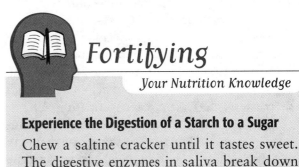

Fortifying
Your Nutrition Knowledge

Experience the Digestion of a Starch to a Sugar

Chew a saltine cracker until it tastes sweet. The digestive enzymes in saliva break down the long chains of sugar molecules to produce glucose and maltose, thus making the cracker eventually taste sweet.

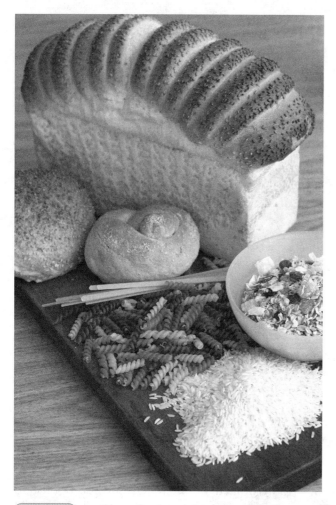

Figure 3.5 Food sources of starch. A variety of grain products, potatoes, and legumes are good sources of starch.

day for women aged 19–50 and older than 50, respectively, and 38 grams and 30 grams per day for men aged 19–50 and older than 50, respectively.[3] These recommendations are based on the fiber intake required to reduce the risk of cardiovascular disease. Unfortunately, the average American consumes only 10–20 grams of fiber per day.[4]

The Food and Nutrition Board, part of a panel convened to evaluate the Dietary Reference Intakes on fiber, proposed new definitions for "dietary fiber," "functional fiber," and "total fiber."[3] These updated definitions evolved from a need to have consistent nutrition labeling regarding fiber because of the creation of new products that behave like fiber but do not meet the former traditional definition of fiber. Many of these new food products have potential health benefits, yet do not meet the previous U.S. definitions for fiber based on analytical methods.[3] The new definitions for fiber include:

- *Dietary fiber:* Consists of nondigestible carbohydrates and lignins that are intrinsic and intact in plants. Examples include cellulose, hemicellulose, pectin, gums, beta-glucans, fibers found in oat and wheat bran, plant carbohydrates, and lignins.
- *Functional fiber:* Consists of isolated, nondigestible carbohydrates that have beneficial physiological effects in humans. Examples include resistant starch, pectin, gums, animal carbohydrates (chitin and chitosan), and commercially produced carbohydrates such as resistant starch, polyols, inulin, and undigested dextrins.
- *Total fiber:* The sum of dietary and functional fiber.

These definitions are not likely to alter the recommended intake levels, but will more clearly define the sources of fiber and the specific potential for health benefits when consumed. Fiber remains intact in the gut and is exposed to the normal bacteria present in the large intestine. Bacteria aid the

soluble fiber A type of indigestible plant carbohydrate that dissolves in water. Soluble fiber has been shown to help lower blood cholesterol levels in some individuals. Sources of soluble fiber are oats, barley, legumes, and some fruits and vegetables.

insoluble fiber A type of non-digestible plant carbohydrate that does not dissolve in water. Insoluble fiber sources are primarily whole grain products, nuts, seeds, and some vegetables.

dietary fiber A complex carbohydrate obtained from plant sources that is not digestible by humans. Although dietary fiber provides no energy for cellular activity, it does help maintain a healthy digestive system, lower blood cholesterol levels, and regulate blood glucose levels.

functional fiber Isolated, non-digestible carbohydrates that have beneficial physiological effects in humans.

total fiber The sum of dietary and functional fiber.

provides no caloric or carbohydrate value when consumed. There are two types of fiber, which are classified based on their solubility in water: soluble and insoluble. **Soluble fibers** are found primarily in oats, barley, legumes (dried beans, peas, lentils), and some fruits and vegetables. **Insoluble fiber** sources are primarily whole grain products, nuts, seeds, and some vegetables. Consuming foods that contain both soluble and insoluble fiber can help prevent high cholesterol and diverticular disease, regulate blood glucose levels, and help prevent and/ or treat constipation. A high-fiber diet also produces an increased satiety level that may aid in weight loss over time by reducing hunger, and thus ultimately decreasing caloric intake. Current recommendations for fiber intake are 25 grams and 21 grams per

gaining the performance edge

Glycogen is the storage form of carbohydrates in muscle cells. It is a readily available source of energy for muscle and is critical for fueling performance in endurance, strength/ power, and team sports.

digestive process and as bacterial metabolism occurs, it produces gas as a by-product. Fiber, when consumed in excess, can cause bloating and flatulence that can be uncomfortable to athletes during training and competition. In addition, undigested fiber increases stool mass and volume, and attracts water in the large intestine. The added weight, feeling of heaviness, and possible complications with diarrhea or constipation are dependent upon water intake and can contribute to uncomfortable workouts and competitions for athletes. Some athletes choose to limit high-fiber foods in their diet for several hours, or up to one day, prior to heavy training or competitions to avoid potential intestinal discomfort. However, because of fiber's health-promoting effects, high-fiber foods should not be completely avoided, and athletes should make an effort to include carbohydrates containing fiber on a regular basis.

gaining the performance edge

Limiting high-fiber foods starting several hours to 1 day prior to competition can help avoid feelings of heaviness, bloating, and/or intestinal discomfort.

Are artificial sweeteners carbohydrates? Are they beneficial or harmful?

As their name indicates, artificial sweeteners provide sweetness to foods but not at the expense of calories. Artificial sweeteners can actually be hundreds of times sweeter than sucrose (see **Table 3.3**). Some artificial sweeteners are derived from carbohydrates, modified with alterations to their molecular structure, making them less digestible and thereby yielding fewer calories when eaten. Other artificial sweeteners, such as aspartame, are not carbohydrates at all and may be derived from amino acids. Because they contain few or no calories, their value in producing better-tasting low-calorie foods and providing sweetness without calories is quite beneficial to those on restricted diets or trying to lose weight. Individuals with diabetes or insulin sensitivity can also enjoy sweetened foods without consuming excess sugars and calories.

Artificial sweeteners are regulated in the United States by the Food and Drug Administration (FDA). Some are on the **Generally Recognized as Safe (GRAS)** list regulated by the FDA, and others are considered food additives. Food additives must be approved for use in food products by the FDA before entering the food supply. The FDA approves and regulates the safety limit of food addi-

Generally Recognized as Safe (GRAS) Substances that have not been conclusively proven to be safe but are generally accepted by experts as being safe for human consumption and therefore can be added to foods by manufacturers.

TABLE 3.3 Sugars and Artificial Sweeteners

Name	Sweetness (relative to sucrose)	ADI (mg/kg/day)	Trade Name	Appropriate for Cooking/Baking
Sucrose	1.0			Yes
Maltose	0.4			Not commonly used
Fructose	1.73			Yes
Tagatose	0.92	Not specified		Yes
Sorbitol	0.6	Not specified		Not commonly used
Xylitol	0.9	Not specified		Not commonly used
Mannitol	0.5	Not specified		Not commonly used
Acesulfame K	130–200	15mg/kg	Sunett; Sweet One	Yes
Aspartame	200	50mg/kg	Nutrasweet; Equal	No
Saccharin	300	5mg/kg	Sweet'N Low; Sugar Twin	Yes
Sucralose	600	5mg/kg	Splenda	Yes
Cyclamate	30	11mg/kg		Yes
Stevia	250–450	2mg/kg	Truvia; Purevia; Sweetleaf	Yes
Neotame	7000–13,000	18mg/kg		Yes

Sources: American Dietetic Association. Position of the American Dietetic Association: Use of nutritive and nonnutritive sweeteners. *J Am Diet Assoc.* 1998;98;580–587; and Bray GA, Nielsen SJ, Popkin BM. Consumption of high-fructose corn syrup in beverages may play a role in the epidemic of obesity. *Am J Clin Nutr.* 2004;79;537–543.

acceptable daily intake (ADI) The FDA-established safety limit for food additives and artificial sweeteners. The ADI is set at approximately 100 times below the level required for toxic or adverse effects.

tives and sets **acceptable daily intakes** (**ADIs**). The ADI is the estimated amount per kilogram of body weight that a person can consume every day over a lifetime without risk.[4] The ADI is conservative and is set at an amount approximately 100 times less than the maximum level at which observed adverse effects occurred in animal studies. Artificial sweeteners such as aspartame, saccharin, acesulfame K, and sucralose have all obtained FDA approval for use in food products. However, some researchers and practitioners remain concerned about the safety of sugar substitutes. Because of the inconsistent results from research studies on the long-term safety of artificial sweetener consumption, intake should be kept to a minimum.

Saccharin was the first of the commercially produced artificial sweeteners; it hit the market in the early 1960s. The safety of saccharin became an issue when it was determined that laboratory rats consuming saccharin had a higher incidence of bladder cancer than rats that did not consume saccharin. In 1991, the FDA withdrew its proposed ban on saccharin and now considers it to be a safe food additive for use in foods and beverages, cosmetics, gums, and candies. Aspartame and acesulfame K are two other common artificial sweeteners that have been approved for use as tabletop sweeteners and use in heat-stable foods such as diet sodas, puddings, gelatins, candies, and gum.

Sucralose and tagatose are relatively new additions to the list of artificial sweeteners. Sucralose is a chemically altered form of sucrose that is manipulated by substituting the sucrose hydroxyl group with chlorine. This produces an intense sweetness—about 600 times sweeter than sucrose.[5] Tagatose attained GRAS status in 2002 and is a low-calorie, full-bulk natural sugar that is 92% as sweet as sucrose.[6] It contains a caloric value of 1.5 kcal/g because only about 15–20% of the product is absorbed in the small intestine. Tagatose provides sensory and textural qualities similar to sugar in many foods, adding to its versatility in the development of new food products with lower calories without a reduction in palatability.

Sugar alcohols, also known as **polyols**, are dissimilar to regular sugars and

polyols A class of food sweeteners that are found naturally in some plants but are not easily digested and thus yield fewer calories. Polyols, also known as sugar alcohols, include xylitol, sorbitol, and mannitol and often are added to sweeten products such as mints, candy, and gum.

sugar substitutes because they are digested and absorbed differently. They are found naturally in plants such as berries and other fruits and some vegetables, but are also produced for commercial use. Sugar alcohols such as xylitol, sorbitol, and mannitol are nutritive sweeteners (contain some calories) and often are added to sweeten products such as mints, candy, and gum. They are not as easily digested or absorbed by the body and therefore contain fewer calories (½ to ⅓ fewer) than sugar. The incomplete absorption does not allow for direct metabolism that would provide the usual 4 calories per gram of carbohydrate.[7] Depending on the type or brand, sugar alcohols generally contain 1.5–3.0 calories per gram. Because sugar alcohols do contain calories, they can have some effect on glucose levels, and if eaten in large amounts can increase blood glucose levels.

All sugar alcohols are regulated by the GRAS list or as food additives. Sugar alcohols must be listed on food labels if a nutrient claim is made, such as "sugar-free" or "reduced sugar." Sugar alcohols are listed on the ingredient list and on the nutrition facts section of the label. Excessive intake of sugar alcohols can have a laxative effect and may cause diarrhea.[7] Food products that contain sugar alcohols can put a warning on the label stating "excess consumption of this product may have a laxative effect." Athletes trying to reduce caloric or carbohydrate intake may consume foods that contain sugar alcohols as artificial sweeteners. However, because of the laxative effect, athletes may need to reduce the amount and type of artificial sweeteners consumed prior to exercise.

There are benefits to using all of the varieties of artificial sweeteners in foods. They provide a sweet taste and several have bulking properties, while contributing fewer calories than sugars. They do not promote tooth decay, and consumption of gum and mints sweetened with sugar substitutes instead of sugars can be beneficial to dental health. Consumers need to be aware, however, that foods containing sugar substitutes and those promoted as "low carbohydrate" are not necessarily low calorie. This misconception may lead to overconsumption of foods with sugar substitutes and therefore an increased overall calorie intake.

gaining the performance edge

Artificial sweeteners can be used by athletes wishing to control body weight; however, because of the laxative effect of some sweeteners, athletes may need to reduce the amount and type of artificial sweeteners consumed prior to competition.

What functions do carbohydrates serve in the body?

Carbohydrates serve several important roles in the body, many of which are critical to optimal sport performance. Carbohydrates are the most important source of energy for the body. Although fat stores supply a large quantity of energy, carbohydrates must be present to metabolize fats at the rapid rates needed to support the caloric demands of exercise and sport competition. Furthermore, the higher the intensity of the activity, the greater the reliance of the body on carbohydrates. In fact, carbohydrates are the only macronutrient that can provide energy for anaerobic activities such as sprinting. Adequate carbohydrate intake also helps spare muscle tissue. If an athlete's carbohydrate intake is low, his or her body will turn to the breakdown of muscle protein to make up for the deficit in needed carbohydrates. Finally, carbohydrates are the primary energy source for the nervous system. Nerve cells do not store carbohydrates like muscle cells do; their source for carbohydrates is the bloodstream. When blood glucose levels fall, nerve cell function suffers, which can have a dramatic effect on exercise and sport performance.

gaining the performance edge

Cutting carbohydrates from an athlete's diet leads to "performance suicide." Carbohydrates are the "master fuel" for all sports.

How can carbohydrates affect overall health?

It is widely recognized that a diet moderate to high in carbohydrates is important for optimal daily training, high energy levels, and overall good health. Carbohydrate-rich foods contain not only energy for working muscles, but also nutrients required for proper body functioning such as fiber, vitamins and minerals, and various **phytochemicals**.

phytochemicals A large class of biologically active plant chemicals that have been found to play a role in the maintenance of human health.

What role does fiber play in health?

Fiber is a complex carbohydrate that the body cannot digest or absorb. Most fibers are made up of long chains of sugar units and thus are classified as polysaccharides. However, unlike starch, fiber polysaccharides cannot be broken down by human digestive enzymes into small enough units for the body to absorb. Thus, fiber, with the exception of some resistant starches, does not contribute energy to the body as do other digestible carbohydrates. Even though it is a minimal energy source, fiber promotes good health in many ways.

When we eat plant foods, the indigestible fiber portion adds bulk to the intestinal contents. It does so by attracting water into the intestines, some of which is absorbed by the fiber itself, causing it to expand. The greater the bulk of the intestinal contents, the greater the peristaltic actions of the smooth muscles in the intestinal walls and the faster the passage of foods through the digestive system. The water drawn in by the fiber also helps soften the stools for easy passage out of the system. If fiber intake is low, there is less water and less intestinal bulk, which results in stools that are small and hard, and that pass more slowly through the length of the intestines. Constipation and hemorrhoids can occur more readily when stools are hard and when fiber intake is low. Constipation produces an uncomfortable full feeling, often with gas, and is particularly uncomfortable during exercise.

Active individuals who eat adequate fiber and consume adequate fluids will have fewer problems with constipation than nonexercisers. Physical exercise not only strengthens the muscles used during exercise, but also tends to produce a healthier gastrointestinal tract that moves food and fluids efficiently and quickly through the system. This is just another example of the importance of combining exercise with good nutrition.

Choosing foods rich in fiber may help reduce the risk of some types of cancers. The link between fiber and colon cancer has received much attention recently. Controversy exists in the research as to whether fiber has a positive or a neutral effect on the risk for colon cancer. Some studies support a positive correlation between high fiber intakes and colon cancer risk reduction[8,9] whereas others do not support this finding.[10–12] The theory behind fiber's potential ability to decrease colon cancer risk is that the higher bulk of insoluble fibers may "dilute" toxins in the intestinal tract plus speed the passage of toxins out of the body. This decreased transit time may reduce the amount of contact between potential cancer-causing agents and the intestinal mucosal cells. More research, especially studies that control for type of fiber and food intake, needs to be conducted to determine whether there is a direct correlation between high fiber intake and a lowered incidence of colon cancer. Regardless of future findings, eating a diet rich in complex carbohydrates including fruits, veg-

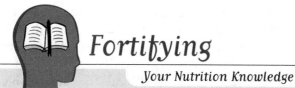
Carbohydrate Descriptors: What Do "Low Carb" and "Net Carb" Mean?

The FDA regulation for nutrient content claims allows manufacturers to highlight and make health-related claims on their food labels regarding certain nutrients or dietary substances in their products. However, the FDA permits only specified nutrients or substances to have these nutrient content claims. The FDA has not established a set of values for descriptors identifying carbohydrates. Food manufacturers can put quantitative statements on labels such as "6 grams of carbohydrates" as long as they are factual. However, they cannot make a statement such as "only 6 grams of carbohydrates" because that implies the food is carbohydrate-reduced or a low-carbohydrate food. If the label "characterizes" the level of a nutrient, then it is considered a nutrient content claim. Therefore, a claim of "low carbohydrate" cannot be used on food labels because it characterizes the amount of carbohydrates in that food.

Although there are no official definitions of low carbohydrate, the FDA is gathering evidence and developing a statement outlining carbohydrate food-labeling guidelines. Guidelines are likely to be similar to those established for such terms as "low fat" or "reduced sugar or fat." These will list the number of grams of carbohydrates to be considered "low" and probably will include definitions of reduced carbohydrates as well.

The term *net carbs* has become the latest catchphrase for the diet- and weight-conscious consumer. *Net carbs* is not a term that has been found in the scientific literature or nutritional sciences research, nor is it an allowable nutrient content claim. However, a trip to the grocery store shows that food manufacturers are labeling their products "net carbs" with abandon. The net carbs as determined by food manufacturers is the total amount of carbohydrates in a serving of the food minus the total fiber grams and any sugar alcohol grams. The remaining grams of carbohydrates are considered the net carbs for the product.

This description is based on the premise that only the net carbs have an impact on blood glucose and insulin levels. Indeed, fiber generally contributes negligible energy as it passes through the intestinal tract unabsorbed. However, sugar alcohols do contain some calories despite their reduced effect on blood glucose levels. The FDA is likely to address the net carb definition when it publishes guidelines on food labeling for carbohydrates.

etables, whole grains, and legumes provides a healthful diet and can aid in the prevention of many other disease conditions (see Figure 3.6).

Soluble fiber appears to play a significant role in reducing the risk of heart disease. Several studies have shown that diets high in soluble fiber decrease blood cholesterol levels. Soluble fiber may help reduce serum cholesterol levels by binding bile acids in the gastrointestinal tract, thus preventing their reabsorption. This is significant because bile acids are made from cholesterol in the liver and are secreted into the intestinal tract to aid with fat absorption. In addition, short-chain fatty acids, produced from bacterial fermentation of fiber in the large intestine, may inhibit cholesterol synthesis.

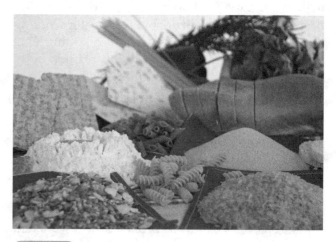

Figure 3.6 Food sources of fiber. Whole grains are a good source of fiber.

Foods rich in complex carbohydrates may indirectly help with weight loss or maintenance of a healthy weight. Fruits, vegetables, whole grains, and starchy legumes are usually low in total fat and calories. A diet that contains adequate portions of these lower calorie foods may replace higher calorie foods, thus producing a caloric deficit. Because of their bulk, these foods provide a feeling of fullness that lasts longer when compared with less complex carbohydrate foods. High-fiber foods take longer to digest and absorb; thus the full feeling lasts longer, and individuals may eat less often.

What role do simple sugars have in health?

In contrast to the benefits of high complex carbohydrate and fiber intake, simple carbohydrates—specifically refined sugars—may have some negative health consequences. Highly sugared foods and those that are sticky and stay in the mouth longer may produce more dental caries (cavities). Sugar, sugared soda and fruit drinks (especially when sipped slowly throughout the day), crackers, and chewy candies that get caught in teeth have a greater likelihood of producing cavities than do less sticky, sweet foods. Bacteria in the mouth react with sugar and produce acids. These acids erode the tooth enamel and produce cavities. Choosing low-sugar foods and rinsing the mouth after eating sugary or sticky foods can help reduce the risk of dental caries.

Recently, sugar, specifically in the form of high fructose corn syrup (HFCS), has been purported to be one of the reasons for the rise in obesity and related disease rates in the United States.[13,14] Much of the research has focused on the correlation between increased consumption of sodas, and other sugar-sweetened beverages containing HFCS, and weight gain.[15-17] However, not all studies have shown a direct link, especially in humans.[18] A proposed metabolic theory explaining the mechanism by which fructose causes weight gain is through the suppression of insulin and leptin production.[13,19] More research is needed to elucidate a cause and effect relationship as well as to develop associated intake recommendations.

From a practical standpoint, weight gain may be associated with the consumption of high-sugar foods as a result of the typical high calorie value of these items. However, it may not be simply the sugar that makes the foods high calorie. Many sweet foods contain significant amounts of fat as well. All carbohydrates, simple sugars or complex, contain 4 calories per gram. Fats contain 9 calories per gram. Foods such as cookies, cakes, ice cream, and many chocolate candies contain both simple sugars and fat. The fat often contributes as many (or more) calories to these products as sugars do.

Sugar and foods made with significant amounts of sugar are often low in total nutrients, lack fiber, and are calorie-dense. Choosing these foods regularly makes it difficult to meet individual needs for vitamins, minerals, and other nutrients because they can take the place of nutrient-dense foods. This, combined with a higher incidence of dental caries, the caloric density of high-sugar foods contributing to weight problems, and the low amount of fiber found in individuals consuming a high-sugar diet, suggests that reducing refined sugar intake in foods and beverages is the best option for better health.

How much carbohydrates should be consumed daily?

The quantity of carbohydrate needed on a daily basis varies among athletes based on several factors including current body weight, total energy needs, the specific metabolic demands of their sport, and their stage of training or competition schedule. The primary role of carbohydrates is to provide energy to cells, particularly the brain, which is the only carbohydrate-dependent organ in the body. The RDA for carbohydrates recommends at least 130 grams per day for adults and children, based on the average minimum amount of glucose utilized by the brain.[20] The Acceptable Macronutrient Distribution Range (AMDR) for carbohydrates for males and females age 9 and older is 45–65% of daily calories.[20]

What is the relationship between current body weight and carbohydrate intake?

Carbohydrate needs can be determined based on current body weight. Five to 10 grams of carbohydrate per kilogram (kg) of body weight is a general recommendation for calculating daily carbohydrate needs for athletes.[21-23] This method shows clearly that individual carbohydrate needs can vary greatly. An athlete who weighs 60 kg requires 300–600 grams of carbohydrates per day versus a 90-kg athlete whose estimate reaches the range of 450–900 grams. The large range in recommendations allows for changes in exercise intensity, environmental conditions, and personal preferences, as well as type and quantity of daily physical activity. Recreational athletes who are exercising three to five times per week will require amounts at the low end of the range. Competitive athletes and recreational athletes training 6 to 7 days per week, and sometimes multiple workouts a day, will require carbohydrate intakes at the higher end of the range.

How can carbohydrate needs be determined based on a percentage of total calories?

The recommended range of 45–65% of calories coming from carbohydrates is quite large. The level of carbohydrate in this range can be chosen for each individual based on medical conditions, training regimen, and personal food preferences. This range provides enough carbohydrates for the general population to maintain energy levels. For athletes, the higher end of this percentage range is usually recommended. As training volume increases, or for endurance athletes preparing and tapering for competition, the percentage of calories from carbohydrates can increase beyond the recommended range to as high as 70–75%. For recreational athletes or individuals with certain medical conditions, such as diabetes, carbohydrate intake at the middle to low end of the range is typically appropriate.

The following provides an example of how to calculate carbohydrate needs based on a percentage of total calories:

Assume a recreational athlete requires 2500 calories daily and 55% of total calories from carbohydrates:

1. *Calculate the number of total calories contributed by carbohydrates based on the goal percentage:* 2500 × 0.55 (55% of calories from carbohydrates) = 1375 calories from carbohydrates
2. *Convert calories from carbohydrates to grams of carbohydrates daily:* 1375 calories ÷ 4 calories/gram = 344 grams of carbohydrates daily (see **Training Table 3.1**).

It is important to calculate and compare the grams of carbohydrates based on both current body weight and the percentage of calories coming from carbohydrates. It can be misleading to follow only one formula or the other. For example, a 70-kg middle-distance runner who consumes 4000 calories per day, of which 50% are carbohydrate calories, will consume approximately 500 grams of carbohydrates. At 70 kg, 500 grams is approximately 7 grams of carbohydrates per kilogram of body weight. If the quantity of carbohydrates was evaluated solely on the percentage of total calories contributed by carbohydrates, it might be perceived as falling on the low end of the recommendations. However, 7 grams of carbohydrate per kilogram of body weight

Training Table 3.1: Sample Meal Plan Providing 340–350 Grams of Carbohydrate

Food/Beverage	Grams of Carbohydrate
Breakfast	
1½ cups of raisin bran cereal	62
1 cup skim milk	12
1 cup sliced strawberries	11
Lunch	
Grilled cheese sandwich	28
2 cups of vegetable soup	24
10 saltine crackers	20
Pear	26
Dinner	
1½ cups of spaghetti with marinara sauce	70
+ 3 oz ground turkey	0
1 cup mixed vegetables	15
2 cups skim milk	24
1 cup frozen yogurt with ⅓ cup mixed nuts	54
Total Carbohydrate Intake	**346 grams**

falls well within the 5–10 g/kg recommendation, and therefore both guidelines are met.

Another important consideration is to calculate the percentage of calories contributed by carbohydrates and compare it to daily protein and fat needs. In cases such as weight loss, total calories may be restricted slightly and therefore carbohydrate estimates based on current body weight may launch the percentage from carbohydrates into the 75–85% range. This high percentage makes it challenging, if not impossible, to include adequate levels of proteins and fats in the daily meal plan without exceeding total calorie needs. It is important to always balance carbohydrate, protein, and fat needs relative to total calorie estimates to ensure that athletes are properly fueled while meeting their goals of weight loss, maintenance, or gain.

Recommendations as high as 70–75% have been suggested as optimal for some athletes, especially during long-duration and high-intensity training sessions and competitive events.[21] Athletes competing in the Race Across America, a nonstop cycling race from coast to coast, may consume as much as 70–80% of their calories from carbohydrates during the event.

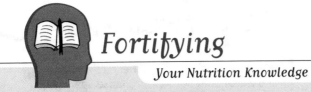

Fortifying
Your Nutrition Knowledge

Heather's Experience as the Dietitian for Team 70+ in the Race Across America

The Race Across America is a nonstop cycling event from the West Coast to the East Coast of the United States. I had the pleasure of planning and executing the nutrition plan for the 70+ Team—a four-man team of athletes over the age of 70—in August of 1996.

We met as a team in April of that year to begin planning. During this meeting, I gathered background information on each individual—their food likes and dislikes, the type of beverages and food usually consumed during cycling, estimates of their sweat rates, food allergies and intolerances, medications, and much more. Between April and August, I calculated the daily energy, carbohydrate, protein, and fat needs for all four riders. The estimates were based on the system of two riders performing an 8-hour shift: riding 1 hour, and resting for 1 hour in the van following the riders. The average distance and time ridden in one day, based on an estimate of the riders pedaling at 15 mph, was 60–90 miles, or 4 to 6 hours a day. The average total calorie needs for the riders was approximately 5000–5500 calories a day, with at least 65% of the total calories coming from carbohydrate.

I devised a daily regimen that included several meals, many snacks, and lots of fluid. Meals were eaten during a rider's 8-hour shift off, in which the riders would be delivered to the roaming motor home following the team. In the motor home, the riders would eat a solid meal, get a massage, and sleep. Snacks were consumed during the rider's rest hour in the van during his 8-hour shift. Fluids were consumed throughout the day, with a focus on sports drinks while cycling. The meals consisted of high-carbohydrate, moderate-protein foods including items such as spinach lasagna, turkey chili, and yogurt and cheese stuffed potatoes. As the week progressed, the riders' tastes changed, requiring slight modifications to the menu items. The most requested food combination was baked potatoes with raisins, salt, and milk. I would have never guessed that this combination would be so appealing!

The men ate a wide variety of foods throughout the week, supplying a perfect balance of carbohydrate, protein, fat, and fluids. Through daily food records, weigh-ins before and after shifts, and monitoring urine color and quantity, I ensured the men stayed energized and hydrated. The 70+ Team completed the race in 9 days, 2 hours, and 27 minutes. This achievement granted them the recognition of the first team of men 70 years and older to ever successfully finish the Race Across America.

What impact does the stage of training or competition schedule have on carbohydrate intake?

For most athletes, carbohydrate needs will increase slightly as training volume increases or when approaching a competition. Specific recommendations for varying carbohydrate needs throughout the year will be discussed in Chapters 12, 13, and 14. However, in general during the off-season or recovery periods, total calorie needs may be lower and therefore total carbohydrate needs will also decline. As pre-season conditioning begins and training volume and intensity are on the rise, carbohydrate needs will increase. During the competitive season, carbohydrate needs remain high in preparation for hard workouts or events. Later in this chapter, the concept of car-

bohydrate loading, or supercompensation, which involves increasing the intake of carbohydrates in the days leading up to a competition, is discussed.

Some athletes, such as body builders, maintain a moderate amount of carbohydrate intake during training but decrease carbohydrate intake in the days and weeks leading up to a competition, to create a more lean or "cut" look. This pattern of eating will be discussed further in Chapter 13.

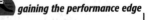

gaining the performance edge

Carbohydrate needs are determined based on a variety of factors including total body weight, percentage of total calories, stage of training, and individual health conditions. Consider all of these factors when advising athletes on an appropriate level of daily carbohydrate intake.

What are the various sources of dietary carbohydrates?

Carbohydrates are found within each food group of the MyPlate food guidance system. The richest sources of carbohydrates are found in the grains, fruits, and vegetables. Most dairy/alternative products as well as beans, legumes, and nuts from the protein foods group provide moderate amounts of carbohydrates. Sweets, desserts, and sodas—part of the empty calories allowed in the new MyPlate system—provide carbohydrates mainly in the form of simple sugars. Even though carbohydrates are found universally within each food group, it is imperative that athletes choose the most nutrient-dense options within each category for optimal performance and health.

What are the best carbohydrate choices within the grains group?

Most of the foods found in the grains section of MyPlate are excellent sources of complex carbohydrates, fiber, and B vitamins (see **Training Table 3.2**). The key is to choose whole grain products that are more nutrient-dense and sustain energy longer than refined carbohydrates. **Table 3.4** lists a variety of healthy whole grain options to choose most often, as well as refined starches to be incorporated sparingly.

What are the best carbohydrate choices within the fruit and vegetable groups?

In addition to carbohydrates, fruits and vegetables are ideal for athletes because they contain:
- Soluble and insoluble fiber
- Vitamin C, potassium, and beta carotene
- A variety of antioxidants and phytochemicals

TABLE 3.4	The Goodness of Whole Grains
Whole Grains to Choose Often	**Refined Grains to Choose Sparingly**
Whole wheat bread	White bread
Whole grain cereals	High-sugar cereals
Brown rice	White rice
Whole wheat pasta	White pasta
Barley	Crackers
Bulgur wheat	Croissants
Oatmeal	
Quinoa	
Spelt berries	
Wheat pita bread	
Wheat berries	
Whole grain tortillas	
Whole wheat couscous	

- Fewer calories than other carbohydrate sources, for those attempting to lose weight

Fruits and vegetables can be consumed in many forms (see **Training Table 3.3**). There are benefits and

Training Table 3.3: Incorporating Carbohydrate-Rich Fruits and Vegetables into Meals/Snacks

- Keep fresh fruit on hand for quick snacks and complements to breakfast, lunch, or dinner.
- Freeze slightly overripe fruits to blend into smoothies (see Soccer Smoothie recipe) made with other ingredients such as milk, yogurt, peanut butter, or juices.
- Add sautéed vegetables to spaghetti sauce or canned soups.
- Purchase precut vegetables for snacks, stir-fry, salads, or stews.

Soccer Smoothie

1 frozen banana*
8 oz skim or soy milk
1 scoop chocolate-flavored protein powder
1–2 tbsp peanut butter
Place all ingredients in a blender and mix until smooth.
* Peel overripe banana, place in a plastic bag, and freeze overnight beforehand.
Serving Size: 2 cups (Recipe makes one serving)
Calories: 373 kcals
Protein: 32 grams
Carbohydrates: 44 grams
Fat: 10 grams

Training Table 3.2: Incorporating Carbohydrate-Rich Whole Grains into Meals/Snacks

- Cook a mixture of old-fashioned oatmeal and bulgur wheat with skim or soy milk and top with dried fruit and nuts.
- Toast whole wheat, spelt, or millet bread and top with peanut butter.
- Stir-fry lean meats or tofu with vegetables and serve over brown rice, whole wheat couscous, or wheat berries.
- Make a complete meal with a dish of whole wheat pasta, garbanzo beans, and roasted/steamed vegetables mixed lightly with olive oil and Italian seasonings.

drawbacks to each form: fresh, frozen, canned, dried, and juices. **Table 3.5** outlines the reasons to choose or not to choose each form for a variety of different situations and preferences.

What are the best carbohydrate choices within the dairy/alternative group?

Dairy/alternative foods and beverages provide a convenient mix of carbohydrates and proteins (see **Training Table 3.4**). Most choices from this group are good sources of calcium. Milk is unique because it is an excellent source of calcium as well as vitamin D. Calcium and vitamin D are essential nutrients, especially to athletes participating in weight-bearing sports, providing strength and structure to bones.

Dairy foods are produced from a variety of sources, most commonly from the milk of cows. Soy and other grain-derived milk, yogurt, and cheese products are an excellent alternative for those choosing to avoid animal products or for individuals who struggle with lactose intolerance. The soy/grain products tend to be low in saturated fat, have no cholesterol, and provide a good source of carbohydrates and proteins. However, the plant sources of dairy

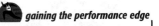
gaining the performance edge

Athletes should be educated on the benefits and drawbacks of different forms of fruits and vegetables. However, the bottom line is to encourage athletes to eat more fruits and vegetables, in any form they find convenient!

TABLE 3.5	Pros and Cons of Various Forms of Fruits and Vegetables		
Form	**Benefits**	**Drawbacks**	**When to Include in the Meal Plan**
Fresh	Can be enjoyed raw or cooked. Retains nutrients if eaten soon after purchasing. Very flavorful.	Spoils within 7–14 days of purchase. Produce shipped from other countries may lose some nutritional value between being harvested and served at the table.	Anytime! Raw fruits and vegetables are perfect for snacking. Fruits and vegetables should compose about $\frac{1}{3}$–$\frac{1}{2}$ of each meal.
Frozen	Frozen soon after harvesting, thus retaining most nutrients. Can be stored in the freezer for 3–6 months for convenience and availability year-round.	May not be sustainable for dishes calling for fresh fruits/vegetables or in salads.	Fruits can be used in smoothies or thawed and eaten with yogurt or cereals. Vegetables make quick meals by thawing and heating thoroughly on the stove or in the microwave. Perfect for soups, stews, lasagna, and casseroles.
Canned	Canned soon after harvesting, thus retaining most nutrients. Can be stored for 6–12 months for convenience and availability year-round. Do not have to be refrigerated.	Fruits may be canned with added sugars. Look for fruits canned in their own juice. Vegetables are typically canned with sodium or other preservatives. Rinse canned vegetables before serving.	Canned fruits are perfect to keep in a desk drawer or in the car for a quick, easy snack, any time. Canned vegetables can be used for any dish calling for cooked vegetables, or added to sauces, soups, or stews for a vegetable boost.
Dried	Do not require refrigeration. Can be stored for 6–12 months or more. Concentrated source of calories.	May not be appropriate for all recipes. High in calories for a small amount of food compared to fresh fruits and vegetables; therefore, may not be the best form for individuals attempting to lose weight.	Add to nuts for a trail mix snack. Keep on hand for a fruit source when fresh fruits are not available. Great for traveling.
Juices	Quick and easy source of fruits and vegetables. Concentrated source of vitamins and minerals compared to whole fruits and vegetables.	Contains significantly more calories per serving than fresh fruits and vegetables. Minimal to no fiber is found in juices.	Ideal for after exercise, providing a dose of fluids, carbohydrates, potassium, vitamin C, and other nutrients. For some, a small amount of juice before exercise settles well and supplies fluid and carbohydrates to sustain effort during exercise.

- Top yogurt with oatmeal, nuts, or dried fruit for a mid-day snack or light breakfast.
- Layer fresh fruit, yogurt, and granola in a tall glass for a yogurt parfait.
- Use milk to make hot cereals, tomato soup, or hot chocolate.
- Thinly slice or shred cheese for salads, chili, and sandwiches.

alternative products are typically not naturally high in calcium and vitamin D; therefore, look at the Nutrition Facts label on each dairy alternative product to ensure that it has been fortified with these nutrients.

What are the best carbohydrate choices within the protein foods group?

Beans, lentils, nuts, seeds, and soy products are included in the protein foods group and are excellent sources of carbohydrates (see **Training Table 3.5**). These foods are also a good source of protein, iron, zinc, and fiber. Beef, chicken, fish, eggs, and other animal meats do not contain carbohydrates.

Can foods containing simple sugars or artificial sweeteners be used as a source of carbohydrates?

Some sugary or sweet foods can serve as sources of carbohydrates (see **Training Table 3.6**). Candies, desserts, jellies, and regular sodas contain carbohydrates in the form of simple sugars but are otherwise void of nutrient value. These foods complement other foods to make meals and snacks more flavorful and enjoyable. Sweets and sodas do not need to be permanently excluded from the diet but should be used sparingly. Diet sodas, desserts, and snacks replace sugar with artificial sweeteners, thus providing minimal or no carbohydrates. Diet foods can be incorporated into a healthy diet, but should also be used sparingly to make room for carbohydrate-rich and nutrient-dense foods.

gaining the performance edge

Dietary carbohydrates can be obtained from a variety of foods throughout the MyPlate food guidance system. Each food group provides a unique blend of carbohydrates and other nutrients. Athletes should focus on the most nutrient-dense carbohydrate sources including whole grains, fruits, vegetables, low-fat dairy/alternatives, beans/legumes, and nuts.

Training Table 3.5: Incorporating Carbohydrate-Rich Protein Foods into Meals/Snacks

- Use extra-firm tofu for spaghetti sauce or casseroles.
- Keep canned beans on hand to toss into salads or pasta dishes.
- Make hummus (see Handball Hummus recipe) from garbanzo, canellini, or black beans for a quick sandwich spread or dip for vegetables.
- Spread peanut butter on whole grain bread, bagels, or crackers.

Handball Hummus

1 15 oz can of garbanzo beans, drained; reserve liquid
1–2 tbsp liquid from the can of garbanzo beans
1–2 tbsp tahini (sesame seed paste)
1–2 tbsp lemon juice
1 tsp ground cumin
1/2 tsp ground coriander
1/4 tsp ground black pepper
Place all ingredients in a food processor. Blend until smooth. Serve with pita bread, raw vegetables, or as a sandwich spread.
Serving Size: 1/4 cup (Recipe makes eight servings)
Calories: 110 kcals
Protein: 5 grams
Carbohydrates: 16 grams
Fat: 3 grams

Training Table 3.6: Incorporating Moderate Amounts of Carbohydrate-Rich Sweets into Meals/Snacks

- Use 1–2 teaspoons of jelly on toasted whole grain bread or muffins.
- Enjoy 1–2 small cookies with milk as a bedtime snack.
- Bake oatmeal cookies with a few chocolate chips.
- Savor a bite-sized candy bar instead of a full-size bar after a meal.

What are the "glycemic index" and "glycemic load" and how can they be used in sports nutrition?

There has been much interest in the lay and scientific literature about the glycemic index of foods. In the quest for the optimal diet for sport performance, researchers have been discovering information about the different types of carbohydrate foods and the timing of these foods that may be beneficial to athletes. The glycemic index and the glycemic load can provide guidance to athletes to help them make appropriate carbohydrate choices. These concepts, combined with other solid nutrition practices, have the potential to improve sport performance.

The **glycemic index** (GI) indicates how much a certain food raises blood glucose levels when consumed in isolation. The index is calculated by measuring the incremental area under the blood glucose curve following ingestion of a test food that provides 50 grams of carbohydrates, compared with the area under the curve following an equal carbohydrate intake from a reference food.[24] Glucose and white bread are most often used as the food standard, given a GI value of 100, to which all other foods are compared. Accordingly, a GI of 70 indicates that consuming 50 grams of the food in question provides an increase of blood glucose 70% as great as that for ingesting 50 grams of pure glucose.[25] Glycemic index testing occurs after an overnight fast. The GI ranking of specific foods is based on the measurement of the blood glucose response 2 hours after the sample food is ingested. Information in **Table 3.6** is excerpted from Foster-

glycemic index (GI) An index for classifying carbohydrate foods based on how quickly they are digested and absorbed into the bloodstream. The more quickly blood glucose rises after ingestion, the higher the glycemic index.

| TABLE 3.6 | Glycemic Index and Glycemic Load of Common Foods |

Food	Glycemic Index (Glucose = 100)	Glycemic Index (White Bread = 100)	Glycemic Index Category*	Serving Size (g)	g CHO/ Serving	Glycemic Load
White bread, Wonder	73±2	105±3	High	30	14	10
White rice, boiled	64±7	91±9	High	150	36	23
Couscous	65± 4	93±6	High	150	35	23
Gatorade	78±13	111	High	250 mL	15	12
Ice cream	61±7	87±10	High	50	13	8
Sweet potato	61±7	87±10	High	150	28	17
Baked potato, russet	85±12	121±16	High	150	30	26
Cranberry juice cocktail	68±3	97	High	250 mL	36	24
Grapenuts	71±4	102±6	High	30	21	15
Cornflakes	81±3	116±5	High	30	26	21
Blueberry muffin	59	84±8	High	57	29	17
Power bar	56±3	79±4	Med	65	42	24
Honey	55±5	78±7	Med	25	18	10
White rice, long grain	56±2	80±3	Med	150	41	23
Coca-Cola	58±5	83±7	Med	250 mL	26	16
Sweet corn	54±4	78±6	Med	80	17	9
Carrot	47±16	68±23	Med	80	6	3
New potato	57±7	81±10	Med	150	21	12
Banana	52±4	74±5	Med	120	24	12
Orange juice	50±4	71±5	Med	250 mL	26	13
Chickpeas	28±6	39±8	Low	150	30	8
Kidney beans	28±4	39±6	Low	150	25	7
Xylitol	8±1	11±1	Low	10	10	1
Lentils	29±1	41±1	Low	150	18	5
Chocolate cake, frosted	38±3	54	Low	111	52	20
Fructose	19±2	27±4	Low	10	10	2
Tomato juice	38±4	54	Low	250 mL	9	4
Skim milk	32±5	46	Low	250 mL	13	4
Smoothie, raspberry	33±9	48±13	Low	250 mL	41	14
Apple	38±2	52±3	Low	120	15	6

* Category = High (>85); Medium (60–85); Low (<60) using GI white bread = 100.

Source: Adapted from Foster-Powell K, Holt SHA, Brand-Miller JC. International table of glycemic index and glycemic load values. *Am J Clin Nutr.* 2002;76:5–56.

Powell et al.'s extensive compilation of data on the GI of foods.[26] Their research, published between 1981 and 2001, contained nearly 1300 entries of more than 750 different types of foods. Table 3.6 provides a small sample of foods that have had GI testing completed.

The glycemic index can be altered or affected by any of the following factors:

- *Type of carbohydrate:* Unfortunately, the glycemic index of individual carbohydrate foods cannot be determined based simply on their classification as a mono-, di-, or polysaccharide. For example, baked russet potatoes have a high glycemic index whereas new potatoes and corn have a moderate glycemic index. The GI is different, but all are considered polysaccharides. Similarly, it is too simplistic to instruct people to eat more complex carbohydrates than simple carbohydrates to help keep glycemic response low. The assumption is still held by many health professionals and consumers that simple carbohydrates produce a higher glycemic response than do starches; however, the data do not completely support this assumption. For example, white bread and most types of potatoes have been shown to produce a higher GI than sucrose. In contrast, fructose has been found to have a GI far lower than that of most of the starches.[27] Indeed, many foods thought of as "simple sugars" such as candy and soda do have a high glycemic index, but a surprising number of complex carbohydrates also have moderate to high glycemic index scores.

- *Fiber content of foods:* A high fiber content in foods can cause the item to digest more slowly and may delay the time it takes for blood glucose to rise, thus lowering GI. However, not all high-fiber foods have a low GI. Foods containing soluble fiber, such as apples or legumes, tend to have a low GI because they are soluble in water, become viscous in the intestinal tract, and thus slow digestion. Conversely, sources of insoluble fiber that have been finely milled, such as wheat bread, are not soluble in water, do not become viscous in the intestinal tract, and therefore digest more rapidly.

- *Protein and fat content of foods:* Protein and fat foods do not have GI rankings because they do not raise blood glucose appreciably. Combining protein and fat in meals along with carbohydrates can delay gastric emptying and thus potentially increase the time it takes for blood glucose levels to rise. Therefore, carbohydrate foods that also contain protein or fat, such as higher protein breads and baked goods, may cause vast differences in GI response from product to product.

- *Liquid versus solid form of the food:* In general, liquids are digested and absorbed more quickly than solids are, thus potentially increasing blood glucose levels more rapidly. For example, liquid carbohydrates such as juices are absorbed quickly into the bloodstream whereas some whole fruits containing fiber take longer to digest, be absorbed, and then be transported into the bloodstream as glucose.

- *Timing of the meal:* Most individuals eat three or more times within 24 hours. Timing of the foods eaten can affect GI greatly. If an individual consumes a meal 2 hours prior to eating a high-GI candy, the GI effect for that person may be different than the GI for someone who hasn't eaten for 6 or 8 hours.

- *Combination of foods consumed at the same time:* The glycemic index gives individuals an accurate assessment of the amount a single food raises blood glucose levels. Using the GI to make food choices may be confusing because humans usually eat a combination of foods and often eat more or less than 50 grams of carbohydrates at one time. Researchers are starting to do GI testing on combination foods that may be more beneficial to consumers because it more appropriately reflects daily food consumption patterns.

- *Total amount of carbohydrates consumed:* A greater amount of total carbohydrates consumed will presumably have a greater effect on glucose and insulin levels. The GI only reflects the blood glucose effect of one specific food. We may consume two or more different carbohydrate foods in the same meal or snack, such as fruit juice with graham crackers. When foods with differing GI are consumed together, the GI of the meal depends on their combined blood glucose response, or glycemic load.

The glycemic index of foods appears to be much more complex than initially thought and is not an easy way to categorize food. However, it is an additional way to obtain information about the carbohydrate content of foods. The GI, used in conjunction with food-labeling information and food preferences, can be an effective way to help athletes make healthy carbohydrate choices.

glycemic load A way of assessing the overall glycemic effect of a diet based on both the glycemic index and the number of carbohydrates provided per serving for each food ingested.

What is glycemic load?

The concept of **glycemic load** was introduced in 1997 to determine whether the overall glycemic effect of a diet, not just the carbohydrate content, is related to disease risk.[28] Researchers defined dietary glycemic load as the product of the GI of food and the amount of carbohydrates in a serving. Therefore, an individual food that has an established glycemic index and a known amount of carbohydrates in the serving size tested can also have a glycemic load number. Table 3.6 contains both the glycemic index and glycemic load values for selected foods. By summing the glycemic load of individual foods consumed throughout one day, the overall glycemic load of the whole diet can be calculated.[29] Thus, glycemic load looks at the impact of carbohydrate consumption, taking the glycemic index into consideration.

Glycemic Load = (GI × carbohydrate content per serving) / 100

Brand-Miller and colleagues studied 30 lean, healthy volunteers to test the assumptions that (1) portions of different foods calculated to the same glycemic load produce similar blood glucose responses and (2) stepwise increases in glycemic load produce proportionate increases in both glycemia and insulinemia.[29] The subjects were split into two groups to research these two assumptions separately.

In the first study, 10 different food portions having the same glycemic index as one slice of white bread (GI of 70, 15 grams of carbohydrates) or a glycemic load of 10.5 were compared. Ten subjects consumed each food portion on different occasions in random order several days apart. The test foods were selected to provide a wide range of carbohydrate content and glycemic index. The foods tested were white bread, rice, spaghetti, cornflakes, yogurt, jellybeans, bananas, lentils, baked beans, and orange juice. The glucose responses to 9 out of 10 foods fed at the same glycemic load as one slice of white bread did not differ. However, lentils resulted in an unexpectedly lower response than the other foods.

The second study used the other 20 volunteers who consumed two sets of five foods, one of which was white bread, to determine dose–response relationships for four variables: subject, dose, food,

and order. The foods in the two different sets in this study were the same as those in the first study. Increasing the glycemic load (dose level) affected the glucose response within both sets of food and also had a significant influence on insulin response. The authors suggest that these findings provide the first evidence of the physiological validity of the glycemic load concept because, with one exception (lentils), the 10 foods fed at the same glycemic load as one slice of white bread produced relatively similar glycemic responses. Stepwise increases in glycemic load (from the GI equivalent of one to six slices of bread, regardless of food source) gave predictable increases in glycemia and insulinemia. These findings are relevant to the assumption that the overall glycemic and insulinemic effect of a diet can be calculated from the GI and the amount of carbohydrates per serving.

The authors of this combined study noted that glycemic load remains controversial because it is a mathematical calculation based on an already controversial approach to classifying foods, the glycemic index. However, much more research into the glycemic index has been done since then, and many more foods have been tested and assigned a GI value. So, despite its controversial beginnings, the GI is now widely recognized as a reliable, physiologically based classification of foods according to their postprandial glycemic effects.[26] In fact, the 2002 Dietary Reference Intake (DRI) report on macronutrients extensively refers to the glycemic index because many studies have been conducted using this classification system.[20]

As mentioned, the glycemic load can be calculated for any food that has a GI value. However, there are many influences that affect individual responses to the glycemic load, including factors that could slow carbohydrate absorption, the total glycemic load of a meal or several meals throughout the day, and the differences in single serving sizes that people typically consume that may be very different from the portions tested to establish a GI for individual foods. The glycemic load data should be used cautiously to account for these variances, and health professionals and researchers should calculate their own glycemic load based on the types of foods and portion sizes consumed.

Does glycemic kinetics affect the glycemic index?

Closer study into the glycemic effects of foods indicates that the glycemic index value of specific foods may not be just an indication of how quickly the carbohydrate source is digested and absorbed into the bloodstream. Emerging research into glucose kinetics reveals that glucose levels in the blood are dependent not only on the rate of appearance of glucose from the gut, but also on the rate of disappearance based on uptake by cells. Schenk et al.[30] compared the effects of low- and high-glycemic breakfast cereals on blood glucose levels, blood insulin levels, and glucose uptake rates for 3 hours after ingestion. Six healthy males consumed high-GI cornflakes (CF) and low-GI bran cereal (BC) containing 50 grams of carbohydrates on separate days. After ingestion, the plasma glucose concentration was significantly lower for BC (low-GI) than CF (high-GI). In fact, the GI for CF was more than twice that for BC. Although on first blush this finding seems to support the fact that high-GI foods release glucose more quickly into the blood, glucose kinetic measures of glucose appearance rates did not support this thought. The appearance rate of glucose into the bloodstream was not different between the high- and low-GI cereals. However, a difference was found in the plasma insulin levels and glucose uptake rates. It is interesting to note that insulin levels in the blood were actually 76% higher and glucose uptake rates were 31% greater after ingestion of the low-GI BC compared to the high-GI CF cereal, thus the reason for the lower GI. These findings indicate that GI values are not merely an indicator of how quickly different carbohydrates are digested and released from the gut into the bloodstream. Whether the glucose kinetics of the cereal foods used in this study are representative of other carbohydrate foods is unknown, and other studies will have to be performed. However, it is important for sports nutrition professionals to be aware of growing developments regarding the glycemic index, what it means, and how it can be used. Knowledge of the current ambiguities regarding the glycemic index will prevent overuse or abuse of the index in sports and will, it is hoped, prevent the abandoning of sound dietary advice for athletes.

How does the glycemic index relate to exercise?

The extensive amount of information about the GI has led researchers to test whether the GI of foods is helpful to active individuals. Because carbohydrates are a primary fuel for athletes, especially during high-intensity or long-duration exercise, it has been suggested that manipulating the diet using GI information may improve sport performance. The goal of using the GI is to optimize carbohydrate availability before, during, and after exercise.

Preexercise meals with a low GI may be best for athletes. When DeMarco et al. compared trained cyclists who had either a high-GI or low-GI meal prior to a 2-hour cycling bout and exercise to exhaustion, the low-GI group had higher glucose levels at 120 minutes and cycled significantly longer in the exhaustion test.[31] Other researchers have studied the effects of the consumption of a single low-GI food on long-duration exercise and found similar results.[32–34] Recent studies reporting an enhanced performance after consuming a low-GI meal often attribute the gains to an increase in fat oxidation compared to the consumption of a high-GI meal.[35,36] However, not all research has been able to establish a direct link between metabolic changes caused by a low-GI meal and increased work output or time to exhaustion during performance tests.[33,37,38] More information is needed before precise recommendations regarding the GI of preexercise meals for athletes can be formulated.

During exercise, muscles depend on the quick delivery of ingested carbohydrates for the continuation of high-intensity or long-duration efforts. Therefore, carbohydrate-rich foods and/or sports drinks of moderate to high GI are the most appropriate. Consuming low-GI foods during exercise may lead to decreased performance and early cessation of exercise.

After exercise, the focus is placed on nutrition for optimal recovery. Carbohydrate consumption immediately after exercise is critical for glycogen replenishment. Consumption of medium- and high-GI foods can help athletes replenish carbohydrate stores as quickly as possible. It has been suggested that athletes should consume 50–100 grams of high-GI carbohydrates immediately following intense, glycogen-depleting exercise.[39] Although studies have supported this recommendation, it appears that differences in recovery are found primarily in the 6–24 hours postexercise.[40] After 24 hours, glycogen replenishment from low- and high-GI meals may be similar.[41]

Using the GI of foods to help athletes improve sport performance appears to have some merit. However, there are also some limitations. Most GI studies have been conducted using human subjects who are not exercise trained. The responses to GI in trained versus untrained individuals could be very different. In general, trained individuals have more muscle mass and are more insulin sensitive than are untrained individuals. In addition, not all research reports a direct correlation between the GI of foods consumed before, during, and after exercise and enhanced athletic performance.[42]

Not all foods have been tested and ranked in the GI system. Many factors affect the glycemic index and can ultimately influence the glucose and subsequent insulin response in the bloodstream. Glycemic load and glycemic kinetics are newer concepts that may in the future help to determine more clearly how different foods, timing of meals, and the amount of carbohydrates affect the glucose response.

In practical terms, a variety of low-, moderate-, and high-GI foods contain a variety of nutrients, soluble and insoluble fiber, and phytochemicals that are beneficial to the body. Educating athletes about these health benefits, while incorporating recommendations on carbohydrate intake for sport performance, will help athletes stay healthy and perform optimally. The glycemic index can be used to help improve knowledge about foods that contain carbohydrates, but its limitations in practical daily eating need to be recognized. Further information and research on the effects and validity of the GI will help athletes make decisions concerning the best types of carbohydrates to consume for health, sport performance, and recovery. Scientific research, theory, and practical applications of glycemic index, load, and kinetics are still evolving. As more research and practice in the athletic arena occurs, it is likely that research will provide more definitive and specific recommendations on using the glycemic index of foods to enhance health and sport performance.

How are carbohydrates utilized during exercise?

Whether an athlete is engaging in long-duration endurance activities, intermittent exercise, or short-duration, high-intensity power sports, carbohydrates are needed to supply fuel to the muscles and brain. In regard to oxygen consumption, carbohydrates produce energy in a more efficient manner than fats or proteins. Athletes who eat lower levels of carbohydrates find that workouts become harder to complete, mental focus is more difficult, energy levels drop, and muscles feel fatigued.

The body prefers to use carbohydrates as fuel during exercise. Depending on the intensity of the exercise, carbohydrates may be broken down for energy via aerobic or anaerobic means (see Chapter 2). At low to moderate exercise levels, carbohydrates are primarily aerobically metabolized for energy. Each glucose molecule passes through glycolysis, where it

is broken down to pyruvate. From there the pyruvate is converted to acetyl coenzyme A (CoA) and enters into the citric acid cycle. The citric acid cycle strips hydrogens off the carbon structure of the acetyl CoA, leaving the carbon atoms to bind with oxygen to form CO_2. The hydrogens are carried to the electron transport chain, where they are used to create energy in the form of adenosine triphosphate (ATP). In the process of transferring hydrogens, water is formed (see Figure 3.7).

At rest and during low exercise intensities (<20% of aerobic capacity), fatty acids play a major role in energy production along with carbohydrates. However, when exercise intensities increase to 40–60% of VO_2max, carbohydrates become the major source of energy. The point at which carbohydrates take over as the primary energy source is called the **crossover point**.[43] As depicted in Figure 3.8 , activities to the

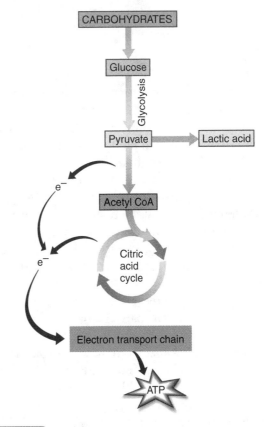

Figure 3.7 Carbohydrate metabolic pathways. The citric acid cycle strips hydrogen from the carbon structure of the acetyl CoA, leaving the carbon atoms to bind with oxygen to form CO_2. The hydrogen is then carried to the electron transport chain, where it is used to create energy in the form of ATP.

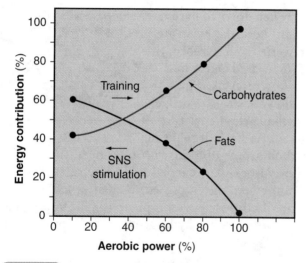

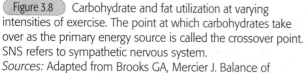

Figure 3.8 Carbohydrate and fat utilization at varying intensities of exercise. The point at which carbohydrates take over as the primary energy source is called the crossover point. SNS refers to sympathetic nervous system.
Sources: Adapted from Brooks GA, Mercier J. Balance of carbohydrate and lipid utilization during exercise: the "crossover" concept. *J Appl Physiol.* 1994;76(6):2253–2261. American Physiology Society.

left of the crossover point rely primarily on fats for energy. Endurance training causes adaptations in the body that cause the crossover point to move to the right. In other words, trained endurance athletes can exercise or perform at higher intensities and rely more on fats than carbohydrates for energy than untrained individuals. This is important because the body's carbohydrate stores are limited and when the muscles deplete their glycogen stores, they fatigue. Because endurance training increases the body's ability to use fats for energy, it helps to spare glycogen and thus delays fatigue, which improves endurance performance.

During the most intense activities, such as an all-out sprint, carbohydrates are the only macronutrient that can be metabolized fast enough to provide energy. The energy comes from the anaerobic breakdown of glucose to lactic acid (see Figure 3.7). This metabolic pathway is capable of producing energy very rapidly and thus can supply the energy needed in activities that require rapid production of ATP. Because most sports require bursts of intense activity that draw energy from anaerobic metabolism, restricting carbohydrates from an athlete's diet is tantamount to performance suicide.

How much carbohydrate is stored within the body?

As previously discussed, carbohydrates are stored in the body as glycogen. Unfortunately, compared to fats, the other major source of energy in the body, very little glycogen is stored. The body may be able to store a total of only 400–600 grams of carbohydrates in the liver and muscle.[44] This amounts to about 1600–2400 kcal (4 kcal per gram of carbohydrate) depending on body size, time of day, and dietary intake. Although 1600 to 2400 kcals sounds like a lot, it should be noted that only about 400 to 500 kcals are actually directly available to be used for maintaining blood glucose levels. The remaining 1200 to 1900 calories from glycogen are found in the muscle cells, which are very stingy about sharing their glycogen. In other words, muscle cells are not capable of releasing stored glucose directly into the bloodstream. Unlike in liver cells, which can release glucose back into the blood to help to maintain glucose levels between meals, once glucose is taken into the muscle cell, it cannot be directly released back into the bloodstream. Therefore, once the liver is depleted of glycogen, blood glucose levels begin to decrease. Conversely, fat cells, known as **adipocytes**, store an estimated 90,000 kcals of energy and are capable of sharing their stored energy with the rest of the body. Because carbohydrates are such an important fuel for the exercising muscle and so little is stored in the body, individuals need to be aware of ways to improve both circulating and storage forms of carbohydrates for success during training and competition.

adipocyte A single fat cell.

Why are carbohydrates an efficient fuel source?

There are several reasons why carbohydrates are a good source of rapid energy, which is particularly important during intense exercise. One reason is that carbohydrates are actually stored in the muscle cells themselves. This means they are readily available to provide energy at the very outset of exercise, unlike most fats that are stored at remote sites in the body and must be delivered via the bloodstream.

Another reason carbohydrates are such an efficient fuel is that they can provide energy for a short period of time without the need for oxygen. To get energy for exercise or sports from fats, our cells must have oxygen. Without adequate amounts of oxygen being delivered to the muscles, fats and, to a lesser extent, proteins cannot produce enough energy to support intense exercise. Fortunately, not only are carbohydrates readily available for energy, but also muscle cells can break down carbohydrates for energy without oxygen being present. This is known as anaerobic metabolism (see Chapter 2).

Finally, when carbohydrates are broken down in the presence of adequate oxygen, because of the chemical makeup of carbohydrates compared to fats, less oxygen is needed. A person's aerobic exercise rate is limited by how fast oxygen can be delivered to muscle cells, so it is better to rely on carbohydrates because less oxygen is needed.

Does carbohydrate intake enhance performance?

There is no question about the importance of carbohydrates in sport performance. In fact, any athlete who practices a diet that restricts carbohydrates for a long period of time is severely hindering their preparation for and performance in his or her sport. A review of the earlier section on the role of carbohydrates gives hints to this fact. Regardless of the sport or its energy requirements, a positive mental attitude and energetic approach to training are required on an ongoing basis if improved sport performance is the goal. Depleted muscle glycogen levels and low blood glucose levels lead to loss of mental focus, feelings of weakness, and thus ineffective training.

Does carbohydrate intake delay fatigue?

The answer to this question is a resounding yes, if the fatigue is the type experienced by many endurance athletes. As noted earlier in this chapter (see the section "What functions do carbohydrates serve in the body?"), carbohydrates, namely glucose, are an important source of energy during exercise. Because carbohydrates are an important energy source, the body stores them as glycogen in the liver and muscles. Liver glycogen is important for maintaining blood glucose levels between meals and during exercise, thereby providing a relatively constant supply of energy to muscles and other tissues. The muscle glycogen stores serve as readily available energy sources for muscle during activity. Exercise and/or diet can greatly affect glycogen levels (see Figure 3.9). A diet high in carbohydrates can lead to increased glycogen stores in both the liver and the muscle, whereas one that is low in carbohydrates can decrease glycogen levels. Depletion of glycogen stores at either of these locations can negatively affect performance. Figure 3.9 clearly indicates that the carbohydrate composition of a diet affects initial muscle glycogen levels and that high glycogen levels can significantly increase the amount of time until exhaustion in an exercising athlete. In fact, this is

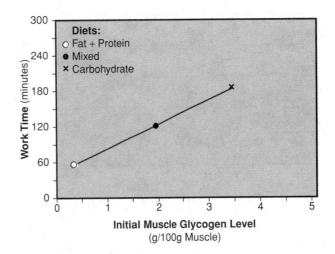

Figure 3.9 Diet composition, muscle glycogen levels, and time to fatigue. The muscle glycogen stores serve as readily available energy sources for muscle during activity. Exercise and/ or diet can greatly affect glycogen levels.
Source: Data from Astrand PO. Diet and athletic performance. *Federation Proc.* 1967; 26:1772–1777.

the main reason why carbohydrate loading is practiced by endurance athletes in the days leading up to an event. It is not that extra glycogen in the muscle cells makes endurance athletes faster; it just enables them to maintain their race pace for a longer period of time, which translates into faster race times.

Ingestion of carbohydrates during activity is also critical for delaying fatigue in endurance sports.[45] Over time the liver's glycogen stores begin to decrease because of the increased demand for glucose. As the liver's glycogen stores near depletion, its ability to maintain blood glucose levels decreases and work output diminishes. If exercise persists after liver glycogen is depleted, muscles will continue to use available blood glucose for energy. Eventually, blood glucose levels will fall below normal levels, causing hypoglycemia (low blood sugar). Signs and symptoms of low blood glucose include hunger, dizziness, shakiness, headache, and irritability. If carbohydrate intake remains insufficient and glucose levels continue to drop, unconsciousness, coma, and death can result.

As shown in Figure 3.10 , after about 90 minutes of exercise, which corresponds to the amount of time it takes to severely diminish liver glycogen stores, blood levels of glucose begin to fall below resting levels (i.e., Time = 0 minutes). However, when a glucose polymer drink was ingested at minute 135, blood glucose increased to levels comparable to those earlier in the exercise session. Helping the body to maintain blood glucose levels through carbohydrate

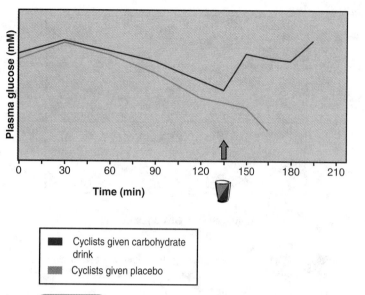

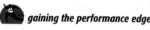

Figure 3.10 Carbohydrate sports drinks and performance. Blood glucose levels begin to fall below resting levels after 90 minutes. Subjects that consumed carbohydrate drinks (135 minutes) dramatically increased blood glucose levels, whereas levels continued to decrease in subjects fed a placebo.
Source: Coggan AR, Coyle EF. Metabolism and performance following carbohydrate ingestion late in exercise. *Med Sci Sports and Exerc.* 1989;21(1):59–65. Reprinted with permission from Wolters Kluwer.

ingestion during exercise can in turn translate into sustained effort and thus enhanced performance.[45] Figure 3.10 clearly demonstrates the importance of consuming carbohydrates during activity and its impact on blood glucose.

Power sports are those that require very short bursts of intense activity. The most extreme examples of power sports are shot put, discus, Olympic weightlifting, and the 100-meter sprint. In power sports, reliance on stored glycogen for energy is very low, and thus glycogen depletion in regard to performance is not necessarily of concern. However, a strong argument can be made for the impact carbohydrates have on the preparation (i.e., the intense training required) for the sport competition. Diets low in carbohydrates combined with frequent intense training can, over time, diminish muscle and liver glycogen levels and lower blood glucose levels. Low blood glucose decreases overall energy level, motivation to train, and the mental focus needed for high-intensity training. In addition, decreased muscle glycogen levels can lead to feelings of chronic fatigue and thus decreased training intensity levels. The end result is suboptimal sport preparation and thus poor competition performance.

What type, how much, and when should carbohydrates be consumed before exercise?

To perform optimally, adequate amounts of carbohydrates need to be supplied to the body prior to exercise. The source, quantity, and timing of the carbohydrates ingested can lead either to a high-energy, high-performance exercise session or to a feeling of staleness and fatigue. Proper nutrition before exercise focuses on the quantity and type of food consumed in the days leading up to a workout or event. Also of importance is the timing between eating and exercise. The key to optimal nutrition before, as well as during and after, exercise is individualization. Each person has likes and dislikes, tolerances and intolerances. There is not one "best" pregame meal, sports beverage, or postexercise snack. However, by following a few guidelines and lots of experimentation, athletes can determine the nutrition plan that best fits their sport and lifestyle.

gaining the performance edge

Listen and learn about athletes' food/beverage likes and dislikes. Encourage them to experiment with a variety of carbohydrate-rich meals, snacks, and sports beverages during training to determine the best option for optimal performance on race day.

What should an athlete eat on the days leading up to an important training session or competition?

It is widely recognized that exercise performance will be enhanced when preceded by several days of a high-carbohydrate diet. It is critical to consume adequate amounts of carbohydrates in the days, as well as the hours, leading up to an exercise session or competition to maximize energy levels and performance.

As mentioned previously, research has shown that by increasing glycogen stores prior to exercise, athletes can increase the time to fatigue and enhance performance during prolonged, strenuous exercise (see Figure 3.9). The term **carbohydrate loading** has traditionally referred to the process of muscle glycogen supersaturation and has been shown to increase glycogen levels above normal, thus allowing athletes to perform longer before fatiguing. For example, the glycogen content of skeletal muscle in an untrained individual, consuming a balanced diet, is typically around 80 mmol/kg of muscle wet weight. An

carbohydrate loading A high-carbohydrate dietary plan commonly used by endurance athletes that is designed to engorge muscle cells with glycogen.

adaptation of regular exercise training is the ability for muscles to store more glycogen. Therefore, trained individuals generally have muscle glycogen levels of ~125 mmol/kg. However, during tapering and carbohydrate loading, when exercise is decreased so that less glycogen is used on a daily basis and carbohydrate intake is simultaneously increased, glycogen stores can be boosted to levels of 175–200 mmol/kg of muscle wet weight.[46]

The concept of carbohydrate loading was first investigated by Bergstrom and colleagues in the late 1960s.[47] Although he found his 6-day regime to be effective at packing the muscle cells with up to two times their normal glycogen concentration, the two exhaustive exercise bouts and the first 3 days of low carbohydrate ingestion were found to be physically and mentally taxing to the athletes. Since then several modified versions of the original (i.e., classical 6-day protocol) have been developed with the intent of making it easier on the athlete and thereby avoiding the unwanted side effects (e.g., muscle soreness, fatigue, poor mental attitude). See **Table 3.7** for de-

tails on a few of the modified carbohydrate loading regimes.

Much of what is known about carbohydrate loading has been derived from studies involving male subjects. It is interesting to note that studies involving carbohydrate loading in females have yielded equivocal results. It appears that for effective carbohydrate loading to occur in females, close attention must be paid to the total energy intake, level of carbohydrate intake, and phase of the menstrual cycle.[48] Female athletes who increased their normal total energy intake by 34%, and at the same time maintained a carbohydrate intake of 75% of total calories, demonstrated muscle glycogen increases comparable to males.[49] It has also been reported that carbohydrate loading is more effective during the luteal phase rather than the follicular phase of the menstrual cycle. The difference in the glycogen loading within the cells seems to be related to the differences in hormonal levels that exist between the menstrual phases.[50] In fact it has been reported that women taking oral contraceptives may have an

TABLE 3.7	Methods of Carbohydrate (CHO) Loading			
CHO Loading Regime	Requires Exhaustive Exercise or Glycogen Depletion	Exercise Protocol	Diet Details	Reference
Classic 6-day	Yes	Day 1 involves an exhaustive bout of exercise; Days 2 and 3 involve moderate submaximal exercise; Day 4 involves another exhaustive exercise bout; No exercise on days 5 and 6	First 3 days low CHO diet (~15% total calories); next 3 days high CHO diet (~70% total calories)	Bergstrom et al.[47]
6-day	No	First 3 days involve intense submaximal exercise of decreasing duration. Day 1 involves 90 minutes of exercise and days 2 and 3 require 40 minutes of exercise. Next 2 days only 20 minutes of submaximal exercise. Last day no exercise.	First 3 days mixed diet (~50% CHO); next 3 days high CHO (~70% of total calories)	Sherman et al.[52]
Classic 3-day	Yes	Exhaustive bout of exercise followed by 3 days of no exercise.	3 days of high CHO intake (~70% total calories)	Ahlborg et al.[53]
Modified 3-day	No	No exercise for 3 days	3 days of high CHO (10g of CHO/kg of body weight per day)	Burke et al.[54]
1-day	No	No exercise for 1 day	1 day of high CHO (10g of CHO/kg of body weight per day)	Burke et al.[55], Bussau et al.[56]

advantage when it comes to carbohydrate loading due to the muting of hormonal differences between the menstrual phases.[48,51]

An athlete must take into consideration that with the process of carbohydrate loading, temporary water weight gain may occur. Muscles store 3 grams of water for every 1 gram of carbohydrate. Some individuals find that the extra water weight contributes to a bloated feeling and a sense of stiffness, which may negatively affect performance. Instead, "loading" the muscles with carbohydrates can be viewed as a daily component of training. If an athlete consumes 55–70% of total calories from carbohydrates daily, muscles may be consistently "topped off," therefore not requiring an alteration to normal eating immediately prior to an event.

What should an athlete eat in the hours leading up to an important training session or competition?

The 24 hours leading up to an important training session or competition are a critical time for carbohydrate-rich meals. By understanding the importance to performance and the general guidelines for intake, athletes can perfect their ideal preexercise meal/snack routine.

4 to 24 hours prior to exercise, training, or competition

Four to 24 hours prior to exercise, foods high in carbohydrates should compose a majority of each meal and snack, providing approximately 60–70% of total calories. Eating high-carbohydrate foods during this time frame will help to "top off" glycogen stores in the muscles and liver, allowing athletes to start an exercise session with a full tank of "energy fuel."

In addition to carbohydrates, proteins and fats play a role in the preexercise meals 4–24 hours before activity. By incorporating protein- and fatcontaining foods, the athlete ensures balance and moderation. Proteins and fats also contribute to the feeling of satiety, preventing the athlete from overeating.

Especially when competing, athletes should consume meals and snacks consisting of familiar foods in the 24 hours prior to the event. There should be no trial-and-error at this time; meals and snacks should be planned weeks in advance after experimentation to find the optimal blend and type of solid foods and liquids. Eating or drinking unfamiliar foods in the 24 hours before an event can lead to unwanted gastrointestinal distress such as indigestion, upset stomach, diarrhea, and cramping. Any of these symptoms will certainly compromise an athlete's ability to perform to his or her potential.

0 to 4 hours prior to exercise

At this point, carbohydrate stores are at their peak prior to exercise, and the focus shifts to foods and beverages that will digest easily and prevent the athlete from feeling hungry at the beginning of a training session or competition (see **Training Table 3.7**). Athletes should strive to consume 1–4.5 grams of carbohydrate per kilogram of body weight in the 1–4 hours prior to exercise.[57–60] Specific recommendations within these ranges will be based on individual tolerance. Athletes should be encouraged to experiment with varying quantities of carbohydrate and timing of intake during training to devise a plan for game day.

In the 1–4 hours prior to exercise, athletes should consider including the following foods:

- *Complex carbohydrates:* Carbohydrates consumed at this time will be used to elevate blood glucose levels for the start of an exercise session. Choose foods that are easy to digest and relatively low to moderate in fiber. Low glycemic index carbohydrates may be best before exercise, to avoid a spike in blood glucose and subsequent blood insulin levels immediately prior to exercise.[31–34]

- *Carbohydrate-rich protein sources:* Protein will help to maintain blood glucose levels by delaying the digestion and absorption of carbohydrates after the meal. Foods that contain both carbohydrates and protein include dairy products, dairy

Training Table 3.7: Carbohydrate-Rich Preexercise Meals (grams of carbohydrate)

- 1.5 cups cereal, 1 cup skim milk, and 1 cup orange juice (86 g)
- 2 pancakes, 3 tbsp syrup, 1/2 cup fresh fruit, and 1 cup skim milk (83g)
- 1 bagel, 2 tbsp peanut butter, 1 tbsp jelly, 0.5 cup unsweetened applesauce (71 g)
- 6 oz yogurt, 1 medium banana, 0.5 cup granola (85 g)
- 3/4 cup oatmeal [dry], 1/4 cup raisins, 2 tbsp walnuts, 1 cup skim milk (83 g)
- Turkey sandwich [2 slices bread, 6 slices turkey], 1 apple, 6 oz yogurt (101 g)
- 1.5 cup spaghetti with marinara sauce, 4 oz chicken, 2 cups garden salad, 2 tbsp salad dressing (87 g)
- Hummus/cheese wrap [4 tbsp hummus, 2 slices cheese, 1 cup lettuce, 1 flour tortilla], 1.5 cup vegetable soup, 10 Saltine crackers, 8 oz apple juice (95 g)
- 4 oz baked ham, 1 cup mashed potato, 1 cup fruit salad (96 g)

alternative products, soy products, and legumes. Legumes should be consumed in small amounts because they are packed with fiber, which can cause gastrointestinal discomfort in some athletes.

- *Fluids:* Approximately 2 cups of fluid should be consumed 2 hours prior to exercise. In addition, aim for 1 cup of fluid 1 hour prior, and 7 ounces of fluid 30 minutes prior to exercise. Water, milk, and juice are the best choices in the 2–4 hours before exercise. Water provides fluid and is absorbed quickly. Milk and juices provide fluid, carbohydrates, and a variety of vitamins and minerals. In general, sports drinks are not the best choice 2–4 hours before exercise, but are ideal during training. Compared to milk and juice, sports drinks have a lower concentration of carbohydrates, vitamins, and minerals. One exception to this rule may be for endurance athletes preparing for a long-duration training or exercise session. Sports drinks will provide fluid and a small amount of carbohydrates before training or competition, generally without gastrointestinal distress. Some individuals find that consuming concentrated fluids such as milk or juices within an hour of exercise causes nausea and cramping. Each athlete is different; trial and error will uncover tolerances and preferences.

In the last 2 hours prior to exercise, light meals, small snacks, and beverages containing carbohydrates are ideal. Small quantities of carbohydrates help to keep blood glucose levels elevated, while minimizing the risk for gastrointestinal upset. Some research has suggested that eating carbohydrates during the 30 minutes immediately prior to exercise can be detrimental to performance. The theory is that ingested carbohydrates will elevate insulin levels, causing a reduction of blood glucose within 15 minutes of the initiation of exercise.[61] However, most studies have failed to demonstrate a reduction in exercise performance during endurance activities resulting from preexercise carbohydrate consumption, especially if carbohydrate consumption is continued during exercise.[62] The bottom line is that each athlete responds differently to the ingestion of carbohydrates immediately prior to exercise, and therefore, individual preferences and tolerances must be built into an athlete's nutrition recommendations.

Some individuals are concerned about eating prior to exercise and are hesitant about consuming any type of food or beverage. In some cases, the athlete has never consumed food or liquid prior to exercise, especially morning exercise, and is doubtful or leery about testing the procedure. These athletes should be encouraged to try a small snack or beverage such as a glass of juice or milk, a piece of fruit, or a slice of toast. The athlete may not consume a full, well-balanced meal, but something is better than nothing. If an athlete becomes nervous or anxious before an event, an upset stomach or intestinal distress will often result. Suggest the athlete eat small amounts at a time of the foods he or she has found agreeable during training. Bites of a bagel, sips of juice, or sports beverages can be used in this situation to provide some fuel without further upsetting the gastrointestinal tract.

Besides the energy that can be provided by carbohydrates ingested prior to exercise, it has also been reported that the presence of carbohydrates in the mouth activates regions of the brain that can improve exercise performance.[63] Merely rinsing the mouth for about 10 seconds with a 6% carbohydrate solution appears to stimulate oral sensory receptors that activate brain areas associated with reward and the regulation of motor activity. Although the mechanisms are not clearly understood, the evidence is convincing that mouth rinsing with carbohydrate solutions immediately prior to or during exercise may be a worthwhile practice.

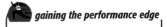

gaining the performance edge

Athletes should strive to consume 1–4.5 grams of carbohydrate per kilogram of body weight in the 1–4 hours prior to exercise. Experimentation during training will help each athlete determine the optimal amount to include in the preexercise meal for performance enhancement.

gaining the performance edge

Remember that each athlete is different. Some people may feel most comfortable eating their preexercise meal 3–4 hours prior to training, and find that waiting longer to eat leads to stomach and intestinal cramping. Others may find that they get too hungry if too much time passes between their last meal/snack and exercise. Individuals should experiment not only with the type of carbohydrate-rich food and beverage, but also with the timing of their meals/snacks prior to exercise.

gaining the performance edge

Performing a 10-second mouth rinse with a 6% carbohydrate solution before and during exercise may improve athletic performance.

What type, how much, and when should carbohydrates be consumed during exercise?

Consuming carbohydrates during exercise has been shown to help delay fatigue in short-duration and long-duration activities.[64–69] The theory is that carbohydrates provided during exercise can either reduce the reliance on the glycogen stored in the muscles and liver for energy or provide an alternative source of carbohydrates when glycogen is depleted. Various forms of carbohydrates have different properties related to digestion, absorption, availability of glucose for oxidation, and taste. Because of their varying characteristics, the type of carbohydrate ingested during activity is of importance. Athletes need to develop a nutrition plan for during activity based on the nature of their sport, the availability of foods/beverages during training or competition, and individual tolerances.

What types of carbohydrates should be consumed during exercise or sport?

Research has shown that glucose, sucrose, glucose polymers/maltodextrins, and starches are absorbed and oxidized at a high rate and therefore are appropriate fuels for during exercise.[70–77] Fructose and galactose are absorbed and oxidized at a slower rate than other carbohydrate sources. Fructose is absorbed half as fast as glucose and has to be converted to glucose in the liver before it can be metabolized. When consumed in large amounts, fructose can cause gastrointestinal distress, cramping, or diarrhea. Therefore, galactose and, more specifically, fructose, are viewed as less desirable fuels during exercise. However, fructose increases the palatability of sports performance products, and therefore a combination of fructose and more desirable sources of carbohydrates are often mixed together. Sports nutrition products can be highly valuable to athletes based on their digestibility and ease of preparation. Most products are formulated with a combination of different carbohydrate sources to create a food or beverage that is easily digestible, is convenient to consume during activities, and tastes good. Common sports nutrition products geared mainly for supplying carbohydrates during exercise include sports beverages, carbohydrate gels, and energy bars (see Table 3.8).

How much carbohydrate should be consumed during exercise or sport?

The quantity of carbohydrates consumed during exercise is determined by considering two factors: (1) the rate of carbohydrate utilization (i.e., oxidation rate) during the activity and (2) the rate at which gastric emptying and intestinal absorption of carbohydrates occurs. The oxidation rate or use of blood glucose for energy by muscle has been estimated to be approximately 1.0 to 1.1 grams of glucose per minute.[78] Several factors such as exercise intensity, muscle glycogen saturation, and fitness level have the

TABLE 3.8	Carbohydrate Content of Commonly Used Sport Drinks, Gels, and Bars			
Sports Drink	Calories	Carbohydrates	% Sugar Solution	Type of Carbohydrates
(all values per 8 fl oz)				
All Sport	70	20 g	8	High fructose corn syrup
Gatorade	50	14 g	6	Sucrose, glucose, fructose
Powerade	70	19 g	8	High fructose corn syrup, maltodextrin
Carbohdyrate Gels				
(all values per one packet)				
Gu Energy Gel	100	25 g		Maltodextrin, fructose
Hammer Gel	90	23 g		Maltodextrin, fructose
PowerBar PowerGel	110	26 g		Maltodextrin, fructose
Energy Bars				
(all values per one bar)				
Clif Bar	240	45 g		Brown rice, oats, evap. cane sugar
Hammer Bar	220	25 g		Date paste, agave nectar
PowerBar	230	45 g		Oats, rice crisps, glucose syrup

potential to alter the use of blood glucose for energy during exercise. However, the magnitude and direction of the effects these factors have on oxidation rates are presently unclear.[78]

On the other hand, research on the effects of the rate of gastric emptying, intestinal absorption, and delivery of glucose to the working muscles during exercise has yielded more consistent findings. It appears that the rate of digestion, absorption, and transport of glucose is the limiting factor to carbohydrate utilization during exercise. A study conducted by Jeukendrup et al.[79] compared varying doses of exogenous carbohydrates during exercise to the appearance of glucose from the gut into the systemic circulation and the subsequent muscle oxidation rates. A low dose of ingested carbohydrates (0.43 grams of carbohydrate per minute) produced an equivalent appearance rate of glucose in the bloodstream (0.43 grams per minute), and the muscle was capable of metabolizing 90–95% of the delivered glucose during exercise. When a high dose of carbohydrates was consumed (3 grams of carbohydrate per minute) the appearance of glucose into the bloodstream was only 33% of the amount ingested (0.96–1.04 grams of carbohydrate per minute), thus indicating that this was the maximum rate of digestion/absorption. It is interesting to note that the muscle was still able to oxidize 90–95% of the delivered glucose for energy. Based on these findings, the authors concluded that glucose entrance into the systemic circulation is the limiting factor for exogenous carbohydrate oxidation during exercise. Ingesting carbohydrates at levels above the rates of absorption would not be beneficial, and any carbohydrates that are not absorbed may continue to move through the gastrointestinal tract and cause cramping or diarrhea. Therefore, following the notion that the absorption of exogenous carbohydrates reaches its maximum at 1.0–1.1 grams of carbohydrate per minute, it is recommended that athletes consume approximately 60–70 grams of carbohydrate per hour during exercise to help maintain energy output while preventing gastrointestinal upset.

Individual variances in the quantity of carbohydrates tolerated during exercise may be great. Some individuals can consume 60–70 grams of carbohydrates per hour without gastrointestinal distress, whereas others start cramping and feeling bloated after ingesting 50 grams of carbohydrates per hour. Experimentation during training will reveal the ideal quantity for each athlete. The form of carbohydrate ingested can affect the quantity an athlete feels com-

fortable consuming. Athletes should try different combinations of sports drinks, bars, gels, and other foods to determine the best mix of solids and fluids to consume during training and competition. The following examples provide 60–70 grams of carbohydrates an hour:

- 1 quart of a sports beverage
- 2 carbohydrate gels
- 1 to 1½ energy bars

Sports beverages provide a convenient means for consuming not only carbohydrate, but also fluid and electrolytes during exercise. Chapter 8 discusses in detail how to choose an appropriate sports beverage. It is generally recommended that athletes choose a sports beverage containing 6–8% carbohydrate (i.e., 14–20 grams of carbohydrate per 8 oz serving) to optimize gastric emptying and fluid absorption during exercise.[80] Beverages containing greater than 8% carbohydrate can be included in the athlete's diet, however, preferably not during training or competition. An exception to this rule is during ultra-endurance activities, which are covered in Chapter 12. These more concentrated carbohydrate beverages can also be useful during carbohydrate loading or for athletes who are struggling to consume enough total calories or carbohydrates.

When should carbohydrates be consumed during exercise or sport?

Limited research has been conducted on a wide range of carbohydrate feeding schedules. The results from recent studies suggest that athletes should begin ingesting carbohydrates early in a training session and continue to consume carbohydrates at a steady rate throughout the exercise period.

One schedule variation that has been investigated is the difference in oxidation rates between a bolus carbohydrate feeding at the start of an exercise session versus the equivalent amount of carbohydrates consumed in repetitive feedings throughout a bout of exercise. Several studies provided subjects with a single glucose load of 100 grams at the onset of exercise lasting 90–120 minutes.[81-83] These studies have shown a similar oxidation pattern: oxidation rates increase during the first 75–90 minutes of exercise, followed by a plateau thereafter. When the equivalent amount of carbohydrates (100 grams) is consumed in repetitive feedings throughout an exercise bout lasting 90–120 minutes, the same oxidation pattern is observed.[84-86] In general, repetitive small feedings are easier to tolerate than one large bolus feeding while exercising. If the oxidation rate is the same, then repetitive feedings may be more desirable if food and beverages are readily available. If not, then infrequent, larger doses of carbohydrates before and during prolonged exercise may provide the same effect for endurance performance.

If an athlete chooses to consume carbohydrates at regular intervals during exercise, the feedings should begin soon after the onset of exercise. A study conducted by McConell et al.[87] investigated the performance effects of consuming carbohydrates throughout exercise versus the ingestion of an equal amount of carbohydrates late in the exercise session. The results revealed a performance benefit versus controls only when carbohydrates were consumed throughout exercise. Ingestion of carbohydrates late in the exercise session did not improve performance despite an increase in circulating glucose and insulin after ingestion. Therefore, the consumption of sports drinks, energy bars, gels, or other sports-related foods and beverages should begin soon after the initiation of exercise to enhance performance during training and competition.

What type, how much, and when should carbohydrates be consumed after exercise?

Muscle and liver glycogen are used partially or completely during moderate-intensity/moderate-duration and high-intensity/long-duration activities, respectively. After exercising, it is critical to feed the muscles with carbohydrates to replenish stores of muscle and liver glycogen to be used in the next exercise session.

Unless sufficient carbohydrates are consumed in the diet after training or competition, muscle glycogen will not normalize on a daily basis and performance will suffer. A study conducted by Costill et al.[88] studied the performance effect of a low-carbohydrate diet fed to runners on successive training days. After 3 days on the low-carbohydrate diet, muscle glycogen was depleted progressively, and sub-

sequently some runners found it difficult to complete the prescribed workouts (see Figure 3.11).

When devising a postexercise recovery nutrition plan for athletes, there are several important factors to consider:

- The timing of carbohydrate ingestion
- The type of carbohydrates and inclusion of other macronutrients
- The quantity of carbohydrates in the postexercise meal or snack

When should carbohydrates be consumed after exercise or sport?

Replenishing glycogen stores used during exercise can take 20 hours or more even when consuming a diet consisting of 60% of total calories from carbohydrates.[89] This relatively slow rate of glycogen replenishment does not pose major problems for recreational athletes or others who train aerobically three to four times per week and ingest adequate carbohydrates because usually there is sufficient time between workouts to allow for glycogen recovery. On the other hand, the slow glycogen recovery rates can pose problems for endurance athletes who train daily or who perform multiple workouts per day. In these cases, the timing and type of carbohydrates ingested are important.

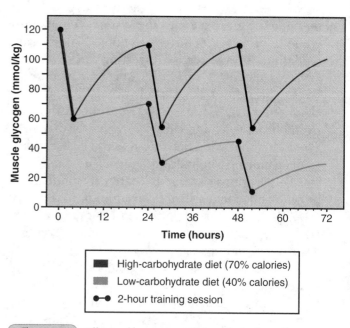

Figure 3.11 Effects of low- versus high-carbohydrate diet on glycogen stores. A high-carbohydrate diet replenishes glycogen stores better than a low-carbohydrate diet does.
Source: Modified from Costill DL, Miller JM. Nutrition for endurance sport: carbohydrate and fluid balance. *Int J Sport Nutr.* 1980;1:2–14.

Research indicates that muscles absorb blood glucose and restore glycogen at higher rates when carbohydrates are ingested within 2 hours after cessation of training/sport performance.[90] Delaying carbohydrate consumption until 4 hours or more after training can cut the glycogen synthesis rate in half compared to when carbohydrates are consumed immediately after exercise.[90] To take advantage of this window of opportunity, athletes should begin consumption of high glycemic index carbohydrate sources as soon as possible—some suggest as soon as 15 minutes after exercise.[91] Eating immediately or as soon as possible after exercise will allow time to digest and absorb the carbohydrates into the bloodstream and shuttle it to the cells.[90] An athlete's nutrition plan should include snacks and beverages that will be available for consumption immediately postexercise. In many cases, athletes are away from home and without refrigeration during this time frame; therefore, nonperishable foods and drinks are the best options.

What type of carbohydrates should be consumed after exercise or sport?

Because the quick delivery of carbohydrates to the muscles is of utmost importance, choosing carbohydrate-rich foods that are digested and absorbed quickly is essential. Several factors have been suggested to enhance glycogen resynthesis after exercise, including high glycemic index foods, liquid forms of carbohydrates, and beverages combining carbohydrates and protein. High glycemic index foods seem to be a desirable carbohydrate source during the postexercise recovery period.[92] High glycemic index foods may digest more quickly, allowing for a fast delivery of carbohydrate to the muscles. Choosing high glycemic index foods may be more relevant when athletes are choosing a small snack after exercise versus a well-balanced meal. If the snack is large enough to supply sufficient amounts of carbohydrate, then the rapid rise in blood glucose can be beneficial for a quick delivery of carbohydrate to hungry muscle cells. However, a well-balanced meal, composed of a variety of foods, can supply a wider range of not only carbohydrates, but also protein, vitamins, and minerals to a depleted body. In this case, choosing high glycemic index foods may have less relevance and importance.

Liquid carbohydrate sources may not necessarily be more beneficial than solids in regard to the rate of glycogen synthesis. Several studies have found similar glycogen restoration rates after the inges-

tion of an equal amount of carbohydrates in liquid and solid form.[93,94] Because no differences between liquids and solids exist, individual preferences can determine the form of carbohydrates ingested after exercise. Some athletes are ready for a full meal after training, and therefore, a balanced meal with sufficient carbohydrates will be appropriate. Other athletes have a small appetite after exercising, so a liquid meal has more appeal. The *Soccer Smoothie* recipe in Training Table 3.3 provides an example of a liquid source of carbohydrates as well as other nutrients. Depending on the size of the athlete and the duration of exercise, foods or beverages in addition to the smoothie might be required to supply sufficient amounts of carbohydrates to the body after a training session or a competition.

It has recently been suggested by some researchers that the combination of carbohydrates and protein in a postexercise beverage enhances glycogen storage beyond that of a carbohydrate-only product. One of the first studies to report this phenomenon was completed by Zawadzki and colleagues.[95] They reported an impressive 39% greater rate of glycogen repletion with a combined carbohydrate-protein versus carbohydrate-only supplement after exercise. However, the results are difficult to interpret because the carbohydrate-protein supplement provided 43% more energy than the carbohydrate-only supplement. Other studies have not been able to replicate the differences reported in the Zawadzki study when supplying isoenergetic beverages of varying macronutrient content.[96–98] It appears that both carbohydrate-only and carbohydrate-protein supplements can enhance glycogen resynthesis postexercise to a similar extent.[99] Therefore, at this time it can be concluded that the energy content of a postexercise beverage is more critical than macronutrient content is in determining the glycemic and insulin response as well as the extent of muscle glycogen resynthesis.

How much carbohydrate should be consumed after exercise or sport?

To maximize glycogen synthesis, athletes should consume carbohydrates at a rate of 1.2 grams per kilogram of body weight per hour for 3–4 hours postexercise.[30] For example, Sue is a soccer player. She weighs 150 pounds (68.2 kg). After a 1–2 hour prac-

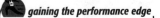
gaining the performance edge

Consuming carbohydrates after exercise accelerates the recovery process. A carbohydrate intake of 1.2 grams per kilogram of body weight per hour for 3–4 hours postexercise will ensure a complete restoration of glycogen levels.

tice or game, her carbohydrate needs are 82 grams of carbohydrates (68.2 kg × 1.2 grams of carbohydrate per kilogram of body weight = 82 grams of carbohydrates) to be consumed within 15–30 minutes of the end of her training session/competition, and then again every hour for 2–3 hours. Eighty-two grams of carbohydrates can be supplied by consuming:

- A banana and 8 ounces of yogurt
- 6–8 ounces of juice and a bagel
- 8 ounces of milk and 1 to 1½ cups of cereal

What are some examples of good meals/snacks for after exercising?

Meals and snacks postexercise should supply adequate amounts of carbohydrates as well as other nutrients. The best way to obtain a balance of all required postexercise nutrients is to consume whole foods. **Table 3.9** presents a variety of ideas for postexercise meals/snacks that provide 50–100 grams of carbohydrates.

TABLE 3.9	Quality Food and Beverage Choices for Postexercise Carbohydrate Replenishment

Meals and Snacks Supplying 50–75 Grams of Carbohydrates

Food/Beverage	Serving Size	Quantity of Carbohydrates
Juice	8 fl oz	27 g
Bagel w/peanut butter	1 medium + 2 tbsp	45 g
Tomato juice	12 fl oz	16 g
Turkey sandwich	2 slices bread + 3 oz meat	24 g
Cottage cheese w/pineapple	1 cup + ½ cup	25 g
Dried apricots	5 halves	11 g
Bran muffin	1 small	24 g
Yogurt (with fruit)	6 oz	33 g
Soccer Smoothie	1 smoothie	50 g
Veggie chili	8 oz	25 g
Corn bread	1 piece	29 g

Meals and Snacks Supplying 75–100 Grams of Carbohydrates

Food/Beverage	Serving Size	Quantity of Carbohydrates
Raisin bran	1 cup	47 g
Skim milk	8 fl oz	12 g
Apple	1 medium	21 g
Whole wheat toast and jam	1 slice + 1 tbsp	27 g
Banana	1 medium	27 g
Yogurt	6 oz	33 g
Macaroni and cheese	2 cups	80 g
Green salad	1½ cups	7 g
Skim milk	8 fl oz	12 g
Spaghetti	1½ cups	60 g
Marinara sauce	¾ cup	18 g
Mixed vegetables	¾ cup	18 g

The Box Score

Key Points of Chapter

- Adequate carbohydrate intake is essential for optimal sport performance. Carbohydrate intake should be in the range of 5 to 10 grams per kilogram of body weight per day, which should amount to approximately 55% to 70% of total daily calories.

- Athletes may not consume adequate calories to meet training and competition needs. Encouraging athletes to consume adequate calories during training and competition will help ensure appropriate carbohydrate intake.

- Carbohydrates are synthesized by plants via a process known as photosynthesis. Photosynthesis is an energy-requiring process that relies on the sun's light energy to combine water and carbon dioxide to make carbohydrates.

- Carbohydrates are commonly classified as simple or complex based on their chemical composition and structure. Both simple and complex carbohydrates provide energy, but have different nutrient profiles related to vitamins, minerals, fiber, and phytochemicals.

- Glucose is the most abundant simple carbohydrate found in nature and serves as an important energy source for cells in the human body.

- The storage form of carbohydrates in plants and animals is starch and glycogen, respectively.

- Fiber is a plant form of carbohydrates that is indigestible by the body and therefore provides minimal to no energy. However, fiber is an important part of a normal diet and helps to prevent high cholesterol, diabetes, and constipation.

- Artificial sweeteners can be derived from carbohydrates, amino acids, and other substances but are less digestible, thus limiting their caloric value to the body. Athletes may use artificial sweeteners to help control caloric intake; however, overuse can be unhealthy and detrimental to athletic performance.

- Carbohydrates are the sole energy source during very intense physical activity and thus are a key source of energy for many sport activities. Failure to ingest adequate amounts of carbohydrates not only robs the athlete of energy, but also can affect mental focus.

- The timing and type of carbohydrates consumed in the days and hours leading up to competition can be critical to performance. Experimenting with new foods or beverages on competition day can be disastrous. Always experiment weeks ahead of time for the best combination, types, and amounts of carbohydrates to consume.

- The richest sources of carbohydrates are grains, fruits, and vegetables. These nutrient-dense foods make up over half of the entire MyPlate food guidance system.

Dairy/alternatives and legumes, nuts/seeds, and soy products from the protein foods group also provide quality sources of carbohydrates. Carbohydrates obtained from sweets, desserts, and sodas are part of empty calories of the MyPlate food guidance system and should be moderated because they lack other nutrients important for optimal health and performance.

- The glycemic index of foods can be used to help identify the glucose response of a single food. However, the concepts of glycemic index, glycemic load, and glucose kinetics are still under investigation, and the limitations in practical daily eating need to be recognized.

- The body stores limited amounts of carbohydrates (approximately 400–600 grams), which is why athletes must pay particular attention to carbohydrate intake in their diet. Failure to replace glycogen stores used during training or competition can lead to low energy levels and decreased motivation, both of which can spell disaster for an athlete.

- Diets consisting of 60% to 70% of total calories from carbohydrates have been shown to increase resting muscle glycogen levels. High muscle glycogen levels have been shown to delay the time to fatigue in endurance athletes, which is one of the primary reasons endurance athletes carbohydrate-load in the week leading up to a competition.

- There is no one best precompetition meal, sports beverage, or postexercise snack that fits everyone's likes or tolerances. Athletes should follow the general guidelines of carbohydrate intake and experiment prior to competition with different meals, snacks, and/or drinks to find which best suits their unique requirements.

- Glucose polymer drinks and other carbohydrate-rich foods consumed during sport performance can increase blood glucose levels and delay onset of fatigue.

- Muscles are most receptive to uptaking blood glucose to replenish glycogen stores within 2–4 hours of exercise or competition. As a result, postgame snacks or meals should contain high-carbohydrate foods and should be consumed as soon as possible after the cessation of exercise.

Study Questions

1. Explain why restricting carbohydrates in the diets of athletes is detrimental.

2. Briefly discuss where carbohydrates come from and how they are formed in nature.

3. What roles do carbohydrates play in the body and how do these roles relate to athletic performance?

4. How many calories are derived from ingested carbohydrates that are classified as dietary fiber? What are the different types of fiber and what role do they play in the body?

5. What are the basic building blocks of carbohydrates? Based on the number of building blocks, how are different carbohydrates classified?

6. What is the difference between starch and glycogen?

7. Name and briefly discuss four of the commonly used artificial sweeteners. Are artificial sweeteners carbohydrates? What are some of the positives and negatives associated with using artificial sweeteners?

8. Discuss the various sources of carbohydrates in our diet. Which sources of carbohydrates should predominate in our diet? Which sources of carbohydrates should be limited, and why?

9. Discuss how knowledge of the glycemic index of foods can be used by athletes to optimize performance during sport. What about its application in regard to recovery?

10. Jason is an elite cross-country athlete who is currently training 5 days per week. He weighs 135 pounds. Based on his body weight, what should his daily carbohydrate intake be? Defend your answer.

11. What is carbohydrate loading? Which athletes would benefit most from it, and why?

12. Describe the "crossover concept" and its relevance to sport performance.

13. Jim is excited to be competing in his first half-marathon (13.1 miles) and comes to you for dietary advice for during the race. What advice regarding intake of carbohydrates might you give him to improve his chances of having a successful race?

14. Sarah is an elite triathlete who is currently training twice a day. What nutritional advice would you give her in regard to optimizing her recovery between workouts?

References

1. Duyff RL. *American Dietetic Association's Complete Food and Nutrition Guide*. Minneapolis, MN: Chronimed Publishing; 1996.

2. Insel P, Turner RE, Ross D. *Nutrition*. Sudbury, MA: Jones and Bartlett Publishers; 2002.

3. Institute of Medicine. Dietary, functional, and total fiber. In: *Dietary Reference Intakes for Energy, Carbohydrate, Fiber, Fat, Fatty Acids, Cholesterol, Protein, and Amino Acids (Macronutrients)*. Washington, DC: The National Academy Press; 2002:265–334.

4. Alaimo K, McDowell MA, Briefel RR, Bischof AM, Caughman CR, Loria CM, Johnson CL. Dietary intake of vitamins, minerals and fiber of persons ages 2 months and over in the United States; Third National Health and Nutrition Examination Survey, Phase 1, 1988–91. National Center for Health Statistics. 1994. Available at: http://www.cdc.gov/nchs/data/ad/ad258.pdf. Accessed January 23, 2011.

5. Henkel J. Sugar substitutes: Americans opt for sweetness and lite. *FDA Consumer Magazine*. 1999;33(6):12–17.

6. Levin GV. Tagatose, the new GRAS sweetener and health product. *J Med Food*. 2002;5(1):23–36.

7. American Dietetic Association. Position of the American Dietetic Association: use of nutritive and nonnutritive sweeteners. *J Am Diet Assoc*. 2004;104:255–275.

8. Cummings JH, Bingham SA, Heaton KW, Eastwood MA. Fecal weight, colon cancer risk and dietary intake of non-starch polysaccharides (dietary fiber). *Gastroenterology*. 1992;103:1783–1789.

9. Howe GR, Benito E, Castelleto R, et al. Dietary intake of fiber and decreased risk of cancers of the colon and rectum: evidence from the combined analysis of 13 case-control studies. *J Natl Cancer Inst*. 1992;84:1887–1896.

10. Schatzkin A, Lanza E, Corle D, et al. Lack of effect of a low-fat, high-fiber diet on the recurrence of colorectal adenomas. *New Engl J Med*. 2000;342:1149–1155.

11. Alberts DS, Marinez ME, Kor DL, et al. Lack of effect of a high-fiber cereal supplement on the recurrence of colorectal adenomas. *New Engl J Med*. 2000;324:1156–1162.

12. Bonithon-Kopp C, Kronborg O, Giacosa A, Rath U, Faivre J, for the European Cancer Prevention Organization Study Group. Calcium and fibre supplementation in prevention of colorectal adenoma recurrence: a randomized intervention trial. *Lancet*. 2000;356:1300–1306.

13. Bray GA, Nielsen SJ, Popkin BM. Consumption of high-fructose corn syrup in beverages may play a role in the epidemic of obesity. *Am J Clin Nutr*. 2004;79:537–543.

14. Gross LS, Li L, Ford ES, Liu S. Increased consumption of refined carbohydrates and the epidemic of type 2 diabetes in the United States: an ecologic assessment. *Am J Clin Nutr*. 2004;79:774–779.

15. Berkey CS, Rockett HRH, Field AE, Gillman MW, Colditz GA. Sugar-added beverages and adolescent weight change. *Obes Res*. 2004;12:778–788.

16. Welsh JA, Cogswell ME, Rogers S, Rockett H, Mei Z, Grummer-Strawn LM. Overweight among low-income preschool children associated with the consumption of soft drinks: Missouri 1999–2002. *Pediatrics*. 2005;115:e223–229.

17. Schulze MB, Manson JE, Ludwig DS, et al. Sugar-sweetened beverages, weight gain, and incidence of type 2 diabetes in young and middle-aged women. *JAMA*. 2004;292:927–934.

18. Drewnowski A, Bellisle F. Liquid calories, sugar, and body weight. *Am J Clin Nutr*. 2007;85:651–661.

19. Teff KL, Elliott SS, Tschop M, et al. Dietary fructose reduces circulating insulin and leptin, attenuates postprandial suppression of ghrelin, and increases triglycerides in women. *J Clin Endocrinol Metab*. 2004;89:2963–2972.

20. Institute of Medicine. *Dietary Reference Intakes for Energy, Carbohydrate, Fiber, Fat, Fatty Acids, Cholesterol, Protein, and Amino Acids (Macronutrients)*. Food and Nutrition Board. Washington, DC: National Academy Press; 2002.

21. Burke LM, Cox GR, Culmmings NK, Desbrow B. Guidelines for daily carbohydrate intake: do athletes achieve them? *Sports Med*. 2001;31(4):267–299.

22. Position of the American Dietetic Association, Dietitians of Canada, and the American College of Sports Medicine: nutrition and athletic performance. *J Am Diet Assoc*. 2000;100:1543–1556.

23. Walberg-Rankin J. Dietary carbohydrate as an ergogenic aid for prolonged and brief competition in sport. *Int J Sport Nutr*. 1995;5(suppl):S13–S28.

24. Jenkins DJ, Wolever TM, Taylor RH, et al. Glycemic index of foods: a physiological basis for carbohydrate exchange. *Am J Clin Nutr*. 1981;34:362–366.

25. Rankin JW. Glycemic index and exercise metabolism. *Sports Science Exchange*. 1997;10(1):SSE# 64.

26. Foster-Powell K, Holt SHA, Brand-Miller JC. International table of glycemic index and glycemic load values: 2002. *Am J Clin Nutr*. 2002;76(1):5–56.

27. Daly M. Sugars, insulin sensitivity, and the postprandial state. *Am J Clin Nutr*. 2003;78(4):865S–872S.

28. Salmeron J, Ascherio A, Rimm EB, et al. Dietary fiber, glycemic load, and risk of NIDDM in men. *Diabetes Care*. 1997;20:545–550.

29. Brand-Miller JC, Thomas M, Swan V, Ahmad ZI, Petocz P, Colagiuri S. Physiological validation of the concept of glycemic load in lean young adults. *J Nutr*. 2003;133:2728–2732.

30. Schenk S, Davidson CJ, Zderic TW, Byerley LO, Cole EF. Different glycemic indexes of breakfast cereals are not due to glucose entry into blood but to glucose removal by tissue. *Am J Clin Nutr*. 2003;78(4):742–748.

31. DeMarco HM, Sucher KP, Cisar CJ, Butterfield GE. Pre-exercise carbohydrate meals: application of glycemic index. *Med Science Sports Exerc*. 1999;31(1):164–170.

32. Thomas DE, Brotherhood JR, Brand JC. Carbohydrate feeding before exercise: effect of glycemic index. *Int J Sports Med*. 1991;12:180–186.

33. Thomas DE, Brotherhood JR, Brand JC. Plasma glucose levels after prolonged strenuous exercise correlate inversely with glycemic response to food consumed before exercise. *Int J Sports Med*. 1994;4:361–373.

34. Kirwan JP, O'Gorman D, Evans WJ. A moderate glycemic meal before endurance exercise can enhance performance. *J Applied Physiol*. 1998;84(1):53–59.

35. Stevenson EJ, Williams C, Mash LE, Phillips B, Nute ML. Influence of high-carbohydrate mixed meals with different glycemic indexes on substrate utilization during subsequent exercise in women. *Am J Clin Nutr*. 2006;84:354–360.

36. Wu CL, Nicholas C, Williams C, Took A, Hardy L. The influence of high-carbohydrate meals with different glycaemic indices on substrate utilization during subsequent exercise. *Br J Nutr*. 2003;90:1049–1056.

37. Febbraio MA, Stewart KL. CHO feeding before prolonged exercise: effect of glycemic index on muscle glycogenolysis and exercise performance. *J Appl Physiol*. 1996;81:1115–1120.

38. Sparks MJ, Selig SS, Febbraio MA. Pre-exercise carbohydrate ingestion: effect of the glycemic index on endurance performance. *Med Sci Sports Exerc*. 1998;30:844–849.

39. Manore MM. Using glycemic index to improve athletic performance. Gatorade Sports Science Institute News Online. Available at: http://www.gssiweb.com/Article_Detail.aspx?articleid=623. Accessed January 23, 2011.

40. Burke LM, Collier GR, Hargreaves M. Muscle glycogen storage after prolonged exercise: effect of the glycemic index of carbohydrate feedings. *J Appl Physiol*. 1993;75:1019–1023.

41. Kiens B, Raben AB, Valeur AK, Richter EA. Benefit of simple carbohydrates on the early post-exercise muscle glycogen repletion in male athletes (Abstract). *Med Sci Sports Exerc*. 1990;22(suppl 4):S88.

42. Burke LM, Collier GR, Hargreaves M. Glycemic index—a new tool in sport nutrition? *Int J Sport Nutr*. 1998;8:401–415.

43. Brooks GA, Mercier J. Balance of carbohydrate and lipid utilization during exercise: the "crossover" concept. *J Appl. Physiol*. 1994;76(6):2253–2261.

44. Felig P, Wahren J. Fuel homeostasis in exercise. *New Engl J Med*. 1975;293(21):1078–1084.

45. Coggan AR, Coyle EF. Metabolism and performance following carbohydrate ingestion late in exercise. *Med Sci Sports Exerc*. 1989;21:59–65.

46. Maughan RJ. *Nutrition in Sport*. London: Blackwell Science; 2000.

47. Bergstrom J, Hermansen L, Hultman E, Saltin B. Diet, muscle glycogen and physical performance. *Acta Physiol Scand*. 1967;71:140–150.

48. Sedlock DA. The latest on carbohydrate loading: a practical approach. *Curr Sports Med Rep*. 2008;7(4):209–213.

49. Tarnopolsky MA, Zawada C, Richmond LB, Carter S, Shearer J, Graham T, Phillips SM. Gender differences in carbohydrate loading are related to energy intake. *J Appl Physiol*. 2001;91:225–230.

50. McLay RT, Thomson CD, Williams SM, Rehrer NJ. Carbohydrate loading and female endurance athletes: effect of menstrual-cycle phase. *Int J Sport Nutr Exerc Metab*. 2007;17:189–205.

51. James AP, Lorraine M, Cullen D, Goodman C, Dawson B, Palmer TN, Fournier PA. Muscle glycogen supercompensation: absence of a gender-related difference. *Eur J Appl Physiol*. 2001;85:533–538.

52. Sherman WM, Costill DL, Fink WJ, Miller JM. Effect of exercise–diet manipulation on muscle glycogen and its subsequent utilization during performance. *Int J Sports Med*. 1981;2(2):114–118.

53. Ahlborg B, Bergstrom J, Brohult J, Ekelund LG, Maschio G. Human muscle glycogen content and capacity for prolonged exercise after different diets. *Forsvarsmedicin*. 1967;3:85–99.

54. Burke LM, Hawley JA, Schabort EJ, Gibson ASC, Mujika I, Noakes TD. Carbohydrate loading failed to improve 100-km cycling performance in a placebo-controlled trial. *J Appl Physiol*. 2000;88:1284–1290.

55. Burke LM, Angus DJ, Cox GR, Cummings NK, Febbraio MA, Gawthorn K, Hawley JA, Minehan M, Martin DT, Hargreaves M. Effect of fat adaptation and carbohydrate restoration on metabolism and performance during prolonged cycling. *J Appl Physiol*. 2000;89(6):2413–2421.

56. Bussau VA, Fairchild TJ, Rao A, Steele P, Fournier PA. Carbohydrate loading in human muscle: an improved 1 day protocol. *Eur J Appl Physiol*. 2002;87:290–295.

57. Dunford M. *Sports Nutrition: A Practice Manual for Professionals*. Chicago, IL: American Dietetic Association; 2006.

58. Sherman WM, Peden MC, Wright DA. Carbohydrate feedings 1 hour before exercise improves cycling performance. *Am J Clin Nutr*. 1991;54:866–870.

59. Sherman WM, Brodowicz G, Wright DA, Allen WK, Simonsen J, Dernbach A. Effects of 4 hour pre-exercise carbohydrate feedings on cycling performance. *Med Sci Sports Exerc*. 1989;12:598–604.

60. Febbraio MA, Keenan J, Angus DJ, Campbell SE, Garnham AP. Pre-exercise carbohydrate ingestion, glucose kinetics and muscle glycogen use: effect of the glycemic index. *J Appl Physiol*. 2000;89:1845–1851.

61. Foster C, Costill DL, Fink WJ. Effects of pre-exercise feedings on endurance performance. *Med Sci Sports Exerc*. 1979;11(1):1–5.

62. Febbraio MA, Chiu A, Angus DJ, Arkinstall MJ, Hawley JA. Effects of carbohydrate ingestion before and during exercise on glucose kinetics and performance. *J Applied Physiol*. 2000;89:2220–2226.

63. Chambers ES, Bridge MW, Jones DA. Carbohydrate sensing in the human mouth: effects on exercise performance and brain activity. *J Physiol*. 2009;587(8):1779–1794.

64. Coggan AR, Coyle EF. Reversal of fatigue during prolonged exercise by carbohydrate infusion or ingestion. *J Applied Physiol*. 1987;63:2388–2395.

65. Coggan AR, Coyle EF. Metabolism and performance following carbohydrate ingestion late in exercise. *Med Sci Sports Exerc*. 1989;21:59–65.

66. Coyle EF, Coggan AR, Hemmert MK, Ivy JL. Muscle glycogen utilization during prolonged strenuous exercise when fed carbohydrate. *J Applied Physiol*. 1986;61(1):165–172.

67. Hargreaves M, Costill DL, Coggan AR, Fink WJ, Nishibata I. Effect of carbohydrate feedings on muscle glycogen utilization and exercise performance. *Med Sci Sports Exerc*. 1984;16(3):219–222.

68. Ivy JL, Costill DL, Fink WJ, Lower RW. Influence of caffeine and carbohydrate feedings on endurance performance. *Med Sci Sports Exerc*. 1979;11(1):6–11.

69. Ivy JL, Miller W, Dover V, et al. Endurance improved by ingestion of a glucose polymer supplement. *Med Sci Sports Exerc*. 1983;15(6):466–471.

70. Decombaz J, Sartori D, Arnaud MJ, Thelin AL, Schurch P, Howald H. Oxidation and metabolic effects of fructose and glucose ingested before exercise. *Int J Sports Med*. 1985;6(5):282–286.

71. Hawley JA, Dennis SC, Nowitz A, Brouns F, Noakes TD. Exogenous carbohydrate oxidation from maltose and glucose ingested during prolonged exercise. *Eur J Applied Physiol*. 1992;64(6):523–527.

72. Leijssen DPC, Saris WHM, Jeukendrup AE, Wagenmakers AJ. Oxidation of orally ingested [13C]-glucose and [13C]-galactose during exercise. *J Applied Physiol*. 1995;79(3):720–725.

73. Massicotte D, Peronnet F, Allah C, Hillaire-Marcel C, Ledoux M, Brisson G. Metabolic response to [13C] glucose and [13C] fructose ingestion during exercise. *J Applied Physiol*. 1986;61(3):1180–1184.

74. Massicotte D, Peronnet F, Brisson G, Bakkouch K, Hillaire-Marcel C. Oxidation of a glucose polymer during exercise: comparison with glucose and fructose. *J Applied Physiol*. 1989;66(1):179–183.

75. Moodley D, Noakes TD, Bosch AN, Hawley JA, Schall R, Dennis SC. Oxidation of exogenous carbohydrate during prolonged exercise: the effects of the carbohydrate type and its concentration. *Eur J Applied Physiol*. 1992;64(4):328–334.

76. Rehrer NJ, Wagenmakers AJM, Beckers EJ, et al. Gastric emptying, absorption and carbohydrate oxidation during prolonged exercise. *J Applied Physiol*. 1992;72(2):468–475.

77. Saris WHM, Goodpaster BH, Jeukendrup AE, Brouns F, Halliday D, Wagenmakers AJ. Exogenous carbohydrate oxidation from different carbohydrate sources during exercise. *J Applied Physiol*. 1993;75(5):2168–2172.

78. Jeukendrup AE, Jentjens R. Oxidation of carbohydrate feedings during prolonged exercise. *Sports Med*. 2000;29(6):407–424.

79. Jeukendrup AE, Wagenmakers AJ, Stegen JH, Gijsen AP, Brouns F, Saris WH. Carbohydrate ingestion can completely suppress endogenous glucose production during exercise. *Amer J Physiol*. 1999;276:E672–E683.

80. Convertino VA, Armstrong LA, Coyle EF, et al. Exercise and fluid replacement. *Med Sci Sports Exerc*. 1996;28(1):i–vii.

81. Guezennec CY, Satabin P, Duforez F, Merino D, Peronnet F, Koziet J. Oxidation of corn starch, glucose and fructose ingested before exercise. *Med Sci Sports Exerc*. 1989;21(1):45–50.

82. Krzentowski G, Jandrain B, Pirnay F, et al. Availability of glucose given orally during exercise. *J Applied Physiol*. 1984;56(2):315–320.

83. Pirnay F, Lacroix M, Mosora F, Luyckx A, Lefebvre P. Effect of glucose ingestion on energy substrate utilization during prolonged muscular exercise. *Eur J Applied Physiol*. 1977;36(4):247–254.

84. Burelle Y, Peronnet F, Charpentier S, Lavoie C, Hillaire-Marcel C, Massicotte D. Oxidation of an oral [13C] glucose load at rest and during prolonged exercise in trained and sedentary subjects. *J Applied Physiol*. 1999;86(1):52–60.

85. Massicotte D, Peronnet F, Brisson G, Boivin L, Hillaire-Marcel C. Oxidation of exogenous carbohydrate during prolonged exercise in fed and fasted conditions. *Int J Sports Med*. 1990;11(4):253–258.

86. Massicotte D, Peronnet F, Adopo E, Brisson GR, Hillaire-Marcel C. Effect of metabolic rate on the oxidation of ingested glucose and fructose during exercise. *Int J Sports Med*. 1994;15(4):177–180.

87. McConell G, Kloot K, Hargreaves M. Effect of timing of carbohydrate ingestion on endurance exercise performance. *Med Sci Sports Exerc*. 1996;28(10):1300–1304.

88. Costill DL, Bowers R, Branam G, Sparks K. Muscle glycogen utilization during prolonged exercise on successive days. *J Applied Physiol*. 1971;31(6):834–838.

89. Costill DL, Miller JM. Nutrition for endurance sport: carbohydrate and fluid balance. *Int J Sports Med*. 1980;1:2–14.

90. Ivy JL, Katz AL, Cutler CL, Sherman WM, Coyle EF. Muscle glycogen synthesis after exercise: effects of time of carbohydrate ingestion. *J Applied Physiol*. 1988;64(4):1480–1485.

91. Storlie J. The art of refueling. *Training and Condition*. 1998;8:29–35.

92. Parco MS, Wong SHS. Use of the glycemic index: effects on feeding patterns and exercise performance. *J Physiol Anthropol Appl Human Science*. 2004;23:1–6.

93. Keizer HA, Kuipers J, van Krandenburg G, Geurten P. Influence of liquid and solid meals on muscle glycogen resynthesis, plasma fuel hormone response and maximal physical work capacity. *Int J Sports Med*. 1986;8(2):99–104.

94. Reed MJ, Brozinick JT, Lee MC, Ivy JL. Muscle glycogen storage post-exercise: effects of mode of carbohydrate administration. *J Applied Physiol*. 1989;66(2):720–726.

95. Zawadzki KM, Yaspelkis BB, Ivy JL. Carbohydrate–protein complex increases the rate of muscle glycogen storage after exercise. *J Applied Physiol*. 1992;72:1854–1859.

96. Carrithers JA, Williamson DL, Gallagher PM, Godard MP, Schulze KE, Trappe SW. Effect of post-exercise carbohydrate–protein feedings on muscle glycogen restoration. *J Applied Physiol*. 2000;88:1976–1982.

97. Roy BD, Tarnopolsky MA. Influence of differing macronutrient intakes on muscle glycogen resynthesis after resistance exercise. *J Applied Physiol*. 1998;84:890–896.

98. Wojcik JR, Walberg-Rankin J, Smith L, Gwazdauskas FC. Comparison of carbohydrate and milk-based beverages on muscle damage and glycogen following exercise. *Int J Sport Nutr Exerc Metab*. 2001;11(4):406–419.

99. Tarnopolsky MA, Bosman M, MacDonald JR, Vandeputte D, Martin J, Roy BD. Postexercise protein–carbohydrate and carbohydrate supplements increase muscle glycogen in men and women. *J Applied Physiol*. 1997;83(6):1877–1883.

Additional Resources

Bergstrom J, Hermansen L, Hultman E, Saltin B. Diet, muscle glycogen and physical performance. *Acta Physiol Scand*. 1967;71(2):140–150.

Bergstrom J, Hultman E. Muscle glycogen synthesis after exercise: an enhancing factor localized to the muscle cells in man. *Nature*. 1967;210(33):309–310.

Blom PCS, Hostmark AT, Vaage O, Kardel KR, Maehlum S. Effect of different post-exercise sugar diets on the rate of muscle glycogen synthesis. *Med Sci Sports Exerc*. 1987;19(5):491–496.

Casa DJ, Armstrong LE, Hillman SK, et al. National Athletic Trainers' Association position statement: fluid replacement for athletes. *J Athletic Train*. 2000;35(2):212–224.

Cummings JH. Microbial digestion of complex carbohydrates in man. *Proc Nutr Soc*. 1984;43(1):35–44.

Giovannucci E, Ascherio A, Rimm EB, Stampfer MJ, Colditz GA, Willett WC. Intake of carotenoids and retinal in relation to risk of prostate cancer. *J Natl Cancer Inst*. 1995;87:1767–1776.

Ivy J. Glycogen resynthesis after exercise: effect of carbohydrate intake. *Int J Sports Med*. 1998;19(supplement):S142–S145.

Ivy JL, Lee MC, Brozinick JT, Reed MJ. Muscle glycogen storage after different amounts of carbohydrate ingestion. *J Applied Physiol*. 1988;65(5):2018–2023.

McBurney MI, Thompson LU. Fermentative characteristics of cereal brans and vegetable fibers. *Nutr Cancer*. 1990;13(4):271–280.

Siu PM, Wong SH. Use of the glycemic index: effects on feeding patterns and exercise performance. *J Physiol Anthropol Appl Human Science*. 2004;23(1):1–6.

U.S. Food and Drug Administration. Chapter IV—nutrition labeling (editorial revision). Center for Food Safety and Applied Nutrition. 1999. Available at: http://www.fda.gov/Food/GuidanceComplianceRegulatoryInformation/GuidanceDocuments/DietarySupplements/DietarySupplementlabelingguide/ucm070597.htm. Accessed January 23, 2011.

U.S. Food and Drug Administration. Chapter V—ingredient list. Center for Food Safety and Applied Nutrition. 1999. Available at: http://www.fda.gov/Food/GuidanceComplianceRegulatoryInformation/GuidanceDocuments/DietarySupplements/DietarySupplementlabelingguide/ucm070611.htm. Accessed January 23, 2011.

U.S. Food and Drug Administration. Chapter VI—definitions of claims. Center for Food Safety and Applied Nutrition. 2004. Available at: http://www.fda.gov/Food/GuidanceComplianceRegulatoryInformation/GuidanceDocuments/DietarySupplements/DietarySupplementlabelingguide/ucm070613.htm. Accessed January 23, 2011.

U.S. Food and Drug Administration. Food additives permitted for direct addition to food for human consumption: aspartame. *Fed Register*. 1984;49:6672–6677.

U.S. Food and Drug Administration. Food additives permitted for direct addition to food for human consumption: sucralose. Code of Federal Regulations Title 21, 172.63.

Van Munster IP, deBoer HM, Jansen MC, et al. Effect of resistant starch on breath–hydrogen and methane excretion in healthy volunteers. *Am J Clin Nutr*. 1994;59:626–630.

CHAPTER

4

Fats

Shelley is a marathoner from Austin, Texas. She has been competing in marathons for more than 5 years and is the type of person who enjoys taking on new physical challenges. Although she is not an experienced swimmer, she has agreed to join some friends in tackling the challenge of swimming the English Channel. The plan is to train for a year and then make an attempt at swimming the Channel. Because of the energetic demands of her sport, she is extremely lean and in excellent cardiovascular shape. She loves the warm temperatures in the South and gets chilled easily, which is a concern of hers because she knows the water temperatures in the Channel are very cold.

Question

- What nutrition recommendations would you give Shelley in regard to fat intake to address both her physical and dietary needs over the next 12 months as she trains for the swim? Include suggestions for fat intake before, during, and after the actual Channel swim.

What's the big deal about fats?

Fats, similar to carbohydrates, are an important nutrient for both athletes and nonathletes. They serve as a primary energy source at rest and during light- to moderate-intensity exercise. In addition, dietary fat provides essential fatty acids required for normal physiological functioning of the body, adds flavor to foods, and is a calorie-dense nutrient capable of meeting the high daily energy needs of athletes.

However, fat is an often maligned nutrient because of the well-known association of cholesterol and saturated fats with heart disease. The thought of body fat also raises negative feelings, particularly in athletes who are aware of the potential impact excessive levels of body fat can have on sport performance. In some instances, extreme behaviors are adopted to maintain or decrease body fat levels. The purpose of this chapter is to provide the reader with the knowledge required to keep a healthy and informed perspective on an essential nutrient that is often feared and shrouded in misconceptions.

What are fats?

Fats are molecules that belong to a group of compounds known as lipids. Lipids are organic, carbon-containing compounds that are **hydrophobic** (water insoluble), **lipophilic** (fat soluble), and have a physical characteristic of feeling greasy to the touch. The fact that lipids are not water soluble affects how they are digested, absorbed, and transported throughout the body compared to the other macronutrients such as carbohydrates and proteins (see Chapter 2). Calorically, lipids are an energy-rich nutrient yielding 9 calories per gram, compared to only 4 calories per gram for both carbohydrates and proteins.

Similar to other nutrients, lipids are obtained from foods and beverages. Lipids are found in foods of both plant and animal origin. In addition, nonlipid molecules can be converted into lipids within the body. For example, if carbohydrates or proteins are consumed in excess, they will be converted into lipids (i.e., fats) and stored in adipose tissue for later use as energy.

How are lipids (fats) classified?

A number of different chemical compounds are found in food and within the body that are classified as lipids. However, the most important ones fall into three main categories based on their molecular structure: triglycerides, phospholipids, and sterols. Although all three of these are lipids, each plays a significantly different role in the body.

Triglycerides make up the majority of lipids found within the body and in foods and beverages. In fact, triglycerides provide much of the flavor and texture in foods. **Phospholipids** are found in both plants and animals and have a unique molecular structure that allows them to be both fat and water soluble. Phospholipids constitute the cell membranes of various tissues found throughout the body. In addition, because they are water soluble, phospholipids help suspend other hydrophobic lipids in water. Finally, a very small percentage of fats in the body exist as **sterols**. Sterols are quite different from both triglycerides and phospholipids in their structure and function. The most commonly known sterol is cholesterol. Triglycerides, phospholipids, and sterols are discussed in more detail in the following sections.

What are triglycerides?

Triglycerides are commonly occurring fats that are more accurately classified as simple lipids. Triglycerides, also referred to as **triacylglycerols**, are the predominant form of fats found in the human diet. An estimated 98% of dietary fats are triglycerides.[1] In addition, triglycerides are the most common type of fat found in the human body. Triglycerides serve as a major energy reserve and are stored primarily in adipocytes located throughout the body. Triglycerides are also stored in lesser amounts in the liver and muscle, where they are more readily available for use as energy during exercise. Because triglycerides make up the overwhelming majority of fats found in the diet and body, the terms *triglycerides* and *fats* are used interchangeably throughout this chapter and the text.

What is the molecular structure of a triglyceride?

The structure of a triglyceride is a combination of **glycerol** and three fatty acids. The glycerol "backbone" of a triglyceride molecule is

hydrophobic Term used to describe molecules or compounds that are water-insoluble. Lipids are hydrophobic substances.

lipophilic Substances that are fat soluble.

phospholipid A type of lipid that consists of a glycerol backbone, two fatty acids, and a phosphate group. Phospholipids are derived from both plant and animal sources and are both water and fat soluble. Phospholipids constitute the cell membranes of tissues throughout the body.

sterols A category of lipids that possess carbon rings in their structure rather than carbon chains. Cholesterol is the most commonly known sterol.

triacylglycerols A category of lipids more commonly referred to as triglycerides (see triglycerides, defined in Chapter 2).

glycerol A three-carbon molecule that makes up the backbone of mono-, di-, and triglycerides.

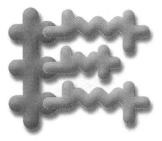

Figure 4.1 Generic triglyceride structure.

always constant; however, the three fatty acids attached to the glycerol may differ (see Figure 4.1). During triglyceride breakdown, one fatty acid may be removed, leaving a diglyceride, or two fatty acids may be removed, leaving a monoglyceride. The fatty acids cleaved from the glycerol backbone become what are known as free fatty acids (see "What are fatty acids?" later in this chapter) and are available for use by the body as needed. When all three fatty acids have been stripped from the triglyceride, the remaining glycerol backbone can be metabolized for energy or used to form blood glucose in the liver.

What are some of the functions of triglycerides in the body?

As noted earlier, triglycerides are the predominant form of fat found in the body. Fats perform a variety of critical roles and thus are considered essential nutrients. The following are the six main functions of fats in the body; the functions of other lipids in the body, primarily phospholipids and sterols, are discussed later in this chapter.

1. *Triglycerides serve as an important source of energy at rest and during exercise.* At rest, in well-fed individuals, dietary and stored fats can supply approximately 60% to 80% of the body's energy needs. During exercise, both fats and carbohydrates serve as fuel sources, with fats being the predominant energy source during low to moderate exercise intensities (see Chapter 2).

2. *Fat serves as an abundant energy reserve for the body.* In athletic populations, fat tissue accounts for approximately 8–12% and 18–22% of body weight in males and females, respectively. Some is stored as visceral fat (i.e., in adipocytes surrounding the internal organs), but most fat is stored subcutaneously (i.e., beneath the surface of the skin). Small amounts of fat are stored in muscle, where it serves as a readily available energy source. In total, as much as 80,000–100,000 calories can be stored as fat in a 70-kilogram man

who is within a healthy body fat range. These fats are available to provide fuel when energy intake is lower than expenditure.

Energy stored as fat in the body is advantageous for two reasons. First, fats yield more than twice the number of calories per gram (9 kcal/gram) than proteins or carbohydrates (4 kcal/gram). In other words, fats are a concentrated storage form of energy in that twice the calories can be stored for an equivalent increase in body weight resulting from stored carbohydrates as glycogen. Second, because fats are hydrophobic, they are stored with much less water than carbohydrates. Carbohydrates are hydrophilic—each gram of stored carbohydrate (i.e., glycogen) is associated with 3 grams of water. Therefore, fats not only yield twice the energy, but also are a much lighter storage form of energy for the body (see **Table 4.1**).

3. *Visceral and subcutaneous fat provide protection to vital organs and serve as a thermal and electrical insulator in the body.* Visceral fat stores act like gel-packing used to protect fragile materials during shipping. Essentially, their gel-like consistency helps to cushion internal organs, thus preventing damage during falls, jarring types of activities, and contact sports. Visceral fat is relatively inert and is less likely to be utilized as an energy source unless adipose tissue is depleted. Subcutaneous fat provides a layer of protection

TABLE 4.1	Difference in Weight with Fat Versus Carbohydrate Storage
Average calories stored in body fat = 80,000–100,000 calories	
Fat	**Carbohydrate**
80,000 calories	80,000 calories
÷ 9 kcal/gram	÷ 4 kcal/gram
8889 grams	20,000 grams
× 0.1 grams water stored/gram fat	× 3 grams water stored/gram carbohydrate
889 additional grams	60,000 additional grams
889 + 8889 = 9778 grams of energy stored as fat	60,000 + 20,000 = 80,000 grams of energy stored as carbohydrate
9778 ÷ 454 g/lb =	80,000 ÷ 454 g/lb =
21.5 lb	**176 lb**

for skeletal muscles and also acts as a thermal insulator for the body. Fat keeps heat from transferring away from the body, especially in cold weather and water sports. This is critical because maintenance of body temperature is important for normal internal organ and cellular function. In the case of distance swimmers, body fat not only serves as an energy source and insulator, but also buoys the swimmer in the water, thus decreasing drag, which can potentially increase performance. Finally, fats are also used in the formation of myelin, a fatty substance that serves as insulation for nerve cells. This fatty myelin insulation helps speed conduction of electrical signals along the appropriate neural pathway and prevents unwanted spread of electrical activity to adjacent nerves. In other words, myelin is analogous to the plastic sheath found on electrical wires that directs the electrical flow along the length of the wire but prevents it from spreading to any other wires that may be lying beside it.

4. *Fats play an important role as carriers of substances into the body and within the bloodstream.* Fats carry fat-soluble vitamins A, D, E, and K; carotenoids; and other fat-soluble phytochemicals. Without fat in the diet, fat-soluble vitamins would not be absorbed and deficiencies would result. Fats also aid in the absorption of other fat-soluble substances such as lycopene. Lycopene, a phytochemical, is absorbed more readily when tomato-based products contain some fat. For example, canned tomatoes mixed with an olive oil vinaigrette dressing will enhance the absorption of lycopene. When fat is removed from a product such as skim milk, the fat-soluble vitamins are removed as well. Therefore, as indicated on the label, nonfat milk is "Vitamin A and D fortified" because the fat-soluble vitamins need to be added back into the product.

5. *Fats enhance the sensory qualities of foods.* Chemicals within the fat molecules of food provide flavor, odor, and texture. Cooking fatty foods or frying foods in fat releases the odors and seals in flavor. Fats in baked goods provide products with a moist and light texture and a flaky structure. Fats also offer a creamy, smooth mouthfeel to many products, thus enhancing their appeal.

6. *Fat consumption during meals or snacks can enhance satiety level.* Fats are calorically dense compared to carbohydrates or proteins. Fats take longer to digest and can provide a physical

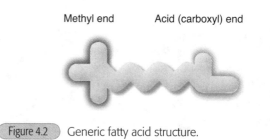

Methyl end   Acid (carboxyl) end

Figure 4.2   Generic fatty acid structure.

feeling of satiation for a longer time between meals.

What are fatty acids?

Fatty acids are basically carbon atoms linked in a chainlike fashion. All fatty acids have an organic acid group or a carboxyl acid (COOH) at one end and a methyl (CH_3) group at the other end (see Figure 4.2). The carboxyl group is referred to as the alpha end, and the methyl group makes up the omega end of the fatty acid. Paying attention to the different ends of the fatty acid chain is important because it provides for a consistent way of classifying fatty acids based on chain length and the number and location of single and/or double bonds. These differences determine not only the type of fatty acid, but also its physical characteristics, how it is digested and assimilated, and the role it will play within the body.

What is the effect of fatty acid chain length?
As mentioned earlier, the carbon chains of fatty acids vary in length. The number of carbons in a chain affect how the fatty acid is digested, absorbed, and used in the body. Short-chain fatty acids (SCFAs) consist of 2 to 4 carbons in a chain, medium-chain fatty acids (MCFAs) contain between 6 and 10 carbons, and long-chain fatty acids (LCFAs) contain 12 or more carbons (see Figure 4.3). The shorter the carbon chain, the more liquid the fat is at room temperature and the more soluble it is in water. SCFAs and MCFAs are digested and absorbed more quickly than LCFAs. Rarely are SCFAs found naturally in food sources, with the exception of butyric acid, found in milk fat. The SCFAs are a by-product of bacterial fermentation of undigested food in the large intestine. Most commonly, bacteria work on soluble fiber in the colon and produce SCFAs. The short-chain fatty acids that are produced in this process are absorbed by the colon cells and used as an energy source. The fermentation process is anaerobic; thus less energy is recovered from fiber than the 4 calories/gram recovered from other carbohydrates.[1] The number of actual calories is still unclear,

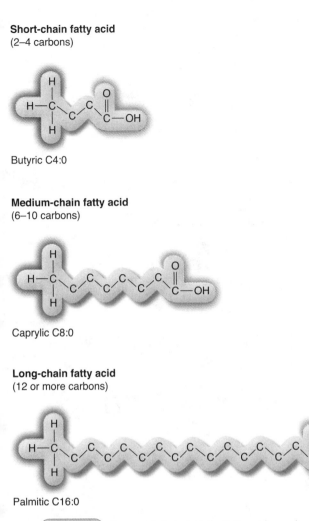

Short-chain fatty acid
(2–4 carbons)

Butyric C4:0

Medium-chain fatty acid
(6–10 carbons)

Caprylic C8:0

Long-chain fatty acid
(12 or more carbons)

Palmitic C16:0

Figure 4.3 Fatty acid chain length. Fatty acids can be classified by their chain length as short-, medium-, and long-chain fatty acids.

but it is likely that the energy yield is 1.5–2 calories per gram.[2,3] Some research suggests that butyric acid stimulates colon cells to suppress cancer growth, a finding that may explain how dietary fiber, when bacteria attack fiber and release other SCFAs, may aid in the prevention of colon cancer.[4]

What does fatty acid saturation level indicate?
Each carbon in a fatty acid carbon chain has four bonds. The bonds between the carbons can be either single bonds or double bonds. The remaining bonds that branch from the carbon backbone can be filled by other atoms. Hydrogen is the atom commonly filling the other bonds in fatty acids (see Figure 4.4). When the carbons in a chain are linked by single bonds and the remaining two bonds are filled with hydrogen, the fatty acid is termed **saturated**. This means that all bonds are full (saturated) with hydrogen atoms. **Unsaturated fatty acids** have one or more

double bonds between carbons in the chain. With unsaturated fats, the carbons attached by the double bond can accept only one hydrogen atom. A **monounsaturated fatty acid (MUFA)** has one double bond in its carbon chain, whereas a **polyunsaturated fatty acid (PUFA)** has two or more double bonds (see Figure 4.4).

Hydrogenation is a chemical process in which hydrogen atoms are added to unsaturated fatty acids. The introduction of the hydrogen atoms breaks some of the double bonds between carbons and thus causes the previously unsaturated fat to become more saturated. This artificial hydrogenation process allows foods containing unsaturated fats to take on the somewhat desirable physical properties of saturated fats. As the saturation content of the fat in food increases, the food becomes harder at room temperature. For example, stick margarine is produced through the hydrogenation of unsaturated vegetable oils. Vegetable oil is liquid at room temperature, but it becomes solid after hydrogenation, making it more desirable for baking and cooking.

Although foods are often labeled as containing either saturated or unsaturated fatty acids, it is important to realize that foods actually contain a combination of unsaturated and saturated fats. Plant foods generally are lower in saturated fats than foods from animal sources. However, food labels can help individuals identify the total and saturated fat content of foods. **Table 4.2** lists common foods that contain fat and their respective amounts of saturated and unsaturated fats.

Information regarding the total fat content and the type of fat in foods is important because saturated fats have been implicated in cardiovascular disease. They have been found to contribute to **atherosclerosis**, the buildup of fatty plaques on the interior arterial walls, particularly in the arteries of the heart and neck. Reducing saturated fat intake by reducing total fat intake and substituting mono- and

saturated fatty acid A fatty acid in which all hydrogen-binding sites are filled, and thus no double bonds exist in its hydrocarbon chain.

unsaturated fatty acid A fatty acid whose hydrocarbon chain contains one or more double bonds.

monounsaturated fatty acid A fatty acid whose hydrocarbon chain contains one double bond.

polyunsaturated fatty acid A fatty acid whose hydrocarbon chain contains two or more double bonds.

hydrogenation A chemical process in which hydrogen atoms are added to unsaturated fatty acids. Hydrogenation of fatty acids leads to the formation of trans fatty acids, which are a growing health concern in regard to cardiovascular disease.

atherosclerosis The progressive narrowing of the lumens of arteries caused by fatty deposits on their interior walls. Over time these fatty plaques can block blood supply to vital tissues, causing poor delivery of oxygen; complete blockage results in cell death.

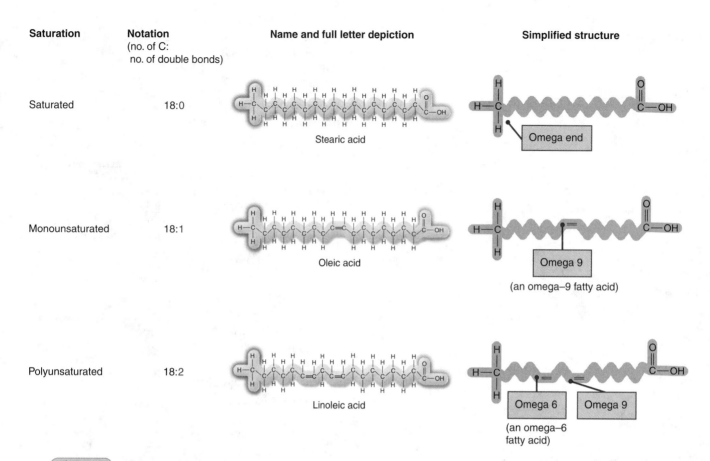

Saturation	Notation (no. of C: no. of double bonds)	Name and full letter depiction	Simplified structure
Saturated	18:0	Stearic acid	Omega end
Monounsaturated	18:1	Oleic acid	Omega 9 (an omega–9 fatty acid)
Polyunsaturated	18:2	Linoleic acid	Omega 6 Omega 9 (an omega–6 fatty acid)

Figure 4.4   Saturation of fatty acids. Saturated, monounsaturated, and polyunsaturated fatty acids. Hydrogens saturate the carbon chain of saturated fatty acids. Unsaturated fatty acids are missing some hydrogens and have one (mono) or more (poly) carbon–carbon double bonds.

isomer Compounds like unsaturated fats that may have the exact same molecular makeup as another compound but exist in a different geometric shape.

cis A type of molecular configuration in which the atoms surrounding a double bond are arranged on the same side of the molecule. Most naturally occurring unsaturated fatty acids exist in the cis configuration.

trans A type of molecular configuration in which the atoms surrounding a double bond are arranged on opposite sides of the molecule. Trans fatty acids are not common in nature but are formed during the process of hydrogenation.

polyunsaturated fats in the diet are recommended to reduce cardiovascular disease risk.

What is a trans fatty acid?
Unsaturated fatty acids that are identical in molecular makeup but exist in different geometric forms (i.e., shapes) are known as **isomers**. The location of the hydrogen atoms on each side of the double bond in the fatty acid determines whether the fat is in the **cis** or **trans** position. In the cis position, the hydrogen atoms on either side of the double bonds are on the same side of the carbon chain. This causes the fatty acid to bend slightly. In the trans position, the hydrogen atoms on either side of the double bond are on opposite sides of the car-

bon chain, and thus the fatty acid is straight rather than bent (see Figure 4.5). Fatty acids in nature are almost exclusively found in the cis formation; however, the commercial processing of foods has increased the occurrence of trans fats in our diets.

The commercial process of hydrogenation adds hydrogen at some of the double bond locations creating the trans positioning at one or more of the bonds. Most trans fatty acids are monounsaturated (contain one double bond) and are found in foods such as stick margarine, solid vegetable shortenings, snack items, and packaged foods. The problem with trans fats is that recent studies have implicated them with raising blood cholesterol levels.

What are omega fatty acids?
The methyl end of a fatty acid is the omega end. The double bond that occurs closest to this end identifies the omega classification. Because there are double bonds in all of these classifications, the omega fatty acids are all unsaturated fatty acids. There are omega-3, -6, and -9 classifications that signify the first double bond location from the omega end at the

TABLE
4.2
Fat Content of Various Foods

Food Item	Serving Size	Total Fat (grams)	Saturated Fat (grams)	Monounsaturated Fat (grams)	Polyunsaturated Fat (grams)
Grains					
Oatmeal, dry	½ cup	2.5	0.5	1.0	1.0
English muffin	1 muffin	1	0.1	0.2	0.5
Pasta, cooked	1 cup	0.9	0.1	0.1	0.4
Brown rice	1 cup	1.8	0.4	0.6	0.6
Whole wheat bread	1 slice	1.2	0.3	0.5	0.3
Whole wheat pita	1 pita (6½")	1.7	0.3	0.2	0.7
Blueberry muffin, made from a mix	1 muffin	6.2	1.2	1.5	3.1
Biscuit	1.2 oz	4.6	0.9	2.8	0.2
Fruits/Vegetables					
Pear	1 medium	1	<0.1	0.1	0.2
Orange	1 medium	0	0	0	0
Watermelon	1 cup	0.7	0.1	0.2	0.2
Banana	1 medium	0.5	0.2	<0.1	0.1
Spinach, raw	½ cup	0	0	0	0
Broccoli, cooked	½ cup	0.1	<0.1	<0.1	<0.1
Carrots, cooked	½ cup	0.1	<0.1	<0.1	<0.1
Avocado	1 medium	27	5.3	14.8	4.5
Dairy/Alternative					
Skim milk	8 oz	0.5	0.4	0.2	<0.1
1% milk	8 oz	2.6	1.6	0.7	0.1
2% milk	8 oz	4.7	2.9	1.4	0.2
Whole milk	8 oz	8	5.1	2.4	0.3
Cottage cheese, 2%	¼ cup	4.4	2.8	1.2	0.1
Swiss cheese	1 oz	8	5.0	2.1	0.3
Soy milk	8 oz	5	0.5	1.0	3.0
Protein Foods					
Ground beef, lean	3 oz	13.2	5.2	5.8	0.4
Chicken with skin	3 oz	9	2.4	3.4	1.9
Chicken without skin	3 oz	3.1	0.9	1.1	0.7
Turkey, white meat, without skin	3 oz	3	1.0	0.6	0.9
Turkey, dark meat, without skin	3 oz	6	2.2	1.5	2.0
Pork chop	3 oz	6.9	2.5	3.1	0.5
Salmon, pink	3 oz	4	1.0	0.8	0.6
Orange roughy	3 oz	1	<0.1	0.5	<0.1
Veggie burger	1 patty	0.5	0.1	0.3	0.2
Almonds	1 oz	15	1.1	9.5	3.6
Oils					
Margarine, stick	1 tbsp	11	2.1	5.2	3.2
Butter	1 tbsp	12	7.2	3.3	0.4
Olive oil	1 tbsp	14	1.8	9.9	1.1
Salad dressing, ranch	2 tbsp	18	2.5	NA	NA
Salad dressing, reduced calorie ranch	2 tbsp	5	0.4	NA	NA

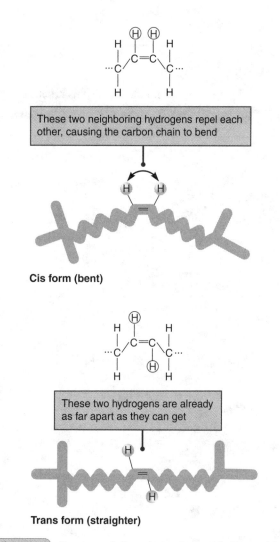

These two neighboring hydrogens repel each other, causing the carbon chain to bend

Cis form (bent)

These two hydrogens are already as far apart as they can get

Trans form (straighter)

Figure 4.5   Structure of cis and trans fatty acids. Fatty acids with the cis form are more common in food than those in the trans form.

third, sixth, or ninth carbon in the chain. A common omega-3 fatty acid is linolenic acid; linoleic acid is the most commonly known omega-6 fatty acid, and oleic acid is the most common omega-9 fatty acid.

There can be more than one double bond in the omega fatty acid chain; the classification merely signifies the first double bond from the omega end. All of these omega fats are utilized as an energy source. However, these fatty acids may be used to synthesize other compounds, and they can have quite different functions in the body. For example, omega-3 fatty acids are used to form localized hormones known as **eicosanoids** that cause dilation of blood vessels and reduce inflammation and blood clotting. On the other hand, eicosanoids formed from omega-6 fatty acids do the opposite. They promote the inflamma-

eicosanoids A group of localized, hormone-like substances produced from long-chain fatty acids.

tory process, increase blood clotting, and cause vasoconstriction. Therefore, the presence and ratio of omega-3 to omega-6 fatty acids in the diet is attracting the attention of researchers because of the possible negative role that higher levels of omega-6 fatty acids play in cardiovascular disease.

Which fatty acids are considered essential?
Linoleic acid (an omega-6 fatty acid) and linolenic acid (an omega-3 fatty acid) are considered **essential fatty acids** because the body cannot manufacture these fats. The body can make saturated and omega-9 fatty acids; therefore, they are considered **nonessential fatty acids**. However, nonessential does not mean unimportant; it simply means it is not essential to consume these fats in the diet. The body can produce an adequate supply of the nonessential fatty acids as demand occurs.

Linoleic acid is found primarily in vegetable oils such as safflower, soy, corn, sunflower, and peanut oils. Linolenic acid is found in leafy greens, soy products, seafood, nuts, seeds, and canola oil. Dietary recommendations for adequate intake of essential fatty acids are met if fat comprises approximately 5% of total calorie intake. The Adequate Intake (AI) for linoleic acid is 17 g/day for men 19–50 years of age (14 g/day for 50+ years) and 12 g/day for women 19–50 years of age (11 g/day for 50+ years); the AI for linolenic acid is 1.6 g/day and 1.1 g/day for men and women 19 years of age and older, respectively.[1]

essential fatty acids Fatty acids that must be obtained from the diet. Linoleic acid and linolenic acid are considered essential fatty acids.

nonessential fatty acid A fatty acid that can be made by the body and thus does not have to be consumed in the diet.

What are phospholipids?

Phospholipids are another classification of lipids, although they are not as abundant in the body and diet as triglycerides. Phospholipids are found in a small number of specific foods such as egg yolks, liver, soybeans, and peanuts. Fortunately, phospholipids are not essential in the diet because the body can readily synthesize them when needed.

Phospholipids have the same glycerol backbone as triglycerides but with only two fatty acids attached to it rather than three (see Figure 4.6). The third site on the glycerol is attached to a phosphate group. The unique structure of phospholipids allows them to be both water and fat soluble. The fatty acids in the structure attract and attach to fat-soluble substances, and the phosphate/nitrogen compound attracts and attaches to water-soluble substances. Phospholipids

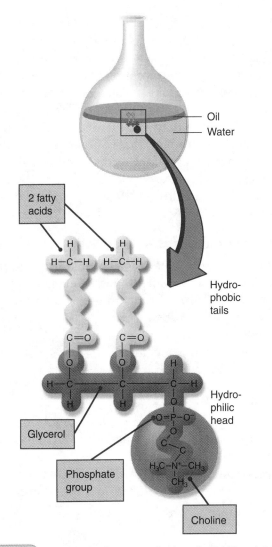

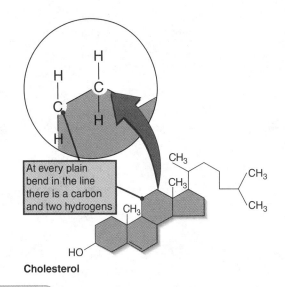

Phospholipids are a major component of cell membranes, which consist of a double layer of phospholipids. The hydrophilic glycerol and phosphate heads line up adjacent to the watery environments of both the outside and the inside of the cell. The inside of the double phospholipid layer contains the fatty acid tails that are hydrophobic.

Phospholipids also provide transport functions in the body. Their ability to combine with water and fatty substances allows them to break fats in the stomach into smaller particles during digestion; bile contains phospholipids that help produce emulsifying effects. Phospholipids also coat the surface of lipoproteins that carry lipid particles to their destinations in the body.

What are sterols?

Sterols are a category of lipids found in both plants and animals. Although sterols are classified as lipids, they differ significantly from triglycerides and phospholipids in structure and function. Unlike the other lipids discussed thus far, most sterols do not contain fatty acid chains. Instead, sterol molecules consist of multiple rings made primarily of carbon and hydrogen atoms that are attached to each other. Despite their different molecular makeup, they have the same hydrophobic and lipophilic characteristics as triglycerides.

Cholesterol is a sterol consisting of a hydrocarbon with a multiple-ring structure (see Figure 4.7). Although it is much maligned because of its relation-

Figure 4.6 Phospholipid structure. A phospholipid is soluble in both oil (i.e., fat) and water. This is a useful property for transporting fatty substances in the body's watery fluids.

are located primarily in the cell membranes of tissues throughout the body.

What functions do phospholipids serve both inside and outside of the body?

Because of their unique structure, phospholipids are ideal emulsifiers. Emulsifiers keep fat-soluble substances suspended in a watery environment. Emulsification is a process that allows two substances that normally do not mix (water and fat in this case) to mix. Phosphatidylcholine, or lecithin, is an emulsifier found naturally in foods of animal origin and in the body. Lecithin is a food additive that can also be derived from plant oils. Lecithins in foods help keep fats from separating, such as the water and oil in dressings, and keep fats in suspension and dispersed in foods such as canned soups, chili, and frozen entrees.

Figure 4.7 Structure of cholesterol. Sterols are multi-ring structures. Cholesterol is the best known sterol because of its role in heart disease.

How are lipids (fats) classified? **107**

ship to heart disease, cholesterol serves some critical roles in the body. It is essential for:

- Proper structure of cell membranes, especially in nerve and brain tissues
- Producing vitamin D in the body; cholesterol is the precursor to the vitamin
- Forming steroid hormones such as progestins, glucocorticoids, androgens, and estrogen
- Manufacturing bile acids

Approximately 0.5–2 grams of cholesterol are produced in the liver, small intestine, and walls of arteries daily, so it is therefore not considered an essential nutrient in the diet.

Two compounds that are similar in structure to cholesterol but also are very different from cholesterol are the plant sterols and plant stanols. The plant sterols and stanols are found only in plants, whereas cholesterol is found in animals and humans. Plant sterols are found naturally in small quantities in many vegetables, fruits, nuts, seeds, legumes, cereals, and vegetable oils. Plant stanols are found naturally in similar foods but in much lower quantities than the plant sterols. Both plant sterols and stanols are found in greater quantities in certain margarines and dressings as well as in some dietary supplements.

Both plant sterols and stanols have cholesterol-lowering effects in the body. With consumption of adequate amounts, the most prominent effect on blood lipid levels is the lowering of low-density lipoprotein (LDL) cholesterol. The maximum cholesterol-lowering benefits are achieved at doses of 2–3 grams/day.[5-7] To achieve this level of plant sterols and stanols, consumption of certain margarines and dressings and/or supplements is necessary because the quantities naturally found in food are significantly lower than the therapeutic dosage. The food labels of products that contain at least half the amount per serving of the recommended daily doses of the stanols and sterols include a health claim that describes the health benefits of plant sterols and stanols in reducing the risk of heart disease.

Is there such a thing as artificial fats?

Because of an increase in the public demand for low-fat and lower calorie foods, food manufacturers have responded by formulating artificial fats, better known as **fat substitutes**.
Fat substitutes are popular in a variety of foods including "luxury" foods such as ice cream, salad dressings, and desserts. The goal of using fat substitutes is to decrease calories while maintaining the texture and taste functions of fat in foods. Fat substitutes can be made from carbohydrates, proteins, or fats. **Table 4.3** provides examples of some of the more common fat substitutes found in the U.S. food supply.

fat substitutes Artificial fats derived from carbohydrates, proteins, or fats that provide foods with the same texture and taste functions of fat but with fewer calories.

TABLE 4.3	Common Fat Substitutes				
Fat Substitute Name	Main Ingredient	Calories	Typical Uses	Approval	Comments
Oatrim	Whole oats with beta-glucan	4 calories/gram	Sauces, gravies, baked goods	GRAS	Can be used in baked products as a substitute for some or all of the fat; consumers can alter the amount substituted to meet acceptable texture.
Simplesse	Whey protein	1–4 calories/ gram depending on water content	Frozen desserts, dressings, and spreads	GRAS	Not as versatile as other substitutes because it cannot be used in heated products.
Benefat	Glycerol and fatty acids	5 calories/gram	Reduced-fat candies, baked goods	GRAS	Variety of uses in many types of candies; can also be used in heated products but not in high-temperature frying.
Olean	Sucrose and fatty acids	0 calories/gram	Fried snack foods	FDA-approved for use in select fried snack foods only	Can bind fat-soluble vitamins; therefore A, D, E, K are added; may cause oily diarrhea and abdominal cramping, especially if too much product is consumed.

The common carbohydrate-based fat substitutes are made from starches, fibers, and gums. They typically reduce calories because carbohydrates contain only 4 calories per gram versus 9 calories per gram of fat. Carbohydrate-based fat substitutes bind water in the product, increasing moisture and thickness and thereby creating the same smooth mouthfeel as fats but with fewer calories. These substitutes are used primarily in baked goods such as cookies, cakes, biscuits, and muffins. Oatrim is a carbohydrate-based fat substitute that is a flour-like product extracted from whole oats (see Table 4.3). It is used as a replacement for half the amount of fat in baked goods and can also be used to thicken sauces, gravies, and salad dressings.

Proteins can also be modified to produce similar qualities to fats but with fewer calories. Typically whey protein from dairy or egg whites is the protein used to produce these protein-based fat substitutes. Proteins are generally broken down by high heat; therefore, fat substitutes made from protein are not heat stable. Simplesse is a patented, multifunctional dairy ingredient made from whey protein concentrate that undergoes a unique microparticulation process. It is approved for use as a thickener or texturizer in frozen desserts, but it is not heat stable and cannot be used in baking or frying (see Table 4.3).

Specialty fats have been produced to provide the market with fat substitutes that are more heat stable and have more of the qualities of whole fats. These are engineered molecular structures that manipulate the degree of saturation and fatty acid chain length to produce similar qualities in food products as fats and oils. Olestra and salatrim are two such fat substitutes that have gained popularity in the last decade (see Table 4.3). Benefat is the trade name for salatrim, which is made of a triglyceride blend of short- and long-chain fatty acids. Benefat contains 5 kcal/gram instead of the 9 kcal/gram in traditional fat. It provides the same creaminess and mouthfeel as fat and maintains these sensory qualities in baking, but not during high-temperature frying.

Olestra (trade name Olean) is a unique combination of sucrose and fat. Instead of the glycerol backbone with three fatty acids, as in a triglyceride, olestra is a sucrose polyester that has a sucrose backbone with six to eight fatty acids attached. Different fatty acids can be attached to the sucrose backbone, altering olestra's characteristics to produce fat-like qualities in foods. The arrangement of olestra prevents hydrolysis and therefore olestra is nondigestible and not absorbed, making olestra calorie-free.

Olestra is also highly heat stable and has been approved for use in limited amounts of fried snack foods such as potato and corn chips.

How much fat is recommended in an athlete's diet?

Fat is an essential nutrient in the diet; however, no Recommended Dietary Allowance (RDA) or AI is set for total fat intake because there is insufficient data to determine a defined level of fat intake at which risk of inadequacy or prevention of chronic disease occurs.[1] The Acceptable Macronutrient Distribution Range (AMDR) for fat intake has been set at 20–35% of total energy for adults.[1] The American Heart Association promotes a slightly stricter range, recommending a total fat intake of 30% or less of total energy intake for decreasing cardiovascular disease risk. The National Cholesterol Education Program (NCEP) recommends less than or equal to 30% of total calories from fat with 10% polyunsaturated, 10% monounsaturated, and a range of 7–10% saturated fat, keeping individuals with high cholesterol levels at or below 7%. The newest guidelines recommended by the NCEP and listed in the Adult Treatment Panel III report[8] were developed as treatment guidelines for individuals with high LDL cholesterol levels. These guidelines may not be appropriate for athletes unless they have higher than recommended cholesterol and LDL cholesterol levels.

In general, athletes report an average fat intake of 35% of total calories; however, fat intake varies among athletes in different sports.[9] Endurance athletes tend to have lower fat and higher carbohydrate intake than sprinters and short distance runners.[9] Athletes dieting for weight loss and those involved in sports requiring weigh-ins or judging on appearance also tend to have lower fat intakes. Appearance sport athletes such as ice skaters, divers, cheerleaders, and gymnasts may become so fixated on low fat/low caloric intake that in some cases they may exhibit disordered eating habits that can lead to more serious conditions such as anorexia nervosa or bulimia nervosa.[10,11] Conversely, collegiate athletes, many of whom are living away from home, may consume too much dietary fat because of an overreliance on fast foods. Overconsumption of fats usually leads to ingesting too many calories. Excessive calories can lead to increases in body fat deposition, and in most cases this has detrimental effects on sport performance. Clearly, athletes must be aware of their dietary fat intake to ensure optimal energy levels, body composition, and ultimately sport performance.

Athletes should focus not only on the total amount of fat in their diet, but also on the type of fat consumed. Saturated and trans fats should be kept to a minimum. These fats have been shown to be the most detrimental to cardiovascular health because they increase cholesterol levels. Saturated fats are found mainly in meat and high-fat dairy products. Trans fats are widespread in processed, packaged foods. Athletes should look for "hydrogenated" or "partially hydrogenated" oils within the ingredients listing of the food label because these terms indicate trans fats. Monounsaturated and polyunsaturated fats are beneficial to health, leading to more favorable cholesterol levels and possibly aiding in the prevention of cancer and arthritis. Monounsaturated fats are found mainly in plant foods including olives, olive oil, canola oil, nuts, seeds, and avocados. Polyunsaturated fats can be further broken down into omega-3 and omega-6 fatty acids.

Recently, the omega-3 fatty acids have received attention for their beneficial effects on the cardiovascular system. Research thus far has suggested that these fatty acids are protective by lowering triglyceride levels, blood pressure, growth of atherosclerotic plaque, and inflammation.[12] Because of these positive effects and since most Americans are deficient, athletes are encouraged to increase their intake of omega-3 fatty acids. As mentioned previously in this chapter, the AI for linolenic acid is 1.1 g/day and 1.6 g/day for women and men 19 years of age and older, respectively. This recommendation can be further broken down to 0.3 to 0.5 g/day of eicosapentaenoic acid (EPA) and docosahexaenoic acid (DHA) combined (marine-derived omega-3 fatty acids), plus 0.8 to 1.1 g/day of alpha-linolenic acid (plant-derived omega-3 fatty acids).[12] As with many nutrients, it appears that focusing on food sources of omega-3 fatty acids, versus supplements, is the best approach. The American Heart Association recommends that individuals consume at least two servings of fish per week (providing EPA + DHA), as well as vegetable sources of omega-3 fatty acids (providing alpha-linolenic acid).[12] Vegetable sources of these fats include walnuts, flaxseed, soybeans, and canola oil. Americans appear to be consuming plenty of omega-6 fatty acids, which are found in corn, sunflower, and safflower oils. These oils can be included in a healthy diet but should not be emphasized as heavily as omega-3 fatty acids. By focusing mainly on plant sources of fats, athletes

will consume mainly beneficial fats, leading to good health and optimal performance. Although there is no direct evidence that omega fatty acids enhance athletic performance, there is some evidence to suggest that omega-3 fatty acids may decrease inflammation and improve blood flow during exercise.[13] Clearly, decreasing muscle pain due to inflammation and improving blood flow during exercise can both positively affect athletic performance; however, much more research regarding the impact of omega fatty acids in athletic performance is needed before specific recommendations can be made.

Can a diet be too low in fat?

Because dietary fat contributes a significant amount of calories per gram, low fat intakes can affect energy balance. Low dietary fat intake combined with low total caloric, carbohydrate, and protein intake can lead to negative energy balance in individuals. For athletes, negative energy balance is counterproductive except in athletes for whom weight loss is indicated. However, when energy balance is negative, training often suffers. Therefore, athletes need to balance their fat and calorie intake with general health and weight-loss goals.

Essential fatty acid deficiency is rare in the United States. A lack of the essential omega-6 fatty acid, linoleic acid, is characterized by rough, scaly skin and dermatitis. Lack of essential and other fatty acids decreases the body's ability to transport fat-soluble vitamins and phytochemicals throughout the body. The omega-3 essential fatty acid, linolenic acid, can be converted to EPA and DHA, which have been shown to be beneficial in reducing vascular disease. A lack of linolenic acid could decrease the amount of converted EPA or DHA, thus reducing these positive health benefits.

Can a diet be too high in fat?

Consuming too much fat can lead to the over-consumption of total calories, resulting in weight gain in the form of body fat. Excess body fat in athletes inhibits performance in most sports. Body fat is a less active tissue and does not produce energy for exercise as easily as stored carbohydrates. Because fat tissue does not help produce movement, it acts as "dead weight." In sports such as track, gymnastics, basketball, volleyball, and many others, the over-fat athlete is weighted down by excess fat, and his or her performance can be hindered. Yet in some sports, higher body weights are beneficial. Athletes in football or other throwing and contact sports may benefit from some additional body fat weight (as well as muscle tissue) to provide extra mass for their activities.

Which foods contain fat?

Fats are found within most food groups of the My-Plate food guidance system. The richest sources of fat are found within the oils. Some grain products as well as certain vegetables provide a small to moderate amount of fat. Fruits provide minimal or no fat. Dairy/alternative products and protein foods products can vary from low to high in fat. Because the type of fat consumed is important for overall health and performance, it is imperative that athletes choose the healthiest selections within each food group to include a variety of fat sources in sufficient, but not excessive, amounts each day.

How much fat is in the grains group?

Many of the foods within the grains group of My-Plate are very low in fat, although specific selections can be very high in fat. Whole grains, such as oatmeal, barley, bulgur wheat, millet, and spelt, contain less than 1–3 grams of fat per serving. The fat in these grains is mainly unsaturated. At the other end of the fat spectrum are foods such as biscuits and croissants. These foods are high in fat, with a larger percentage coming from saturated and trans fats, and therefore intake should be minimized. Table 4.2 earlier in the chapter lists a variety of bread, cereal, rice, and pasta options and their respective fat content. **Training Table 4.1** provides some tips on including low-fat grains in meals.

How much fat is in the fruit and vegetable groups?

In general, fruits and vegetables contain minimal to no fat. However, certain vegetables, such as avocados and olives, contain a considerable amount of fat, although mainly unsaturated. The higher-fat vegetables should be included in a well-balanced diet, in moderate amounts, because of their favorable fat profile. Table 4.2 lists a variety of fruits and vegetables and their respective fat content. **Training Table 4.2** provides some tips on using fruits and vegetables rich in unsaturated fats.

How much fat is in the dairy/alternative group?

Dairy/alternative foods and beverages span both ends of the spectrum in regard to fat content. Full-fat dairy products, such as whole milk or hard cheeses, may contain 8–10 grams of fat per serving, with a high percentage coming from saturated fat. Low-fat or nonfat dairy products, such as skim milk, low-fat yogurt, and cottage cheese, may have only 1–4 grams of fat or less per serving. To help minimize the intake of saturated fats, as well as overall fat, low-fat and nonfat dairy products are the preferred choice.

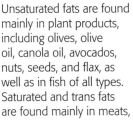

gaining the performance edge

Unsaturated fats are found mainly in plant products, including olives, olive oil, canola oil, avocados, nuts, seeds, and flax, as well as in fish of all types. Saturated and trans fats are found mainly in meats, high-fat dairy products, cheeses, butter, margarine, desserts, and snack foods. Athletes should focus mainly on unsaturated fats while minimizing saturated fats.

Training Table 4.1: Meal Planning Tips for Using Low-Fat Grains

- Cook bulgur wheat with oatmeal for a hot cereal in the morning, topped with fresh fruit.
- Use kamut or wheat berries for stir-fry and casseroles.
- Make a pilaf with couscous, canned beans, chopped tomatoes, and fresh parsley for a light summer lunch.
- Add dry oatmeal to pancake batter for fluffier and heartier pancakes.

Training Table 4.2: Meal Planning Tips for Using Fruits and Vegetables Rich in Unsaturated Fats

- Toss olives on top of fresh green salads.
- Make homemade guacamole for burritos or a chip dip (see *Goalie Guacamole* recipe).
- Include olives in pasta primavera.
- Slice avocado for sandwiches or burgers.

Goalie Guacamole

2 avocados, peeled and chopped
2 tomatoes, chopped
1 tsp chili powder
½ tsp garlic salt
1–2 tsp chopped cilantro
juice of one lime

Mash the avocados in a medium-sized mixing bowl. Stir in the tomatoes and mash together slightly. Add the remaining ingredients, mixing well. Serve with chips, tacos, or burritos.

Serving Size: 3–4 tbsp (Recipe makes 4 servings)

Calories: 165 kcal

Protein: 2.4 grams

Carbohydrates: 9.2 grams

Fat: 15.0 grams (12.75 grams unsaturated)

Most soy, rice, or other dairy alternative products contain approximately 1–6 grams of fat per serving. The fats in dairy alternative choices are mainly unsaturated fats, and therefore are excellent substitutes for full-fat dairy products.

If fortified, the low-/nonfat dairy/alternative products contain the equivalent amounts of calcium and vitamin D as their full-fat counterparts. Therefore, athletes should choose the lower-fat options to gain the proteins, carbohydrates, calcium, and vitamin D benefits of dairy/alternative foods, without the drawback of higher fat and saturated fat consumption. Table 4.2 lists a variety of dairy/alternative products and their respective fat content. **Training Table 4.3** provides tips on including low-fat dairy/alternative products in meal planning.

How much fat is in the protein foods group?

Foods in this group vary greatly in regard to the quantity of fat per serving as well as the type of fat predominating in the product. In general, beef contains a higher quantity of fat and a higher percentage of saturated fat than most other foods in this group. Therefore, athletes should focus mainly on lean cuts of beef. Chicken, turkey, and pork contain moderate amounts of total fat and saturated fat. Some fish are very lean, such as orange roughy, whereas other choices are higher in fat, such as salmon. However, a majority of the fat in fish is unsaturated, and the higher-fat fish are a rich source of omega-3 fatty acids.

Eggs are relatively low in fat, especially the egg white. Nuts and seeds contain higher levels of fat, but similar to fish, contain mainly unsaturated fats. Legumes are very low in fat and the little they do contain is unsaturated. Soy products range from low-fat choices such as tofu to higher-fat choices such as soy nuts, but also consist mainly of unsaturated fats. Table 4.2 lists a variety of protein foods and their respective fat content. **Training Table 4.4** provides meal-planning tips for using low-fat protein foods.

Training Table 4.3: Meal Planning Tips Using Lower-Fat Dairy/Alternatives

- Choose 1%, skim, or soy milk for cereal.
- Replace half the fat in a recipe with low-fat yogurt.
- Order a latte or café mocha with skim or soy milk.
- Substitute low-fat yogurt for a portion or all of the sour cream in dips or sauces. (See *Volleyball Veggie Dip* recipe.)

Volleyball Veggie Dip

1 cup plain low-fat yogurt
1 cup nonfat sour cream
1 10 oz package frozen spinach, thawed and drained
¼–½ cup chopped green onions
¼ tsp salt
¼ tsp ground black pepper
2 tbsp fresh dill or 1 tbsp dried dill

Mix all ingredients together and refrigerate for several hours to chill. Serve as a dip for crackers or raw vegetables.

Serving Size: ¼ cup (Recipe makes 16 servings)

Calories: 28 kcal

Protein: 2.0 grams

Carbohydrates: 4.9 grams

Fat: 0.3 grams

Training Table 4.4: Meal Planning Tips for Using Lower-Fat Protein Foods

- Choose 90–95% lean ground beef for sloppy joes and meatloaf.
- Cook salmon on the grill and serve with a couscous pilaf.
- Scramble 2–3 egg whites together and add low-fat cheese.
- Use tempeh or texturized soy protein for a barbeque sandwich. (See *Baseball Barbeque Sandwiches* recipe.)

Baseball Barbeque Sandwiches

1 package of tempeh, cut into cubes
½–¾ cup barbeque sauce
2 whole wheat buns

Preheat oven to 350 degrees F. Mix cubed tempeh and barbeque sauce together in a small mixing bowl. Transfer tempeh to a lightly greased baking dish. Bake in the oven for 10–15 minutes. Serve tempeh on buns for an open face or closed sandwich.

Serving Size: one sandwich (half tempeh mixture and one bun)

Calories: 498 kcal

Protein: 27.7 grams

Carbohydrates: 69.6 grams

Fat: 12.7 grams

How much fat is in the oils?

This category contains the richest sources of fat. The best choices include the unsaturated oils such as olive, canola, flax, and sesame oils. Saturated and trans fatty acids found in butter, margarine, snack items, desserts, and other fried or processed foods should be kept to a minimum. Table 4.2 lists a variety of fats, sweets, and oils and their respective fat content. **Training Table 4.5** provides some healthier options within the oils.

How can the percentage of calories from fat be calculated for specific foods?

The Institute of Medicine, the American Heart Association, and even the NCEP have all published recommendations for daily fat consumption. The fat intake recommendation is often stated as a percentage of total calories rather than an absolute number. Many athletes wonder, "What does the percentage mean, and how do I figure out the percentage of fat in the foods I eat?" This section explains how to interpret the percentage and how to calculate the percentage of calories from fat in specific foods. For general health, it has been suggested that total fat intake should remain at or below 30–35% of total calories per day. Saturated and trans fat combined should contribute no more than 10% of total calories per day. For most athletes, total fat intake should range from 20% to 30%, leaving plenty of room in the diet for carbohydrates and proteins. Therefore, all athletes should be aware of how to calculate the percentage of calories from fat in various foods in order to make healthy food choices (see Figure 4.8). The percentage of total calories from fat, saturated fat, or trans fat for any food item can be calculated by the following basic formula:

$$\% \text{ calories from fat} = (\text{calories from fat} / \text{total calories}) \times 100$$

In order to complete the equation, an athlete will need to do some fact finding on the food label and also know how to calculate the calories from total, saturated, or trans fat. The total calories per serving

Training Table 4.5: Meal Planning Tips for Healthier Food Flavoring with Oils

- Dip whole grain bread in olive oil for an appetizer.
- Use 1–2 tbsp of sesame oil in tofu or chicken stir-fry.
- Spread peanut butter or almond butter on toast, English muffins, pita bread, or homemade bran muffins.
- Marinate vegetables for the grill in a mixture of olive oil, balsamic vinegar, and spices.

Nutrition Facts

| Serving Size: | | 1 Cup (30g) |
| Servings Per Container | | About 15 |

Amount Per Serving	Cereal	with ½ cup Skim Milk
Calories	100	140
Calories from Fat	5	10

	% Daily Value*	
Total Fat 0.5g	1%	1%
Saturated Fat 0g	0%	0%
Trans Fat 0g		
Cholesterol 0mg	0%	1%
Sodium 125mg	5%	8%
Potassium 230mg	7%	12%
Total Carbohydrate 24g	8%	10%
Dietary Fiber 13g	52%	52%
Sugars 0g		
Other Carbohydrates 11g		
Protein 2g		

| Vitamin A 0% | • | Vitamin C 15% |
| Calcium 6% | • | Iron 25% |

* Percent Daily Values are based on a 2,000 calorie diet. Your daily values may be higher or lower depending on your calorie needs:

	Calories:	2000	2,500
Total Fat	Less Than	65g	80g
Sat Fat	Less Than	20g	25g
Cholesterol	Less Than	300mg	300mg
Sodium	Less Than	2,400mg	2,400mg
Total Carbohydrate		300g	375g
Dietary Fiber		25g	30g

Calories per gram:
Fat 9 • Carbohydrate 4 • Protein 4

Total calories
Calories from fat

Figure 4.8 Calculating the percentage of total calories from fat using the food label. Athletes need to know how to calculate the percentage of fat in foods they consume. The food label lists the total number of calories and the total number of calories from fat in one serving, which can be used to calculate this percentage. In this example, the calculation is $(5/100) \times 100 = 5\%$, meaning 5% of the total calories are contributed from fat.

and total calories from fat are listed at the top of the Nutrition Facts label on any food product. Divide the calories from fat by the total calories and then multiple by 100 to calculate the percentage.

If the calculated percentage is less than 35%, the athlete knows the product fits within healthy eating guidelines. However, athletes should keep in mind that the recommendation for 20–35% of total calories coming from fat is a guideline for the overall diet—not necessarily for every individual food eaten in the diet. Sometimes athletes will take this recommendation too far and exclude all foods that do not fall into this category. However, this approach is not necessary and can steer athletes away from healthy choices. An example of a very healthy food that does not fall into the 20–35% range is peanut butter. By studying the label, the consumer can see that the percentage of calories from fat can range from 50% to 80%. Therefore, peanut butter does not fall into the 20–35% goal. However, if an athlete has a peanut butter sandwich on whole wheat bread with an apple and a cup of yogurt, then the percentage of calories from the whole meal is less than 30%, which would be classified in the healthy category. Plus, nuts are full of other nutrients such as fiber, protein, and zinc, and the fat in nuts is mainly unsaturated fat. Use the percentage of calories from fat, along with other nutritional benefits or drawbacks, to fully evaluate a food or beverage in the context of an entire meal. If the athlete is calculating the percentage of calories from saturated fat or trans fat or is obtaining nutrition information about a product through means other than the food label, the only information needed is:

1. Total calories per serving
2. Total grams of fat, saturated fat, or trans fat per serving

One extra step is required before the numbers can be plugged into the same equation as listed previously: *Multiply the number of grams of fat, saturated fat, or trans fat by 9 (because there are 9 calories per gram of any type of fat) to obtain the total number of calories from fat.* For example, if a package of crackers has 130 total calories per serving and 1 gram of saturated fat, the calculation would be as follows:

1 gram saturated fat × 9 = 9 calories from saturated fat
(9 calories from saturated fat / 130 total calories) × 100 = 6.9% of total calories from saturated fat

As stated previously, if the percentage of saturated fat, as well as monounsaturated and polyunsaturated fat, is approximately 7–10%, the athlete will know the product fits within healthy eating guidelines. Trans fats should be kept to a minimum.

The Food and Drug Administration approved a regulation in 2003 that all food labels must list the amount of trans fats contained in the product.[14] The trans fats must be listed in grams and shown on all food labels directly below the listing for saturated fats. Trans fats, similar to saturated fats and dietary cholesterol, can raise LDL cholesterol levels, potentially increasing risk for cardiovascular disease. Currently, there is not an RDA for trans fats and no specific recommendations for the maximum number of grams of trans fat to consume daily. Therefore, trans fats will not have a Percent Daily Value (%DV) listed on the food label. However, athletes who want to limit trans and saturated fats can use the gram amounts listed on the food label. By combining the grams of saturated fat and trans fat on the food label, similar products can be compared for their fat content. Athletes should choose the product with the least amount of these two fats combined.

Athletes need to be careful not to confuse the percentages listed under the Percent Daily Value column as the respective percentage of calories from fat. The %DV is based on a 2000-calorie diet. At this calorie level, the FDA recommends consuming no more than 65 grams of total fat and 20 grams of saturated fat. Therefore, the %DV is providing the relationship between eating one serving of a product and how that compares to total daily needs. Refer to the label of the package of instant oatmeal in Figure 4.9 for an example.

Another common labeling statement that often creates questions is when foods are labeled "95% fat-free." An athlete might assume that 95% fat-free means that only 5% of the total calories come from fat and that this would be a healthy choice. However, these statements are based on the total weight of the food product, not on the total calorie content of the product. Some foods have higher water contents, and therefore the amount of fat compared to the total weight will be small; however, the percentage related to total calorie content may be moderate or high. For example, these statements are commonly found at the meat counter describing options for ground meats. A 95% fat-free meat does not mean that only 5% of the total calories are coming from fat. These meats can still have a significant amount of fat and saturated fat compared to the calorie content of one

Nutrition Facts

Serving Size: 1 cup (28g)
Servings Per Container: About 18

Amount Per Serving

Calories 160   Calories from fat 20

	% Daily Value*
Total Fat 2g	3%
Saturated Fat 0g	0%
Trans Fat 0g	
Cholesterol 0mg	0%
Sodium 300mg	13%
Total Carbohydrate 29g	10%
Dietary Fiber 1g	4%
Sugars 2g	
Other Carbohydrates 26g	
Protein 6g	

Vitamin A 15%	•	Vitamin C 25%
Calcium 0%	•	Iron 45%

* Percent Daily Values are based on a 2,000 calorie diet. Your daily values may be higher or lower depending on your calorie needs:

		Calories:	2,000	2,500
Total Fat	Less Than		65g	80g
Sat Fat	Less Than		20g	25g
Cholesterol	Less Than		300mg	300mg
Sodium	Less Than		2,400mg	2,400mg
Total Carbohydrate			300g	375g
Dietary Fiber			25g	30g

Calories per gram:
Fat 9 • Carbohydrate 4 • Protein 4

Figure 4.9 Difference in the percentage of calories from fat and the Percent Daily Value for fat. A serving of cereal may have 160 total calories with 20 calories coming from fat, which equals 12.5% of the total calories from fat. The label lists the %DV associated with total fat as 3%. This means 2 grams is 3% of the total daily recommendation of 65 grams, not that the product has 3% of its total calories from fat. Therefore, use the %DV as an indication of how much fat one serving contributes to total daily needs; use the numbers indicated for Total Calories and Calories from Fat to determine whether the product is low-fat.

serving of meat. However, these statements can still be a good tool for decision making, regardless of whether they help an athlete determine exactly how much fat is in a product. An athlete should look for a product labeled as a higher percentage fat-free, which indicates a leaner item and thus a healthier choice. For example, a meat product labeled as 98% fat free is leaner than a 95% fat-free product.

What's the big deal about cholesterol?

As mentioned several times earlier in this chapter, it is recommended that fat intake be kept at a moderate level for the prevention of cardiovascular disease. So, what is the connection between dietary fat and an increased risk of the disease? On the basis of ongoing research in the area of cardiovascular health, blood cholesterol has been strongly associated with a higher risk for cardiovascular disease. Therefore, blood cholesterol levels have been targeted as one of the first lines of defense in the prevention of the disease. One of the most influential ways to modify blood cholesterol levels is to adapt lifestyle factors such as exercise and diet, specifically dietary fat, saturated fat, and cholesterol.

What is cholesterol, and which foods contain it?

As mentioned earlier in this chapter, cholesterol is a sterol. Cholesterol is found only in animal products (see **Table 4.4**). All meats contain cholesterol, with organ meats having the highest amounts. Eggs and dairy products also contain cholesterol, with nonfat dairy options having the least. Some breads, muffins, and baked goods will have cholesterol if they were made with eggs and/or dairy products.

Plant products, such as fruits, vegetables, whole grains, legumes, and soy, are cholesterol-free. These foods do contain plant sterols, however, which have a similar ring structure to cholesterol. Plant sterols or stanols have recently been researched for their potential effects as cholesterol-lowering substances. Plant sterols and stanols are poorly absorbed by humans and, therefore, may reduce the amount of cholesterol absorbed in the intestinal tract.

How is blood cholesterol classified?

Cholesterol is measured by taking a sample of blood and analyzing the levels of total cholesterol, high-density lipoprotein (HDL), and low-density lipoprotein (LDL). Each component can provide unique information regarding an individual's risk for heart disease (see **Table 4.5**). Several other cholesterol components can be tested to contribute additional information, such as triglycerides, very low-density lipoproteins, and lipoprotein(a). Blood cholesterol measurements are most accurate after a 9- to 12-

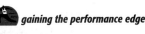
gaining the performance edge

Athletes should aim for 20–35% of their total calories from fat. The percentage can be calculated from information provided within the Nutrition Facts panel on the food label. Athletes should keep in mind that the 20–35% guideline is for the overall diet, not necessarily for every individual food. A specific food should be evaluated based on both its total fat percentage and its overall nutrient contribution to a healthy diet.

TABLE 4.4 Cholesterol Content of Various Foods

Food Item	Serving Size	Cholesterol Content (mg)
Grains		
Bran flakes	¾ cup	0
Bagel	1 bagel	0
Spelt	½ cup	0
Fruits/Vegetables		
Apple	1 medium	0
Plum	1 medium	0
Acorn squash	½ cup	0
Olives	10 medium	0
Dairy/Alternative		
Skim milk	8 fl oz	4
1% milk	8 fl oz	10
2% milk	8 fl oz	18
Whole milk	8 fl oz	33
Low-fat yogurt	6 oz	10
Cheddar cheese	1 oz	30
Soy milk	8 fl oz	0
Protein Foods		
Ground beef, lean	3 oz	82
Chicken breast with skin	3 oz	82
Chicken breast without skin	3 oz	73
Turkey, white meat, without skin	3 oz	69
Turkey, dark meat, without skin	3 oz	85
Pork chop	3 oz	79
Salmon, pink	3 oz	20
Orange roughy	3 oz	22
Whole egg	1 large	212
Egg white	1 egg white	0
Veggie burger	1 patty	0
Almonds	1 oz	0
Oils		
Margarine, stick	1 tbsp	0
Butter	1 tbsp	33
Olive oil	1 tbsp	0
Salad dressing, ranch	2 tbsp	5
Salad dressing, reduced calorie ranch	2 tbsp	10

let of blood to be quickly analyzed. These results should be verified by also taking a test completed after a fast.

Athletes are inherently helping to lower their cholesterol levels because of their active lifestyles. However, many athletes are not focused on dietary approaches that are protective and therapeutic. Physical activity alone is not enough to keep cholesterol levels in the desirable range; a healthy diet is also critical.

What is total cholesterol?
Total cholesterol is a measurement that combines the levels of HDL, LDL, and triglycerides in the blood. It can provide a general estimate of risk, but is not as informative as the breakdown of the various lipoproteins. The National Cholesterol Education Program recommends a total cholesterol level below 200 mg/dL. A level between 200 and 239 mg/dL is considered borderline high, and ≥ 240 mg/dL is considered high; both require changes to lower the level to the desirable range. Total cholesterol can be lowered by making dietary and physical activity changes that will decrease LDL and triglycerides.

What is HDL?
HDL is often referred to as the "good" cholesterol. HDL has a higher protein content and a smaller triglyceride and cholesterol content than LDL. HDL is a "scavenger," picking up cholesterol from the bloodstream and arteries, and delivering it to the liver to be packaged into bile and excreted from the body. Because of this action, HDL often is considered protective against cardiovascular disease. However, through research, it has not been conclusively determined that alterations to HDL through modifications to diet and exercise lead to reduced risk of disease. More research is required before firm dietary and physical activity guidelines can be set based on a proven track record of protection. In the meantime, individuals should focus on the lifestyle factors that have been shown to increase HDL—weight management and regular exercise. In terms of the diet influence on HDL, very low-fat eating plans can lead to a lowering of HDL levels. Therefore, individuals should follow a moderate-fat diet, with 20–35% of total calories coming from fat, and a strong emphasis should be placed on the unsaturated fats. The desirable level for HDL set by the NCEP is ≥ 60 mg/dL. A level of <40 mg/dL is considered low, requiring lifestyle modifications.

hour fast. Total cholesterol can be estimated with portable machines, often used at health fairs, which require only a finger stick to obtain a small drop-

TABLE 4.5	National Cholesterol Education Program: Classification of Lipoprotein Levels			
Lipoprotein	Desirable	Borderline	Undesirable
Total cholesterol	<200 mg/dL	200–239 mg/dL	≥240 mg/dL
Low-density lipoprotein	<100 mg/dL	130–159 mg/dL	≥160 mg/dL
High-density lipoprotein	≥60 mg/dL	40–59 mg/dL	<40 mg/dL

Source: U.S. Department of Health and Human Services, National Institutes of Health, National Heart, Lung, and Blood Institute (2001). National Cholesterol Education Program. ATP III At-A-Glance: Quick Desk Reference. Available at: www.nhlbi.nih.gov/guidelines/cholesterol/atglance.htm. Accessed January 21, 2011.

What are VLDL and lipoprotein(a)?

VLDLs, very low-density lipoproteins, contain a triglyceride-rich core.[15] Lipoprotein lipase digests some of the triglycerides from the VLDL, leaving an intermediate-density lipoprotein (IDL). The IDL travels through the bloodstream to the liver, where it is converted into LDL. VLDL can be measured in a blood test similar to HDL and LDL. However, the NCEP has not established a guideline for screening, prevention, or treatment of VLDL.

Lipoprotein(a) has been receiving more attention over the years as an indicator of risk for heart disease. Lipoprotein(a) is structurally similar to LDL and has been linked to heart disease because of its involvement in atherogenesis and thrombogenesis. Similar to VLDL, a recommended level of lipoprotein(a) is not carved in stone. More research is needed to determine the recommended levels of lipoprotein(a) for use in screening individuals as well as the influence of diet and exercise to modify VLDL and lipoprotein(a) levels over time.

What is LDL?

LDL is the rival to HDL and is termed the "bad" cholesterol. This cholesterol-rich lipoprotein delivers cholesterol to the cells of the body to be used for a variety of functions. The problems begin when cells, specifically those in the arterial walls, are damaged as a result of a variety of environmental factors, genetics, disease states, and/or medical conditions. White blood cells rush to the areas of damage and bind to LDL, which releases its cholesterol, leading to a buildup on the arterial wall and eventually escalating into atherosclerosis (see Figure 4.10). Because of this action of LDL and the large volume of evidence linking LDL to greater risk for cardiovascular disease, LDL has become the primary target of therapy. Ideally, LDL should

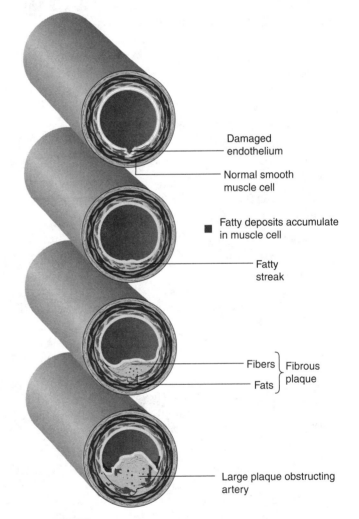

Figure 4.10 Buildup in an artery leads to atherosclerosis. High LDL cholesterol levels can contribute to plaque formation in artery walls and atherosclerosis.

be <100 mg/dL, with levels of 100–129 mg/dL considered near optimal/above optimal, 130–159 mg/dL borderline high, 160–189 mg/dL high, and ≥190 mg/dL very high.

LDL increases when saturated fats, trans fats, and cholesterol are consumed in excess through the diet. LDL can be lowered by substituting polyunsaturated and monounsaturated fats for saturated fats and increasing soluble fiber, plant sterols/stanols, and soy protein intake. Weight loss, for those who are overweight, can also decrease LDL levels.

The National Cholesterol Education Program (NCEP) has developed a list of dietary recommendations for lowering LDL blood levels and preventing cardiovascular disease. See **Fortifying Your Nutrition Knowledge** for an explanation of the NCEP plan for "therapeutic lifestyle changes." Also listed in **Training Table 4.6** are two diets—a typical American diet high in fat and cholesterol, and an example of a cholesterol-lowering diet plan. Recognizing the difference in these meal plans can help athletes achieve their nutrient needs while minimizing cholesterol intake.

How can fats affect daily training and competitive performance?

Fats are a major fuel source for muscle cells. Fats are the primary source of energy at rest, during low- to moderate-intensity activities (see Figure 3.8), and in periods of recovery between intense bouts of activity. Endurance training improves the body's ability to utilize fats for energy, which shifts the crossover point in Figure 3.8 to the right. This right shift of

Fortifying
Your Nutrition Knowledge

The National Cholesterol Education Program's Therapeutic Lifestyle Recommendations

In May 2001, the National Cholesterol Education Program (NCEP) released the Third Report of the Expert Panel on Detection, Evaluation, and Treatment of High Blood Cholesterol in Adults (Adult Treatment Panel III). The series of seven steps posted in the report provides a framework for detecting risk for heart disease and treating those who have heart disease or who present significant risk factors for developing heart disease. Also included in the report are therapeutic lifestyle changes that can be implemented to lower LDL cholesterol levels in the blood.

The therapeutic lifestyle changes suggested are as follows:

- *Consume a diet with <7% of total calories from saturated fat:* Saturated fat comes mainly from animal products such as meats and full-fat dairy. The only vegetable oils containing a significant amount of saturated fat are coconut, palm, and palm kernel oils.
- *Keep dietary cholesterol intake to <200 mg per day:* Cholesterol is found only in animal products such as meats and higher-fat dairy products.
- *Increase soluble fiber to 10–25 grams per day:* Soluble fiber is found only in plant products such as oats, oat bran, legumes, and some fruits and vegetables.
- *Consider consuming plant stanols/sterols (2 grams per day) to help lower cholesterol:* Derived from plant foods, plant stanols/sterols can be found in commercial products such as Take Control or Benecol margarines and have been shown to actively aid in lowering blood cholesterol.
- *Maintain a healthy body weight:* Balance calorie intake (diet) with calorie expenditure (exercise, training, competition, and daily movement) on a daily basis.
- *Increase physical activity:* Achieve at least 30 minutes, preferably 60 minutes, of physical activity every day of the week.

For more information on the Third Report of the Expert Panel on Detection, Evaluation and Treatment of High Blood Cholesterol in Adults, visit www.nhlbi.nih.gov/guidelines/cholesterol/atglance.htm. In 2004, the NCEP updated the report based on the results from new clinical trials. The updates applied to moderately high and high-risk patients only and thus will not be discussed. However, to get the updated information, go to www.nhlbi.nih.gov/guidelines/cholesterol/atp3upd04.htm.

Training Table 4.6: How Can the Cholesterol Guidelines Be Applied to a Daily Meal Plan?

High-Fat, High-Cholesterol Diet	Cholesterol-Lowering Diet
Breakfast	*Breakfast*
2 eggs scrambled with 2 tbsp cheddar cheese	2 cups bran flakes with 1 cup skim milk and ½ cup strawberries
2 pieces of toast with 2 tsp butter	2 pieces toast with 2 tbsp peanut butter
Banana	12 oz orange juice
12 oz 2% milk	
	Snack
Snack	Banana
2 oz pretzels	
	Lunch
Lunch	3 oz turkey sandwich on whole wheat bread with 2 tsp mustard
3 oz roast beef sandwich on white bread with 1 tbsp mayonnaise	1½ cups black bean soup
1.5 oz bag of potato chips	Pear
20 oz diet soda	
	Snack
Snack	8 oz low-fat yogurt
Protein sports bar	2 tbsp raisins
	Dinner
Dinner	6 oz chicken stir-fry with 2 cups of broccoli, carrots, and mushrooms, and 1 cup brown rice
9 oz steak	2 cups green salad with 2 tbsp olive oil and vinegar dressing
1.5 cups mashed potatoes	12 oz skim milk
½ cup green beans	2 oatmeal cookies
12 oz 2% milk	
2 cups ice cream	*Daily Totals*
	Calories: 3130
Daily Totals	Fat: 71 grams (20% of total calories)
Calories: 3400	Saturated fat: 16 grams
Fat: 148 grams (39% of total calories)	Trans fat: 6 grams
Saturated fat: 63 grams	Cholesterol: 223 mg
Trans fat: 24 grams	
Cholesterol: 871 mg	

the crossover point occurs because endurance training enhances the body's ability to mobilize fats from adipocytes, thus making more fatty acids available to the working muscle.[16] In addition, endurance training improves the working muscle's capacity to oxidize the fats that are delivered. Increased muscle blood flow, improved transport of fats into the muscle cells, larger and more numerous mitochondria, and increased quantities of enzymes involved in fat metabolism are adaptations that help explain the enhanced ability of trained muscles to utilize fats for energy.[17,18] Clearly, the adaptations that occur with endurance training indicate the importance of fats as an energy source.

However, despite the body's abundant fat reserves and ability to increase fat utilization in response to endurance training, fats are still not the most efficient fuel for working active muscles, par-

ticularly at higher levels of exercise intensity. The limitation of fat utilization for energy during exercise is the relatively slow rate of adenosine triphosphate (ATP) production as compared to carbohydrates. As discussed in Chapter 2, fats must be aerobically metabolized to produce ATP. There must be adequate availability of oxygen to the muscle cells for fats to be broken down, not to mention that fat metabolism is a complicated process involving three metabolic pathways (see Figure 4.11). Finally, although some fats are stored within the muscles, research evidence to date does not support the contention that these fats provide much energy during exercise.[19,20] This means that the fats must be released from adipocytes and then delivered to the working muscles via the blood. Taking all of this into account, the delivery and metabolic disassembly of fats for energy is not only slower than that of carbohydrates at respond-

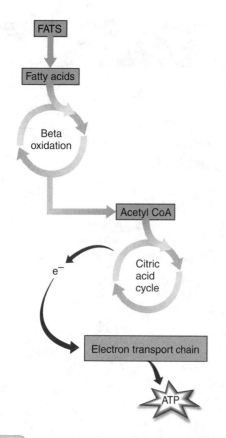

Figure 4.11 Metabolic mill for fats. The metabolic mill for fats can produce nearly limitless amounts of ATP; however, the delivery and metabolic disassembly of fats to the working muscle are slow.

ing to changes in activity, but also slower at producing ATP. The advantage of fat utilization is that the metabolic mill for producing ATP from fats can produce almost limitless amounts of ATP. If fats could be made more readily available to muscle via dietary manipulation, then conceivably endurance sport performance could be enhanced. The following discussions explore what is currently known about dietary fat intake and sport performance.

What type, how much, and when should fats be consumed before exercise?

Current research has focused on the potential of dietary fat to enhance performance, mainly in endurance activities.[21–25] Some information suggests that an increase in dietary fat in the weeks leading up to a competition, sometimes referred to as fat loading, can enhance the body's ability to utilize fat and therefore spare glycogen and prolong exercise. Others claim that a permanent shift to higher fat intakes allows the body to burn more fats for fuel, decreasing adipose stores and therefore improving

an athlete's body composition. The following sections will explore the ability of fat to enhance performance in a single high-fat meal prior to exercising, a short-term pattern of high-fat meals and snacks, and a long-term diet plan consisting of high-fat foods. In conclusion, recommendations will be stated for fat intake prior to exercise based on the research and information presented.

Is a single high-fat meal prior to exercise beneficial?

Previous research has demonstrated that the rate of fat utilization for energy during exercise increases as the availability of fatty acids in the blood increases.[26,27] In other words, the more fat that is delivered or made available to a working muscle, the more fat the working muscle will metabolize for energy. Therefore, it has been proposed that a high-fat meal prior to competition would increase fatty acid levels in the blood and in turn enhance endurance performance compared to a high-carbohydrate meal. Some studies have provided meals to athletes with as high as 60–75% of total calories from fat in the 4 hours prior to exercise. Others have experimented with ingestion of medium-chain (6–10 carbons) and long-chain ($\geq$ 12 carbons) fatty acids with the hope of increasing fatty acids in the blood by providing a fat source that is readily broken down and absorbed. Unfortunately, to date the majority of studies have not found any benefit to ingesting high-fat meals prior to competition when compared to high-carbohydrate meals.[27,28] In fact, many athletes find that a meal high in fat in 1–4 hours prior to an exercise session, or especially a competition, leads to gastrointestinal distress including bloating, diarrhea, stomach cramping, and a sense of fullness.[29] Therefore, it is not recommended that athletes eat a high-fat meal immediately prior to exercise.

gaining the performance edge

It is not recommended that athletes eat a high-fat meal immediately prior to exercise because of the potential for gastric upset.

Is a short-term pattern of eating high-fat meals beneficial to exercise performance?

"Short-term" for the purposes of this question includes periods of time less than 2 weeks. As mentioned in Chapter 3, carbohydrate stores in the body are limited and can be depleted by 3 hours or less of continuous exercise. The significance of depleting carbohydrate stores is that it results in fatigue and decreases exercise performance. On the other hand, fat stores on even very lean individuals are ample enough to fuel activity for several days. A theory has developed that if an athlete consumes a relatively high-fat diet in the 1 to 2 weeks prior to an important training session or competitive event, the body will adjust to the higher fat intake and become more efficient at using fat for fuel during exercise. This has been termed "fat adaptation." In other words, if an athlete is able to shift to a heavier reliance on fat for energy, carbohydrate usage declines, thus delaying the depletion of carbohydrate stores and increasing the time to exhaustion.

Several studies have shown an increase in fat oxidation during submaximal exercise after fat adaptation.[30–32] Fat intakes in these studies have ranged from 60–70% of total calories, and the exercise tests are generally conducted at 60–70% of maximal oxygen uptake for relatively short periods of time. Unfortunately, when the effects of a short-term dietary manipulation of fat intake on athletic performance are examined, the switch to a high-fat diet does not appear to increase time to exhaustion. In fact, the majority of studies involving short-term alteration of fat intake show the opposite effect, causing a decreased time to exhaustion, increased perceived exertion, and an impaired ability to metabolize carbohydrates for energy.[27,32–34] However, several studies do exist that report an increase in endurance performance after a high-fat diet adaptation,[35,36] and therefore more research with consistent methodology is warranted in this area. At this time, however, short-term high-fat intake does not appear to be an effective practice for improving athletic performance.

gaining the performance edge

Short-term (i.e., 2 weeks or less) high-fat diets do not appear to be effective for improving endurance performance.

Is a long-term pattern of eating high-fat meals beneficial to exercise performance?

For the purposes of this question, "long-term" includes patterns of eating followed for longer than 2 weeks. Although short-term high-fat diets to date have not consistently panned out as a good dietary practice for endurance athletes, it has been suggested that 2 weeks or less is not enough time for the body to make sufficient metabolic adjustments. Numerous studies investigating the effects of long-term, high-fat dietary interventions have been published.[37–39] Overall, no benefit has been found over balanced, high-carbohydrate, moderate-protein, low- to moderate-fat diets.[40] It appears that although high-fat diets can cause favorable shifts in fat metabolism, they also lead to lower muscle glycogen stores. Unfortunately, the improvement in fat utilization is not enough to offset the effect of diminished glycogen stores. Even in cases when adaptation to a high-fat diet is followed by a short carbohydrate loading period, suboptimal endurance performance persists, suggesting deleterious effects of a high-fat diet beyond carbohydrate availability.[38] In addition, high-fat diets have resulted in higher perceived exertion ratings despite maintaining comparable training intensities.[37] This also can have negative ramifications if the athletes are not as motivated to train during the high-fat dietary period. Only a few studies have explored the effects of a long-term high-fat diet on high-intensity activities. Fleming et al.[37] performed 30-second Wingate anaerobic tests on subjects following a high-fat diet (61% of total calories) for 6 weeks. Peak power output decreased in the high-fat group as compared to the low-fat control group. More research on high-intensity activities needs to be conducted to determine the short- and long-term effects on athletic performance.

Typically, athletes' diets containing 20–30% fat are recommended to allow adequate carbohydrate intake and to assist weight management when needed. Specific recommendations for fat intake should be individualized and based on body size, weight, and body composition goals, as well as the sport played and sport performance goals. Using the broader AMDR recommendation of 20–35% of calories from fat provides flexibility in the amount of fat intake to meet specific total macronutrient needs of individual athletes with varying training schedules and performance goals.

gaining the performance edge

Long-term (i.e., more than 2 weeks) high-fat dietary intakes are not recommended as a means to improve athletic performance.

What are the recommendations for fat intake prior to exercise?

As with any macronutrient, athletes need to experiment with the best preexercise meal for their digestive system and sport. Fat will create a feeling of satiety to prevent an athlete from feeling hungry before exercising. However, consuming too much fat 4 hours or less prior to exercise can cause bloating, intestinal cramping, or diarrhea. Therefore, meals and snacks within 4 hours of training sessions and/or competitions should be low in fat, focused mainly on the unsaturated fats. An athlete should determine his or her personal upper limit of fat ingestion for the 1–4 hours prior to exercise. Encourage athletes to start conservatively in their experimentation, limiting fat to small quantities. A "small amount" of fat may be obtained by consuming peanut butter (1 tbsp) on toast or olive oil (1–2 tsp) on a salad. These quantities are generally well tolerated before exercise, but individual tolerances will vary.

If the athlete finds that he or she becomes hungry before starting exercise, have the athlete try eating the same meal closer to exercise or add a little more fat to the same meal in the same time frame. For example, if an athlete eats a breakfast of toast with 1 tablespoon of peanut butter and a banana 3 hours before training, ask the athlete to test: (1) eating the same meal 1½ to 2 hours before training, or (2) adding 2 tablespoons of peanut butter to the toast instead of one. The breakfast, lunch, or snack options in **Training Table 4.7** contain a small amount of fats, while maintaining a balance of carbohydrates and proteins.

What type, how much, and when should fats be consumed during exercise?

Our bodies use fat for energy during exercise. The fat stored in adipose tissue is burned relatively slowly as compared to intramuscular fats. Recent studies have explored ways to increase the amount of fat burned during exercise and/or to increase the body's reliance on fat for energy, thus sparing carbohydrates. In the previous section, it was determined that at this point, existing research does not consistently reveal a benefit to consuming high-fat meals in the hours, days, or months leading up to exercise or

competition. But what about if fat is consumed during exercise? Would the body then rely more heavily on fats for fuel versus carbohydrates? To answer these questions, studies have focused on the effects of long-chain triglycerides (LCTs) and medium-chain triglycerides (MCTs).

As mentioned earlier in this chapter, LCTs (dietary fats) are composed of three long fatty acid chains connected to a glycerol backbone. They are digested by bile acids in the liver and by lipase from the pancreas. The absorption rate of LCTs is slow, and therefore consuming high-fat foods during exercise is not beneficial. Athletes can include small amounts of fat in their preexercise meal or snack but should avoid consuming fat while exercising.

Conversely, the theory surrounding the proposed beneficial effects of MCTs is based on the fact that unlike LCTs, MCTs are easily digested, readily absorbed into the blood, and oxidized rapidly.[41,42] MCTs are broken down into medium-chain fatty acids (MCFAs), which are water-soluble and therefore do not delay gastric emptying and are absorbed rapidly through the intestinal wall into the bloodstream. MCFAs are then delivered to muscle cells, where they pass through the plasma membrane and enter the mitochondria for oxidation. MCTs are oxidized in the first 30 minutes of exercise and can be absorbed across the mucosal membrane, similar to glucose. For these reasons, MCTs have spurred interest in the potential benefit of including MCTs in sports beverages, foods, or other products to delay fatigue.

Early studies regarding MCTs' effects on performance involved consuming small amounts (~30 grams) of MCTs before exercise.[43,44] These studies reported no effect on carbohydrate or lipid oxidation. Therefore, subsequent studies increased the MCT dosage to determine whether the quantity ingested was a limiting factor on changes in metabolism.[45,46] Researchers reported that intakes of ~45–85 grams of MCTs either before or during exercise can affect metabolism, shifting away from a reliance on carbohydrates and thus improving time trial performance. However, more recent studies on MCT ingestion have not reproduced these positive results.[40] When a carbohydrate-rich meal is consumed several hours prior to exercise and MCT ingestion, the glycogen-sparing effects and performance improvements have not been shown.[47–49] In

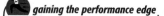
Training Table 4.7: Examples of Preexercise, Well-Balanced Meals Containing Small Amounts of Fat (grams of fat)
• 1½ cups cold cereal, 1 cup 1% milk, 1 cup orange juice (3 g)
• 2 pancakes, 2 tbsp syrup, 6 oz fruited low-fat yogurt (4 g)
• Grilled chicken sandwich [1 bun, 3 oz chicken, lettuce, tomato], 2 tsp light mayonnaise (7 g)
• Granola bar or sports bar (6 g)

many MCT studies, subjects complain of moderate to severe gastrointestinal distress, thus hindering athletic performance.

What type, how much, and when should fats be consumed after exercise?

Unlike carbohydrates and proteins, it is not essential to replace fats used during exercise by consuming certain quantities or types of fat immediately following training or competition. The body's stores of fat are so great that they will not be depleted in an exercise session, even after prolonged endurance events. Carbohydrates and proteins are the main priorities after exercising to replace, restore, and replenish muscles. Therefore, fats should be kept to a minimum immediately after exercise. Fats cause the stomach to empty more slowly than do carbohydrates and proteins, which could potentially delay the delivery of nutrients to the muscles in a timely fashion. However, fats add flavor to foods and create a sense of satiety, and therefore can be included in small amounts in the postexercise meal or snack.

Consuming fats in meals after exercise has received much less research attention in the sports arena than has consuming carbohydrates and proteins. In one small study, seven active individuals were studied to determine the effect of adding fat calories to meals after exercise and its effects on glucose tolerance.[50] They found that the addition of approximately 1500 calories as fat after exhaustive exercise did not alter muscle glycogen resynthesis or glucose tolerance the next day. The subjects consumed the same amount of carbohydrates in a low-fat versus high-fat postexercise diet trial. The high-fat diet increased intramuscular triglyceride storage after exercise. Because the study's purpose was to determine the effect of high- or low-fat diets on glucose tolerance, it is not clear whether there are implications to the increased intramuscular triglycerides as an attempt at improving postexercise recovery or utilization of more intramuscular triglycerides in subsequent exercise bouts. **Training Table 4.8** provides some examples of postexercise meals that contain small amounts of fats.

gaining the performance edge

The dietary guidelines for fats that pertain to daily meal planning can also be applied to the postexercise meal. The focus should be placed on unsaturated fats, in small quantities. As discussed in the carbohydrates chapter, the postexercise meal should be consumed as soon as possible after exercise.

Training Table 4.8: Examples of Postexercise Meals Containing Small to Moderate Amounts of Fat (grams of fat)

- 6 oz. low-fat yogurt, 2 tbsp mixed nuts, 1/4 cup oatmeal (12 g)
- Scrambled tofu [3 oz tofu, 1/4 cup onions, 1/4 cup peppers, 2 tbsp sunflower seeds], 1 slice toast, 1 tbsp jelly (14 g)
- Turkey sandwich [2 slices whole wheat bread, 2 oz turkey, 1 slice tomato, 2 slices cucumber, 2 slices avocado] (11 g)
- Chicken and bean burrito, 1/4 cup salsa, 2 tbsp guacamole (12 g)

The Box Score

Key Points of Chapter

- Fats are an important nutrient for athletes. Not only are dietary fats a primary energy source during rest, light to moderate exercise, and recovery, but they also provide the body with essential fatty acids, serve as vitamin carriers, and provide taste and texture to food.

- Fats belong to a group of compounds known as lipids and can be obtained in the diet from both plants and animals.

- Fats are classified based on their molecular structure. Triglycerides make up the majority of fats in the body; however, other classifications include phospholipids and sterols.

- Triglycerides are composed of a glycerol backbone with three attached fatty acid chains. The fatty acid chains vary in length and saturation level.

- Fatty acids are carbon atoms linked in a chainlike fashion. They can be short (≤4 carbons), medium (6–10 carbons), or long chains (≥12 carbons). In addition, fatty acids can be classified as saturated or unsaturated, and essential or nonessential.

- Fat substitutes have been formulated from carbohydrates, proteins, or fats and offer fewer calories without sacrificing the texture and taste of food. Examples include Oatrim, Benefat, Simplesse, and Olestra.

- No RDA or AI has been set for total dietary fat because of insufficient data to determine a defined level of fat intake at which risk of inadequacy or prevention of chronic disease occurs. The acceptable Macronutrient Distribution Range for fat intake has been set at 20–35% of total energy for adults.

- The formula for calculating the percentage of calories from fat equals the total fat calories divided by the total calories; then multiply by 100.

- Cholesterol serves several vital functions in the body. However, high levels of cholesterol in the blood are related to an increased risk for cardiovascular disease. Of particular concern in regard to cardiovascular disease is the level of low-density lipoprotein (LDL) in the blood, which optimally should be <100 mg/dL.

- Fats are an important energy source during endurance activities. However, high-fat diets either weeks before or hours before competition have not been shown to improve endurance performance.

- Fat consumption during exercise, particularly in ultra-endurance sports, has garnered research interest because of the extreme caloric demands of the sports. However, recent research has not supported the practice of fat intake during exercise. Performance decrements and gastrointestinal distress make fat intake during exercise a dietary practice to avoid. Care must be taken when ingesting MCTs during exercise because MCTs can cause gastrointestinal upset.

- Fat intake after exercise is not as critical as carbohydrate and protein intake because of the body's ample stores of fat; however, small amounts of fats in the postexercise meal or snack can add taste and create a sense of satiety.

Study Questions

1. How do fats differ from carbohydrates both structurally and energetically (i.e., in the number of calories they yield)?

2. What functions do fats serve in the body?

3. What is cholesterol, and what is its role in the body?

4. Discuss the advantages and disadvantages of "fat substitutes."

5. Would cutting out all dietary fat be an appropriate recommendation for an athlete wanting to decrease body fat? Defend your answer.

6. What is the difference between unsaturated, saturated, and hydrogenated fatty acids?

7. Explain how to find and calculate the percentage of calories from saturated fat in a particular food.

8. What would be an appropriate suggestion for fat intake prior to a morning exercise session for an athlete who does not like nuts or seeds?

9. How would you counsel/respond to an endurance athlete who enjoys eating potato chips during long-duration training sessions because they taste salty?

References

1. Institute of Medicine. *Dietary Reference Intakes for Energy, Carbohydrate, Fiber, Fat, Fatty Acids, Cholesterol, Protein, and Amino Acids (Macronutrients)*. Food and Nutrition Board. Washington, DC: National Academy Press; 2002.

2. Livesey G. Energy values of unavailable carbohydrate and diets: an inquiry and analysis. *Am J Clin Nutr*. 1990;51:617–637.

3. Smith T, Brown JC, Livesey G. Energy balance and thermogenesis in rats consuming nonstarch polysaccharides of various fermentabilities. *Am J Clin Nutr*. 1998;68:802–819.

4. Archer SY, Meng S, Shei A, Hodin RA. p21(WAF1) is required for butyrate-mediated growth inhibition of

human colon cancer cells. *Proc Natl Acad Sci USA*. 1998;95(12):6791–6796.

5. Jones PJ, Ntanios FY, Raeini-Sarjaz M, Vanstone CA. Cholesterol-lowering efficacy of a sitostanolcontaining phytosterol mixture with a prudent diet in hyperlipidemic men. *Am J Clin Nutr*. 1999;69(6):1144–1150.

6. Miettinen TA, Puska P, Gylling H, Vanhanen H, Vartiainen E. Reduction of serum cholesterol with sitostanolester margarine in a mildly hypercholesterolemic population. *New Engl J Med*. 1995;333(20):1308–1312.

7. Jones PJ, Raeini-Sarjaz M, Ntanios FY, Vanstone CA, Feng JY, Parsons WE. Modulation of plasma lipid levels and cholesterol kinetics by phytosterol versus phytostanol esters. *J Lipid Res*. 2000;4:697–705.

8. Expert Panel on Detection, Evaluation, and Treatment of High Blood Cholesterol in Adults. Executive summary of the Third Report of the National Cholesterol Education Program (NCEP) Expert Panel on Detection, Evaluation and Treatment of High Blood Cholesterol in Adults (Adult Treatment Panel III). *JAMA*. 2001;285(19):2486–2497.

9. Hawley JA, Dennis SC, Lindsay FH, Noakes TD. Nutritional practices of athletes: are they sub-optimal? *J Sports Sci*. 1995;13:S75–S81.

10. Sundgot-Borgen J. Risk and trigger factors for the development of eating disorder in female elite athletes. *Med Sci Sport Exerc*. 1994;26(4):414–419.

11. Powers P, Johnson C. Targeting eating disorders in elite athletes. Part 1. *Eating Disord Rev*. 1996;7:4.

12. Kris-Etherton PM, Harris WS, Appel LJ. Fish consumption, fish oil, omega-3 fatty acids, and cardiovascular disease. *Circulation*. 2002;106:2747–2757.

13. Spano M. Functional foods, beverages, and ingredients in athletics. *Strength Cond J*. 2010;32(1):79–86.

14. Food and Drug Administration. Food labeling: trans fatty acids in nutrition labeling. *Federal Register*. July 11, 2003; 68 FR 41433.

15. Insel P, Turner RE, Ross D. *Nutrition*. Sudbury, MA: Jones and Bartlett Publishers; 2002.

16. Issekutz B, Miller HI, Paul P, Rodahl K. Aerobic work capacity and plasma FFA turnover. *J Appl Physiol*. 1965;20:293–296.

17. Kiens B. Effect of endurance training on fatty acid metabolism: local adaptations. *Med Sci Sports Exerc*. 1997;29:640–645.

18. Martin WH III. Effect of acute and chronic exercise on fat metabolism. *Exerc Sport Sci Rev*. 1996;24:203–231.

19. Kiens B, Richter EA. Utilization of skeletal muscle triacylglycerol during postexercise recovery in humans. *Am J Physiol*. 1998;275(2):E332–E337.

20. Bergman BC, Butterfield GE, Wolfel EE, et al. Net glucose uptake and glucose kinetics after endurance training in men. *Am J Physiol*. 1999;277:E81–E92.

21. Goedecke JH, Christie C, Wilson G, et al. Metabolic adaptations to a high-fat diet in endurance cyclists. *Metab*. 1999;48:1509–1517.

22. Helge JW. Adaptation to a fat-rich diet: effects on endurance performance in humans. *Sports Med*. 2000;30(5):347–357.

23. Helge JW. Long-term fat diet adaptation effects on performance, training capacity, and fat utilization. *Med Sci Sports Exerc*. 2002;34(9):1499–1504.

24. Kiens B, Helge JW. Effect of high-fat diets on exercise performance. *Proc Nutr Soc*. 1998;57(1):73–75.

25. Okana G, Sato Y, Takumi Y, Sugawara M. Effect of 4h pre-exercise high carbohydrate and high fat meal ingestion on endurance performance and metabolism. *Int J Sports Med*. 1996;17(7):530–534.

26. Hawley JA. Fat metabolism during exercise. In: R. Maughan, ed. *Nutrition in Sport*. Oxford: Blackwell Scientific; 2000:184–191.

27. Jeukendrup AE, Saris WH, Wagenmakers AJ. Fat metabolism during exercise: a review—part III: effects of nutritional interventions. *Int J Sports Med*. 1998;19(6):371–379.

28. Hawley JA. Effect of increased fat availability on metabolism and exercise capacity. *Med Sci Sport Exerc*. 2002;34(9):1485–1491.

29. Rehrer NJ, van Kemenade M, Meester W, Brouns F, Saris WH. Gastrointestinal complaints in relation to dietary intake in triathletes. *Int J Sport Nutr*. 1992;2(1):48–59.

30. Burke LM, Angus DJ, Cox GR, et al. Effect of fat adaptation and carbohydrate restoration on metabolism and performance during prolonged cycling. *J Appl Physiol*. 2000;89:2413–2421.

31. Staudacher HM, Carey AL, Cummings NK, Hawley JA, Burke LM. Short-term high-fat diet alters substrate utilization during exercise but not glucose tolerance in highly trained athletes. *Int J Sports Nutr Exerc Metab*. 2001;11:273–286.

32. Stepto NK, Carey AL, Staudacher HM, Cummings NK, Burke LM, Hawley JA. Effect of short-term fat adaptation on high-intensity training. *Med Sci Sports Exerc*. 2002;34:449–455.

33. Burke LM, Hawley JA. Effects of short-term fat adaptation on metabolism and performance of prolonged exercise. *Med Sci Sports Exerc*. 2002;34(9):1492–1498.

34. Stellingwerff T, Spriet LL, Watt MJ, et al. Decreased PDH activation and glycogenolysis during exercise following fat adaptation with carbohydrate restoration. *Amer J Physiol Endocrinl Metab*. 2006;290:E380–E388.

35. Lambert EV, Gordecke JH, van Zyl C, et al. High-fat diet versus habitual diet prior to carbohydrate loading: effects on exercise metabolism and cycling performance. *Int J Sports Nutr Exerc Metab*. 2001;11:209–225.

36. Lambert EV, Speechly DP, Dennis SC, Noakes TD. Enhanced endurance in trained cyclists during moderate intensity exercise following 2 weeks adaptation to a high fat diet. *Eur J Appl Physiol*. 1994;69:287–293.

37. Fleming J, Sharman MJ, Avery NG, et al. Endurance capacity and high-intensity exercise performance responses to a high-fat diet. *Int J Sports Nutr Exerc Metab*. 2003;13:466–478.

38. Helge JW, Richter EA, Kiens B. Interaction of training and diet on metabolism and endurance during exercise in man. *J Physiol*. 1996;492:293–306.

39. Havemann L, West S, Goedecke JH, et al. Fat adaptation followed by carbohydrate-loading compromises high-intensity sprint performance. *J Appl Physiol*. 2006;100:194–202.

40. Burke LM, Hawley JA. Fat and carbohydrate for exercise. *Clin Nutr Metab Care*. 2006;9(4):476–481.

41. Jeukendrup AE, Saris WH, Van Diesen R, Brouns F, Wagenmakers AJ. Effect of endogenous carbohydrate availability on oral medium-chain triglyceride oxidation during prolonged exercise. *J Appl Physiol*. 1996;80(3):949–954.

42. Jeukendrup AE, Saris WH, Schrauwen P, Brouns F, Wagenmakers AJ. Metabolic availability of medium-chain triglycerides coingested with carbohydrates during prolonged exercise. *J Appl Physiol*. 1995;79(3):756–762.

43. Decombaz J, Arnaud M, Milton H, et al. Energy metabolism of medium-chain triglycerides versus carbohydrates during exercise. *Eur J Appl Physiol*. 1983; 52:9–14.

44. Massicotte D, Peronnet F, Brisson GR, Hillarie-Marcel C. Oxidation of exogenous medium-chain free fatty acids during prolonged exercise: comparison with glucose. *J Appl Physiol*. 1992;73(4):1334–1339.

126   **CHAPTER 4** Fats

45. Satabin P, Portero P, Defer G, Bricout J, Guezennec C. Metabolic and hormonal responses to lipid and carbohydrate diets during exercise in man. *Med Sci Sports Exerc*. 1987;19(3):218–223.

46. Van Zeyl CG, Lambert EL, Hawley JA, Noakes TD, Dennis SC. Effects of medium-chain triglyceride ingestion on fuel metabolism and cycling performance. *J Appl Physiol*. 1996;80(6):2217–2225.

47. Goedecke JH, Elmer-English R, Dennis SC, Schloss I, Noakes TD, Lambert EV. Effects of medium-chain triacylglycerol ingested with carbohydrate on metabolism and exercise performance. *Int J Sports Nutr*. 1999; 9:35–47.

48. Jeukendrup AE, Thielen JJHC, Wagenmakers AJM, Brouns F, Saris WHM. Effect of MCT and carbohydrate ingestion during exercise on substrate utilization and subsequent cycling performance. *Am J Clin Nutr*. 1998;67(3):397–404.

49. Goedecke JH, Clark VR, Noakes TD, et al. The effects of medium-chain triacylglyceral and carbohydrate ingestion on ultra-endurance exercise performance. *Int J Sport Nutr Exerc Metab*. 2005;15:15–28.

50. Fox AK, Kaufman AE, Horowitz JF. Adding fat calories to meals after exercise does not alter glucose tolerance. *J Appl Physiol*. 2004;97:11–16.

Additional Resources

Institute of Medicine. *Dietary Reference Intakes for Water, Potassium, Sodium, Chloride, and Sulfate*. Food and Nutrition Board. Washington, DC: National Academy Press; 2004.

Miller SL, Wolfe RR. Physical exercise as a modulator of adaptation to low and high carbohydrate and low and high fat intakes. *Eur J Clin Nutr*. 1999;53(Suppl):S112–S119.

CHAPTER 5

Proteins

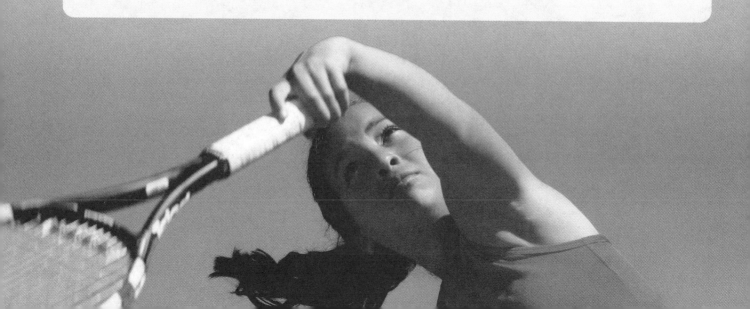

Jamar is a 17-year-old high school junior who has a chance of starting as a linebacker on the football team his senior year. He is 6 feet tall and weighs 175 pounds. His coach has recommended that he gain 10 to 15 pounds over the next 8 months, but not at the sacrifice of his speed and quickness. Jamar eats home-cooked, well-balanced meals for breakfast and supper. At breakfast he also drinks a mega-protein supplement that contains 56 grams of protein. For school, he packs his own lunches, which usually include two tuna or chicken sandwiches with potato chips and milk. He also has a mid-morning and mid-afternoon snack, which typically consists of a protein bar (24 grams of protein/bar). He works out in the high school weight room two to three times per week in the late afternoon. When he arrives home, he studies until the family eats supper, around 7 p.m. His final snack of the day occurs just before bedtime, when he consumes another mega-protein supplement that contains 56 grams of protein.

Questions

- Is Jamar getting enough dietary protein to achieve his goals?

- What are the recommended guidelines for protein intake for an athlete wanting to gain weight?

- Is it detrimental to consume a diet containing too much protein?

Why is protein important to athletes?

If the tissues of the body had an ingredient list similar to the ones on food labels, for most, proteins would be second on the list after water. Most athletes are well aware of the importance of proteins, particularly in regard to muscle, and tend to be concerned that they may not be consuming adequate amounts to meet the body's demands for protein resulting from training/competition. The protein–muscle mass connection is just one of many reasons protein is an essential nutrient to athletes and untrained individuals alike.

Proteins are constantly being turned over in the body. In other words, they are continuously being broken down, transformed, and/or rebuilt. They also can be metabolized for energy, which is of particular concern to athletes involved in energy-demanding endurance sports, such as triathlons or marathons. Any part of the molecular protein structure that is not used is excreted from the body. As a result, proteins, which are a macronutrient, must be replaced on a daily basis through proper diet. Research suggests that athletes engaged in endurance, strength/power, or team sports have higher protein requirements than their sedentary counterparts; however, this does not mean that protein supplementation of their diet is required. This chapter explores proteins, their constituent amino acids, their functions in the body, and specifics about food sources, supplements, and protein needs before, during, and after training.

What are proteins?

Proteins consist of a series of amino acids. Individual

amino acid A molecule that serves as the basic building block for proteins. Amino acids are composed of atoms of carbon (C), hydrogen (H), oxygen (O), and nitrogen (N).

amino acids are molecules composed of atoms of carbon (C), hydrogen (H), oxygen (O), and nitrogen (N). The different amino acids have similar basic structures (see Figure 5.1). All amino acids contain a central carbon atom that is bound to an amino group (NH₂), a carboxylic acid group (COOH), a carbon side chain, and a hydrogen atom. The presence of the nitrogen-containing amino group and the carboxylic acid group in the chemical structure of these molecules accounts for why they are called "amino acids." The carbon side chain gives each amino acid its unique structure, physical characteristics, and specific name. The side chains vary in shape, size, electrical activity, and pH. When two or more amino acids link to form a protein, it is the side chain characteristics of

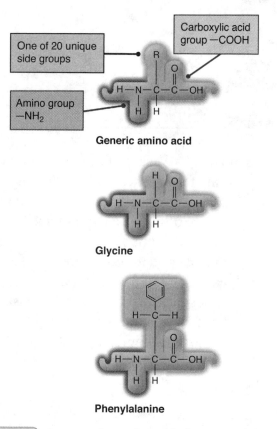

Figure 5.1 Structure of an amino acid. All amino acids have a similar structure. Attached to a carbon atom is a hydrogen (H) atom, shown here but not in later illustrations of amino acids; an amino group (NH₂); a carboxylic acid group (COOH); and a side group (R). The side group gives each amino acid its unique identity.

the amino acids that determine the protein's specialized function and shape.

The amino acids that make up a protein are held together via **peptide bonds**. The peptide bonds that link amino acids are formed when the amine group of one amino acid connects with the acid group of another amino acid (see Figure 5.2). In the course of peptide bond formation, a water molecule is formed. The process in which water is created during the formation of a chemical bond is known as **condensation**. Conversely, if large amounts of protein are consumed in the diet, the body must break the peptide bonds between amino acids holding the dietary proteins together. To do so, a process known as **hydrolysis**, which is the opposite of condensa-

peptide bond A type of chemical bond that links the amine group of one amino acid to the acid group of another amino acid when forming a protein.

condensation A chemical process that results in the formation of water molecules. Condensation occurs when peptide bonds are formed between amino acids.

hydrolysis A chemical process that requires utilization of water to break the chemical bond between elements or molecules. Hydrolysis is required to break peptide bonds between amino acids.

<table>
<tr><td>

essential amino acid An amino acid that must be obtained from the diet because the body is unable to make it on its own.

nonessential amino acid A type of amino acid that can be made by the body from other amino acids or compounds and thus does not need to be supplied by diet.

conditionally essential amino acid An amino acid that under normal conditions is not considered an essential amino acid, but because of unusual circumstances (e.g., severe illness) becomes essential because the body loses its ability to make it.

tion, must occur. Hydrolysis uses water in the process of breaking the peptide bonds of the ingested proteins. As a result, the digestion of high-protein diets can contribute to water loss resulting from hydrolysis and eventually lead to dehydration if fluid intake is not maintained.

Twenty different amino acids are available for use in the human body. Nine of these are considered **essential amino acids** because they cannot be produced in the body. Therefore, they must be consumed in adequate amounts through dietary intake. Eleven additional amino acids are considered **nonessential**. They can be produced in the body and therefore do not need to be consumed in the diet (see **Table 5.1**). Two of the nonessential amino acids, tyrosine and cysteine, can become essential amino acids under certain conditions. They are considered **conditionally essential.** Under normal conditions the body makes tyrosine from phenylalanine and makes cysteine from methionine. If intake of phenylalanine and methionine (both essential amino acids) is low, the body will need exogenous tyrosine and cysteine from the diet, and thus they

TABLE 5.1	Essential and Nonessential Amino Acids
Essential Amino Acids	**Nonessential Amino Acids**
Leucine*	Alanine
Isoleucine*	Arginine
Valine*	Asparagine
Histidine	Aspartic acid
Lysine	Cysteine
Methionine	Glutamic acid
Phenylalanine	Glutamine
Threonine	Glycine
Tryptophan	Proline
	Serine
	Tyrosine

*Branched chain amino acids

become essential. Arginine may also be considered conditionally essential during serious illness, stress, and growth spurts in young individuals.

Although the main role of amino acids is to build proteins needed by the body, they can also be metabolized in the liver and muscle for energy. However, to be used for energy, most amino acids must be converted to glucose via gluconeogenesis in the liver and then delivered via the blood to the working muscle. The branched chain amino acids (BCAAs), which are essential amino acids, can be metabolized for energy directly within the muscle itself. BCAAs make up approximately one-third of the protein content of muscle and include the amino acids leucine, isoleucine, and valine. The BCAAs have garnered recent research attention because of their role as an energy source during exercise and because they also may play a role in regulating muscle protein synthesis. Branched chain amino acids are relatively abundant in whole foods. Dairy products, meat, wheat protein, soy, and whey protein isolates are rich sources of BCAAs.

Proteins are chains of amino acids that are linked in a very specific sequence (see Figure 5.3). The specific sequence of the amino acids in the chain gives the protein not only its physical characteristics, but also its three-dimensional shape. The shape of the protein in many instances dictates its function in the body, which is particularly true for those proteins that serve as enzymes or hormones.

Proteins can be classified according to the length of their amino acid chain. When two

dipeptide A simple protein consisting of two amino acids linked via peptide bonds.

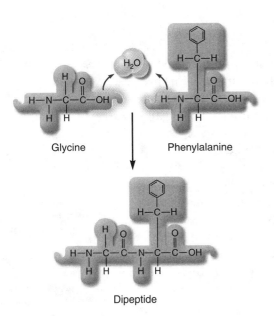

Figure 5.2 Peptide bond formation. When two amino acids join together, the carboxylic acid group of one amino acid is matched with the amino group of another.

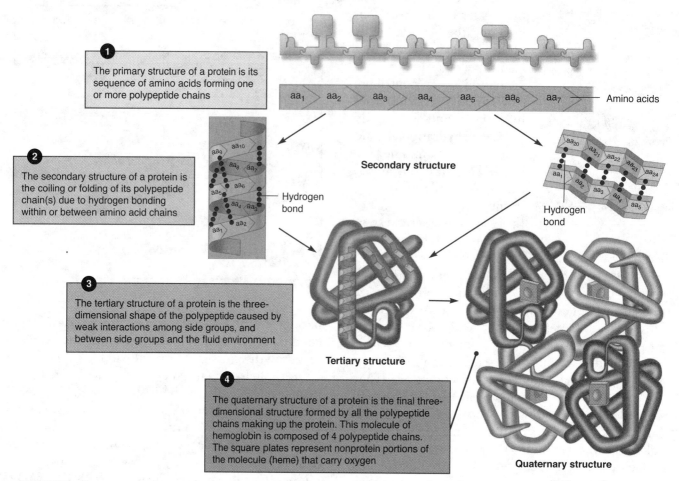

Primary structure

1 The primary structure of a protein is its sequence of amino acids forming one or more polypeptide chains

aa_1 aa_2 aa_3 aa_4 aa_5 aa_6 aa_7 — Amino acids

2 The secondary structure of a protein is the coiling or folding of its polypeptide chain(s) due to hydrogen bonding within or between amino acid chains

Secondary structure

Hydrogen bond

Hydrogen bond

3 The tertiary structure of a protein is the three-dimensional shape of the polypeptide caused by weak interactions among side groups, and between side groups and the fluid environment

Tertiary structure

4 The quaternary structure of a protein is the final three-dimensional structure formed by all the polypeptide chains making up the protein. This molecule of hemoglobin is composed of 4 polypeptide chains. The square plates represent nonprotein portions of the molecule (heme) that carry oxygen

Quaternary structure

Figure 5.3   Primary protein structure. Each protein becomes folded, twisted, and coiled into a shape all its own. This shape defines how a protein functions in your body. The simplest depiction of a protein reveals its unique sequence of amino acids.

tripeptide A protein molecule made up of three amino acids linked via peptide bonds.

oligopeptide A protein molecule made up of 4 to 10 amino acids that are linked via peptide bonds.

polypeptide A protein molecule made up of more than 10 amino acids that are linked via peptide bonds.

amino acids are linked, the result is a **dipeptide** protein. A **tripeptide** is a protein made of three amino acids. There are also **oligopeptides** (chains of 4–10 linked amino acids) and **polypeptides** (chains with more than 10 amino acids). Most proteins found in the body and in foods are polypeptides made up of hundreds of amino acids. Foods eaten daily must provide the amino acids required to maintain these complex polypeptides found in the body.

What is the difference between a "complete" and an "incomplete" protein?

Consuming protein-rich foods on a daily basis is necessary to obtain appropriate amounts of the es-

sential amino acids. Protein is found in both animal- and plant-based foods. The terms *complete* and *incomplete* often are used to categorize protein sources. It should be noted that these terms should not be inferred to mean "superior" and "inferior." Each food provides a unique profile of proteins and amino acid content, as well as other health benefits, and therefore a variety of protein sources should be consumed throughout the day.

Animal proteins, such as eggs, dairy products, meat, and fish, contain all of the essential amino acids in high amounts and therefore are considered **complete proteins**. Animal proteins are also commonly referred to as **high-quality proteins**. A high-quality protein (1) con-

complete protein A protein source that supplies the body with all of the essential amino acids in high amounts.

high-quality protein Source of protein that contains a full complement of all the essential amino acids, has extra amino acids that are available for nonessential amino acid synthesis, and has good digestibility.

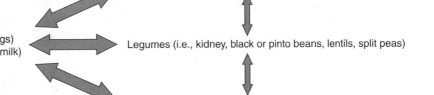

Grains (i.e., whole grain bread, cereal, rice, pasta)

Animal products (i.e., meat, dairy, eggs)
Soy products (i.e., tofu, tempeh, soy milk)

Legumes (i.e., kidney, black or pinto beans, lentils, split peas)

Nuts and Seeds (i.e., peanuts, almonds, walnuts, flaxseeds, sunflower seeds)

Figure 5.4 Complementary protein combinations. Because animal and soy products contain high levels of all essential amino acids, they can be consumed with any grain, legume, or nut/seed. Grains are complemented by legumes, and legumes are complemented by nuts/seeds. Grains are not a complementary match to nuts/seeds, but these two groups make a tasty combination in recipes.

incomplete protein Sources of proteins that do not contain the full complement of essential amino acids.

limiting amino acid The essential amino acid that is in short supply in an incomplete protein source.

complementing proteins A group of two or more incomplete protein foods that when eaten together provide the full complement of essential amino acids.

tains all of the essential amino acids, (2) has extra amino acids available for nonessential amino acid synthesis, and (3) has good digestibility. Animal proteins provide all of the essential amino acids, as well as extra nonessential amino acids, and are about 95% digestible (as compared to plant proteins, which are 85% digestible); animal proteins thus deserve the high quality rating.

An **incomplete protein** source lacks one or more essential amino acids. The essential amino acid that is in short supply in a specific food is called the **limiting amino acid**. All plant products (grains, beans, vegetables, fruits, nuts, and seeds), with the exception of soy, are categorized as incomplete proteins. Soy is unique in that it is the only plant product that provides a full profile of essential amino acids in high amounts, similar to animal proteins; thus, soy is considered a complete protein. In regard to other plant proteins, a variety of foods should be consumed daily to consume all the amino acids in sufficient amounts. Consuming proteins from a variety of food sources so that the diet contains all the essential amino acids in a meal or within a day is called **complementing proteins**. If two different foods are eaten in the same meal or in the same day, one food may contain all but one essential amino acid in sufficient amounts while the other may provide this limiting amino acid, thus complementing both foods. For example, grains' limiting amino acid is lysine, but grains are high in the amino acid methionine. Therefore, grains match well with legumes, which are low in methionine but high in lysine. Refer to **Figure 5.4** for examples of complementary protein combinations. Examples of plant-

based meals combining complementing proteins include the following:

- Stir-fried vegetables and tofu over rice (soy and grains)
- Vegetable chili with cornbread (legumes and grains)
- Barbecued tempeh on whole wheat bun (soy and grains)
- Oatmeal with nuts and soy milk (grains, nuts, and soy)
- Spinach salad with vegetables, garbanzo beans, and sunflower seeds (legumes and seeds)

Table 5.2 provides the protein content of a variety of plant-based foods.

TABLE 5.2	Protein Content of Plant-Based Foods
Protein Source	**Protein Content (g)**
Grains	
Brown rice, 1 cup	5
Wheat bread, 2 slices	6
Spaghetti, 1 cup	6.7
Legumes	
Lentils, 1 cup	7.9
Kidney beans, 1 cup	15.4
Chickpeas, 1 cup	14.5
Nuts/Seeds	
Peanut butter, 2 tbsp	9
Walnuts, 1 oz	6.9
Sunflower seeds, 1 oz	6.5
Soy Products	
Soy milk, 1 cup	7
Tempeh, ½ cup	16
Soybeans, 1 cup cooked	26
Soy nuts, ¼ cup	8

gaining the performance edge

For health and optimal sport performance, the body requires adequate amounts of essential amino acids on a daily basis. Athletes can meet protein needs by consuming a variety of protein-rich foods from both plant and animal sources.

Complementing proteins also can occur when combining a plant food with an animal product. The bottom line is that variety is best. Adequate protein can be consumed through all animal foods, all plant foods, or a combination of the two. The variety of protein sources and the daily meal plan developed for athletes should be derived from their preferences and tolerances for various protein sources.

The term *incomplete* given to most plant protein sources is often misinterpreted as meaning "inadequate" or "useless" because of the concept of a limiting amino acid. Not only can sufficient amounts of all amino acids be obtained by consuming a variety of plant protein sources throughout the day, but also additional health benefits can be derived from focusing heavily on a plant-based diet. Plant proteins contain fiber, are low in fat, contain no cholesterol, and are usually lower in calories than animal proteins. They also contain antioxidants and phytochemicals that can provide protection against heart disease and some cancers.

What are the main functions of proteins in the body?

Proteins have a role in almost all major body functions. They provide structure to muscles and other tissues, act as regulators of cell functions, assist in maintaining fluid and acid-base balance, help transport substances throughout the body, and serve as an energy source when needed. Overall health and sport performance can be impaired if protein intake is too low or if protein catabolism is too high.

Proteins make up the constituent parts of many structures, including bones, ligaments, tendons, hair, fingernails/toenails, muscles, teeth, and organs. Without adequate protein intake, these structures, particularly muscle, cannot be maintained, much less strengthened, in response to training. Thus the end result of chronic low dietary protein intake is decreased sport performance and increased risk for injury.

enzymes A group of complex proteins whose function is to catalyze biochemical reactions in the body.

Dietary proteins are also used by the body to make **enzymes**. Enzymes serve as catalysts for a variety of bio-

chemical reactions. Every cell contains and/or produces many types of enzymes, each with its own purpose. Digestive enzymes are produced and released by cells found in the stomach, intestines, and pancreas to break down carbohydrates, proteins, and fats into monosaccharides, amino acids, and fatty acids, respectively, so that they can be absorbed and utilized by the body. In regard to sport performance, all of the bioenergetic pathways responsible for the formation of adenosine triphosphate (ATP), which is the ultimate energy source for muscles, are dependent on enzymes. Without adequate dietary intake of protein, the body cannot maintain enzyme levels, and critical body functions begin to decline.

Many of the body's hormones are structurally derived from proteins. Most hormones are produced by specialized glands located throughout the body and serve a variety of regulatory functions. The pancreas produces insulin and glucagon, protein-derived hormones that help regulate blood glucose levels. Hormones also stimulate certain tissues to assist the body in meeting physical challenges. For example, the adrenal glands produce epinephrine and norepinephrine, which are protein-derived hormones that play a large role in preparing and helping the body to perform physical activity. These hormones stimulate the heart to beat faster and more forcefully so that more blood can be delivered to working muscles. They also stimulate enzymes in fat cells to release fatty acids into the bloodstream, supplying the muscles with energy. Hormones clearly play an important role in the athlete's ability to perform, and thus dietary proteins are required to ensure normal hormone production.

Proteins also are important to the body's immune function. Protein-derived antibodies attack and destroy bacteria, viruses, and other foreign substances. Immunizations such as the flu shot include inactive viruses. When injected into the body, these viruses stimulate the body to develop antibodies to the specific virus. The antibodies "remember" the virus to which they were exposed. If an individual is exposed to the virus again, the body initiates its defense mechanism and produces more antibodies to fight off the infection. If dietary protein needs are not met, the immune system can be compromised and the athlete's risk for illness is increased.

Circulating proteins in the blood play a role in maintaining the body's fluid balance. Proteins cannot diffuse freely through cell membranes, so they help establish an osmotic pressure within the blood. To maintain equilibrium, fluids must be moved back

intracellular A term used to describe structures, fluids, or other substances found inside the cell.

extracellular A term used to describe structures, fluids, or other substances found outside of the cell.

and forth between the blood and the **intracellular** (inside the cells) or **extracellular** (outside the cells) spaces. Albumin is the major blood protein that helps maintain fluid balance between the tissues and the blood. If inadequate blood protein levels occur, the osmotic pressure within the blood is high, and fluid "leaks" into the surrounding tissues, causing swelling or edema.

Proteins also help control the acidity level (i.e., pH balance) within the body. Under normal conditions the body's fluids are close to neutral, neither acidic nor basic. However, during exercise, lactic acid is produced. Lactic acid increases the acidity of body fluids, and if not buffered can cause fatigue within the muscle. Proteins buffer the lactic acid and thus delay the onset of fatigue, which is critical to an athlete's performance.

Many of the body's transporter molecules also are made of protein. A prime example is hemoglobin. Hemoglobin is a protein-derived carrier molecule that transports oxygen in the blood to tissues throughout the body. If hemoglobin levels are low, less oxygen is delivered to muscle cells, greatly reducing exercise capacity and endurance.

Although not a major source of energy, protein can be used as energy during or following exercise.

gaining the performance edge

Without adequate protein intake, many key enzymes, hormones, and other compounds cannot be made by cells. In addition, body structures, such as muscle, cannot be maintained, repaired, or strengthened with intense training. Athletes should consume protein-rich foods daily to ensure overall health, optimize performance, and prevent athletic-related injuries.

The body prefers to burn carbohydrates and fats for energy at rest and during exercise; however, if carbohydrate stores are low, energy expenditure is high, and/or calorie intake is inadequate, proteins can be converted to glucose and used for energy (see "How does carbohydrate intake affect protein metabolism?" in Chapter 2). This is one of the reasons why endurance athletes must ensure that they consume adequate carbohydrate and protein in their diet (see Chapter 12).

What is nitrogen balance?

Because proteins in the body are constantly breaking down and have to be resynthesized, daily input of new amino acids into the body's amino acid pool is required. The goal of any dietary plan should be to supply enough amino acids to support the increase in protein synthesis resulting from training and competition, while at the same time meeting the body's basic maintenance needs. One way to determine whether an individual's protein needs are being met is through the measurement of **nitrogen balance**.

Nitrogen balance occurs in the body when dietary input of nitrogen (i.e., protein gain) equals the output of nitrogen (i.e., protein loss).

nitrogen balance A way of monitoring nitrogen status in the body. When dietary input of nitrogen (i.e., protein gain) equals the output of nitrogen (i.e., protein loss), then nitrogen balance has been achieved.

The state of nitrogen balance can be calculated using the following equation:

(nitrogen in) – (nitrogen out) = nitrogen status

Because dietary protein is the main source of nitrogen, the amount of "nitrogen in" can be estimated by monitoring daily protein intake. Determining "nitrogen out" is much more complicated.

Proteins are constantly being lost from the body. Some proteins are lost from the external surface of the body as a result of mechanical wear (e.g., sloughed off skin, broken fingernails, lost hair), but the majority are lost via cellular metabolism. When amino acids are broken down internally, the nitrogen group is cleaved from the molecule. The released nitrogen can be lost from the body via the formation of urea in the liver or, to a much lesser extent, as ammonia. By measuring the urea levels in urine and sweat, it is possible to estimate nitrogen loss. If the body is in nitrogen balance, then the difference between nitrogen in (i.e., dietary protein intake) and nitrogen out (i.e., urea excreted) is zero.

A positive nitrogen balance indicates that dietary protein intake (nitrogen in) is greater than protein loss (nitrogen out). When nitrogen is being retained by the body, it indicates that it is being used to make lean tissue.[1] A positive nitrogen balance can occur in an athlete who is weight training to build muscle mass and is consuming adequate calories along with a high, but appropriate, protein intake.[1] Conversely, some athletes may find themselves in negative nitrogen balance. For exam-

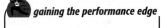
gaining the performance edge

By consuming adequate daily calories and protein, athletes can maintain nitrogen balance or even achieve positive nitrogen status. A positive nitrogen balance indicates that an athlete is in a "protein-building state" versus one of protein breakdown, which can negatively affect athletic performance.

ple, an endurance athlete who is training intensely but not eating enough food to meet her or his daily caloric needs will start mobilizing proteins for energy and thus increase nitrogen loss.[2] A negative nitrogen status is not desirable because it is an indication that lean body tissue is being metabolized by the body. At a minimum, the goal for any athlete is to maintain nitrogen balance; ideally, he or she should try to achieve a positive nitrogen balance.

How much protein should athletes consume daily?

It is clear that protein is critical for optimal athletic performance. It is also known that athletes have higher protein needs than their sedentary counterparts. However, even among athletes, protein recommendations are not one-size-fits-all. Recommendations exist for different categories of athletes, with variances in individual protein requirements based on a variety of factors. Current body weight, total energy intake, desire to lose or gain weight, carbohydrate availability, exercise intensity and duration, training status, quality of dietary protein, and the age of the individual all need to be considered when calculating protein recommendations and developing a dietary plan for athletes.

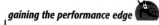

gaining the performance edge

Current research indicates that athletes have higher protein needs than nonathletes.

How can protein requirements be calculated based on body weight?

The easiest and most reliable way to determine individual protein needs is to calculate daily requirements based on current body weight. The Recommended Dietary Allowance (RDA) for the general public is 0.8 grams of protein per kilogram of body weight (0.8 g/kg).[3] The adult Acceptable Macronutrient Distribution Range (AMDR) for protein is 10–35% of daily calories.[3] Current research suggests that athletes need more protein than the general public, but the recommended ranges are still under debate.

A majority of the recent research has focused on the amount of protein required to keep strength athletes in positive nitrogen balance despite the breakdown of muscle tissue and the subsequent increased protein synthesis during and after resistance training. The current daily protein recommendations for strength athletes range from 1.4 g/kg to 2.0 g/kg.[4–7] Some recommendations suggest an upper limit as high as 2.5 g/kg. The exact upper limit of protein

intake that is safe and effective for athletes has yet to be determined. Intakes of 1.4–2.0 g/kg mean that the percentage of total calories coming from protein will typically range from 15–20%, which is well within the AMDR range. Refer to Chapter 13 for example calculations of protein needs for strength and power athletes.

Endurance athletes also have increased daily needs for dietary protein. Because of factors such as repetitive muscle contractions, high-impact activities, increased demand for mitochondria and enzymes involved in aerobic metabolism, and some oxidation of amino acids during aerobic exercise, it is suggested that endurance athletes consume at least 1.2 g/kg of protein daily.[8–13] Individual needs can range up to 2.0 g/kg, especially for the ultra-endurance athlete who trains 4–6 hours or more a day. Because calorie needs for endurance and ultra-endurance athletes can range from 3000–6000 or more per day, the relative contribution of protein at levels of 1.2–2.0 g/kg will typically fall between 12% and 18% of total calories. See Chapter 12 for example calculations of protein needs for endurance athletes.

Research regarding the protein needs of team sport athletes is sparse. Because of the nature of most team sports, which use a combination of strength/power and endurance, it can be assumed that protein needs would fall in the middle of the ranges for both strength and endurance athletes. Therefore, the current protein recommendation for team sport athletes ranges from 1.2–1.6 g/kg daily. This amount of dietary protein typically contributes 12–16% of the total calories ingested per day. Chapter 14 provides several sample calculations of protein needs for various team sport athletes. **Table 5.3** provides a summary of the protein needs for various athletes.

TABLE 5.3	Daily Protein Recommendations for Athletes	
Type of Athlete	Daily Grams of Protein/ Kilogram Body Weight	Percentage of Total Calories Contributed by Protein
Sedentary individual	0.8 g/kg	12–15%
Strength athlete	1.4–2.0 g/kg	15–20%
Endurance athlete	1.2–2.0 g/kg	12–18%
Team sport athlete	1.2–1.6 g/kg	12–16%
Weight gain/loss	1.6–2.0 g/kg	16–20%

As already stated, protein intake for athletes should contribute approximately 12–20% of total calories. After calculating an estimated range of protein requirements (in grams) for an athlete based on body weight, always compare the recommendation to total calorie requirements. The percentage of total calories from protein is calculated as follows:

total grams of protein × 4 calories per gram of protein =
total calories from protein
(total calories from protein ÷ total calorie requirements) × 100 =
% of total calories contributed by protein

For example, a team sport athlete who weighs 82 kg requires 98–131 grams of protein per day (1.2–1.6 g/kg). If this individual consumes 2800–3300 calories per day, protein will be contributing 14–16% of total calories:

98 × 4 = 392 calories from protein
(392 ÷ 2800) × 100 = 14% of total calories from protein

or

131 × 4 = 524 calories from protein
(524 ÷ 3300) × 100 = 16% of total calories from protein

Calculating the percentage of total calories from protein is an excellent way to double-check the accuracy and appropriateness of estimated individual protein recommendations. Ideally, protein should contribute at least 12–20% of total calories. Although no tolerable upper limit (UL) has been set for protein, it is suggested that all Americans, including athletes, consume no more than 30–35% of total calories from protein to decrease the risk of chronic disease.[3]

How do various dietary and training factors affect protein recommendations?

As mentioned previously, individual protein requirements will vary based on a variety of factors. When calculating daily protein needs for a specific athlete, begin with the recommended ranges stated in the previous section, based on the sport. Then consider the following factors to ultimately determine whether protein requirements will be calculated at the low or high end of the recommended ranges.

Total energy intake

If an athlete is consuming an adequate number of calories, protein requirements can be calculated in the middle of the recommended range. Adequate energy intake, particularly in the form of carbohydrates, spares muscle protein and promotes protein synthesis. In general, athletes who consume adequate calories tend to have adequate protein intakes as well, even meeting their increased needs for training and competition.[14] However, it is not always easy for athletes to maintain an adequate calorie and protein intake. For example, athletes who train one or more times a day and those involved in endurance sports have higher calorie and protein needs. It is often difficult for these athletes to have the time, energy, desire, and appetite to eat the number of calories needed to maintain nitrogen balance. Athletes should focus on consuming calorie-dense foods and fluids, along with additional snacks, during intense training sessions and long-duration exercise to spare protein.

Desire to lose or gain weight

Many athletes have the goal of either gaining or losing weight. In both of these situations, protein needs are increased and should be calculated at the high end of the recommended range. For example, a football player may be working intensely in the weight room during preseason training to increase muscle mass, which requires a higher level of protein to ensure proper recovery from training and to assist the body in synthesizing new muscle tissue. Conversely, a triathlete may be aiming to lose 5–10 pounds during off-season training, which typically consists of weekly swim, bike, and run workouts with long-duration sessions of each discipline, plus an emphasis on strength training in the weight room. More protein is required not only to recover from the workouts, but also to ensure that the athlete stays in positive nitrogen balance when calorie intake is lower than normal.

In either scenario, adequate daily calories should be consumed in order to maximize the use of ingested protein. If caloric intake is inadequate, proteins will be increasingly relied upon to provide energy both at rest and during exercise. When amino acids become an energy source, it is at the expense of being used for their primary purposes such as making enzymes and hormones, repairing and developing structural tissues, and providing transport needs. In addition, low calorie and protein intake can lead to a loss of muscle mass, which will ultimately decrease an athlete's strength, power, endurance, and

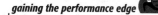
metabolism. It is imperative that sports nutrition professionals counsel athletes on the detrimental impact of not meeting total energy needs, on the consequences of following a very low calorie diet, and on athletes' ability to meet their weight goals as well as to recover from and adapt to physical training.

Carbohydrate availability

In Chapter 3, we discussed how carbohydrates are the primary fuel for working muscles at moderate and high exercise intensities. Carbohydrates are the only fuel that can be metabolized anaerobically and thus become the primary source during intense aerobic activity. Because of their energetic value and their role in maintaining blood sugar levels, if carbohydrate stores become depleted, the body will begin manufacturing carbohydrates (i.e., glucose) from proteins. Adequate daily carbohydrate intake keeps carbohydrate stores at an optimal level and thus spares proteins. In short, as carbohydrate availability increases, protein metabolized for energy decreases, thus moderating protein requirements.

Exercise intensity and duration

Training intensity and duration both increase protein requirements. Exercise intensity refers to how much effort is being put forth to perform an exercise. In other words, as the intensity of exercise increases, so does an athlete's rating of perceived exertion. Duration refers to how long the exercise bout lasts. Although the role of protein in the body is more functional and structural than energetic, whenever the body's metabolism increases, the energetic role of proteins in the body also increases. Protein utilization appears to be positively related to both the intensity and the duration of exercise. This is particularly the case with endurance-type exercise and is exacerbated when carbohydrate stores are depleted or low during exercise. Increasing the duration of exercise begins to deplete glycogen reserves in the liver and muscle, and, as already noted, whenever carbohydrate levels fall in the body, protein utilization increases. This is often seen when athletes exercise in an already glycogen-depleted state or when carbohydrate stores become depleted during a single bout of long-duration or highly intense exercise.

Unlike endurance training, single sessions of resistance exercise, regardless of the length or intensity of the workout, do not appear to increase the use of protein during the workout itself. However, amino acid uptake after the resistance training session does increase, indicating that the amino acids are being used for muscle repair and construction rather than for energy. The additional use of protein for energy in endurance athletes, and for muscle repair and synthesis with intense resistance training, explains the recommendations for increased daily protein intakes.

Training state/fitness level

Protein utilization appears to be higher for athletes who are less fit. When endurance training is initiated, nitrogen balance may be negative for the first 2 weeks. When strength training is first initiated, protein requirements may be higher in the first weeks to support new muscle growth.[4] As both strength- and endurance-focused athletes continue their training, nitrogen balance becomes neutral or positive. After 1 to 2 weeks on the program, the utilization of protein decreases as the body adapts to the training. The take-home message is that protein needs appear to increase during the first couple weeks of a new training regimen and return to baseline levels soon thereafter. Based on this knowledge, temporarily increasing the protein intake of individuals starting a new training program or athletes starting a new phase in their training cycle (i.e., from off-season training to in-season training) may be a practice worth considering.

Dietary protein quality

Athletes need to consume adequate amounts of all essential amino acids to sustain protein functions. Athletes who consume animal proteins (complete proteins) will have all the essential amino acids available for protein functions. Vegetarian athletes have slightly higher protein needs because of the intake of incomplete proteins, and therefore protein intake levels should be calculated at the high end of the recommended range. Vegetarians may also need to plan more diligently to consume adequate levels of daily protein through complementary plant protein sources. Whether athletes consume animal or plant proteins, variety is the key to consuming all of the essential amino acids.

Age

The RDAs for young people are 0.95 g/kg/day for 4–13-year-olds and 0.85 g/kg/day for 14–18-year-olds.[3] Youth and teenage athletes have a slightly higher RDA for protein for several reasons. Body growth and development increase greatly around puberty, which place tremendous energy and protein demands on the body. When combined with the physiologic energy and protein demands imposed by training and sport participation, the concern regarding calorie and protein intake becomes evident. The concern surrounding young athletes is further exacerbated by their typically poor dietary habits, particularly in the teenage group. Young athletes need to focus on achieving adequate energy and protein intakes for growth and development, as well as for the added energy demands of sport training/competition. Doing so will help spare body proteins needed not only for growth and development, but also for recovery and adaptive purposes.

The number of older adults (i.e., individuals 65 years of age and older) exercising and/or competing in sports is rising. Unlike young athletes, protein needs caused by growth and development are not an issue; however, this does not mean that protein intake is inconsequential. Research clearly indicates that older individuals can tolerate and respond to exercise training. Their tissues retain the ability to adapt by becoming larger and stronger. For example, Esmark et al. found a 25% increase in mean muscle fiber area in elderly males after a 12-week resistance training program.[15] This program also included a protein/carbohydrate supplement (10 grams protein + 7 grams carbohydrate) immediately after resistance training to aid in muscle recovery and construction. Amino acids are needed to meet older adults' adaptive needs, similar to younger athletes. Unfortunately, elderly individuals often have poor nutritional habits, may lack an appetite, or lack the knowledge to purchase and prepare high-quality, nutrient-dense foods. Sports nutrition professionals should pay close attention to total calories consumed and protein intake of older athletes. Despite previous misconceptions, the bodies of older adults are capable of adapting to training regardless of age. Educating older adult athletes on the importance of consuming adequate total calories and nutrient-dense protein sources is essential.

Can too much protein be harmful?

Although adequate protein consumption is of great importance to athletes, more is not always better. Based on the AMDR for protein, individuals should not exceed 35% of total calories from protein. Protein is a hot topic for athletes, particularly strength/power athletes and those attempting to lose weight. Many of these athletes consume more than 35% of their total calories from protein. Although these athletes believe they are enhancing their performance, very high levels of protein can actually hinder health and performance. All athletes need to understand the potential safety and health concerns associated with excessive protein intake.

A considerable number of questions have been raised about the effects of high protein intake on kidney function. The kidneys filter waste from the liver, including urea, which is one of the waste products of protein metabolism. When protein intake exceeds the body's ability to use it, the excess protein is stripped of its amine group and the remaining carbon skeleton is used for energy or converted to fat. The nitrogen-containing amine group forms urea, which is then carried via the blood to the kidneys for excretion in the urine. As a result, high-protein diets can place additional stress on the kidneys to remove urea. Although a concern, the increased strain on the kidneys does not appear to affect athletes with normal kidney function—at least short term.[4,10] Long-term studies on the effects of high protein intakes on healthy athletes are currently not available. However, athletes with kidney disease or chronic conditions that may lead to kidney malfunction, such as diabetes or high blood pressure, should avoid excessive protein consumption, maintaining an adequate but moderate intake of protein daily.

Dehydration also can be a result of a high-protein diet. The breaking of peptide bonds during digestion of proteins requires water. In addition, the excretion of urea resulting from protein degradation

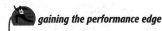

increases body water loss in the form of urine. If athletes consume excessive amounts of protein via food or through supplementation, the body's fluid needs are increased. Failure to meet fluid needs results in dehydration, which can jeopardize not only athletic performance, but also the athlete's health and safety.

The fat and total calorie content typically associated with high protein intake is also of concern. Many high-protein foods, such as full-fat meat and dairy products, are a significant source of total fat, saturated fat, and cholesterol. All of these factors have been associated with an increased risk of cardiovascular disease and some cancers. If high-protein food selections are also high in total calories, weight gain is possible, which will negatively affect health and performance.

Often an emphasis on high-protein foods displaces other lower calorie, nutrient-dense foods such as fruits, vegetables, whole grains, and plant proteins. More research is needed to identify the specific role of protein in chronic diseases and weight management versus other nutritional factors. Until that information becomes available, adequate but not excessive intake of protein is recommended.

High protein consumption increases the excretion of calcium from the bones. A large amount of acid is generated when excessive amounts of protein are consumed, requiring the body to either excrete or buffer the acid to maintain pH balance. When acid levels rise, the body responds by leaching calcium, a buffering agent, from the bones.[16] Over time, this can contribute to bone mineral losses, potentially increasing the risk of osteoporosis. This leaching effect has been documented to be more profound with the excessive consumption of animal versus plant proteins.[17] Therefore, athletes should be encouraged to consume appropriate amounts of protein, including a variety of protein sources, while also obtaining adequate levels of calcium daily. Sports nutrition professionals need to screen athletes for potentially excessive protein intakes. Athletes should be encouraged to achieve adequate protein intake through whole foods versus supplements. Additional protein intake, if needed, should not be at the expense of other macro- and micronutrients. If protein intake is increased, athletes should be counseled to also increase fluid intake to prevent any potential for dehydration.

gaining the performance edge

The recommended protein intake is 1.4–2.0 g/kg for strength athletes, 1.2–2.0 g/kg for endurance athletes, and 1.2–1.6 g/kg for team sport athletes.

Which foods contain protein?

Proteins are found within most food groups of the MyPlate food guidance system (see Chapter 1). The richest sources of protein are found in the dairy/alternative and protein foods groups. Grain products as well as vegetables provide a small to moderate amount of protein. Fruits and oils provide minimal to no protein. Because protein is not found universally within each food group, it is imperative that athletes include a variety of protein sources in sufficient amounts daily for optimal performance and health.

Which foods in the grains group contain protein?

Foods from the grains group are moderate sources of protein. The grains are considered an incomplete protein source because they contain lower levels of lysine. The key is to consume whole grain products in conjunction with legumes, nuts, or seeds throughout the day to balance the intake of amino acids. **Table 5.4** lists a variety of healthy whole grain options and their respective protein levels. **Training Table 5.1** provides some menu ideas for including whole grain sources of protein in the diet.

Which foods in the fruit and vegetable groups contain protein?

Vegetables contain a small amount of protein, contributing approximately 1–2 grams of protein per serving. Fruits contain minimal amounts of protein and therefore should not be considered a protein source. However, both fruits and vegetables contribute valuable nutrients such as fiber, vitamins, minerals, and water that high-protein foods are often lacking. One vitamin that is of particular importance when eating high-protein foods is vitamin C. The non-heme iron present in beans and grains can be absorbed much more readily when consumed with vitamin C. Therefore, fruits and vegetables should accompany plant-based protein sources in meals. Table 5.4 lists a variety of vegetables and their

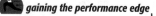

gaining the performance edge

Fruits and vegetables round out any meal, providing carbohydrates, vitamins, minerals, and phytochemicals. Therefore, a high-protein-containing food should be paired with a fruit and/or a vegetable at every meal.

TABLE 5.4 — Protein Content of Various Foods

Protein Source	Protein Content (g)
Grains	
Whole wheat bread, 1 slice	3
Brown rice, ½ cup	3
Pasta, ½ cup	3.5
Fruits/Vegetables	
Apple, 1 medium	0.3
Banana, 1 medium	1.2
Carrots, ½ cup	1
Broccoli, ½ cup	1.3
Dairy/Alternative	
Skim milk, 8 fl oz	8
Low-fat yogurt, 6 oz	6
Cheddar cheese, 1 oz	7
Soy milk, 8 fl oz	5
Soy yogurt, 6 oz	7
Protein Foods	
Beef, 3 oz	25
Chicken, 3 oz	27
Turkey, 3 oz	26
Pork, 3 oz	24
Tuna, 3 oz	22
Black beans, 1½ cup	23
Lentils, 1½ cup	27
Tofu, ½ cup	20
Tempeh, ½ cup	16
Mixed nuts, 1 oz	5

Source: Adapted from Pennington JA, Douglass JS. *Bowes & Church's Food Values of Portions Commonly Used*. 18th ed. Philadelphia, PA: Lippincott Williams and Wilkins; 2005.

respective protein levels. **Training Table 5.2** includes menu ideas for including protein-containing fruits and vegetables in the diet.

Which foods in the dairy/alternative group contain protein?

Dairy/alternative foods and beverages provide an excellent source of protein. Most dairy and soy products contain approximately 6–8 grams of protein per serving. However, some dairy/alternative products, other than soy, may not be excellent sources of protein. Rice and other grain or nut milks often provide only 2–3 grams of protein per serving, but, if fortified, are still good sources of calcium and

vitamin D. Low-fat dairy products contain lower levels of saturated fat and cholesterol compared to their full-fat dairy counterparts while contributing

Training Table 5.1: Menu Ideas for Grain Sources of Protein

- Beans and rice make a balanced, hearty meal. (See *Badminton Beans and Rice* recipe.)
- Pack an almond butter and wheat bread sandwich for long days away from home.
- Make a beef barley soup with extra vegetables for a hot dinner in the winter months that also freezes well for quick meals during the week.
- Add ground turkey to marinara sauce and serve over whole wheat pasta.

Badminton Beans and Rice

1 cup brown rice, uncooked
1–2 tbsp olive oil
1 medium onion, chopped
2 cloves of garlic, minced
4 oz can of chopped green chilies
1½ tsp chili powder
2 tsp cumin powder
2 tbsp chopped fresh cilantro
juice of 1–2 limes
4 cups canned pinto beans, drained and rinsed

Cook brown rice according to package directions. Sauté onion, garlic, and green chilies in oil until onions are translucent. Add the lime juice and seasonings; cook several minutes to blend the seasonings. Add the beans to the onion mixture and cook over low to medium heat for 10–15 minutes. Serve over brown rice.

Serving Size: 2¼ cups (Recipe makes four servings)

Calories: 316 kcals

Protein: 15 grams

Carbohydrate: 53 grams

Fat: 6 grams

Training Table 5.2: Menu Ideas for Combining Fruits and Vegetables with Protein Foods

- Drink a glass of orange juice with an iron-fortified cereal and milk.
- Add onions, carrots, and extra tomatoes to a meat and bean chili.
- Include spinach in a meat lasagna.
- Alternate chicken and peppers, squash, and/or mushrooms for grilled kabobs.

- Drink a cold glass of milk with lunch and dinner.
- Top tomatoes or potatoes with ½ cup cottage cheese.
- Keep yogurt on hand to have as a midday snack.
- Sprinkle parmesan or romano cheese on top of cooked vegetables.

equivalent levels of protein. Table 5.4 lists a variety of dairy/alternative products and their respective protein levels. **Training Table 5.3** includes menu ideas for how to include dairy/alternative sources of protein in the diet.

Which foods make up the protein foods group?

Meat, fish, poultry, eggs, and soy products are excellent sources of a complete protein, containing the highest level of protein per serving within the My-Pylate food guidance system. Legumes, nuts, and seeds are also rich in protein; however, these should be combined with grains, soy, meat, or dairy throughout the day to obtain high levels of all amino acids. A 3-ounce serving of food within this group provides approximately 20–30 grams of protein. Table 5.4 lists a variety of protein foods and their respective protein levels. **Training Table 5.4** contains menu ideas for incorporating protein foods.

gaining the performance edge

Athletes should focus on protein sources from the "heavy hitters" in the dairy/alternative and meat and protein foods groups. Grains and vegetables make up the "second string," while fruits are "bench warmers" in regard to sources for daily protein.

Which foods in the oils contain protein?

Foods in this category do not contain protein. However, these foods complement other protein-rich foods to make meals and snacks more flavorful and enjoyable. Sweets, highly sugared, and high-fat foods make up empty calories and will have variable amounts of protein depending on the food item. Sugars and artificial sweeteners are often found in protein supplements, including bars, powders, and drinks. **Training Table 5.5** contains menu ideas for combining fats with protein-rich foods.

Are protein supplements beneficial?

A variety of protein supplements are heavily marketed to athletes; these purport to increase muscle-

Training Table 5.4: Menu Ideas for Protein Food Sources

- Coat chicken breast with breadcrumbs, bake with marinara sauce, and serve alone or over pasta. (See *Cross-Country Chicken Parmesan* recipe.)
- Order salads in restaurants with grilled lean meats and lots of extra vegetables.
- Try a tofu sandwich with cheese, lettuce, and cucumber— flavored, baked tofu tastes the best for sandwiches.
- Make a weekend omelet with spinach and peppers, and serve with whole wheat toast topped with peanut butter.

Cross-Country Chicken Parmesan

4 chicken breasts
3 egg whites
½–1 cup Italian-flavored breadcrumbs
32 oz jar of spaghetti sauce
8–12 oz dry pasta, any shape
Grated parmesan cheese

Preheat oven to 400°F. Place breadcrumbs in a shallow bowl. Lightly beat the egg whites with a fork in a separate bowl. Dip the chicken breasts in the egg whites, then the breadcrumbs to coat on both sides, and repeat. Place chicken breasts in a greased 9" × 13" pan and cover with spaghetti sauce. Cover the pan with foil and bake in the oven for 30–40 minutes or until the centers of the breasts are no longer pink. Cook pasta according to the package directions. Serve one chicken breast plus sauce over 1–2 cups of cooked pasta. Sprinkle parmesan cheese on top.

Serving Size: 1 chicken breast, 1–2 cups pasta (Recipe makes four servings)

Calories: 740 kcals

Protein: 58 grams

Carbohydrate: 89 grams

Fat: 16 grams

Training Table 5.5: Menu Ideas for Including Oils with Protein Foods

- Sauté beef or chicken and vegetables in 1–2 tbsp of olive oil for a stir-fry.
- Brush chicken or pork with a sweet barbeque sauce while cooking on the grill.
- Use 1–2 tbsp of sesame oil in an oriental salad including grains, lentils, and vegetables.
- Mix honey with orange juice as a glaze for a roast.

building capacity, enhance endurance performance, and speed recovery from exercise. Intact protein and amino acid supplements come in a variety of forms including bars, shakes, powders, and pills. Before choosing to use or not to use a protein supplement, athletes should consider the following:

- What is the quantity of protein or amino acids in the product? Is the supplement necessary?
- What is the supplement's cost?
- Will the supplement enhance performance?
- Are there any risks associated with taking the supplement?

What is the quantity of protein or amino acids in the product? Is the supplement necessary?

Most athletes consume plenty of protein to meet their needs through their daily diet, if they are consuming enough total calories. Similar to carbohydrates and fats, adequate protein intake is essential to optimal sport performance; however, if protein is consumed in quantities greater than daily needs, the excess calories will lead to fat weight gain. A common misconception is that consuming large quantities of protein, often through supplements, will lead to greater gains in muscle mass. Protein intake and overall nutrition are certainly part of the muscle growth equation, but are not the sole reason for muscle mass gains. The other components of the formula include the athlete's strength training program and genetic predisposition for muscle mass. Protein supplements may be indicated for an athlete with huge calorie and protein needs, but for most athletes, the focus should be placed on whole foods. **Table 5.5** provides a comparison of various types of protein

TABLE 5.5 Protein Supplement Comparison*

Supplement Product	Calories per Serving (kcal)	Protein per Serving (g)	Protein Source	Carbs per Serving (g)	Fat per Serving (g)	Other Ingredients
Designer Whey Protein Powder	90	18	Whey	3	2	Artificial flavors, acesulfame K, sucralose
Optimum Nutrition 100% Egg Protein	100	22	Egg	3	0.5	Artificial flavor, sucralose
MuscleTech NITRO-Tech Hardcore	110	20	Whey	3	1.5	Artificial flavors, acesulfame K, aspartame
Naturade 100% Soy Protein	110	25	Soy	0	1	Soy lecithin, natural flavors
Optimum Nutrition 100% Soy Protein	120	25	Soy	2	1.5	Natural and artificial flavors, lecithin, sucralose, acesulfame K
Met-Rx Protein Plus	210	46	Milk, casein, egg, whey	3	1.5	Artificial flavors, aspartame, partially hydrogenated oil
EAS Myoplex Ready to Drink Shakes	310	42	Milk, casein, whey	20	7	Artificial flavors, 19 vitamins/minerals, sucralose
EAS Myoplex Deluxe	330	53	Whey, casein	28	4.5	MCT, conjugated linoleic acid, fortified with 22 vitamins/minerals, sucralose
Cytosport Muscle Milk	350	32	Whey, casein	12	18	Fortified with 20 vitamins/minerals, MCT, L-carnitine, creatine, acesulfame K, sucralose
Prolab N-Large 2	600	52	Whey	86	6	Artificial flavors
Champion Nutrition Heavyweight Gainer 900	630	35	Beef, whey, egg	101	9.5	Fortified with 20 vitamins/minerals, MCT, aspartame, acesulfame K
ABB XXL Weight Gainer	1040	42	Whey, casein, egg	208	4	Artificial flavors, vitamins/minerals, acesulfame K, MCT

*Nutrition information obtained from manufacturers' Web sites.

supplements. The quantity of protein or amino acids can vary greatly from one product to another. As a result, athletes should look for the Supplement Facts label on protein supplement products, which provides information similar to that found on food labels.

Protein supplements can be used when athletes are traveling or do not have easy access to food or refrigeration, and before or after training or competitions. For example, a dry protein powder can be mixed with water and poured over cereal when a cooler or refrigerator is not available for fluid milk. However, when athletes have access to other food sources, protein supplements should not be used preferentially over whole foods.

The Supplement Facts label on protein supplement products will list the grams of protein or milligrams of amino acids in one serving of the product (see Figure 5.5). Often, the quantity of protein supplied in a bar or shake is equivalent to a well-balanced meal. Athletes should be aware when reviewing the label of amino acid supplements that the content will most likely be expressed in milligrams versus grams. For example, a product might contain 500 milligrams of an amino acid, or 0.5 grams. One ounce of beef, chicken, or turkey contains 7 grams, or 7000 milligrams, of amino acids in the form of whole proteins. Obviously, in this example, if an athlete is aiming to consume more amino acids and protein, the food option would be a better choice than the amino acid supplement.

A variety of protein sources is used in protein supplements. Whey protein is quite popular and is heavily promoted as an ideal protein source for athletes. Soy, casein, and egg proteins or combinations of any of these proteins and/or amino acids are also commonly found in protein supplements. Some supplements contain specific single amino acids, or they may contain primarily BCAAs. Manufacturers often trademark (™) their specific formulation of protein and use that formulation in their products. Although there are differences in the absorption rate of the various proteins used in supplements, the actual gram amount of protein in supplements is important to review when choosing a supplement. Food sources of protein can provide as many or more

Roast Turkey

Nutrition Facts

Serving Size: 3oz

Amount Per Serving

Calories	134	
Calories from Fat	27	
		% Daily Value*
Total Fat 3g	1%	
Saturated Fat 1g	0%	
Trans Fat 0g	0%	
Cholesterol 59mg	3%	
Sodium 54mg	13%	
Total Carbohydrate 0g	0%	
Sugars 0g		
Protein 25g		

*Percent Daily Values are based on a 2,000 calorie diet. Your daily values may be higher or lower depending on your calorie needs:

	Calories	2,000	2,500
Total Fat	Less than	65g	80g
Sat Fat	Less than	20g	25g
Cholest	Less than	300mg	300mg
Sodium	Less than	2,400mg	2,400mg
Total Carb		300g	375g
Fiber		25g	30g

L-Tyrosine, 500 mg
100 Capsules

Supplement Facts

Serving Size: 1 Capsule
Servings Per Container: 100

	Amount Per Serving	% Daily Value*
L-Tyrosine	500 mg	

*Percent Daily Values are based on a 2,000 calorie diet. Certified Free of: Yeast, Wheat, Corn, Milk, Eggs, Soy, Glutens, Sugar, Starch, Artificial Colors, and Added Preservatives

Other Ingredients: Magnesium Stearate, Gelatin (Capsule).

Recommended Use: As a Dietary Supplement, take 1–3 Capsules Daily, or as Directed by your Qualified Health Consultant.

Figure 5.5 Supplement vs. sliced turkey nutrition labels. Amino acid supplements often have far fewer amino acids and less total protein than protein-rich foods.

grams of protein than many supplements. Whether soy or whey, casein or amino acids, many whole food sources provide a complement of amino acids that meets protein needs for muscle maintenance, repair, and growth.

What is the cost of protein supplements?

Protein supplements are often much more expensive than whole foods. Products will vary greatly in cost. Examine the Supplement Facts labels carefully to determine the number of servings in one container and then calculate the cost per serving. In general, by choosing whole foods, athletes can obtain protein, plus many other nutrients, for a significantly lower cost. See **Table 5.6** for a comparison of various protein sources and their respective costs per serving.

Will protein supplements enhance performance?

Research based on monitoring changes in nitrogen balance has shown that athletes have higher protein needs than the sedentary population. Other studies have examined changes in body composition (i.e., lean body mass) in response to training while ma-

nipulating dietary protein intake and have indicated that higher protein intakes may be beneficial, particularly when using supplements that contain essential amino acids. However, no studies have been conducted directly investigating the effects of protein supplements on sport performance. Any protein supplement claims related to performance are based on the positive impact supplementation has on protein synthesis, which may or may not ultimately affect physical capabilities. Furthermore, there is little to no research showing a conclusive benefit of engineered protein supplements over whole food products.

Some athletes find it challenging to meet their protein needs through only whole food in the diet because of the large volume of total calories and protein required in one day. In this case, a supplement that supplies the protein lacking in the diet, hence preventing a deficiency, may enhance performance. However, a poorly planned and executed diet should not be remedied by relying on a supplement; focus should first be placed on consuming a well-balanced diet, and then if needs are still not being met, a protein supplement can be considered.

TABLE 5.6	Cost Comparison of Protein Supplied from Protein Supplements Versus Whole Foods			
Protein Source	Grams of Protein per Serving	Cost per Serving	Cost per 8 Grams of Protein	
Supplement Products				
EAS Precision Protein Whey Protein Powder, 25.5 g	20 g	$1.26	$0.50	
Genisoy UltraSoy-XT Protein Powder, 20 g	17 g	$1.00	$0.47	
Optimum Nutrition 100% Egg Protein Powder, 29.4 g	22 g	$1.10	$0.40	
BioProtein Bar, 1 bar	21 g	$1.29	$0.49	
PowerBar Protein Plus Bar, 1 bar	24 g	$2.59	$0.86	
Meso-tech Bar, 1 bar	25 g	$2.69	$0.86	
Prolab Amino 2000 (tablets), 6 tablets	12 g	$0.59	$0.39	
Twinlab Amino Fuel Liquid, 3 tbsp	15 g	$1.23	$0.66	
PBL Liquid Muscle, 2 tbsp	10 g	$0.94	$0.75	
Whole Food Items				
Chicken breast, 3 oz	26 g	$0.47	$0.14	
Turkey (white meat), 3 oz	26 g	$0.47	$0.14	
Ground beef, 3 oz	24 g	$0.75	$0.25	
Salmon, 3 oz	22 g	$1.31	$0.48	
Whole egg, 3	19 g	$0.59	$0.25	
Skim milk, 8 oz	8 g	$0.20	$0.20	
Tofu, 1 cup	20 g	$0.78	$0.31	
Lentils, 1½ cups	27 g	$0.42	$0.13	
Walnuts, 1 oz	4 g	$0.39	$0.79	

---

gaining the performance edge

The need for a protein supplement should be evaluated on an individual basis. Adequate protein consumption is particularly important to individuals beginning a new exercise program or athletes who have increased the intensity or volume of their training.

Are there any risks associated with taking the supplement?

The risks associated with taking any supplement will be discussed in greater depth in Chapter 9. However, there are a few specific precautions related to protein supplementation. Look at the ingredients listing closely. Many protein supplements will include artificial flavors, sweeteners, or colorings that may cause allergic reactions in some individuals. Supplements can also include other substances that are purported to "increase muscle size and strength," such as creatine or androstenedione. These substances, as well as other chemicals or additives, can cause unwanted side effects. Without a close review, athletes can potentially be putting themselves at risk for disqualification if a substance in a consumed supplement is on their sport's list of banned agents. Also, consuming large amounts of one amino acid may affect the absorption of other amino acids in the digestive tract. Because amino acids share carriers for absorption, excess consumption of one amino acid may impair the absorption of other amino acids that share the same carriers in the digestive tract. However, the actual risk of consuming excessive amounts of one single amino acid is currently unknown.

Why is protein essential for daily training?

As discussed in earlier chapters, carbohydrates and fats provide the main sources of energy for training and competition. Protein, conversely, is not a significant source of energy during most forms of exercise because of the slow conversion of amino acids to glucose or ATP. Protein has been shown to contribute as little as 5% of the energy used during exercise. The percentage can increase to 15–18%, but only during prolonged exercise. The small amount of amino acids used can be converted into energy through oxidation as well as by providing the substrates for gluconeogenesis.[18] Proteins complement carbohydrates and fats in providing the resources for growth and maintenance of muscles and other tissues, enzymes, hormones, and hemoglobin, as well as sustaining normal functioning of the immune system.

Sufficient dietary protein is required to maximize protein synthesis in the body in response to daily training. Exercise induces changes in protein and amino acid metabolism, which translate into a greater need for protein. Training and competition cause an increased breakdown of protein resulting from microtrauma sustained by muscle tissue.[19] If an athlete does not consume adequate amounts of protein, the body will rely on endogenous sources of protein for repair and resynthesis, ultimately leading to protein loss. If this process continues over time, performance will decline and illness may ensue.

Low dietary protein intake is one of several purported causes of what is referred to as **sports anemia**. Sports anemia is not considered a real clinical condition; however, it gives the appearance of anemia in that hemoglobin concentration in the blood is decreased.[20] The appearance of sports anemia is more prevalent in untrained individuals who are beginning exercise or in athletes who have undergone a recent increase in the intensity or volume of their training.[20] If protein intake is inadequate during these new or adjusted training bouts, then a competition between tissues for amino acids occurs.[3,21] The available amino acids are used to synthesize more myoglobin, mitochondrial proteins, and muscle proteins that are essential for oxygen utilization in the muscle during exercise, instead of being used to make more hemoglobin.[22] In addition, endurance training, particularly in untrained individuals, causes blood plasma volume to increase, sometimes by as much as 20%.[23,24] The expanded plasma volume decreases hemoglobin concentration, despite the fact that hemoglobin levels are relatively unchanged. Therefore, the combination of increased plasma volume and little to no change in hemoglobin levels gives the appearance of anemia. The ramifications of this apparent sports anemia appear to be relatively benign, and the decreased hemoglobin concentration does not significantly alter aerobic capacity or endurance performance. In addition, hemoglobin levels begin to return to normal levels after the body has had several weeks to adjust to the new training.

For the body to maximize its utilization of daily protein intake, total calorie and carbohydrate needs

sports anemia A condition caused by the combination of intense training and poor protein intake; it results in reduced levels of hemoglobin in the blood.

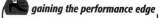
gaining the performance edge

Protein has many roles in the body; however, it is particularly important for handling the stress of daily training and competition. Adequate protein consumption not only will lead to optimal performance, but also will prevent adverse health conditions such as sports anemia.

should also be met. If an athlete is consuming too few calories or restricting intake of carbohydrates, the body will increase protein catabolism. Maintaining an appropriate total calorie intake will ensure that protein is not being used for energy on a daily basis. Adequate carbohydrate intake will decrease amino acid oxidation as well as spare dietary and muscle protein, ultimately leading to improved athletic performance.

What type, how much, and when should protein be consumed before exercise?

Much of the research concerning the optimal preactivity/competition diet has focused on the importance of carbohydrates. However, recent studies investigating methods to manipulate the diet to enhance muscle building have provided insight into the role of protein in preactivity meal planning.

Several reports by Lemon,[25] Wolfe,[26] and Tipton[27] have demonstrated that muscle building is optimized when amino acids are consumed prior to training and thus circulating in the blood while exercising. The amino acids aid in:

- Providing energy for the muscle cells; however, as discussed earlier, only minimal amounts of energy are supplied by amino acids during exercise
- Decreasing catabolism of protein in muscle tissue
- Increasing protein synthesis in muscle tissue

An additional benefit of consuming protein prior to training or competition relates to the speed of digestion. Protein-rich foods take slightly longer to empty from the stomach than do carbohydrates, thus providing a satiety effect and a more gradual delivery of nutrients to the bloodstream. These actions will prevent an athlete from getting hungry before training, which can be mentally distracting, and will sustain energy levels for a longer duration, potentially increasing the amount of work an athlete can perform before fatiguing.

To allow time for the longer digestion of proteins and absorption of amino acids into the bloodstream, protein-containing foods need to be consumed 1–4 hours prior to the onset of exercise. Keep in mind that the preactivity meal should be a combination of proteins, carbohydrates, and fats. Carbohydrate foods should be predominant in the meal or snack, while protein foods are the complement. Athletes should always experiment with the timing of the preexercise meal to determine the ideal quantity and

timing of food and beverage consumption before training or competition.

There is some evidence that it is best to ingest protein at least 3 hours prior to exercise to avoid unnecessary elevations in respiratory exchange ratio and perceived exertion during higher intensity activities. A study conducted by Wiles et al.[28] tested individuals running on a treadmill at 60, 80, 90, and 100% of VO_2max after consuming a protein beverage 1 hour or 3 hours prior to exercise compared to the ingestion of only water. The results of the study revealed that the ingestion of the protein beverage, containing 0.4 g protein/kg body weight, led to a higher VO_2 level and perceived exertion at all exercise intensities. The explanation of this finding focused on the increased metabolism, or thermic effect of food, in the hours immediately following protein ingestion. The authors noted that only a small increase in the thermic effect of food was noted after 3 hours; therefore, it can be implied that an athlete should consume a meal containing protein at least 3 hours prior to exercise. This notion requires more investigation before exact recommendations can be established.

What type and how much protein should be consumed 4–24 hours prior to training or competition?

Similar to the guidelines for daily protein intake, athletes should choose lean protein sources such as lean cuts of beef, chicken, turkey, fish, low-fat dairy, or soy products in the 4–24 hours prior to training or a competition. Athletes should plan a meal that contains 3–6 ounces of a lean protein or 8–12 fl oz of dairy/alternative, as well as a significant source of carbohydrates and a small amount of fat. Legumes, which are very high in fiber, should be limited or consumed in small amounts in the 24 hours leading up to an important training session or competition. The extra fiber may cause gastrointestinal distress for some athletes. However, individuals who eat beans, lentils, and other legumes on a regular basis can generally tolerate these foods without consequence.

What type and how much protein should be consumed 1–4 hours prior to training or competition?

Small amounts of lean protein sources (2–4 oz) can be consumed in the 4 hours prior to exercise. However, the focus should be placed mainly on carbohydrate-rich foods during this period. Athletes need to find a balance between consuming enough carbohydrates and proteins to enhance performance, while mod-

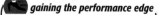
erating the quantity of food and total calories ingested to avoid nausea, vomiting, cramping, or diarrhea. Individuals should plan meals with at least three different food groups, one of which is a protein-rich food and one of which is a carbohydrate-rich food.

Protein sources that are higher in fat, such as high-fat cuts of meat, full-fat dairy, nuts, and seeds, should be consumed in minimal amounts, if not eliminated, in the hours directly leading up to an exercise session. These foods take longer to digest and therefore can disrupt performance because of a sense of a "full stomach" or intestinal distress. In daily training, nuts and seeds are an excellent choice because of their favorable protein, fiber, and fat profile. However, instead of eating nuts and seeds prior to training, athletes can pack a small bag for a great postexercise snack. **Training Table 5.6** contains some ideas for protein-rich foods to eat prior to competition.

What type, how much, and when should protein be consumed during exercise?

In the last couple of decades, the role of exogenous amino acids administered during exercise has garnered research attention. Amino acids ingested during exercise have been hypothesized to improve sport performance in several ways. Most of the current research has focused on the use of amino acids for energy production during exercise and the potential role of the branched chain amino acids in attenuating central fatigue.

Amino acids can be used as a source of energy during exercise. They can be transported via the blood to the liver, converted to glucose via gluconeogenesis, and released into the bloodstream. Thus, glucose formed from amino acids can help to prevent hypoglycemia (low blood glucose) during exercise and continue to provide glucose for sustained physical effort. Unfortunately, this gluconeogenic avenue for deriving energy from amino acids is a slow, involved process that lacks the ability to support the rapid energy needs of intense exercise or sport competition.

As discussed in the previous paragraph, most amino acids must be transported to the liver, converted into substrates or intermediates in the liver, and then transported through the blood back to the active muscle cells where they can finally be used for energy. The exceptions to this rule are the BCAAs, which are leucine, isoleucine, and valine. These amino acids are different because they can be metabolized for energy in the muscle itself (see Figure 5.6) instead of needing to be processed by the liver. Therefore, the energy supplied by BCAAs can be used directly in the muscle cell.

BCAAs started receiving more attention, especially for endurance sports, when researchers discovered that after 3 hours of exercise, BCAA levels in the blood drop dramatically.[29] During long-duration aerobic exercise, the activity of the enzyme responsible for the catabolism of BCAAs, keto acid dehydrogenase, increases. The activity of this enzyme is greatest when carbohydrate stores are low, thus supporting the theory that BCAAs may be providing energy to the active muscles.[19] In addition, falling levels of BCAAs in the blood have been linked to central nervous system fatigue,[30] which leads to decreased sport performance. Accordingly, ingestion of BCAAs may prevent the decrease of BCAAs in the blood, and thus be potentially beneficial, especially during prolonged endurance exercise. Unfortunately, stud-

---

Training Table 5.6: Menu Ideas for Precompetition Protein Foods (grams of protein)

- 1½ cups cereal, 1 cup skim milk/soy milk, ½ cup blueberries, 1 slice wheat toast, 2 tbsp peanut butter (24 g)
- 2 scrambled eggs, 1 English muffin, 2 slices cheddar cheese, 8 oz orange juice (29 g)
- Ham sandwich [2 slices rye bread, 6 slices ham], banana, 6 oz low-fat yogurt (22 g)
- Large salad [2 cups romaine lettuce, ½ cup red pepper, ½ tomato, ½ cup cottage cheese, 3 slices turkey, ¼ cup garbanzo beans, 2 tbsp fat-free dressing], 1 cup skim milk (32 g)

Branched Chain Amino Acid Metabolism

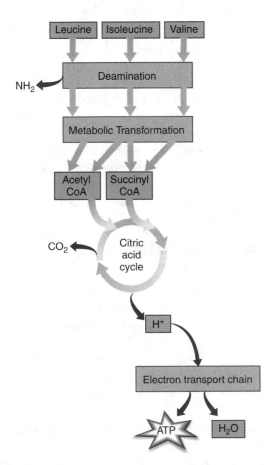

Figure 5.6 Metabolism of BCAAs for energy. Branched chain amino acids are unique because they can be metabolized for energy within the muscle itself instead of needing to first be processed by the liver.

ies involving endurance athletes ingesting BCAAs during exercise have not yielded consistent results, and in fact, most have shown little to no positive effect on endurance. Although more investigation on the role of BCAAs during exercise is indicated, recommending the ingestion of BCAAs to improve performance is not currently warranted.

What type, how much, and when should protein be consumed after exercise?

Protein is a critical nutrient for the postexercise recovery process in muscle. After exercise, protein breakdown diminishes while protein synthesis increases, resulting in a positive muscle protein balance (i.e., an anabolic state). The success of achieving a positive muscle protein balance appears to be dependent on the amino acid composition of the food ingested, the amino acid concentration of the blood supplying the muscle cells, and the timing of the protein feeding.[4]

Which type of protein or amino acid source is most beneficial to consume after exercise?

The availability of amino acids to the muscles positively influences muscle protein synthesis. Food sources that cause **hyperaminoacidemia** (i.e., high blood amino acid levels) have been shown to increase amino acid delivery to the muscle and transport into the muscle, thereby increasing the intracellular availability for muscle protein synthesis.[26,31] Contrary to the belief of some athletes, hyperaminoacidemia is not solely dependent on the ingestion of free-form amino acid supplements. Consuming complete proteins, such as whey and casein, has been shown to increase amino acid levels in the blood, thus aiding in the recovery process.[25,32]

The amino acid composition of foods ingested following both resistance and endurance exercise appears to affect hyperaminoacidemia and subsequent muscle protein synthesis. Ingesting foods or supplements supplying essential amino acids, rather than nonessential amino acids, is necessary for the greatest positive influence on muscle protein synthesis.[27,33,34] Whey and casein proteins are high-quality proteins that contain essential amino acids. In addition, whey protein has a relatively high proportion of BCAAs.[29,35] Soy protein is another postworkout protein option that also provides all the essential amino acids for muscle rebuilding and repair.[36] Several studies have been conducted comparing soy protein and milk protein on muscle protein anabolism during the first few hours of recovery with varying results.[37–39] Additional research in the area of the type of protein to promote optimal muscle anabolism and recovery is warranted.

Research has focused not only on the importance of essential amino acids for triggering hyperaminoacidemia, but also on the form in which essential amino acids are consumed. Studies have investigated the potential difference in protein absorption, synthesis, and catabolism after exercise between various protein and amino acid sources. In general, intact proteins are digested and absorbed more slowly than are **hydrolyzed proteins**. Hydrolyzed protein

hyperaminoacidemia A condition describing abnormally high levels of amino acids in the blood.

hydrolyzed protein A source of protein that is usually in supplement form and contains proteins that have undergone a predigestion process, breaking the more complex proteins into smaller di- and tripeptide complexes.

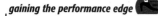
sources are usually in supplement form and contain proteins that have undergone a predigestion process, breaking the more complex proteins into smaller di- and tripeptide complexes. The hydrolyzed proteins are also absorbed slightly faster than are supplements composed primarily of free amino acid mixtures.[40] The differences in absorption of these protein sources are most noticeable in special circumstances, such as when athletes are fasting or following a low-calorie diet, and are least noticeable in individuals who are generously well-fed, which is the case for most athletes. When various proteins are consumed without other energy sources such as carbohydrates or fats, whey proteins and amino acid mixtures appear to be absorbed more quickly than casein proteins. However, when any of these proteins or amino acids are ingested with carbohydrates or fats, the differences in absorption are diminished.[41] The bottom line is that the consumption of essential amino acids should be of greatest importance, regardless of the exact form in which they are ingested. Athletes should be encouraged to consume whole foods, containing essential amino acids, to provide the protein and other important nutrients for muscle recovery and synthesis.

Is there a recovery benefit of combining carbohydrates and proteins after exercise?

Some literature has suggested that consuming a combination of proteins and carbohydrates, versus only carbohydrates or only proteins, enhances the recovery process. A study conducted by Zawadzki et al.[42] compared the effects of carbohydrate, protein, and carbohydrate–protein beverages after 2 hours of cycling. The researchers found that the combination beverage produced the greatest circulating levels of insulin, which in theory would enhance protein and carbohydrate intake into the muscle cells and promote protein synthesis, thus improving the recovery process. Another study by Miller et al.[43] reported that ingesting both proteins and carbohydrates together within 3 hours after exercise resulted in the greatest uptake of amino acids compared to ingesting proteins or carbohydrates alone. Timing of the ingestion of the postexercise carbohydrate–protein recovery drink or meal is important. Berardi et al.[44] found that carbohydrate plus protein supplements given early after exercise enhance glycogen resynthesis relative to carbohydrate only or placebo given later in recovery. Other studies have focused on other substances in the blood, such as levels of growth hormone or creatine kinase, and have also found positive results from a carbohydrate–protein combination after exercise. Taken together, it appears that ingesting carbohydrates and proteins as soon as possible and at least within 3 hours after exercise would be a prudent dietary practice for athletes.

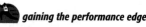
How much protein should be consumed after exercise?

Ingestion of as little as 6 grams of essential amino acids, both with and without carbohydrates, has been shown to increase muscle protein synthesis.[27,33] Nonessential amino acids, in and of themselves, do not appear to have the same protein synthesis effect. Although the availability of essential amino acids does increase protein synthesis, there appears to be a ceiling to the dose response, above which increasing levels of essential amino acids do not increase protein synthesis.[45] When net protein synthesis was compared between athletes consuming 20 grams or 40 grams of essential amino acids, there was no difference in synthetic rates between groups after resistance training.[45] To date, the threshold and ceiling doses of essential amino acids (i.e., the ideal range) needed for optimal protein synthesis have not been determined and are most likely specific to the individual.

However, based on current research, ingesting approximately 6–20 grams of essential amino acids in the postexercise meal will aid in the recovery process. Combining proteins with carbohydrates maximizes glycogen synthesis, causes hormones favorable for muscle growth to be secreted, and enhances protein synthesis. Six to 20 grams of essential amino acids, along with a source of carbohydrates, can be obtained by consuming any one of the following (total grams protein, grams of essential amino acids):

- 6 oz lowfat yogurt, ¼ cup mixed nuts, 1 cup strawberries (14 g, 6 g)
- 3 oz tofu, 1½ cups mixed vegetables, 1 cup brown rice (20 g, 8 g)
- 2 hard-boiled eggs, 1 slice wheat toast with 1 tbsp peanut butter, 8 oz orange juice (22 g, 8 g)

- 2 cups pasta, ½ cup marinara sauce, 3 oz lean ground beef, 1 cup broccoli (49 g, 16 g)
- 4 oz chicken breast sandwich with 1 oz mozzarella cheese, 1 pear, 8 oz skim milk (55 g, 22 g)

When should protein or amino acids be consumed after exercise?

The timing of protein feeding after exercise is also important. Several studies have demonstrated the importance of essential amino acids in stimulating muscle protein synthesis within 3 hours of exercise.[27,33,34,43] Eating protein sources as soon as possible after physical activity takes advantage of the increased blood flow and hormonal milieu (i.e., potential increases in growth hormone and testosterone) caused by the previously performed exercise. Therefore, in practical terms, postexercise protein consumption should occur within 3 hours or less of exercise and include protein sources that provide all the essential amino acids.

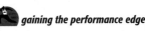
gaining the performance edge

Ingest a minimum of 6–20 grams of protein containing essential amino acids immediately after exercise for optimal recovery. Consuming carbohydrates in addition to this amount of protein appears to further enhance exercise recovery.

The Box Score

Key Points of Chapter

- The protein–muscle mass connection is just one of many reasons protein is an essential nutrient to athletes and untrained individuals alike. Proteins also provide structure to many parts of the body, are needed for building and repairing body tissues, serve as enzymes that initiate cellular processes, and form hormones that help regulate a variety of processes in the body.

- Proteins are chains of amino acids that are linked via peptide bonds in a very specific sequence. The specific sequence of the amino acids in the chain gives the protein not only its physical characteristics, but also its three-dimensional shape. The shape of the protein in many instances dictates its function in the body.

- There are 20 different amino acids used by the body to make proteins. Nine are essential and must be obtained from diet. Complete, high-quality proteins tend to come from animal sources and provide all the essential amino acids needed by the body. However, plant-derived complementary protein sources can also provide all essential amino acids.

- Monitoring nitrogen status is one way of determining whether dietary protein intake is adequate to meet protein needs. When dietary input of nitrogen (i.e., protein gain) equals the output of nitrogen (i.e., protein loss), then nitrogen balance has been achieved. At a minimum, the goal for any athlete is to maintain nitrogen balance and, in most cases, to achieve a positive nitrogen balance.

- Current research suggests that athletes have higher protein needs than nonathletes. The recommended daily protein intake is 1.4–2.0 g/kg for strength athletes, 1.2–2.0 g/kg for endurance athletes, and 1.2–1.6 g/kg for team sport athletes.

- The protein needs of athletes can vary depending on their current body weight, training status, total caloric intake, desire to lose or gain weight, carbohydrate intake, quality of protein sources consumed, type of training, intensity of training, duration of training, and age.

- The richest sources of dietary protein are found in the dairy/alternative and protein foods groups. Grain products as well as vegetables provide a small to moderate amount of protein, while fruits provide little to none.

- The need for a protein supplement should be evaluated on an individual basis. Athletes should focus first on obtaining plenty of protein-rich foods in their daily diet; if protein needs are still not being met, then an appropriate and safe supplement can be considered.

- Protein has many roles in the body; however, it is particularly important for enduring the stress of daily training and competition. Adequate protein consumption not only will lead to optimal performance, but also will prevent adverse health conditions such as sports anemia.

- The pregame or preactivity meal should include a combination of proteins, carbohydrates, and fats. The carbohydrate foods should predominate in the preevent meal, whereas protein foods should serve as a complement. To allow time for digestion, the preevent foods should be consumed 1–4 hours prior to the onset of exercise.

- Protein ingestion during sport competition or training has not consistently been shown to enhance performance. Deriving energy from amino acids is a slow, involved metabolic process that lacks the ability to support the rapid energy needs of intense exercise or sport competition.

- Consumption of high-quality proteins that elevate blood levels of amino acids within 1–3 hours after competition or training has been shown to increase protein synthesis. Research suggests that ingesting carbohydrates along with proteins after exercise may actually enhance the recovery process.

Study Questions

1. How do proteins differ from carbohydrates and fats in regard to their molecular structure?

2. Discuss the various roles of proteins in the body. How does each of these roles apply to training, recovery, and/or sport performance?

3. How would the nitrogen balance of an athlete be determined? Once determined, what does nitrogen balance indicate?

4. What are "complete proteins," and what food sources provide them? What are the ramifications of eating foods that do not provide complete sources of protein?

5. What are "incomplete proteins," and what food sources provide them? Give several examples of complementary incomplete protein sources that provide all essential amino acids.

6. What are branched chain amino acids? What relationship, if any, do they have to athletic performance?

7. Discuss the relationship between carbohydrate intake and protein requirements.

8. What are the recommended protein intake levels for athletes? Discuss reasons why requirements are higher than for sedentary individuals.

9. What dietary protein intake recommendations would you make to an elite athlete training for a marathon? How would those recommendations compare to recommendations for an Olympic weightlifter training 12–15 hours a week?

10. What factors should be considered when determining the protein needs of an athlete?

11. Provide two suggestions for well-balanced preactivity meals containing protein, as well as two examples of quick and easy postexercise snacks containing 6–20 grams of protein.

References

1. Brooks GA, Fahey TD, Baldwin KM. *Exercise Physiology: Human Bioenergetics and Its Applications*. 4th ed. Boston, MA: McGraw-Hill; 2005.

2. Tarnopolsky M. Protein requirements for endurance athletes. *Nutr*. 2004;20:662–668.

3. Institute of Medicine. *Dietary Reference Intakes for Energy, Carbohydrate, Fiber, Fat, Fatty Acids, Cholesterol, Protein, and Amino Acids (Macronutrients)*. Food and Nutrition Board. Washington, DC: National Academy Press; 2002.

4. Tipton KD, Wolfe RR. Protein and amino acids for athletes. *J Sports Sci*. 2004;22(1):65–79.

5. Phillips SM. Protein requirements and supplementation in strength sports. *Nutr*. 2004;20:689–695.

6. Lemon PW. Do athletes need more dietary protein and amino acids? *Int J Sport Nutr*. 1995;5(suppl):S39–S61.

7. Lemon PW, Tarnopolsky MA, MacDougall JD, Atkinson SA. Protein requirements and muscle mass/strength changes during intensive training in novice body builders. *J Appl Physiol*. 1992;73:767–775.

8. Evans WJ. Effects of exercise on senescent muscle. *Clin Orthop Relat Res*. 2002;403(suppl):S211–S220.

9. Lemon PW, Dolny DG, Yarasheski KE. Moderate physical activity can increase dietary protein needs. *Can J Appl Physiol*. 1997;22:494–503.

10. Millward DJ. Inherent difficulties in defining amino acid requirements. In: Committee on Military Nutrition Research, ed. *The Role of Protein and Amino Acids in Sustaining and Enhancing Performance*. Washington, DC: National Academy Press; 1999:169–216.

11. Phillips SM, Atkinson SA, Tarnopolsky MA, MacDougall JD. Gender differences in leucine kinetics and nitrogen balance in endurance athletes. *J Appl Physiol*. 1993;75:2134–2141.

12. Tarnopolsky MA, Atkinson SA, MacDougall JD, Chesley A, Phillips S, Schwarcz HP. Evaluation of protein requirements for trained strength athletes. *J Appl Physiol*. 1992;73:1986–1995.

13. Lamont LS, McCullough AJ, Kalhan SC. Comparison of leucine kinetics in endurance-trained and sedentary humans. *J Appl Physiol*. 1999;86(1):320–325.

14. Lemon PWR. Beyond the zone: protein needs of active individuals. *J Am Coll Nutr*. 2000;19(5,suppl):513S–521S.

15. Esmarck B, Andersen JL, Olsen S, et al. Timing of post-exercise protein intake is important for muscle hypertrophy with resistance training in elderly humans. *J Physiol*. 2001;535:301–311.

16. Barzel US, Massey LK. Excess dietary protein can adversely affect bone. *J Nutr*. 1998;128(6):1051–1053.

17. Itoh R, Nishiyama N, Suyama Y. Dietary protein intake and urinary excretion of calcium: a cross sectional study in a healthy Japanese population. *Am J Clin Nutr*. 1998;67(3):438–444.

18. Rennie MJ, Tipton KD. Protein and amino acid metabolism during and after exercise and the effects of nutrition. *Ann Rev Nutr*. 2000;20:457–483.

19. Rankin JW. Role of protein in exercise. *Clin Sports Med*. 1999;18(3):499–511.

20. McArdle WD, Katch FI, Katch VL. Vitamins, minerals, and water. In: *Exercise Physiology: Energy, Nutrition, and Human Performance*. 5th ed. Philadelphia, PA: Lippincott Williams and Wilkins; 2001:47–81.

21. Chatard JC, Mujika I, Guy C, Lacour JR. Anaemia and iron deficiency in athletes: practical recommendations for treatment. *Sports Med*. 1999;27(4):229–240.

22. Williams MH. *Nutrition for Health, Fitness and Sport*. Boston, MA: WCB McGraw-Hill; 1999.

23. Gledhill N, Warburton D, Jamnik V. Haemoglobin, blood volume, cardiac function, and aerobic power. *Can J Appl Physiol*. 1999;24(1):54–65.

24. Shoemaker JK, Green HJ, Ball-Burnett M, Grant S. Relationships between fluid and electrolyte hormones and plasma volume during exercise with training and detraining. *Med Sci Sports Exerc*. 1998;30(4):497–505.

25. Lemon PW, Berardi JM, Noreen EE. The role of protein and amino acid supplements in the athlete's diet: does type or timing of ingestion matter? *Curr Sports Med Rep*. 2002;1(4):214–221.

26. Wolfe RR, Miller SL. Amino acid availability controls muscle protein metabolism. *Diabetes Nutr Metab*. 1999;12:322–328.

27. Tipton KD, Rasmussen BB, Miller S, et al. Timing of amino acid-carbohydrate ingestion alters anabolic response of muscle to resistance exercise. *Am J Physiol*. 2001;281:E197–E206.

28. Wiles J, Woodward R, Bird SR. Effect of pre-exercise protein ingestion upon VO₂, R and perceived exertion during treadmill running. *Brit J Sports Med*. 1991;25(1):26–30.

29. Mero A. Leucine supplementation and intensive training. *Sports Med*. 1999;27(6):347–358.

30. Davis JM. Carbohydrates, branched-chain amino acids, and endurance: the central fatigue hypothesis. *Int J Sports Nutr*. 1995;5(suppl):S29–S38.

31. Wolfe RR. Protein supplements and exercise. *Am J Clin Nutr*. 2000;72:551S–557S.

32. Ha E, Zemel MB. Functional properties of whey, whey components, and essential amino acids: mechanisms underlying health benefits for active people. *J Nutr Biochem*. 2003;14:251–258.

33. Borsheim E, Tipton KD, Wolf SE, Wolfe RR. Essential amino acids and muscle protein recovery from resistance exercise. *Am J Physiol*. 2002;283:E648–E657.

34. Tipton KD, Borsheim E, Wolf SE, Sanfor AP, Wolfe RR. Acute response of net muscle protein balance reflects 24-h balance after exercise and amino acid ingestion. *Am J Physiol*. 2003;284:E76–E89.

35. Bos C, Gaudichon C, Tome D. Nutritional and physiological criteria in the assessment of milk protein quality for humans. *J Am Coll Nutr*. 2000;19:191S–205S.

36. Endres JG. *Soy Protein Products: Characteristics, Nutritional Aspects, and Utilization*. Champaign, IL: AOCS Press and the Soy Protein Council; 2001.

37. Haub MD, Wells AM, Tarnopolsky MA, Campbell WW. Effect of protein source on resistive training-induced changes in body composition and muscle size in older men. *Am J Clin Nutr*. 2002;76:511–517.

38. Hartman JW, Bruinsma D, Fullerton A, Perco JG, Lawrence R, Tang JE, Wilkinson SB, Phillips SM. The effect of differing post exercise macronutrient consumption on resistance training-induced adaptations in novices. *Med Sci Sports Exerc*. 2004;36(suppl):S41.

39. Wilkinson S, MacDonald J, MacDonald M, Tarnopolsky M, Phillips S. Milk proteins promote a greater net protein balance than soy proteins following resistance exercise. *FASEB J*. 2004;18:Abstract 7548.

40. Rerat A. Nutritional supply of proteins and absorption of their hydrolysis products—consequences on metabolism. *Proc Nutr Soc*. 1993;52:335–344.

41. Dangin M, Boirie Y, Guillet C, Beaufrere B. Influence of the protein digestion on protein turnover in young and elderly subjects. *J Nutr*. 2002;132:3228S–3233S.

42. Zawadzki KM, Yaspelkis BB, Ivy JL. Carbohydrateprotein complex increases the rate of muscle glycogen storage after exercise. *J Appl Physiol*. 1992;72:1854–1859.

43. Miller SL, Tipton KD, Chinkes DL, Wolf SE, Wolfe RR. Independent and combined effects of amino acids and glucose after resistance exercise. *Med Sci Sports Exerc*. 2003;35:449–455.

44. Berardi JM, Price TB, Noreen EE, Lemon PW. Postexercise muscle glycogen recovery enhanced with a carbohydrate-protein supplement. *Med Sci Sports Exerc*. 2006;38(6):1106–1113.

45. Tipton KD, Ferrando AA, Phillips SM, Doyle D, Wolfe RR. Post-exercise net protein synthesis in human muscle from orally administered amino acids. *Am J Physiol*. 1999;276:E628–E634.

Additional Resources

Chandler RM, Byrne HK, Patterson JG, Ivy JL. Dietary supplements affect the anabolic hormones after weight-training exercise. *J Appl Physiol*. 1994;76:839–845.

Stryer L. *Biochemistry*. New York, NY: W.H. Freeman; 1995.

Wagenmakers AJ. Muscle amino acid metabolism at rest and during exercise: role in human physiology and metabolism. *Exerc Sport Sci Rev*. 1998;26:287–314.

Wojcik JR, Walberg-Rankin J, Smith LL. Effect of post-exercise macronutrient intake on metabolic response to eccentric resistance exercise. *Med Sci Sports Exerc*. 1997;29(suppl):294.

CHAPTER 6

Vitamins

You Are the Nutrition Coach

Roger is a starting guard on his college basketball team. He is a leader on his team, stays after practice to work on his shots, and is busy with academic and community life on campus. Because of his hectic schedule, he has little time for meal planning, grocery shopping, and food preparation. Dinner is usually consumed at the athletics training table during the week, and the rest of his meals are consumed either at home or at local restaurants. A 3-day food record kept by Roger recently was analyzed using a nutrition software program. The analysis revealed overall energy intake was not meeting his estimated needs, and vitamins A, C, and folate were consistently low throughout the 3-day period. The rest of the vitamins and minerals met the minimum RDA or AI requirements.

Questions

- What questions should you ask Roger about his typical daily diet?

- What recommendations do you have for Roger to improve his dietary intake of vitamins and his energy intake?

- How can you help Roger meet these recommendations?

What's the big deal about vitamins?

Vitamins play important roles throughout the body and are considered essential; without vitamins, the body could not function. Some vitamins can be synthesized in the body. Many are precursors for different processes, while others are critical for the development of various compounds in the body. For example, vitamin D serves as a precursor molecule in cholesterol formation while beta carotene serves as a precursor for vitamin A.

The role that vitamins play in sport performance has been studied over the years. Although it is clear that vitamins are crucial for body functions, less is known about the potential role they play in improving or hindering sport performance. Many athletes perceive that adequate vitamin intake is crucial to peak performance. Although the performance effect may not be proven, certain athlete populations are more prone to nutrient deficiencies, thus justifying a greater emphasis on a specific vitamin or mineral.[1] For example, female athletes may be more susceptible to iron deficiencies. Therefore, iron, as well as vitamins that enhance iron absorption, such as vitamin C, should receive greater emphasis in the diet. Another example that has recently received more attention is the potential for an increased need for some antioxidant vitamins and phytochemicals for those engaging in high-intensity training of long duration, which may increase oxidative stress within the body.

This chapter discusses the recommended levels of intake for vitamins, antioxidants, and phytochemicals for healthy individuals and for athletes. The functions of these nutrients, their effects on energy systems, deficiency and toxicity symptoms, their importance to sport performance, food sources, and meal-planning tips for athletes are discussed.

What are vitamins?

There are two classifications of vitamins: water soluble and fat soluble. The **water-soluble vitamins** include the B vitamins, vitamin C, and choline. These vitamins dissolve in water and are easily transported in the blood. Because of their water solubility they are also turned over in the body and as a result are not stored in the body in appreciable amounts. Utilization of water-soluble vitamins occurs on an as-needed

water-soluble vitamins A class of vitamins that dissolve in water and are easily transported in the blood. The water-soluble vitamins are the B vitamins, vitamin C, and choline.

basis; excess B vitamins or vitamin C are excreted in the urine. Because little storage of water-soluble vitamins occurs, regular intake of these nutrients is important.

Fat-soluble vitamins do not dissolve easily in water and require dietary fat for intestinal absorption and transport in the bloodstream. Unlike water-soluble vitamins, the fat-soluble vitamins A, D, E, and K are stored in the body, primarily in fat tissue and the liver, as well as in other organs, though in smaller amounts. When taken in excess, stored levels of the fat-soluble vitamins can build up and become toxic to the body. Dietary intake from foods rarely causes a toxic buildup, but intake via high-dosage supplements can quickly and easily build these vitamins to toxic levels.

fat-soluble vitamins A group of vitamins that do not dissolve easily in water and require dietary fat for intestinal absorption and transport in the bloodstream. The fat-soluble vitamins are A, D, E, and K.

gaining the performance edge

Water- and fat-soluble vitamins are vital to human health. An emphasis should be placed on food sources of vitamins, rather than on supplements. These high-vitamin foods should be consumed on a daily basis.

How are the dietary needs for vitamins represented?

The Dietary Reference Intakes (DRIs) include several ways to quantify nutrient needs or excesses of vitamins and minerals. Detailed descriptions of the different DRI categories are included in Chapter 1. As a summary, the DRIs include the Recommended Dietary Allowance (RDA), Estimated Average Requirement (EAR), Adequate Intake (AI), and Tolerable Upper Intake Level (UL). Each vitamin may have one or more of the DRIs established, depending on availability of current research data (see **Table 6.1**). The majority of vitamins have an established RDA or AI, and some have a UL.

What are the water-soluble vitamins?

The water-soluble vitamins include the B-complex vitamins (thiamin, riboflavin, niacin, B_6, B_{12}, folate, biotin, and pantothenic acid), choline, and vitamin C. Water-soluble vitamins are involved in many different processes within the body, including acting as **coenzymes**. A coenzyme is an organic molecule, usually a B vitamin, that attaches to an enzyme and activates or increases its ability to catalyze

coenzymes An organic molecule, usually a B vitamin, that attaches to an enzyme and activates or increases its ability to catalyze metabolic reactions.

156   **CHAPTER 6** Vitamins

TABLE 6.1 Dietary Reference Intakes (DRIs) for Vitamins

Life Stage Group	Vitamin A (µg/d)[1]	Vitamin D (IU/d)[2]	Vitamin E (mg/d)[3]	Vitamin K (µg/d)	Thiamin (mg/d)	Riboflavin (mg/d)	Niacin (mg/d)[4]	Panothenic Acid (mg/d)	Biotin (µg/d)	Vitamin B6 (mg/d)	Folate (µg/d)[5]	Vitamin B12 (µg/d)	Vitamin C (mg/d)	Choline (mg/day)
0–6 mo	400*	400*	4*	2.0*	0.2*	0.3*	2*	1.7*	5*	0.1*	65*	0.4*	40*	125*
7–12 mo	500*	400*	5*	2.5*	0.3*	0.4*	4*	1.8*	6*	0.3*	80*	0.5*	50*	150*
Children														
1–3 years	300	600	6	30*	0.5	0.5	6	2*	8*	0.5	150	0.9	15	200*
4–8 years	400	600	7	55*	0.6	0.6	8	3*	12*	0.6	200	1.2	25	250*
Males														
9–13 years	600	600	11	60*	0.9	0.9	12	4*	20*	1.0	300	1.8	45	375*
14–18 years	900	600	15	75*	1.2	1.3	16	5*	25*	1.3	400	2.4	75	550*
19–30 years	900	600	15	120*	1.2	1.3	16	5*	30*	1.3	400	2.4	90	550*
31–50 years	900	600	15	120*	1.2	1.3	16	5*	30*	1.3	400	2.4	90	550*
51–70 years	900	600	15	120*	1.2	1.3	16	5*	30*	1.7	400	2.4[7]	90	550*
>70 years	900	800	15	120*	1.2	1.3	16	5*	30*	1.7	400	2.4[7]	90	550*
Females														
9–13 years	600	600	11	60*	0.9	0.9	12	4*	20*	1.0	300	1.8	45	375*
14–18 years	700	600	15	75*	1.0	1.0	14	5*	25*	1.2	400[6]	2.4	65	400*
19–30 years	700	600	15	90*	1.1	1.1	14	5*	30*	1.3	400[6]	2.4	75	425*
31–50 years	700	600	15	90*	1.1	1.1	14	5*	30*	1.3	400[6]	2.4	75	425*
51–70 years	700	600	15	90*	1.1	1.1	14	5*	30*	1.5	400	2.4[7]	75	425*
>70 years	700	800	15	90*	1.1	1.1	14	5*	30*	1.5	400	2.4[7]	75	425*
Pregnancy														
≤18 years	750	600	15	75*	1.4	1.4	18	6*	30*	1.9	600	2.6	80	450*
19–30 years	770	600	15	90*	1.4	1.4	18	6*	30*	1.9	600	2.6	85	450*
31–50 years	770	600	15	90*	1.4	1.4	18	6*	30*	1.9	600	2.6	85	450*
Lactation														
≤18 years	1200	600	19	75*	1.4	1.6	17	7*	35*	2.0	500	2.8	115	550*
19–30 years	1300	600	19	90*	1.4	1.6	17	7*	35*	2.0	500	2.8	120	550*
31–50 years	1300	600	19	90*	1.4	1.6	17	7*	35*	2.0	500	2.8	120	550*

This table presents Recommended Dietary Allowances (RDA) and Adequate Intakes (AI). An asterisk (*) indicates AI. RDAs and AIs may both be used as goals for individual intake.

[1] As retinol activity equivalents (RAE).

[2] As cholecalciferol.

[3] As α-tocopherol.

[4] As niacin equivalents (NE).

[5] As dietary folate equivalents (DFE).

[6] In view of evidence linking folate intake with lessening of neural-tube defects in the fetus, it is recommended that all women capable of becoming pregnant consume 400 µg of folic acid from supplements or fortified foods in addition to intake of food folate from a varied diet.

[7] Because 10–30% of older people may malabsorb food-bound vitamin B12, it is advisable for those older than 50 years to meet their RDA mainly by consuming foods fortified with vitamin B12 or a supplement containing vitamin B12.

Source: Data compiled from Institute of Medicine's *Dietary Reference Intakes for Thiamin, Riboflavin, Niacin, Vitamin B6 Folate, Vitamin B12, Pantothenic Acid, Biotin, and Choline.* Food and Nutrition Board. Washington, DC: National Academies Press, 2000; *Dietary Reference Intakes for Vitamin A, Vitamin K, Arsenic, Boron, Chromium, Copper, Iodine, Iron, Manganese, Molybdenum, Nickel, Silicon, Vanadium and Zinc.* Food and Nutrition Board. Washington, DC: National Academies Press, 2001; *Dietary Reference Intakes for Vitamin C, Vitamin E, Selenium, and Carotenoids.* Food and Nutrition Board. Washington, DC: National Academies Press, 2000. Institute of Medicine; *Dietary Reference Intakes for Calcium and Vitamin D.* Food and Nutrition Board. Washington, DC: National Academies Press, 2010.

metabolic reactions. Some of these metabolic reactions are critical for energy production, especially during exercise.

Water-soluble vitamins can be obtained naturally from a large variety of food sources as well as from vitamin-fortified foods and beverages. In general, water-soluble vitamins are destroyed or lost with excessive cooking. To maximize the benefit of eating foods rich in the B-complex and C vitamins, foods should be eaten raw or cooked for short periods of time. The exception to this rule is any meat product. Meats should be cooked thoroughly to prevent foodborne pathogens found in undercooked meats. Because water-soluble vitamins are not stored to any great extent in the body, it is important to eat foods containing these vitamins on a daily basis.

Why is thiamin important to athletes?

Thiamin is also referred to as vitamin B_1. It is absorbed in the small intestine and is stored mainly in skeletal muscle, the liver, the kidneys, and the brain. Thiamin plays a major role in energy production and is also important for developing and maintaining a healthy nervous system. In relation to performance, thiamin is a component of the coenzyme thiamin pyrophosphate that converts pyruvate into acetyl CoA, which then enters into the Krebs cycle during aerobic energy production. Thiamin also plays a role in the conversion and utilization of glycogen for energy as well as the catabolism of branched chain amino acids. Some studies have shown that athletes with low intakes of thiamin have diminished exercise endurance.

What is the RDA/AI for thiamin?

The RDA for thiamin is 1.2 milligrams for males and 1.1 milligrams for females.[2] The RDA is based on the notion that humans need approximately 0.5 milligrams of thiamin per 1000 calories ingested daily. Therefore, thiamin requirements escalate with increased calorie intake. Athletes, who are generally expending more calories through training and competition relative to the sedentary population, will require more thiamin than the RDA on a daily basis. Thiamin is also critical for the proper metabolism of carbohydrates, so as carbohydrate intake increases, so will the requirement for thiamin.

What are the complications of thiamin deficiency?

Thiamin deficiency is typically caused by an athlete consuming very few calories or having a diet composed mainly of processed foods. The signs and symptoms of thiamin deficiency include decreased appetite, mental confusion, headaches, fatigue, muscle weakness, nerve degeneration, and pain in the calf muscles. If a severe deficiency is left untreated for as little as 10 days, the disease Beriberi can develop, which can lead to damage to the heart and nervous system. In regard to performance, studies have found that athletes with low intakes of thiamin and other water-soluble vitamins over the course of 11 weeks suffer decreases in maximal work capacity, peak power, and mean power output.[3,4]

What are the symptoms of thiamin toxicity?

As discussed earlier, water-soluble vitamins tend not to accumulate in the body because any excess is excreted in the urine. As a result, the risk for thiamin toxicity is low, and therefore no upper limit has been set for thiamin intake.

Which foods are rich in thiamin?

Thiamin is found in a variety of foods including whole grains, legumes, wheat germ, nuts, pork, and fortified foods such as refined flours, grains, and breakfast cereals (see Figure 6.1). In the United States, thiamin needs are generally met with a well-balanced diet and adequate total daily calories.

What is a suggestion for a thiamin-rich meal or snack?

Breakfast: One packet of instant oatmeal, made with 8 oz soy milk and topped with ¼ cup sunflower or pumpkin seeds
Total thiamin content = 0.768 milligrams

Do athletes need thiamin supplements?

Research on the ergogenic effects of thiamin supplementation is limited and has provided inconclusive results. Most studies have found that athletes who are restricting intake for the purposes of weight loss could potentially be low in thiamin[3,5] and therefore would benefit from a supplement. However, as with all nutrients, the focus should first be on nutrient-rich foods, and then a supplement if indicated.

Why is riboflavin important for athletes?

Riboflavin is also commonly referred to as vitamin B_2. It is absorbed mainly in the small intestine. Riboflavin is highly involved in the aerobic production of energy (i.e., adenosine triphosphate [ATP]) from carbohydrates, proteins, and fats. The two coenzymes, flavin mononucleotide and flavin adenine dinucleotide, contain riboflavin and are involved in the transport of electrons to the electron transport

THIAMIN

Daily Value = 1.5 mg
RDA = 1.2 mg (males) 1.1 mg (females)

Exceptionally good source			
Sweet potato, cooked	140 g (1 potato)	2.0 mg	
Pork, loin roast, lean only, cooked	85 g (3 oz)	0.76 mg	
Ham, extra lean, cooked	85 g (3 oz)	0.63 mg	
Bagel, plain	90 g (1 4" bagel)	0.48 mg	
Fish, tuna, cooked	85 g (3 oz)	0.43 mg	
Soy milk	240 ml	0.39 mg	
Corn flakes cereal	30 g (1 cup)	0.39 mg	
Cheerios cereal	30 g (1 cup)	0.38 mg	
Fiber One cereal	30 g (1/2 cup)	0.38 mg	
Oatmeal, instant, fortified, cooked	1 cup	0.34 mg	
Spaghetti, enriched, cooked	140 g (1 cup)	0.29 mg	
Wheat germ	15 g (1/4 cup)	0.28 mg	
Orange juice, chilled	240 ml (1 cup)	0.28 mg	
Sesame seeds	30 g (~1 oz)	0.24 mg	
Rice, white, enriched, cooked	140 g (~ 3/4 cup)	0.23 mg	
Salmon, cooked	85 g (3 oz)	0.23 mg	
White bread, enriched	50 g (2 slices)	0.23 mg	
Soybeans, cooked	90 g (~1/2 cup)	0.23 mg	
Black beans, cooked	90 g (~1/2 cup)	0.22 mg	
Pecans	30 g (~1 oz)	0.20 mg	
Grits, corn, enriched, cooked	1 cup	0.20 mg	
Whole wheat bread	50 g (2 slices)	0.20 mg	
Brazilnuts	30 g (~1 oz)	0.19 mg	
Baked beans, canned	130 g (~1/2 cup)	0.19 mg	
Navy beans, cooked	90 g (~1/2 cup)	0.18 mg	
Oysters, cooked	85 g (3 oz)	0.16 mg	
Lentils, cooked	90 g (~1/2 cup)	0.15 mg	

High: 20% DV or more

Good: 10-19% DV

Figure 6.1 Food sources of thiamin. Pork, whole and enriched grains, and fortified cereals are rich in thiamin. Most animal foods, however, contain little thiamin. Note: The DV for thiamin is higher than the current RDA of 1.2 and 1.1 milligrams for males and females, respectively, age 19 and older.
Source: U.S. Department of Agriculture, Agricultural Research Service, 2010. USDA Nutrient Database for Standard Reference, Release 23. Nutrient Data Laboratory home page. Available at: http://www.ars.usda.gov/Services/docs .htm?docid=8964. Accessed January 21, 2011.

chain during aerobic energy production at rest and during exercise.

What is the RDA/AI for riboflavin?

The RDA for riboflavin is 1.3 milligrams for males and 1.1 milligrams for females.[2]

What are the complications of riboflavin deficiency?

Riboflavin deficiency is recognized by symptoms such as red lips, cracks at the corners of the mouth, a sore throat, or an inflamed tongue. In athletics, a riboflavin deficiency may contribute to poor performance. One investigation found that 19% of the young active boys studied had poor riboflavin status. After 2 months of riboflavin supplementation, performance in a maximal bicycle ergometer test improved as compared to presupplementation.[6]

What are the symptoms of riboflavin toxicity?

As with most water-soluble vitamins, there appear to be no adverse effects of high doses of riboflavin because dietary excess is excreted in urine. Therefore, no upper limit has been set for riboflavin.

Which foods are rich in riboflavin?

Figure 6.2 lists some of the foods containing riboflavin. Milk, yogurt, bread, cereal products, mushrooms, cottage cheese, and eggs are all good sources of riboflavin. Similar to thiamin, bread and cereal products in the United States are fortified with riboflavin.

What is a suggestion for a riboflavin-rich meal or snack?

Salad bar creation: 2 cups of romaine lettuce with 1/2 cup each of mushrooms, carrots, and cottage cheese, and 2 tbsp of almonds
Total riboflavin content = 0.661 milligrams

Do athletes need riboflavin supplements?

It is challenging to determine whether athletes need riboflavin supplements. Minimal research has been conducted on the riboflavin status of individuals exercising strenuously[5] or the performance effects of riboflavin supplementation. A study conducted by Winters et al.[7] focused on women 50–67 years of age who exercised for 20–25 minutes, 6 days a week for 4-week periods on a cycle ergometer at 75–85% of their maximal heart rate. Although the investigators found biochemical changes indicating riboflavin depletion, supplemental riboflavin did not enhance exercise performance or endurance. More research is warranted to make a recommendation on whether athletes require more riboflavin than the current RDA. Daily riboflavin needs can typically be met through a balanced and calorically adequate diet.

Why is niacin important for athletes?

Niacin is a general term for two different substances: nicotinic acid and nicotinamide. Some sources might refer to niacin as vitamin B_3. A majority of niacin absorption occurs in the intestines, but a small amount is absorbed through the stomach. Niacin is highly involved in energy production and mitochondrial metabolism, thus affecting muscular and nervous

RIBOFLAVIN

Daily Value = 1.7 mg
RDA = 1.3 mg (males) 1.1 mg (females)

Exceptionally good sources

Food	Amount	Riboflavin
Beef liver, cooked	85 g (3 oz)	2.9 mg
Chicken liver, cooked	85 g (3 oz)	1.96 mg
Wheat bran flakes cereal	30 g (3/4 cup)	1.77 mg

High: 20% DV or more

Food	Amount	Riboflavin
Yogurt, plain, nonfat	225 g (1 8-oz container)	0.53 mg
Yogurt, plain, lowfat	225 g (1 8-oz container)	0.48 mg
Milk, nonfat	240 ml (1 cup)	0.47 mg
Corn flakes cereal	30 g (1 cup)	0.46 mg
Milk, 1%, 2%, whole (3.25%)	240 ml (1 cup)	0.45 mg
Cheerios cereal	30 g (1 cup)	0.43 mg
Fiber One cereal	30 g (1/2 cup)	0.43 mg
Oatmeal, instant, fortified, cooked	1 cup	0.40 mg
Squid, cooked	85 g (3 oz)	0.39 mg
Buttermilk, low-fat	240 ml (1 cup)	0.38 mg
Clams, cooked	85 g (3 oz)	0.36 mg

Good: 10-19% DV

Food	Amount	Riboflavin
Egg, hardcooked	50 g (1 large)	0.26 mg
Soybeans, cooked	90 g (~1/2 cup)	0.26 mg
Mushrooms, cooked	85 g (~1/2 cup)	0.26 mg
Herring, cooked	85 g (3 oz)	0.25 mg
Almonds	30 g (~1 oz)	0.24 mg
Pork, loin chops, lean only, cooked	85 g (3 oz)	0.23 mg
Turkey, dark meat, cooked	85 g (3 oz)	0.21 mg
Spinach, cooked	85 g (~1/2 cup)	0.20 mg
Cottage cheese, 2% milkfat	110 g (~1/2 cup)	0.20 mg
Chicken, dark meat, cooked	85 g (3 oz)	0.19 mg
Beef, porterhouse steak, cooked	85 g (3 oz)	0.18 mg
Ham, extra lean, cooked	85 g (3 oz)	0.17 mg
Soy milk	240 ml (1 cup)	0.17 mg
White bread, enriched	50 g (2 slices)	0.17 mg

Figure 6.2 Food sources of riboflavin. The best sources of riboflavin include milk, liver, whole and enriched grains, and fortified cereals. Note: The DV for riboflavin is higher than the current RDA of 1.3 and 1.1 milligrams for males and females, respectively, age 19 and older.
Source: U.S. Department of Agriculture, Agricultural Research Service, 2010. USDA Nutrient Database for Standard Reference, Release 23. Nutrient Data Laboratory home page. Available at: http://www.ars.usda.gov/Services/docs .htm?docid=8964. Accessed January 21, 2011.

system function. Niacin is a component of two co-enzymes: nicotinamide adenine dinucleotide (NAD+) and nicotinamide adenine dinucleotide phosphate (NADP+). These coenzymes are involved in the transfer of hydrogen ions in the anaerobic and aerobic energy systems. During aerobic exercise, NAD+ can accept a hydrogen ion and become NADH, carrying high-energy electrons to the electron transport chain for the production of ATP. In anaerobic metabolism, NADH is responsible for transferring hydrogen to pyruvate to form lactate during the breakdown of carbohydrates for energy.

What is the RDA/AI for niacin?

The RDA for niacin is 16 milligrams for males and 14 milligrams for females.[2] Niacin is obtained through the diet but can also be formed within the body from the amino acid tryptophan. Therefore, the RDA refers to niacin equivalents (NE) reflecting intake from niacin-rich foods as well as sources of tryptophan that can be converted into niacin. For foods rich in tryptophan, 60 milligrams of tryptophan is equivalent to 1 milligram of niacin.

What are the complications of niacin deficiency?

Niacin is critical for the progression of many metabolic pathways, and therefore a niacin deficiency will affect many bodily systems. Signs and symptoms of niacin deficiency include loss of appetite, skin rashes, mental confusion, lack of energy, and muscle weakness. If the deficiency is left untreated, the deficiency disease pellagra develops. Pellagra is characterized by the three "D's": dementia (mental confusion), diarrhea, and dermatitis (skin rashes). If pellagra is left untreated, there is a fourth "D," death.

What are the symptoms of niacin toxicity?

The upper dietary limit is 35 milligrams per day. Common side effects of high niacin intake include flushing of the face, arms, and chest; itchy skin rashes; headaches; nausea; glucose intolerance; blurred vision; and ultimately, liver complications. Doses several times the RDA are used medicinally for lowering low-density lipoprotein (LDL) cholesterol and raising high-density lipoprotein (HDL) cholesterol. Individuals taking niacin for its cholesterol-lowering effect must be under the supervision of a physician to monitor any potential complications and decrease the risk for liver damage.

Which foods are rich in niacin?

Along with thiamin and riboflavin, refined flours, grains, and cereals are fortified with niacin. Other dietary sources include protein-rich foods such as beef, poultry, fish, legumes, liver, and seafood, as well as whole grain products and mushrooms (see Figure 6.3).

What is a suggestion for a niacin-rich meal or snack?

Dining out—Italian: Chicken Marsala (4 oz chicken in 1 cup mushroom sauce) on 2 cups spaghetti
Total niacin content = 24 milligrams

NIACIN

Daily Value = 20 mg
RDA = 16 mg (males) 14 mg (females)

High: 20% DV or more	Beef liver, cooked	85 g (3 oz)	14.9 mg
	Chicken, light meat, cooked	85 g (3 oz)	10.6 mg
	Chicken liver, cooked	85 g (3 oz)	9.4 mg
	Salmon, cooked	85 g (3 oz)	8.6 mg
	Tuna, canned	55 g (2 oz)	7.3 mg
	Halibut, cooked	85 g (3 oz)	6.1 mg
	Turkey, light meat, cooked	85 g (3 oz)	5.8 mg
	Chicken, dark meat, cooked	85 g (3 oz)	5.6 mg
	Beef, ground, extra lean, cooked	85 g (3 oz)	5.3 mg
	Corn flakes, Cheerios cereals	30 g (1 cup)	5.0 mg
	Fiber One cereal	30 g (1/2 cup)	5.0 mg
	Oatmeal, instant, fortified, cooked	1 cup	4.8 mg
	All Bran cereal	30 g (1/2 cup)	4.8 mg
	Peanut butter	2 Tbsp	4.3 mg
	Pork, loin roast, lean only, cooked	85 g (3 oz)	4.0 mg
	Tomato paste, canned	130 g (~1/2 cup)	4.0 mg
Good: 10-19% DV	Beef, T-bone steak, cooked	85 g (3 oz)	3.9 mg
	Mushrooms, cooked	85 g (~1/2 cup)	3.8 mg
	Salmon, canned, solids + bones	55 g (2 oz)	3.6 mg
	Ham, extra lean, cooked	85 g (3 oz)	3.4 mg
	Beef, porterhouse steak, cooked	85 g (3 oz)	3.2 mg
	Turkey, dark meat, cooked	85 g (3 oz)	3.1 mg
	Barley, cooked	140 g (~1 cup)	2.9 mg
	Sardines, canned, solids + bones	55 g (2 oz)	2.9 mg
	Clams, cooked	85 g (3 oz)	2.9 mg
	Spaghetti, enriched, cooked	140 g (1 cup)	2.3 mg
	Shrimp, cooked	85 g (3 oz)	2.2 mg
	White bread, enriched	50 g (2 slices)	2.2 mg
	Rice, brown, cooked	140 g (~3/4 cup)	2.1 mg
	Cod, cooked	85 g (3 oz)	2.1 mg
	Rice, white, enriched, cooked	140 g (~3/4 cup)	2.0 mg

Figure 6.3 Food sources of niacin. Niacin is found mainly in meats and grains. Enrichment adds niacin as well as thiamin, riboflavin, folic acid, and iron to processed grains. Note: The DV for niacin is higher than the current RDA of 16 and 14 milligrams for males and females, respectively, age 19 and older.
Source: U.S. Department of Agriculture, Agricultural Research Service, 2010. USDA Nutrient Database for Standard Reference, Release 23. Nutrient Data Laboratory home page. Available at: http://www.ars.usda.gov/Services/docs .htm?docid=8964. Accessed January 21, 2011.

Do athletes need niacin supplements?

Although niacin is crucial for facilitating energy production, recent research reviews have concluded that well-nourished athletes do not benefit from niacin supplements. In addition to the lack of apparent benefit of consuming extra niacin, supplements are not recommended because high doses of niacin can:

- Affect fat metabolism by blocking free fatty acid release from adipose tissue,[8–10] increasing the reliance of the body on carbohydrate stores, thus depleting glycogen stores.[11]
- Increase blood flow to the skin, which decreases heat storage. This may be beneficial/ergogenic for some athletes, but more research is needed.[12]

Why is vitamin B_6 important for athletes?

Vitamin B_6 refers to all biologically active forms of vitamin B_6, including pyridoxine, pyridoxal, pyridoxamine, pyridoxine phosphate, pyridoxal phosphate, and pyridoxamine phosphate. Pyridoxine, pyridoxal, and pyridoxamine are the forms most commonly found in foods. All forms of vitamin B_6 are absorbed mainly in the jejunum of the small intestine and are converted in the liver to the most active coenzyme form, pyridoxal phosphate. Vitamin B_6 is important for health and athletic performance in many ways. B_6 is a component of more than 100 enzymes, which facilitate the following:

- *The breakdown of glycogen for energy as well as gluconeogenesis in the liver:* both processes are important during endurance activities.
- *The synthesis of amino acids via transamination:* this process produces amino acids endogenously, meaning that not all amino acids need to be consumed through the diet.
- *The conversion of tryptophan to niacin:* daily niacin requirements are based on a combination of niacin consumed through foods and the amount made by the body from tryptophan.
- *The formation of neurotransmitters:* this is critical for the fine motor movement and control required for various sports.
- *The production of the red blood cells' hemoglobin ring:* hemoglobin is essential for endurance activities that rely on oxygen for energy. A deficiency in B_6 can contribute to microcytic hypochromic anemia (small, low-hemoglobin red blood cells).
- *The production of white blood cells:* this is critical for proper immune function.

Vitamin B_6 has recently been heralded as a dietary protector against heart disease. Research has found that individuals with low intakes of B_6, as well as folate and vitamin B_{12}, have higher blood levels of homocysteine, which is a risk factor for heart disease (see Figure 6.4).

What is the RDA/AI for vitamin B_6?

The RDA for men and women ages 19–50 is 1.3 milligrams.[2] Because of the role of vitamin B_6 in protein metabolism, requirements are based on protein in-

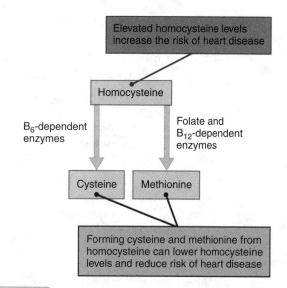

Figure 6.4 Homocysteine and heart disease. Elevated homocysteine levels are linked to an increased risk of heart disease. B_6, B_{12}, and folate-dependent enzymes help lower the amount of homocysteine by converting it to cysteine and methionine.

What are the symptoms of vitamin B_6 toxicity?

The upper limit for vitamin B_6 is 100 milligrams per day. Impaired gait resulting from peripheral nerve damage can be caused by intakes at or slightly above the upper daily limit. Irreversible nerve damage can occur at levels of 1000–2000 milligrams per day.

Which foods are rich in vitamin B_6?

Vitamin B_6 is found in a variety of foods (see Figure 6.5). The richest sources include high-protein foods such as beef, poultry, fish, and eggs. Other significant sources include whole grains, brown rice, wheat germ, white potatoes, starchy vegetables, fortified soy-based meat analogs, and bananas. It should be noted that refined grain products have been stripped of most of their B_6 content. Unlike with thiamin, riboflavin, and niacin, the enrichment process does not replace the lost B_6 in foods.

take. Individuals following a high-protein diet may need to consume more vitamin B_6.

What are the complications of vitamin B_6 deficiency?

Deficiencies in vitamin B_6 in male and female athletes are rare.[13] When athletes fail to ingest adequate vitamin B_6, it is usually explained by low energy intakes and poor food choices.[13] It is interesting to note that even when consuming a diet low in vitamin B_6, one study demonstrated that muscle levels of vitamin B_6 were not depleted.[14] However, if low daily intake persists, or if an athlete is taking diuretics or oral contraceptives, B_6 deficiency is still a possibility. For example, Manore et al.[15] studied three different groups of women, active and sedentary, and found that the elderly groups had low intakes of vitamin B_6 in their daily diets. A vitamin B_6 deficiency can be detected by symptoms such as nausea, impaired immune function (because of low numbers of white blood cells), convulsions, depression (related to the improper functioning of neurotransmitters), skin disorders, mouth sores, weakness, and anemia (because of low levels of red blood cell production).

VITAMIN B_6
Daily Value = 2 mg
RDA = 1.3 mg (males/females)

Exceptionally good source			
Wheat bran flakes cereal	30 g ($^3/_4$ cup)		2.1 mg
All Bran cereal	30 g ($^1/_2$ cup)		1.8 mg
Beef liver, cooked	85 g (3 oz)		0.9 mg
Chicken, light meat, cooked	85 g (3 oz)		0.7 mg
Chicken liver, cooked	85 g (3 oz)		0.6 mg
Garbanzo beans, canned	130 g (~$^1/_2$ cup)		0.6 mg
Banana, fresh	140 g (1 9" banana)		0.5 mg
Corn flakes cereal	30 g (1 cup)		0.5 mg
Fiber One cereal	30 g ($^1/_2$ cup)		0.5 mg
Cheerios cereal	30 g (1 cup)		0.5 mg
Turkey, light meat, cooked	85 g (3 oz)		0.5 mg
Pork, loin roast, lean only	85 g (3 oz)		0.4 mg
Beef, ground, extra lean, cooked	85 g (3 oz)		0.4 mg
Ham, extra lean, cooked	85 g (3 oz)		0.3 mg
Halibut, cooked	85 g (3 oz)		0.3 mg
Potato, baked, w/skin	110 g (1 small)		0.3 mg
Turkey, dark meat, cooked	85 g (3 oz)		0.3 mg
Chicken, dark meat, cooked	85 g (3 oz)		0.3 mg
Beef, porterhouse steak, cooked	85 g (3 oz)		0.3 mg
Herring, cooked	85 g (3 oz)		0.3 mg
Tomato juice, canned	240 ml (1 cup)		0.3 mg
Sweet potato, cooked	110 g (1 small)		0.3 mg
Sesame seeds	30 g (~1 oz)		0.2 mg
Sunflower seeds	30 g (~1 oz)		0.2 mg

High: 20% DV or more

Good: 10-19% DV

Figure 6.5 Food sources of vitamin B_6. Meats are generally good sources of vitamin B_6, as are certain fruits (e.g., bananas) and vegetables (e.g., potatoes, carrots). Note: The DV for vitamin B_6 is higher than the current RDA of 1.3 milligrams for males and females age 19 and older.
Source: U.S. Department of Agriculture, Agricultural Research Service, 2010. USDA Nutrient Database for Standard Reference, Release 23. Nutrient Data Laboratory home page. Available at: http://www.ars.usda.gov/Services/docs .htm?docid=8964. Accessed January 21, 2011.

What is a suggestion for a vitamin B$_6$-rich meal or snack?

Lunch: Egg salad sandwich on whole wheat bread and a banana

Total vitamin B$_6$ content = 0.834 milligrams

Do athletes need vitamin B$_6$ supplements?

The current research on the athletic performance benefits of vitamin B$_6$ supplementation is equivocal. Some studies have found marginal or low vitamin B$_6$ status in physically active individuals.[13,16] When a supplement was provided over several weeks, erythrocyte activity coefficients increased,[16] suggesting that exercise may further decrease vitamin status in active individuals who might already have low intakes of vitamin B$_6$.[17] Much of the exercise-related research has focused on determining the changes in vitamin B$_6$ metabolism during training to establish whether additional vitamin B$_6$ is indicated. Many studies involving short-duration and moderate-intensity exercise have shown an increase in vitamin B$_6$ in the blood within minutes of the onset of exercise and throughout the exercise bout. B$_6$ then shows a slow decline after the cessation of exercise.[15,18] An incremental increase during exercise is plausible in theory because of the increased reliance on gluconeogenesis for energy production, thus requiring more vitamin B$_6$. However, a recent study examining the changes in plasma vitamin B$_6$ in ultra-marathoners observed the opposite result, with postexercise levels lower than preexercise levels, with a further decline 60 minutes after the completion of the ultra-marathon.[19] More research is warranted to determine the exact changes in vitamin B$_6$ metabolism during short-term and long-duration exercise to establish recommendations for supplementation during training or competition.

Why is vitamin B$_{12}$ important for athletes?

Vitamin B$_{12}$ is also commonly referred to as cobalamin. Adequate intake and absorption of this vitamin are of special concern to older athletes as well as vegetarian and vegan athletes. Vitamin B$_{12}$ plays a role in the health and performance of the nervous and cardiovascular systems, the growth and development of tissues, and energy production. Vitamin B$_{12}$ maintains the integrity of the myelin sheath, which is the protective coating surrounding all nerve fibers. Vitamin B$_{12}$ is critical for folate metabolism, which in turn relates to DNA synthesis and tissue growth. Adequate intakes of vitamin B$_{12}$ prevent the onset of pernicious anemia. Vitamin B$_{12}$ is also involved in preparing fatty acid chains to enter the citric acid cycle, thus facilitating energy production.

A health-related task of vitamin B$_{12}$ is the lowering of homocysteine and thus the prevention of heart disease. High levels of homocysteine have recently been accepted as a valid risk factor for cardiovascular disease.[20] Homocysteine is converted to methionine with the coenzyme assistance of vitamin B$_{12}$, thus lowering blood levels of homocysteine and the risk for disease (see Figure 6.4).

What is the RDA/AI for vitamin B$_{12}$?

The RDA for vitamin B$_{12}$ is 2.4 micrograms for adults aged 19–50 years.[2] Older adults have the same requirement; however, many older individuals have a decreased ability to absorb B$_{12}$. The synthetic form of B$_{12}$ can be absorbed more readily than food sources for these individuals; therefore, they should focus on incorporating fortified foods and supplements into their daily diet.

What are the complications of vitamin B$_{12}$ deficiency?

Vitamin B$_{12}$ deficiency is caused by either impaired absorption or decreased intake. Because vitamin B$_{12}$ is found naturally only in animal products, individuals following a vegetarian or especially a vegan diet will need to consume fortified foods or take daily supplements to avoid deficiency problems. The liver stores B$_{12}$, and therefore deficiencies develop gradually over time. Vitamin B$_{12}$ deficiency can result in neurological problems and pernicious anemia. B$_{12}$ is critical for the health of the myelin sheath, so low intake causes the myelin sheath to swell and break down, leading to brain abnormalities and spinal cord degeneration. Pernicious anemia leads to altered red blood cell formation, producing megaloblasts and macrocytes, meaning large, irregular cells. Pernicious anemia may lead to decreased endurance performance, but more research is needed before conclusions can be drawn and recommendations formulated.

In regard to cardiovascular health, a deficiency of vitamin B$_{12}$ can lead to increasing levels of homocysteine and a greater risk for disease. A recent study conducted by Herrmann et al.[21] discovered that 25% of study participants, all recreational athletes, had elevated homocysteine levels that were associated with low levels of both vitamin B$_{12}$ and folate. Engaging in physical activity on a regular basis is a negative risk factor for cardiovascular disease. However, efforts to prevent disease through exercise may be negated if daily nutrition and adequate intake of B_{12} are neglected.

What are the symptoms of vitamin B_{12} toxicity?

Because there are no recognized detrimental effects from high doses of B_{12}, an upper limit has not been set.

Which foods are rich in vitamin B_{12}?

Vitamin B_{12} is naturally found only in animal products such as meats, dairy products, and eggs (see Figure 6.6). For vegetarians and vegans, fortified foods include breakfast cereals, soy milks, and other soy-based products.

VITAMIN B_{12}

Daily Value = 6 µg
RDA = 2.4 µg (males/females)

	Exceptionally good sources		
	Clams, cooked	85 g (3 oz)	84.1 µg
	Beef liver, cooked	85 g (3 oz)	71 µg
	Oysters, cooked	85 g (3 oz)	29.8 µg
	Chicken liver, cooked	85 g (3 oz)	18.0 µg
	Herring, cooked	85 g (3 oz)	11.2 µg
	Crab, Alaska King, cooked	85 g (3 oz)	9.8 µg
	Crab, blue, cooked	85 g (3 oz)	6.2 µg
	Wheat bran flakes cereal	30 g (3/4 cup)	6.2 µg
	All Bran cereal	30 g (1/2 cup)	6.0 µg
High: 20% DV or more	Sardines, canned, solids + bones	55 g (2 oz)	4.9 µg
	Salmon, cooked	85 g (3 oz)	2.6 µg
	Lobster, cooked	85 g (3 oz)	2.6 µg
	Beef, ground, extra lean, cooked	85 g (3 oz)	2.2 µg
	Beef, T-bone steak, cooked	85 g (3 oz)	1.9 µg
	Tuna, canned	55 g (2 oz)	1.7 µg
	Yogurt, plain, nonfat	225 g (8-oz container)	1.4 µg
	Shrimp, cooked	85 g (3 oz)	1.3 µg
	Yogurt, plain, lowfat	225 g (8-oz container)	1.3 µg
	Halibut, cooked	85 g (3 oz)	1.2 µg
Good: 10-19% DV	Milk, 2% milkfat	240 ml (1 cup)	1.1 µg
	Milk, whole 3.25% milkfat	240 ml (1 cup)	1.1 µg
	Squid, cooked	85 g (3 oz)	1.0 µg
	Milk, 1% milkfat	240 ml (1 cup)	1.0 µg
	Milk, nonfat	240 ml (1 cup)	0.9 µg
	Cod, cooked	85 g (3 oz)	0.9 µg
	Frankfurter, beef	55 g (1 each)	0.9 µg
	Bologna, beef	55 g (2 slices)	0.8 µg
	Cottage cheese, 2% milkfat	110 g (~1/2 cup)	0.7 µg
	Pork, loin chops, lean only, cooked	85 g (3 oz)	0.6 µg

Figure 6.6 Food sources of vitamin B_{12}. Vitamin B_{12} is found naturally only in foods of animal origin such as liver, meats, and milk. Some cereals are fortified with vitamin B_{12}. Note: The DV for vitamin B_{12} is substantially higher than the current RDA of 2.4 micrograms for males and females age 14 and older.
Source: U.S. Department of Agriculture, Agricultural Research Service, 2010. USDA Nutrient Database for Standard Reference, Release 23. Nutrient Data Laboratory home page. Available at: http://www.ars.usda.gov/Services/docs .htm?docid=8964. Accessed January 21, 2011.

What is a suggestion for a vitamin B_{12}-rich meal or snack?

Dinner: 3 oz slice of meatloaf with 3/4 cup mashed potatoes, 1 1/4 cups salad, and 12 oz skim milk
Total vitamin B_{12} content = 2.45 micrograms

Do athletes need vitamin B_{12} supplements?

As mentioned previously, vegetarian or vegan athletes may need supplemental B_{12} from fortified vegetarian foods, soy products, or multivitamins. Masters or elderly athletes may also need B_{12} supplements if they have atrophic gastritis and/or low levels of intrinsic factor. Those with diagnosed pernicious anemia will have enhanced performance after consuming higher doses of B_{12}. However, studies following individuals without pernicious anemia who are consuming large doses of vitamin B_{12} through supplements or vitamin B_{12}-rich foods have shown no effect on endurance, VO_2max, or body building. Therefore, a healthy athlete consuming a balanced diet may not benefit from vitamin B_{12} supplements.

Why is folate important for athletes?

The terms *folate* and *folic acid* are often used interchangeably, referring to the same nutrient. However, folate is the form of this vitamin found in whole foods, whereas folic acid is the most stable form or derivative of folate and is therefore used in supplements and fortified foods. The significance of folate for health and well-being is apparent at the moment of conception. Folate is critical for DNA synthesis and cell division, thus playing an important role in the growth and development of a fetus. Adequate folate intake has been recognized as a key in the prevention of neural-tube defects during pregnancy. It is critical for a woman to be consuming enough folate at the time of conception because most neural-tube defects occur within the first month after conception. This discovery was the driving force behind the 1998 Food and Nutrition Board mandate to fortify grains in the United States with folic acid.

Because of its role in cellular development throughout the body, folate also aids in the maturation of red blood cells and the repair of tissues. Adequate folate intake prevents the development of megalo-

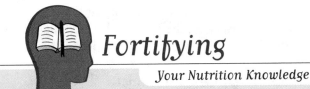

Vitamin B$_{12}$ Absorption

Vitamin B$_{12}$ has a complex progression from ingestion to absorption. For elderly or ill individuals, there are several steps in the digestion pathway that can cause suboptimal absorption:

1. R-protein is produced by the salivary glands in the mouth and travels unconnected to vitamin B$_{12}$ to the stomach.
2. In the stomach, R-protein binds with vitamin B$_{12}$ as a protective mechanism as the complex travels to the small intestine. Intrinsic factor is secreted by the parietal cells of the stomach and travels with the B$_{12}$–R-protein complex to the small intestine. For elderly individuals, the parietal cells become less functional, producing less intrinsic factor and thus affecting vitamin B$_{12}$ absorption in the small intestine.
3. Pancreatic enzymes cleave B$_{12}$ from the R-protein in the small intestine.
4. B$_{12}$ then binds to intrinsic factor and travels to the ileum of the small intestine, where it binds to the brush border and is absorbed and transported throughout the body. For individuals who suffer from chronic diarrhea or sloughing of the brush border because of age, illness, or medications, vitamin B$_{12}$ absorption will be diminished.

Absorption of vitamin B$_{12}$ is a complex process that involves many factors and sites in the GI tract. Defects in this process, especially a lack of intrinsic factor, impair absorption and can result in deficiency.

Salivary glands produce R-protein.

Stomach cells release intrinsic factor.

IF

In the stomach, B$_{12}$ binds with R-protein.

B$_{12}$

R X B$_{12}$

Pancreatic enzymes partially degrade R-protein, releasing B$_{12}$ to bind with intrinsic factor.

B$_{12}$ IF

In the ileum, the B$_{12}$–IF complex binds to an intestinal cell receptor and is absorbed. After 3–4 hours, B$_{12}$ enters circulation bound to transcobalamin, a transport protein.

blastic, macrocytic anemia. This type of anemia is also a result of vitamin B$_{12}$ deficiency; therefore, it is critical to determine which nutrient is the cause of the anemia to establish the appropriate method of treatment. If anemia develops, energy levels for training and competition may suffer. Folate also facilitates muscle tissue repair after strenuous exercise, aiding in recovery.

In addition, folate has recently gained recognition in the area of cardiovascular health. Folate helps to lower levels of homocysteine in the blood, thus potentially lowering the risk for heart disease.

What is the RDA/AI for folate?

The RDA for folate is 400 micrograms per day for adult males and females.[2] The RDA is expressed in Dietary Folate Equivalents (DFE). One DFE equals 1 microgram of folate from food, 0.6 micrograms of folic acid in fortified foods, or 0.5 micrograms of folic acid in supplements taken on an empty stomach.

What are the complications of folate deficiency?

Because of folate's role in basic cell development and division, deficiency of this vitamin affects many components of health and performance. During pregnancy and fetal development, if the mother consumes suboptimal levels of folate, the risk of neural-tube defects increases considerably. The lack of folate causes incomplete and altered neural-tube development within the spine, leading to conditions such as spina bifida. Low folate causes a change in DNA, affecting various cells such as those in the lining of the intestines and causing absorption problems and chronic diarrhea. White blood cell development can also be impaired, contributing to poor immune function.

Insufficient intake of folate can lead to a type of anemia known as megaloblastic anemia. Because of an altered DNA synthesis, division of red blood cells is not normal, producing large, abnormal red blood cells with short life spans. These abnormal cells have a decreased oxygen-carrying capacity, leading to symptoms of anemia such as fatigue, weakness, irritability, and disturbed sleep. Because deficiencies in both B_{12} and folate can cause anemia, it is important to pay attention to all symptoms to prevent misdiagnosis and further complications. For example, if a B_{12} deficiency is mistaken for a folate deficiency, higher levels of folate will repair the megaloblastic anemia, but other neurological problems will continue to develop as a result of the low vitamin B_{12} intake. Low folate intake may also increase the risk for heart disease by allowing homocysteine levels to rise. Folate works with other water-soluble vitamins, B_6 and B_{12}, to reduce homocysteine levels in the blood.

What are the symptoms of folate toxicity?

Folate toxicity is rare because ingesting excessive levels of folate is difficult to do through consumption of foods; in addition, excess folate is excreted in the urine. However, an upper limit has been established for adults at 1000 micrograms. The main reason for the UL is that high levels of folate can hide symptoms of vitamin B_{12} deficiency. Because

athletes have an increased risk for vitamin B_{12} deficiency, observing the UL of folate will help prevent misdiagnosis and resulting complications.

Which foods are rich in folate?

When thinking of folate, think "foliage" or plant foods. Folate-rich foods include many plant-based products such as dark green leafy vegetables, strawberries, oranges, legumes, nuts, brewer's yeast, and fortified grains (see Figure 6.7). Folate fortification of grains and flours was mandated in 1996 and went into effect in 1998 in the United States as a result of a plethora of research showing the importance of adequate folate intake in reducing the incidence of neural-tube defects. Fortification is estimated to

FOLATE

Daily Value = 400 µg
RDA = 400 µg (males/females)

Exceptionally good sources

Chicken liver, cooked	85 g (3 oz)	491 µg
Wheat bran flakes cereal	30 g (1 cup)	417 µg
Product 19 cereal	30 g (1 cup)	400 µg

High: 20% DV or more

All Bran cereal	30 g (½ cup)	393 µg
Beef liver, cooked	85 g (3 oz)	221 µg
Cheerios cereal	30 g (1 cup)	200 µg
Spinach, raw	85 g (~3 cups)	165 µg
Lentils, cooked	90 g (~½ cup)	163 µg
Pinto beans, cooked	90 g (~½ cup)	155 µg
Black beans, cooked	90 g (~½ cup)	134 µg
Asparagus, cooked	85 g (~½ cup)	127 µg
Spinach, cooked	85 g (~½ cup)	124 µg
Romaine lettuce, raw	85 g (~1½ cups)	116 µg
Black-eyed peas, cooked	90 g (~½ cup)	114 µg
Corn flakes cereal	30 g (1 cup)	110 µg
Spaghetti, enriched, cooked	140 g (1 cup)	108 µg
Oatmeal, instant, fortified, cooked	1 cup	101 µg
Turnip greens, cooked	85 g (~⅔ cup)	100 µg
Soybeans, cooked	90 g (~½ cup)	100 µg
Broccoli, cooked	85 g (~½ cup)	92 µg
Rice, white, enriched, cooked	140 g (~¾ cup)	81 µg

Good: 10-19% DV

Collards, cooked	85 g (~½ cup)	79 µg
Sunflower seeds	30 g (~ 1 oz)	71 µg
Beets, cooked	85 g (~½ cup)	68 µg
Mustard greens, cooked	85 g (~⅔ cup)	62 µg
White bread, enriched	50 g (2 slices)	56 µg
Tomato juice, canned	240 ml (1 cup)	49 µg
Orange juice, chilled	240 ml (1 cup)	45 µg
Crab, Alaska King, cooked	85 g (3 oz)	43 µg
Artichokes, cooked	85 g (~½ cup)	43 µg
Kidney beans, canned	85 g (~½ cup)	42 µg
Wheat germ	15 g (¼ cup)	42 µg
Orange, fresh	140 g (1 medium)	42 µg

Figure 6.7 Food sources of folate. Good sources of folate are a diverse collection of foods, including liver, legumes, leafy greens, and orange juice. Enriched grains and fortified cereals are other ways to include folic acid in the diet. *Source:* U.S. Department of Agriculture, Agricultural Research Service, 2010. USDA Nutrient Database for Standard Reference, Release 23. Nutrient Data Laboratory home page. Available at: http://www.ars.usda.gov/Services/docs .htm?docid=8964. Accessed January 21, 2011.

increase the average American's intake of folic acid by approximately 100 micrograms of folic acid per day. This increase in intake was designed to help Americans achieve the RDA of 400 micrograms per day, while not exceeding the upper limit of 1000 micrograms. For more information on folic acid fortification, visit the Food and Drug Administration's Web site at www.fda.gov.

What is a suggestion for a folate-rich meal or snack?

Dinner: Black-eyed peas with Chinese greens (see **Training Table 6.1**)
Total folate content (per serving) = 407 micrograms

Do athletes need folate supplements?

Consuming a variety of plant-based, folate-rich foods should prevent problems such as anemia. Fortified grains should also be included as a significant source of folate for meeting the RDA. A multivitamin can be used for extra insurance of meeting needs. To date, there have been no studies suggesting an increased exercise capacity by consuming extra folate.

Training Table 6.1: Black-Eyed Peas with Chinese Greens

2 cups brown rice

2 tbsp minced ginger root

3 cloves of garlic

1 tbsp peanut oil

1 tbsp sesame oil

2 lbs bok choy or napa cabbage

3 15-oz cans of black-eyed peas

2 tbsp soy sauce

Bring 2 cups of water to a boil. Add the brown rice and cook at a simmer for 30–40 minutes until all the water is absorbed. In the meantime, sauté the ginger and garlic in the peanut and sesame oils in a Dutch oven for 5–10 minutes over medium-high heat. Cut the bok choy or cabbage into ½-in. strips and add to the ginger and garlic; cook for 5–7 minutes. Add the black-eyed peas and soy sauce, and cook for an additional 5 minutes.

Serve over brown rice.

Serving Size: 2 cups (Recipe makes 4–6 servings)

Calories: 540 kcals

Protein: 26 grams

Carbohydrate: 95 grams

Fat: 8 grams

Why is biotin important for athletes?

In the 1920s three similar compounds, bios II, vitamin H, and coenzyme R, were all found to be beneficial to the body. With further investigation, it was recognized that all three compounds were the same nutrient—biotin. Biotin plays a role in synthesizing DNA for healthy cell development and energy production for endurance activities. Biotin is a cofactor for several carboxylase enzymes involved in the metabolism of carbohydrates, proteins, and fats. Biotin also helps produce energy by facilitating gluconeogenesis.

What is the RDA/AI for biotin?

Currently, very little research exists on the biotin requirements for a healthy adult. Therefore, no RDA has been set. The Adequate Intake level for adults is 30 micrograms per day.[2]

What are the complications of biotin deficiency?

Biotin deficiency is rare because so little is required. A few cases of biotin deficiency have been observed in those with a prolonged consumption of raw egg whites and those dependent upon parenteral nutrition without biotin supplementation.[22] Some documented signs and symptoms of biotin deficiency include fatigue, depression, nausea, dermatitis, and muscular pains.

What are the symptoms of biotin toxicity?

No physical or mental signs or symptoms of biotin toxicity have been documented. Biotin appears to be safe even at high levels, so no upper limit has been set.

Which foods are rich in biotin?

Biotin is found in a wide range of different foods. Legumes, cheese, egg yolks, nuts, and green leafy vegetables are all good sources of biotin. Raw egg whites will bind to biotin and may contribute to biotin deficiency if consumed on a regular basis. Cooking of egg whites alleviates this problem and also decreases the risk of sickness caused by foodborne pathogens. Biotin content has not been determined for most foods, and therefore is not listed on most food composition charts.

What is a suggestion for a biotin-rich meal or snack?

Breakfast: 3 scrambled eggs with ¼ cup shredded cheddar cheese and 2 tbsp peanut butter on 1 slice of whole wheat toast
Total biotin content = 57 micrograms

Do athletes need biotin supplements?

Very little research has been conducted on biotin and exercise performance. Because no toxic level has been detected, supplemental biotin may not be harmful to health or performance, but it also may not be necessary.

Why is pantothenic acid important for athletes?

Because of the role pantothenic acid plays in energy metabolism, there is little question that it is important to athletes. Specifically, pantothenic acid is a component of coenzyme A, a molecule critical for the passage of metabolic intermediates from fat, carbohydrate, and protein metabolism into the citric acid cycle. As discussed in Chapter 2, the citric acid cycle is one of the major metabolic pathways involved in the aerobic production of ATP. The key question is whether pantothenic acid supplementation will improve athletic performance. Limited research has been conducted to date; however, pantothenic acid supplementation has not been shown to be beneficial to athletes.[23,24]

What is the RDA/AI for pantothenic acid?

No RDA has been set for pantothenic acid. The Adequate Intake is set at 5 milligrams per day for adults aged 19–50 years.[2]

What are the complications of pantothenic acid deficiency?

Fatigue, sleep disturbances, impaired coordination, nausea, hypoglycemia, and muscle cramps can signal low levels of pantothenic acid. However, deficiencies are very rare.

What are the symptoms of pantothenic acid toxicity?

There appear to be no risks with high intake of pantothenic acid; therefore, no upper limit has been set.

Which foods are rich in pantothenic acid?

Pantothenic acid can be found in beef, poultry, fish, whole grains, dairy products, legumes, potatoes, oats, and tomatoes (see Figure 6.8). Consuming fresh and whole foods is especially beneficial in regard to pantothenic acid because freezing, canning, processing, and refining foods decrease the foods' pantothenic acid content considerably.

PANTOTHENIC ACID

Daily Value = 10 mg
AI = 5 mg (males/females)

High: 20% DV or more			
	Beef liver, cooked	85 g (3 oz)	6.0 mg
	Chicken liver, cooked	85 g (3 oz)	5.6 mg
	Sunflower seeds	30 g (~1 oz)	2.1 mg

Good: 10-19% DV			
	Mushrooms, cooked	85 g (~1/2 cup)	1.8 mg
	Yogurt, plain, nonfat	225 g (1 8-oz container)	1.4 mg
	Yogurt, plain, low-fat	225 g (1 8-oz container)	1.3 mg
	Turkey, dark meat, cooked	85 g (3 oz)	1.1 mg
	Chicken, dark meat, cooked	85 g (3 oz)	1.0 mg

Figure 6.8 Food sources of pantothenic acid. Pantothenic acid is found widely in foods, but it is abundant in only a few sources, such as liver. Note: The DV for pantothenic acid is higher than the current AI of 5 milligrams for males and females age 19 and older.
Source: U.S. Department of Agriculture, Agricultural Research Service, 2010. USDA Nutrient Database for Standard Reference, Release 23. Nutrient Data Laboratory home page. Available at: http://www.ars.usda.gov/Services/docs.htm?docid=8964. Accessed January 21, 2011.

What is a suggestion for a pantothenic acid–rich meal or snack?

Lunch: Baked potato topped with ¾ cup garbanzo beans, ¼ cup salsa, and 2 tbsp melted cheese, and an 8 oz glass of skim milk
Total pantothenic acid content = 2.4 milligrams

Do athletes need pantothenic acid supplements?

Because pantothenic acid is widespread in a balanced diet, and deficiencies are so rare, supplementation for athletes does not appear to be required. In addition, the existing research does not provide enough information to warrant supplementation for enhanced athletic performance.

Why is choline important for athletes?

Choline is a vitamin-like compound, but is not considered a B vitamin. Similar to biotin, choline is not well researched, and therefore limited information is available on its role in health and sport performance. Choline is involved in the formation of the neurotransmitter acetylcholine, which is involved in muscle activation. In theory, higher intakes of choline would maintain higher blood levels of the nutrient and increased levels of acetylcholine in the nerve endings, thus preventing muscle fatigue and/or failure. More research is needed to evaluate this theory, however. Choline has also been shown to help maintain the structural integrity of cell membranes.

What is the RDA/AI for choline?

Because of the lack of research on choline, an RDA has not been set. The Adequate Intake has been set at 550 and 425 milligrams per day for men and women, respectively.[2]

What are the complications of choline deficiency?

The risk for choline deficiency is low because it is found in a wide variety of foods. The human body also makes choline endogenously, further decreasing the risk for deficiency.

What are the symptoms of choline toxicity?

The signs and symptoms of choline toxicity include low blood pressure, diarrhea, and a fishy body odor. The upper limit for choline is set at 3500 milligrams per day, many times the AI level.

Which foods are rich in choline?

Well-balanced diets provide sufficient levels of choline. Some of the richest sources of choline include lecithin, egg yolks, liver, nuts, milk, wheat germ, cauliflower, and soybeans. Choline can be produced in the body from the amino acid methionine. Therefore, ingesting protein-rich foods, which provide methionine, can indirectly contribute to daily choline needs. Very few foods have been tested to determine choline levels, making food value databases containing choline unavailable.

What is a suggestion for a choline-rich meal or snack?

Side dish for dinner: Roasted broccoli and cauliflower (see **Training Table 6.2**). Nutrient databases for choline are incomplete and therefore a nutrient analysis is not available.

Do athletes need choline supplements?

The current research results are equivocal for endurance sports as well as power and strength sports. A recent study by Hongu and Sachan[25] reported that choline supplements given to healthy women promoted **carnitine** conservation and favored incomplete oxidation of fatty acids and disposal of fatty acid carbons in the urine. Earlier studies suggest that this scenario, induced by the choline supplements, might reduce fat mass and increase fat oxidation during exercise.[26,27] However, more research is needed to clarify choline's role in physical activity and whether supplementation would be beneficial to athletes.

carnitine A compound that transports fatty acids from the cytosol into the mitochondria, where they undergo beta-oxidation.

Training Table 6.2: Roasted Broccoli and Cauliflower

½ lb broccoli
½ lb cauliflower
cooking spray
dried basil, oregano, and black pepper

Preheat oven to 500°F. Chop broccoli and cauliflower into 2-inch pieces and spread evenly on a cookie sheet coated with cooking spray. Spray more cooking spray on top of the vegetables and sprinkle with dried basil, oregano, and black pepper. Bake for 10–15 minutes and serve as a side dish to a favorite dinner.

Serving Size: 1½ cups (Recipe makes 2 servings)

Calories: 67 kcals

Protein: 5 grams

Carbohydrate: 13 grams

Fat: 1 gram

Why is vitamin C important for athletes?

Vitamin C is also commonly referred to as ascorbic acid or ascorbate. It has received great attention in the last decade for its **antioxidant** properties. Vitamin C plays several roles in promoting general health. It is critical for the formation of **collagen**, which is a fibrous protein found in connective tissues of the body such as tendons, ligaments, cartilage, bones, and teeth. Collagen synthesis is also important in wound healing and the formation of scar tissue. Vitamin C plays a role in a healthy immune system and enhances iron absorption of nonheme iron, thus protecting the body against iron-deficiency anemia.

Cardiovascular research has indicated that vitamin C's role as an antioxidant seems to be protective against heart disease, especially by preventing the oxidation of LDL, which can lead to atherosclerosis. Atherosclerosis is the progressive narrowing of the lumens of arteries caused by fatty deposits on their interior walls. Over time these fatty plaques can block blood supply to vital tissues, causing poor

antioxidants Compounds that protect the body from highly reactive molecules known as free radicals.

collagen A fibrous protein found in connective tissues of the body such as tendons, ligaments, cartilage, bones, and teeth.

delivery of oxygen; with complete blockage, cell death occurs.

Vitamin C supplementation has recently been promoted to athletes as a potent antioxidant, helping to combat the oxidative damage that can occur during intense exercise. This potential function of vitamin C needs further investigation because current research is contradictory (see the section "Which vitamins or compounds have antioxidant properties?" later in this chapter). Vitamin C also aids in the formation of various hormones and in the production of neurotransmitters such as epinephrine.

What is the RDA/AI for vitamin C?

The RDA for males is 90 milligrams per day and for females is 75 milligrams per day.[28] If an individual smokes regularly, which increases oxidative stress and the metabolic turnover of vitamin C, the RDA increases by 35 milligrams per day.[28]

What are the complications of vitamin C deficiency?

The first signs of vitamin C deficiency are swollen gums and fatigue. If left untreated, the deficiency disease scurvy can develop, causing a degeneration of the skin, teeth, and blood vessels resulting from low collagen production. The physical manifestations of scurvy include bleeding gums, impaired wound healing, and weakness. However, deficiencies in the United States are rare because fruits and vegetables that contain high levels of vitamin C are available year-round. As a protective mechanism, the body stores several grams of vitamin C in case of short periods of low vitamin C intake.

What are the symptoms of vitamin C toxicity?

Vitamin C is a water-soluble vitamin, so it is relatively nontoxic. Intakes of greater than 1500 milligrams a day are not well absorbed, and excesses are excreted in the urine. However, at intake levels greater than the established upper limit of 2000 milligrams daily, side effects can include nausea, abdominal cramps, diarrhea, and nosebleeds. Long-term megadoses of vitamin C can also contribute to kidney stones, decrease the absorption of other nutrients, and may increase the risk for heart disease.

Which foods are rich in vitamin C?

The richest sources of vitamin C include citrus fruits and their juices, tomatoes and tomato juice, potatoes, green peppers, green leafy vegetables, kiwi, and cabbage (see Figure 6.9).

What is a suggestion for a vitamin C–rich meal or snack?

Snack: Fruit salad made with 1 orange, 2 kiwis, and ¾ cup cantaloupe
Total vitamin C content = 269 milligrams

VITAMIN C

Daily Value = 60 mg
RDA = 90 mg (males) 75 mg (females)

Exceptionally good sources

Strawberries, fresh	140 g (~1 cup)	82.3 mg
Orange juice, chilled	240 ml (1 cup)	81.9 mg
Orange, fresh	140 g (1 medium)	74.5 mg
Wheat bran flakes	30 g (³/4 cup)	62.1 mg
Cantaloupe, fresh	140 g (¹/4 medium melon)	51.4 mg
Tomato juice, canned	240 ml (1 cup)	44.5 mg
Mango, fresh	140 g (~³/4 cup)	38.8 mg
Cauliflower, cooked	85 g (~³/4 cup)	37.7 mg
Broccoli, cooked	85 g (~¹/2 cup)	35.7 mg
Spinach, raw	85 g (~3 cups)	23.9 mg
Pineapple, fresh	140 g (~1 cup)	23.7 mg
Watermelon, fresh	280 g (¹/16 melon)	22.7 mg
Sweet potato, cooked	110 g (1 small)	21.6 mg
Mustard greens, cooked	85 g (~²/3 cup)	21.5 mg
Romaine lettuce, raw	85 g (~1¹/2 cups)	20.4 mg
Beef liver, cooked	85 g (3 oz)	19.6 mg
Clams, cooked	85 g (3 oz)	18.8 mg
Cabbage, cooked	85 g (~¹/2 cup)	17.1 mg
Collards, cooked	85 g (~¹/2 cup)	15.5 mg
Soybeans, cooked	90 g (~¹/2 cup)	15.3 mg
Swiss chard, cooked	85 g (~¹/2 cup)	15.3 mg
Okra, cooked	85 g (~¹/2 cup)	13.9 mg
Blueberries, fresh	140 g (~³/4 cup)	13.6 mg
Banana, fresh	140 g (1 9" banana)	12.2 mg
Potato, baked	110 g (1 small)	10.6 mg
Peach, fresh	140 g (2 small)	9.2 mg
Acorn squash, cooked	85 g (~¹/2 cup)	9.2 mg
Spinach, cooked	85 g (~¹/2 cup)	8.3 mg
Green beans, cooked	85 g (~³/4 cup)	8.2 mg
Asparagus, cooked	85 g (~¹/2 cup)	6.5 mg
Corn flakes cereal	30 g (1 cup)	6.4 mg
Cheerios cereal	30 g (1 cup)	6.0 mg

High: 20% DV or more

Good: 10-19% DV

Figure 6.9 Food sources of vitamin C. Vitamin C is found mainly in fruits and vegetables. Although citrus fruits are notoriously good sources, many other popular fruits and vegetables are rich in vitamin C. Note: The DV for vitamin C is lower than the current RDA of 90 milligrams and 75 milligrams for males and females, respectively, age 19 and older.
Source: U.S. Department of Agriculture, Agricultural Research Service, 2010. USDA Nutrient Database for Standard Reference, Release 23. Nutrient Data Laboratory home page. Available at: http://www.ars.usda.gov/Services/docs.htm?docid=8964. Accessed January 21, 2011.

Do athletes need vitamin C supplements?

Some research supports the notion that athletes need higher levels of vitamin C than the RDA because of the oxidative stress of training and competition. Other articles show little or no benefit of vitamin C supplementation on athletic performance. It appears that in athletes with adequate vitamin C status, supplementation with vitamin C does not enhance exercise performance.[29] The U.S. Olympic Committee has approved vitamin C supplements at levels of 250–1000 milligrams per day. Athletes can easily obtain 200–500 milligrams of vitamin C per day through a well-balanced diet including plenty of fruits and vegetables. Supplements used to achieve higher doses of vitamin C should be consumed with caution. As mentioned previously, vitamin C aids in iron absorption. For athletes who are low in iron, this action can be beneficial; however, for those who are more susceptible to hemochromatosis, which is a disorder that results in the excessive absorption of iron, vitamin C supplementation is not recommended and may exacerbate symptoms.

What are the fat-soluble vitamins?

Vitamins A, D, E, and K make up the fat-soluble vitamins. These vitamins require small amounts of dietary fat to help the body absorb, transport, and utilize them. Unlike water-soluble vitamins, these vitamins can be stored in the body, primarily in fat tissues and the liver, but also in other organ tissues in smaller amounts. As a result, the levels of fat-soluble vitamins in the body can build over time, potentially causing toxicity. Dietary intake from food rarely causes toxic buildup of the fat-soluble vitamins, but the risk for accumulating toxic levels in the body increases with the use of supplements containing high levels of these vitamins.

Why is vitamin A important for athletes?

Vitamin A has numerous functions in the body and is found in three different forms—retinol, retinal, and retinoic acid. These three forms are collectively called retinoids. One of the crucial functions of vitamin A in the body is its role in vision (see Figure 6.10). Retinol is transported in the blood to the retina in the eye, where it is converted to retinal. Retinal combines with the protein opsin to form the pigment rhodopsin, which allows humans to see black-and-white images. Iodopsin, another pigment that involves retinal, allows humans to see color images. Light entering the eye stimulates a process of separating retinal from the opsin and iodopsin, causing the proteins to change shape. The change in protein shape stimulates optical receptors in the retina that send electrical impulses to the brain, which in turn enables sight. When vitamin A is deficient, blindness can occur.

Vitamin A also functions in cell differentiation, the process by which stem cells (i.e., cells that possess the capability of dividing and forming any body tissue) develop into specialized cells with specific functions within the body. For example, vitamin A is very important in the differentiation of epithelial cells, which are found throughout the body and form tissues such as the skin and mucous membranes. Epithelial cells also form the linings of internal organs and passageways of the digestive, respiratory, and circulatory systems. Vitamin A actually activates specific genes within the stem cell nuclei that initiate the differentiation of the appropriate tissue type. Adequate vitamin A is essential for athletes to help repair those tissues that may be injured during sporting events. Vitamin A also appears to have a role in immune function by helping to maintain the skin and mucous membranes (i.e., the epithelial tissues), which act as barriers to infection by bacteria and other pathogens. In fact, the maintenance of epithelial tissues in preventing infection is so important that vitamin A has been labeled as the "anti-infection" vitamin. Vitamin A also appears to play a role in bone formation and the maintenance of reproductive health. Finally, vitamin A has shown some promise as an antioxidant that may help prevent cancer and certain chronic diseases. For more information regarding the antioxidant role of vitamin A, see the section "Which vitamins or compounds have antioxidant properties?" later in this chapter.

What is the RDA/AI for vitamin A?

Vitamin A can be consumed in the diet from animal sources as retinoids or from plant sources as

> **retinoids** A class of compounds that have chemical structures similar to vitamin A. Retinol, retinal, and retinoic acid are three active forms of vitamin A that belong to the retinoid family of compounds.

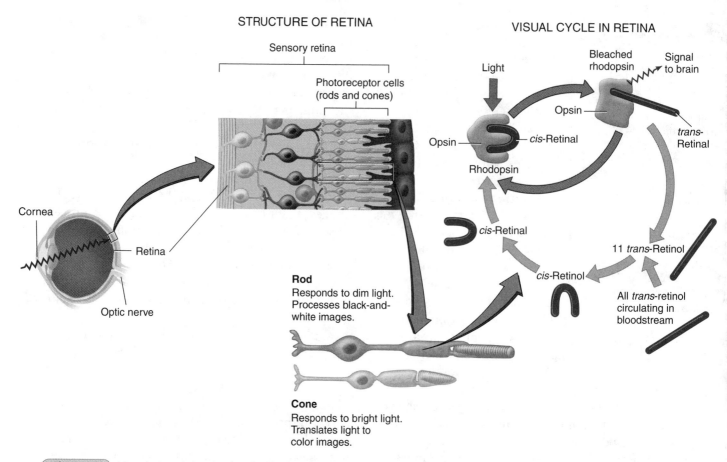

STRUCTURE OF RETINA

Sensory retina

Photoreceptor cells
(rods and cones)

Cornea

Retina

Optic nerve

Rod
Responds to dim light.
Processes black-and-
white images.

Cone
Responds to bright light.
Translates light to
color images.

VISUAL CYCLE IN RETINA

Light

Bleached
rhodopsin

Signal
to brain

Opsin

Opsin — *cis*-Retinal

trans-
Retinal

Rhodopsin

cis-Retinal

11 *trans*-Retinol

cis-Retinol

All *trans*-retinol
circulating in
bloodstream

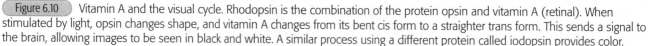

Figure 6.10 Vitamin A and the visual cycle. Rhodopsin is the combination of the protein opsin and vitamin A (retinal). When stimulated by light, opsin changes shape, and vitamin A changes from its bent cis form to a straighter trans form. This sends a signal to the brain, allowing images to be seen in black and white. A similar process using a different protein called iodopsin provides color.

carotenoids. The RDA for vitamin A reflects recommendations based on typical consumption of both plant (carotenoid) and animal (retinoid) sources. However, similar amounts of dietary retinoids and dietary carotenoids do not provide similar amounts of vitamin A. Carotenoids are less biologically active than are retinoids, and therefore greater amounts need to be consumed to meet daily requirements. Because of this difference, the scientific community developed a standardized measurement that can be used for both carotenoid and retinoid consumption in the diet. This standard is the **retinol activity equivalent (RAE).** One RAE is the amount of a given form of vitamin A equal to the activity of 1 microgram of retinol (see Figure 6.11). The RDA for vitamin A for adult males is 900 micrograms RAE and for adult females is 700 micrograms RAE.[30] Although carotenoids may be slightly lacking in their ability to convert to vitamin A, their overall contribution to physical health is expansive. Carotenoids are discussed in more detail in the next section.

Vitamin A content is often expressed in another measurement called **International Units (IU).** This measure is outdated and does not accurately take into consideration bioavailability or absorptive efficiency of the carotenoids. Nonetheless, IU is often the way vitamin A is expressed on the labels of vitamin supplements. When using IU, the recommended intake is 5000 IU daily.

What are the complications of vitamin A deficiency?

Deficiency of vitamin A is rare in the United States, but it does exist in many countries where general

carotenoids A class of colorful phytochemicals that give plants and their fruit the deep colors of orange, red, and yellow. There are hundreds of different carotenoids; however, the ones most identified as vital to health include alpha- and beta-carotene, lycopene, lutein, zeaxanthin, and cryptoxanthin.

retinol activity equivalent (RAE) A unit of measure of the vitamin A content in foods. One RAE equals 1 microgram of retinol.

international units (IU) An outdated system used to measure vitamin activity.

1 retinol activity equivalent (RAE) = 1 μg retinol

= 2 μg supplemental beta-carotene

= 12 μg dietary beta-carotene

= 24 μg dietary carotenoids

Figure 6.11 Retinol equivalents conversion. Retinol activity equivalent (RAE) is a unit of measurement for the vitamin A content of a food. One RAE equals 1 microgram of retinol.

hyperkeratosis A clinical condition resulting from the overproduction of the skin protein known as keratin. Overproduction of keratin plugs skin follicles, thickens the skin surface, and causes skin to become bumpy and scaly. Vitamin A deficiency is related to hyperkeratosis.

malnutrition is found. Blindness is the most common and devastating result of deficiency. Night blindness is often an early symptom of vitamin A deficiency. Early treatment with supplemental vitamin A can reverse these symptoms and prevent further damage to the retina. The skin can develop **hyperkeratosis** from lack of vitamin A. Hyperkeratosis is caused by the overproduction of the protein keratin, which plugs skin follicles, thickens the skin surface, and causes it to become bumpy and scaly. Other epithelial cells are also affected. The mucous-producing cells may not secrete mucus, thus causing dryness in the mucous membranes of the mouth, intestinal tract, female genital tract, male seminal vesicles, and linings of the eyes. This increases the risk of infections and can cause infertility in women and sterility in men.

What are the symptoms of vitamin A toxicity?

Toxicity of vitamin A is rare except in cases of megadoses of vitamin A supplements. Children may be at greater risk of toxicity. Vitamin A toxicity produces a wide range of symptoms including skin conditions, vomiting, fatigue, blurred vision, and liver damage. Vitamin A toxicity can be fatal. The tolerable UL for vitamin A is 3000 micrograms per day of retinol.

Which foods are rich in vitamin A?

Good food sources of the retinoids are liver, fish liver oils (e.g., cod liver oil), and egg yolks (see Figure 6.12). Fruits and vegetables

that contain high amounts of the carotenoids provide substantial vitamin A in the diet when converted to retinol equivalents. Vitamin A–fortified dairy products provide additional sources of vitamin A in the United States.

What is a suggestion for a vitamin A–rich meal or snack?

Lunch: Mix ½ can of salmon (oil-packed), 1 tsp light salad dressing, and chopped onion, celery, and tomato; serve on 2 slices of whole grain bread with ½ cup fresh fruit and 1 cup milk
Vitamin A content: 365 micrograms (RAE)

Do athletes need vitamin A supplements?

Helping athletes meet the RDA for vitamin A from food sources appears to be the most prudent current recommendation. Research on supplementing vitamin A in amounts greater than the RDA to improve sport performance has not shown any ergogenic value. Therefore, encouraging athletes to obtain vi-

VITAMIN A

Daily Value = 5000 IU
RDA = 900 μg (males), 700 μg (females)

Exceptionally good sources

Beef liver, cooked	85 g (3 oz)	22,175 IU
Sweet potato	110 g (1 small)	21,140 IU
Carrots, cooked	85 g (~½ cup)	19,152 IU
Chicken liver, cooked	85 g (3 oz)	12,221 IU

High: 20% DV or more

Spinach, cooked	85 g (~½ cup)	8,909 IU
Spinach, raw	85 g (~3 cups)	7,970 IU
Collards, cooked	85 g (~½ cup)	6,897 IU
Romaine lettuce, raw	85 g (~1½ cups)	4,936 IU
Cantaloupe, fresh	140 g (¼ med. melon)	4,735 IU
Peppers, red, cooked	85 g (~½ cup)	4,265 IU
Broccoli, cooked	85 g (~½ cup)	1,716 IU
Watermelon, fresh	280 g (1/16 melon)	1,593 IU
Oatmeal, instant, fortified, cooked	1 cup	1,252 IU
Tomato juice, canned	240 ml (1 cup)	1,094 IU
Mango, fresh	140 g (~1 cup)	1,071 IU

Good: 10–19% DV

Apricot, dried	40 g (~3 Tbsp)	856 IU
Wheat bran flakes cereal	30 g (¾ cup)	788 IU
Prunes, dried	40 g (~5 prunes)	705 IU
Black-eyed peas, cooked	90 g (~½ cup)	712 IU
Green beans, cooked	85 g (~¾ cup)	595 IU
Corn flakes cereal	30 g (1 cup)	537 IU
All-bran cereal	30 g (½ cup)	524 IU
Milk, 1%, 2%, nonfat	240 ml (1 cup)	500 IU

Figure 6.12 Food sources of vitamin A. Vitamin A is found as retinol in animal foods and as beta-carotene and other carotenoids in plant foods. Units are IU to be consistent with Daily Value definitions.
Source: U.S. Department of Agriculture, Agricultural Research Service, 2010. USDA Nutrient Database for Standard Reference, Release 23. Nutrient Data Laboratory home page. Available at: http://www.ars.usda.gov/Services/docs.htm?docid=8964. Accessed January 21, 2011.

tamin A from food sources rather than supplements to avoid toxicity is recommended.

Why are the carotenoids important for athletes?

The carotenoids are a group of naturally occurring compounds found in plants. They are colorful compounds that give plants and their fruit the deep colors of orange, red, and yellow. Dark green vegetables also contain carotenoids, but the chlorophyll in these plants gives them their green color and masks the carotenoid colors. Carotenoids are not vitamins; however, because some of them can be converted to vitamin A, discussion of these compounds has been included in this chapter. There are approximately 600 different carotenoids identified in plants. The major carotenoids include alpha- and beta-carotene, lycopene, lutein, zeaxanthin, and cryptoxanthin. As discussed previously, some carotenoids are precursors to vitamin A. These provitamin A carotenoids are beta-carotene, alpha-carotene, and beta-cryptoxanthin. Because they have no vitamin A activity in the body, lycopene, lutein, and zeaxanthin are called non-provitamin A carotenoids.

Carotenoids as precursors to vitamin A play a role in vitamin A functions. However, they also have additional functions in the body that are exclusive to carotenoids. They have roles as antioxidants, bolster immune function, aid in cancer prevention, and enhance vision. Beta-carotene and other carotenoids are powerful antioxidants that interfere with **free radical** activity (refer to the "What are free radicals?" section later in this chapter). The carotenoids work primarily to keep free radical production from becoming uncontainable and thus prevent any negative health effects. As an example, two carotenoids, lutein and zeaxanthin, are found in the macula of the eye. The function of the macula is to provide detailed and sharp vision. It is theorized that lutein and zeaxanthin help filter the harmful light entering the macula and scavenge free radicals in the retinal tissues. This theory is reinforced by recent epidemiological studies that have suggested that increased intake of lutein lowers the risk for age-related macular degeneration.

free radicals Highly reactive molecules, usually containing oxygen, that have unpaired electrons in their outer shell. Because of their highly reactive nature, free radicals have been implicated as culprits in diseases ranging from cancer to cardiovascular disease.

What is the RDA/AI for carotenoids?

There are no established RDA/AIs for the carotenoids. However, carotenoid consumption was taken

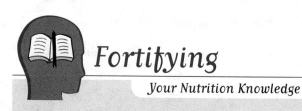

Fortifying
Your Nutrition Knowledge

Tips for Increasing Carotenoid Intake

Athletes can increase their carotenoid intake by:

- Eating 5–9 servings per day of fruits and vegetables.
- Choosing more colorful vegetables and fruits, including reds, yellows, blues, and purples.
- Including at least one vegetable or fruit in each meal and a serving of fruit or vegetables as a snack.
- Drinking 6–8 oz of 100% fruit juice, such as grape, orange, grapefruit, or cranberry, with breakfast.

into consideration when developing the RAE used to establish the RDA and UL for vitamin A. A large body of observational epidemiological evidence suggests that higher blood concentrations of beta-carotene and other carotenoids obtained from foods are associated with lower risk of several chronic diseases.[28] The evidence appears to be consistent in the studies but cannot be used to establish specific RDAs for carotenoids because it is unclear whether the carotenoids alone or other substances in the foods consumed produced the desired effects. Although no DRIs are established for carotenoids, the Food and Nutrition Board recommends eating foods rich in carotenoids and avoiding supplementation.[28]

Which foods are rich in carotenoids?

Most colorful fruits and vegetables contain carotenoids. The best sources include deep red, yellow, and orange fruits and vegetables. Tomatoes and tomato products, red peppers, leafy greens, apricots, watermelon, cantaloupe, pumpkin, squash, sweet potatoes, carrots, and oranges are all excellent sources of carotenoids.

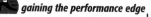
gaining the performance edge

Carotenoids are a unique category of plant-based substances that can positively affect overall health. Some functions, including improved immune function and antioxidant activity, may also be beneficial to athletic performance. Although no DRI has been set for these compounds, a diet rich in dark, colorful fruits and vegetables has been found to be advantageous to health and well-being.

Why is vitamin D important for athletes?

Vitamin D is a unique fat-soluble vitamin because, in general, all of the body's needs for it can be met by synthesis within the body. It is sometimes called the "sunshine vitamin" because the ultraviolet rays of the sun hitting the skin initiate vitamin D synthesis in the body. However, vitamin D may not be produced in high enough quantities in the following instances: in geographic locations where sunlight is marginal; during seasons when sunshine is insufficient; in instances when people are told to stay out of the sun; or in instances when individuals are physically unable or infirm and cannot go outside. It is in these cases that vitamin D, from food or supplemental sources, is essential and, as a result, is considered a vitamin.

The primary role of vitamin D in the body is to control calcium levels in the blood, which in turn affects bone growth and development. However, vitamin D itself is not the active compound that affects the body's calcium levels. It first must be converted through a series of reactions in the liver and then the kidneys to **calcitriol** (see Figure 6.13). Cholecalciferol (from animal foods and sunlight conversion) and ergocalciferol (from plant foods) can both be converted to calcitriol. Sunlight exposure initiates the process by converting 7-dehydrocholesterol in the skin to cholecalciferol. This converted cholecalciferol is carried to the liver, where it and dietary cholecalciferol and ergocalciferol are converted to calcidiol. Calcidiol is then transported to the kidneys, where calcitriol is formed. Calcitriol is the active form of vitamin D in the body. Because calcitriol is produced in one area of the body (the kidneys), carried in the blood, and then exerts effects on tissues in other areas of the body (e.g., bone), it can also be considered a hormone.

calcitriol The active form of vitamin D in the body. It plays a vital role in calcium regulation and bone growth.

The total extent to which vitamin D acts as a hormone is not understood; however, several other tissues have been shown to have receptors that bind calcitriol. The theory is that the calcitriol may regulate cell differentiation and inhibit cell proliferation in the blood, lungs, colon, and elsewhere, thus playing a role in cancer prevention. However, further research is needed to elucidate the extent of its role as an anti-cancer agent.

What is the RDA/AI for vitamin D?

The RDA for vitamin D assumes that no vitamin D is available from synthesis from exposure to sunlight. For men and women aged 19–70 years, the RDA is 600 IU per day.[31] For men and women older than 70, the RDA is 800 IU per day. As they age, individuals have less ability to synthesize vitamin D from sun exposure; therefore, as age increases, the RDA also increases. Similar to vitamin A, international units (IU) are used to express vitamin D recommendations. The IU is presented on food labels and is used as the unit level for % Daily Values.

What are the complications of vitamin D deficiency?

Because of the profound effect vitamin D has on absorption of dietary calcium, vitamin D deficiency can have devastating effects on bone growth and development in children. In children, vitamin D deficiency leads to rickets, which results in poorly formed, weak, and soft bones. In adults, deficiency of vitamin D increases the risk for osteoporosis. Fortunately, the fortification of milk with vitamin D has virtually wiped out deficiency problems in children in the United States. Osteoporosis, on the other hand, is an increasing concern for older adults. Adequate vitamin D intake in food or supplement form is an essential part of prevention and treatment of osteoporosis in the aging population. In elderly individuals who are house-bound and do not receive regular exposure to sunlight, adequate dietary vitamin D intake must be ensured.

What are the symptoms of vitamin D toxicity?

Because it is stored in the body, toxicity of vitamin D can occur. Overexposure to the sun or dietary intake of vitamin D from food sources is unlikely to cause toxicity, but supplementation in high doses can cause problems. The UL for vitamin D for adults over age 19 is 4000 IU. Overdosing with vitamin D causes **hypercalcemia**, or high blood calcium. Hypercalcemia causes a depressed function of the nervous system, muscular weakness, heart arrhythmias, and calcium deposits in the kidneys (i.e., kidney stones), blood vessels, and other soft tissues.

hypercalcemia A clinical condition in which blood calcium levels are above normal.

Which foods are rich in vitamin D?

Food sources of vitamin D come in natural and fortified forms (see Figure 6.14). Fortified forms are included in milk, cereals, and some margarines. Natural sources include fish oils, salmon, sardines, herring, egg yolks, and liver. Plants are poor sources of vitamin D; therefore, strict vegetarians need to rely on the endogenous production of vitamin D from

VITAMIN D: FROM SOURCE TO DESTINATION

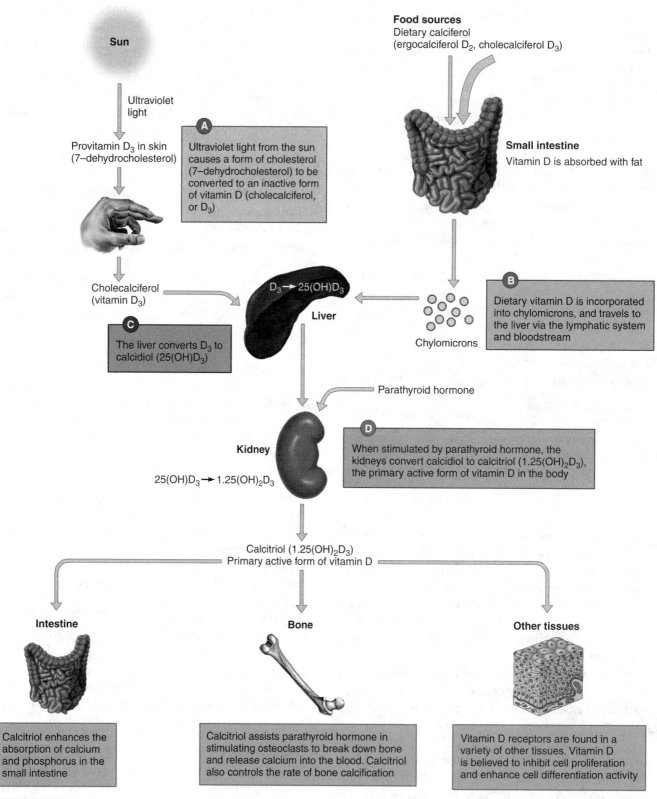

Sun

Ultraviolet
light

Provitamin D₃ in skin
(7–dehydrocholesterol)

A Ultraviolet light from the sun causes a form of cholesterol (7–dehydrocholesterol) to be converted to an inactive form of vitamin D (cholecalciferol, or D₃)

Cholecalciferol
(vitamin D₃)

C The liver converts D₃ to calcidiol (25(OH)D₃)

$D_3 \rightarrow 25(OH)D_3$

Liver

Food sources
Dietary calciferol
(ergocalciferol D₂, cholecalciferol D₃)

Small intestine
Vitamin D is absorbed with fat

B Dietary vitamin D is incorporated into chylomicrons, and travels to the liver via the lymphatic system and bloodstream

Chylomicrons

Parathyroid hormone

Kidney

$25(OH)D_3 \rightarrow 1.25(OH)_2D_3$

D When stimulated by parathyroid hormone, the kidneys convert calcidiol to calcitriol (1.25(OH)₂D₃), the primary active form of vitamin D in the body

Calcitriol (1.25(OH)₂D₃)
Primary active form of vitamin D

Intestine

Calcitriol enhances the absorption of calcium and phosphorus in the small intestine

Bone

Calcitriol assists parathyroid hormone in stimulating osteoclasts to break down bone and release calcium into the blood. Calcitriol also controls the rate of bone calcification

Other tissues

Vitamin D receptors are found in a variety of other tissues. Vitamin D is believed to inhibit cell proliferation and enhance cell differentiation activity

Figure 6.13 Vitamin D: from source to destination. Vitamin D is unique because, given sufficient sunlight, the body can synthesize all it needs. Both dietary and endogenous vitamin D must be activated by reactions in the kidneys and liver. Active vitamin D (calcitriol) is important for calcium balance and bone health, and may have a role in cell differentiation.

VITAMIN D

Daily Value = 400 IU
RDA = 600 IU age 19–70 (males/females)
800 IU age 70+ (males/females)

Exceptionally good source		
Cod liver oil	1 Tbsp	1360 IU
Salmon, canned, solids + bones	55 g (2 oz)	343 IU
Sardines, canned, solids + bones	55 g (2 oz)	150 IU
Milk, nonfat	240 ml (1 cup)	105 IU
Milk, 1%, 2% milkfat	240 ml (1 cup)	102 IU
Milk, whole, 3.25% milkfat	240 ml (1 cup)	98 IU
Fortified, ready-to-eat cereals	30 g	40–50 IU

High: 20% DV or more

Figure 6.14 Food sources of vitamin D. Only a few foods are naturally good sources of vitamin D. Therefore, fortified foods such as milk and some cereals are important, especially for people with limited exposure to the sun. Units are IU to be consistent with Daily Value definitions.
Source: U.S. Department of Agriculture, Agricultural Research Service, 2010. USDA Nutrient Database for Standard Reference, Release 23. Nutrient Data Laboratory home page. Available at: http://www.ars.usda.gov/Services/docs.htm?docid=8964. Accessed January 21, 2011.

sun exposure or the consumption of fortified foods and the use of supplements.

What is a suggestion for a vitamin D–rich meal or snack?

Bedtime snack: 12 oz skim milk and 2 oatmeal raisin cookies
Vitamin D content: 158 IU

Do athletes need vitamin D supplements?

Vitamin D fortification in milk and other foods and the fact that it is manufactured in the body suggest that most individuals maintain adequate amounts of vitamin D. In places where milk is not fortified or where malnutrition, especially in children, is common, vitamin D supplementation is recommended and needed to prevent bone formation abnormalities. Vitamin D in combination with calcium and magnesium can help prevent osteoporosis. Perimenopausal and postmenopausal women may benefit from vitamin D and calcium supplementation to avoid extensive bone loss during menopause. Supplementation and use in athletes are not well studied. Athletes who consume lower or inadequate amounts of calories, or those whose food choices do not include vitamin D–rich sources daily, may need supplementation. Athletes who practice and compete mainly indoors may not get adequate sun exposure to produce the required amounts of vitamin D. In these cases, the following strategies will help ensure adequate vitamin D levels:

- Obtain exposure to the sun for 15 minutes every day. Even exposure on the face and hands is enough to synthesize adequate vitamin D. However, athletes should protect their skin from too much sun exposure and sunburn.
- Drink milk with meals or as a snack.
- Consume fortified cereals with milk for breakfast.
- Try canned or fresh salmon as an alternative to tuna.

Why is vitamin E important for athletes?

Vitamin E is actually a group of compounds that include the tocopherols and the tocotrienols. Both tocopherols and tocotrienols contain four compounds each: the alpha, beta, gamma, and delta configurations. The tocopherols are more widely distributed in nature than tocotrienols and contribute most of the dietary sources of vitamin E. Although all of these compounds can be absorbed in the body, only alpha-tocopherol is considered to have vitamin E activity in the body.[28] It is the alpha-tocopherol configuration of vitamin E that is used to determine the RDA values.

The primary role of vitamin E in the body is as an antioxidant. Antioxidants protect the body from highly reactive molecules known as free radicals (refer to the "What are free radicals?" section later in this chapter). Free radicals are molecules that have unpaired electrons, which give the molecules an electrical charge, thus making them unstable and highly reactive. If not neutralized, free radicals will react with molecules in the body, potentially changing these molecules' structure and/or function. The end result can be an increased risk for damage to tissues such as the skin and other connective tissues. The role vitamin E plays in protecting the skin and its underlying connective tissues is one reason why vitamin E has been advertised as the "anti-aging" vitamin.

Vitamin E not only protects the skin and connective tissues, but also helps to protect the cell membranes and genetic material of virtually all tissues of the body. Free radicals are highly reactive with fatty acids. Because cell membranes are made up of phospholipids (i.e., they contain fats), cell membranes can be attacked by free radicals. Vitamin E protects cell membranes by directly reacting with free radicals, thus preventing them from reacting with the fatty acids in the cell membranes. Free radicals can also react with the genes inside the nuclei of cells, resulting in genetic mutations that could cause aberrant cell growth and/or cancer; vitamin E can help prevent these genetic alterations. Dietary intake of appropriate amounts of vitamin E helps to provide adequate levels of this very important antioxidant vitamin.

What is the RDA/AI for vitamin E?

The RDA for vitamin E is 15 milligrams of alpha-tocopherol for men and women.[28] As with vitamin A, the discontinued International Units (IU) are still found on supplement labels. To convert IU to milligrams of vitamin E, use the following equations:

> 1 IU = 0.67 mg of the natural form of alpha-tocopherol
> 1 IU = 0.45 mg of the synthetic form of alpha-tocopherol

To meet the RDA recommendations of 15 milligrams, the IU equivalent is 23 IU for the natural form and 34 IU for the synthetic form.

What are the complications of vitamin E deficiency?

Overt deficiency of vitamin E is rare because it appears dietary intake is adequate in the general population. Individuals who choose extremely low-fat or fat-free diets could develop vitamin E deficiency over time. Conditions resulting in malabsorption or maldigestion of lipids, such as cystic fibrosis, celiac disease, or hepatic or biliary diseases, may result in poor absorption of vitamin E and thus compromise vitamin E status. Common signs of vitamin E deficiency take time to develop and are related to the breakdown of cell membranes. Muscle weakness and loss of motor coordination can result because of cell membrane damage to muscle and nerve tissue, respectively. In addition, the breakdown of cell membranes of red blood cells results in hemolytic anemia causing lack of energy and decreased physical functioning.

What are the symptoms of vitamin E toxicity?

Vitamin E is less likely than other fat-soluble vitamins such as A and D to become toxic to the body. However, high doses of vitamin E resulting from supplementation can affect vitamin K's blood-clotting functions, leading to excessive bleeding and easy bruising. The UL for adults is 1000 mg of alpha-tocopherol.

Which foods are rich in vitamin E?

Common food sources of vitamin E include both plant and animal products (see Figure 6.15). Plant oils such as corn, safflower, cottonseed, sunflower, soy, and palm oils are good sources of vitamin E. Products made from these oils, such as margarine, shortening, mayonnaise, and salad dressings, also contain vitamin E. Fortified cereals can be a good source of this vitamin; however, not all cereals are fortified with vitamin E. Animal sources such as meat, poultry, and fish are at best moderate contributors to dietary vitamin E.

What is a suggestion for a vitamin E–rich meal or snack?

Nutty black bean salad: Mix together 1 cup black beans; 1 tbsp sunflower seeds; ¼ cup each chopped tomato, corn, and green pepper; 1 tbsp corn oil; and 1 tbsp balsamic vinegar. Serve with whole grain bread and fruit juice.

Total vitamin E content = 27 IU or 18 mg alpha-tocopherol

VITAMIN E

Daily Value = 30 IU
RDA = 15 mg (males/females)

Exceptionally good sources

Wheat bran flakes cereal	30 g (~¾ cup)	41.7 IU
Wheat germ oil	1 Tbsp	30.5 IU
Total cereal	30 g (~¾ cup)	30.2 IU
Product 19 cereal	30 g (~1 cup)	30.2 IU
Sunflower seeds	30 g (~1 oz)	15.5 IU
Almonds	30 g (~1 oz)	11.6 IU
Cottonseed oil	1 Tbsp	7.2 IU
Safflower oil	1 Tbsp	7.0 IU
Special K cereal	30 g (~1 cup)	7.0 IU
Hazelnuts	30 g (~1 oz)	6.8 IU
Tomato paste, canned	130 g (~½ cup)	6.0 IU
Corn oil	1 Tbsp	4.2 IU
Peanuts	30 g (~1 oz)	3.8 IU
Spinach, frozen, cooked	85 g (~½ cup)	3.0 IU

High: 20% DV or more
Good: 10-19% DV

Figure 6.15 Food sources of vitamin E. Nuts and seeds, vegetable oil, and products made from vegetable oil, such as margarine, are among the best sources of vitamin E. Units are IU to be consistent with Daily Value definitions. The DV for vitamin E is higher than the current RDA of 15 milligrams (23 IU) for males and females age 19 and older. Note: USDA tables list vitamin E in mg alpha-tocopherol equivalents. Conversion to IU was done using 1 mg ATE = 1.5 IU.
Source: U.S. Department of Agriculture, Agricultural Research Service, 2010. USDA Nutrient Database for Standard Reference, Release 23. Nutrient Data Laboratory home page. Available at: http://www.ars.usda.gov/Services/docs.htm?docid=8964. Accessed January 21, 2011.

Do athletes need vitamin E supplements?

Much research has been conducted on vitamin E supplementation in hopes of finding an ergogenic effect in athletes. This research has focused on vitamin E's antioxidant effects during exercise. The impact of antioxidants is discussed later in the chapter.

Why is vitamin K important for athletes?

Vitamin K belongs to the quinone family of compounds and is probably the least known of the fat-soluble vitamins. The primary role of vitamin K in the body is in blood clotting. When a laceration or an abrasion occurs, a series of activation reactions involving clotting factors is required to stop the bleeding. Vitamin K is essential in many of the steps of the clotting process. Without vitamin K, even a single cut could be life-threatening from the potential blood loss. Vitamin K is also important to bone health. It assists in the mineralization of bone with calcium, thus keeping bones dense and strong.

What is the RDA/AI for vitamin K?

Because of the lack of data regarding average requirements, no RDA has been established for vitamin K. As a result, AI is used to represent intake levels. The AI for vitamin K for men older than 19 years of age is 120 micrograms; for women older than 19 years of age, the AI is 90 micrograms daily.[30]

What are the complications of vitamin K deficiency?

A deficiency of vitamin K impairs blood clotting and can lead to substantial hemorrhaging. Thus, vitamin K is important to athletes, who are much more likely than the general population to receive cuts, tears, and abrasions as a result of their sport participation. The body needs only small amounts of vitamin K, and it can produce some of the daily requirement through the action of intestinal bacteria. The intestinal bacteria can produce approximately 10–15% of the vitamin K in the body.[32] The vitamin K produced by the body along with dietary vitamin K is absorbed with fat in the intestines, packaged into chylomicrons, and transported via the lymphatic system to the liver. Individuals more prone to vitamin K deficiency include those with fat malabsorptive conditions such as celiac disease, Crohn's disease, and cystic fibrosis and those taking long-term antibiotics that may reduce the intestinal bacteria.

Newborn babies may be at risk for vitamin K deficiency because they lack the intestinal bacteria at birth that produce vitamin K. Breast milk also contains very little vitamin K. Most newborn babies are given a vitamin K injection at birth, and within several weeks the intestinal bacteria will provide adequate vitamin K for the newborn's needs. Individuals using antibiotics for a prolonged period may be at higher risk of deficiency because antibiotics may kill the naturally occurring bacteria in the gut that produce vitamin K.

What are the symptoms of vitamin K toxicity?

Vitamin K is excreted from the body much more readily than the other fat-soluble vitamins, making vitamin K toxicity rare. A UL has not been established because few adverse effects have been reported for individuals consuming high amounts of vitamin K.

Which foods are rich in vitamin K?

Like vitamin D, vitamin K can be made endogenously. However, the body cannot make enough vitamin K to meet all of its needs. The best dietary sources of vitamin K are green leafy vegetables such as spinach and broccoli. Other foods such as milk, eggs, wheat cereals, and some fruits and vegetables contain small amounts of vitamin K (see Figure 6.16).

VITAMIN K

Daily Value = 80 µg
AI = 120 µg (males) 90 µg (females)

	Exceptionally good sources		
	Spinach, raw	85 g (~3 cups)	410 µg
	Turnip greens, raw	85 g (~3 cups)	213 µg
	Cauliflower, raw	85 g (~3/4 cup)	136 µg
	Broccoli, cooked	85 g (~1/2 cup)	120 µg
	Romaine lettuce, raw	85 g (~1 1/2 cups)	87 µg
	Chicken liver, cooked	85 g (3 oz)	68 µg
	Cabbage, raw	85 g (~1 1/4 cups)	51 µg
	Asparagus, cooked	85 g (~1/2 cup)	43 µg
High:	Okra, cooked	85 g (~1/2 cup)	32 µg
20% DV	Prunes, dried	120 g (~1/2 cup)	31 µg
or more	Soybean oil	1 Tbsp.	27 µg
	Blackberries, raw	140 g (~1 cup)	27 µg
	Blueberries, raw	140 g (~3/4 cup)	27 µg
Good:	Green beans, cooked	85 g (~2/3 cup)	14 µg
10-19%	Artichokes, cooked	85 g (~1/2 cup)	13 µg
DV	Tomato, green, raw	85 g (1 small)	8.6 µg

Figure 6.16 Food sources of vitamin K. The best sources of vitamin K are vegetables, especially those in the cabbage family. Liver, eggs, and milk are good sources as well. Note: The DV for vitamin K is lower than the current AI of 120 micrograms and 90 micrograms for males and females, respectively, age 19 and older.
Source: U.S. Department of Agriculture, Agricultural Research Service, 2010. USDA Nutrient Database for Standard Reference, Release 23. Nutrient Data Laboratory home page. Available at: http://www.ars.usda.gov/Services/docs .htm?docid=8964. Accessed January 21, 2011.

What is a suggestion for a vitamin K–rich meal or snack?

Green vegetable salad: 1 cup spinach, ½ cup chopped broccoli, 1 chopped hard-boiled egg, 4 diced scallions, and ¼ cup carrot shreds served with 1 tbsp light ranch dressing
Total vitamin K content = 170 micrograms

Do athletes need vitamin K supplements?

There are no known studies that support an increased need for vitamin K in athletes. Supplementation may be indicated for individuals with risks for deficiency or who present with deficiency symptoms. Supplementation should be provided with physician guidance and supervision, and often requires a prescription. Athletes who are injured and require surgery should inform their physician prior to surgery about any vitamin supplements they use regularly. Most surgeons require their patients to stop taking multivitamins prior to surgery because some vitamins can increase clotting times, increasing the risk of bleeding during surgery.

> **gaining the performance edge**
>
> Fat-soluble vitamins include vitamins A, D, E, and K. Each vitamin has its own function in the body, DRI, complications of deficiency, symptoms of toxicity, unique food sources, and requirements for supplementation. All fat-soluble vitamins are critical to health, and therefore a variety of food sources should be consumed daily to meet the needs of each nutrient.

Which vitamins or compounds have antioxidant properties?

Two of the fat-soluble vitamins, A (including the carotenoids) and E, and the water-soluble vitamin C all have powerful antioxidant properties in the body. As mentioned earlier, antioxidants protect tissues of the body from highly reactive molecules known as free radicals. The following sections discuss free radicals, their association with exercise, and the role that vitamins A, E, and C play in combating them.

What are free radicals?

To understand the antioxidant functions of vitamins and other compounds in the body, it is important to first have a basic knowledge of free radicals, where they come from, and how they are eliminated. Free radicals are highly reactive molecules, usually containing oxygen, that possess unpaired electrons in their structure (see Figure 6.17). The unpaired electrons give free radicals an ionic charge, which makes them reactive with other charged molecules in the body. Free radicals basically cause molecules to give up electrons in a process known as oxidation so that they can match any unpaired electrons and become more stable. Undesirable free radical oxidation may damage DNA, lipids, proteins, and other molecules and thus may be involved in the development of cancer, cardiovascular disease, and possibly nerve degenerative diseases.

Free radicals are produced in the body as by-products of normal cellular metabolism or can be taken into the body from outside sources. Outside sources of free radicals include the breathing of polluted air, such as when runners exercise in congested traffic. Within the body, free radicals produced in the mitochondria of cells as hydrogen ions are transferred to oxygen to form water (H_2O) in the electron transport chain (see Chapter 2). However, occasionally oxygen is not paired with hydrogen ions to form water and instead forms ionically-charged free radical molecules such as superoxide (O_2), hydroxyl (OH), and peroxyl (H_2O_2) radicals. These oxygen-containing molecules are collectively known as **reactive oxidative species (ROS)**. As noted earlier, if these reactive molecules go unchecked in the body, they can be very destructive.

> **reactive oxidative species (ROS)** Free radical molecules that contain oxygen in their molecular formula and that are formed during aerobic metabolism. Commonly occurring reactive oxidative species in the human include superoxidases, hydroxyl radicals, and peroxyl radicals.

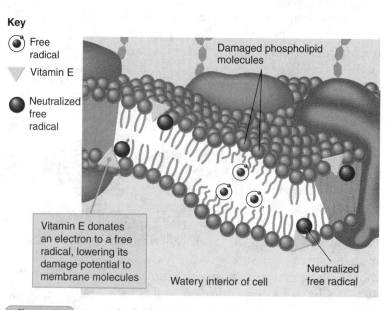

Key
- ◉ Free radical
- ▽ Vitamin E
- ● Neutralized free radical

Damaged phospholipid molecules

Vitamin E donates an electron to a free radical, lowering its damage potential to membrane molecules

Watery interior of cell

Neutralized free radical

Figure 6.17 Free radical damage. Vitamin E helps prevent free radical damage to polyunsaturated fatty acids in cell membranes.

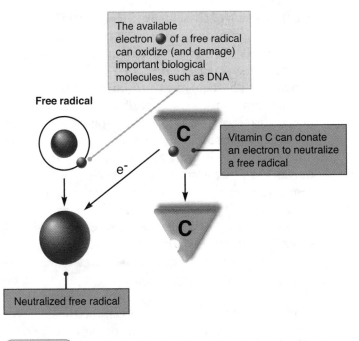

The available electron ● of a free radical can oxidize (and damage) important biological molecules, such as DNA

Free radical

e⁻

Vitamin C can donate an electron to neutralize a free radical

Neutralized free radical

Figure 6.18 Vitamin C minimizes free radical damage by donating an electron to the free radical.

Fortunately, the body has access to compounds that help neutralize the oxidative stresses imposed by free radicals, thereby protecting the body from damage. These protective compounds are collectively known as antioxidants. The body produces a variety of antioxidant enzymes capable of catalyzing reactions that neutralize free radicals. In addition, healthy dietary practices supply the body with antioxidant vitamins such as vitamins A (including the carotenoids), E, and C. These nonenzymatic antioxidants either directly interact with free radicals (see **Figure 6.18**) or work as coenzymes. In summary, the body's antioxidants, whether enzymatic or nonenzymatic, are crucial to helping the body protect itself from free radicals.

lipid peroxidation A chemical reaction in which unstable, highly reactive lipid molecules containing excess oxygen are formed.

An example of the damage that can be caused by free radicals involves a process known as **lipid peroxidation**. During lipid peroxidation the double bond of an unsaturated fatty acid is broken, yielding intermediate compounds that can react with oxygen to form peroxyl free radicals. A peroxyl free radical has one unpaired electron, making it highly reactive with other fatty molecules within the cell membrane. To help decrease the cell membrane damage, vitamin E responds to the free radical by donating an electron, thus preventing it from reacting with other fatty acids in the cell membrane

and causing further damage (see Figure 6.17). At this point, vitamin E needs an electron and is essentially a free radical itself, though not a very reactive one. Vitamin E can get an electron from another antioxidant, such as vitamin C. Vitamin C in turn regains its lost electron from glutathione. To stop this cascading process, the enzyme glutathione reductase restores glutathione to its original form with help from selenium, a mineral. Antioxidant vitamins are commonly referred to independently and do have distinct and independent functions within the body; however, they also work together to keep the body functioning and prevent cellular damage.

What is the relationship between free radicals and exercise?

Free radical production has been shown to increase during exercise, particularly sustained aerobic exercise performed at high intensity.[33–35] The reason for the increase in free radical production with increasing levels of exercise is not well understood but is believed to be related to the increased presence and utilization of oxygen by the mitochondria within the muscle cells to make ATP. As noted earlier, cells continuously produce free radicals as a part of normal metabolism.[36] The free radicals that are produced are usually neutralized by an elaborate antioxidant defense system of enzymatic and nonenzymatic antioxidants. Exercise increases aerobic metabolism and thus may create an imbalance between free radical production and their neutralization by antioxidants.[35,36] Interestingly, it appears that the body's own natural antioxidant defense system is adaptable and up-regulates its response to extended training.[37] This appears to strengthen the body's antioxidant defense mechanism and serves to protect muscle and other tissues from damage during future exercise bouts.

Do athletes need antioxidant supplements?

Antioxidants are beneficial compounds in the human body.[33,38] Without them, oxidation would not be controlled and many processes would suffer. Supplementation with antioxidant vitamins and minerals would appear to make sense for individuals interested in the potential health benefits of antioxidants. Finding ways to prevent the devastation of chronic diseases such as heart disease, cancer, and other illnesses is important for athletes as well as the general population. Although the use of antioxidants is promising, there are still no governing bodies that recommend regular intake of antioxidants at levels higher than the RDA/AIs.

However, there is valid reasoning for the interest in antioxidant supplementation use by athletes.[3,37] If, as noted earlier, exercise training can bolster the body's natural free radical defense mechanism, then why wouldn't nonenzymatic antioxidant supplementation also increase the defense against free radicals? Unfortunately, research into the effects of taking nonenzymatic antioxidant supplements (i.e., vitamins A, C, and E) on free radical levels during exercise is presently unclear. The problem is that free radical levels are difficult to measure directly because they are so highly reactive. Therefore, scientists must rely on markers that might indicate the presence of free radicals, such as cellular damage or other molecules that result because of reactions with free radicals. However, using indirect indicators of free radical activity is prone to error and explains the equivocal research results to date. In addition, some argue that the real issue is the body's 24-hour ability to neutralize free radicals, and that the relatively brief intervals of exercise and their associated increased production of free radicals are just a minor, short-lasting spike in the 24-hour battle against free radicals. The bottom line is that so little is known about the effects of antioxidant supplementation on exercise that making recommendations to well-nourished athletes regarding antioxidant supplementation currently is neither necessary nor advisable.[39] For now, the best nutrition advice is to incorporate more antioxidant-containing foods into the daily diet to ensure adequate intake of a variety of antioxidants and other nutrients.

gaining the performance edge

Antioxidants are beneficial compounds in the human body that are particularly helpful in maintaining overall health and preventing chronic disease. The ergogenic effects of antioxidants have not yet been clearly elucidated but continue to be a focus of exercise science research. Current recommendations call for intakes at the established RDA/AIs, with a strong focus on whole food sources.

What are phytochemicals?

Although phytochemicals are not nutrients, they have important health functions. The term *phytochemicals* comes from the Greek word *phyto*, meaning plant; they are so named because they are chemical substances found in plants. In their 1991 publication, Steinmetz and Potter[40] identified more than a dozen classes of biologically active plant chemicals known as phytochemicals.[40] It is estimated that there are thousands of these plant chemicals that may or may not significantly affect the human body. Approximately 50 phytochemicals are commonly consumed in the American diet. Research on the many benefits of phytochemicals to human health varies for different classes and specific compounds. Evidence clearly supports consumption of a diet rich in fruits, vegetables, and whole grains in helping individuals stay healthy and reduce the risk of cardiovascular disease and cancer.[41,42] However, further research is needed to determine what role specific phytochemicals play in reducing these chronic diseases. The effect of phytochemicals on exercise and sport performance is not well researched.

Dietitians and other health professionals who educate the public about healthful eating must be aware of the different types of phytochemicals in foods.[43–44] Consumers are savvy about the latest research and want more information about how they can benefit by eating more nutrient-dense foods. In a recent study of the effects of one educational session on functional food consumption, 79% of participants expressed intent to eat more tomatoes/tomato products, and 75–77% indicated intent to consume purple grape juice, oats, and broccoli.[45–46] In addition, many consumers may not be aware of the health benefits of consuming more plant-based foods. Fruits, vegetables, and grain products contain many more components than just the vitamins and minerals found in a multivitamin supplement.

This section briefly describes three classifications of phytochemicals that have fairly solid research evidence suggesting a health-protective role. These classifications are the phenolic compounds, organosulfides, and one of the carotenoids, lycopene. More research is required to fully understand phytochemicals' roles in the body, especially in regard to disease prevention. Many of the food sources that contain phytochemicals discussed in the following sections are excellent choices to include in a sports nutrition plan for athletes. Although research has focused on health and disease prevention and not on sport performance, athletes can also reap the benefits of good health by consuming a phytochemical-rich diet. **Table 6.2** provides a summary of a variety of phytochemicals and examples of good food sources of these phytochemicals.

What are phenolic compounds?

The phenolic compounds are a large and varied group of phytochemicals that are found in many different foods. The majority of the research on phe-

TABLE 6.2	Phytochemicals in Foods
Phytochemical	**Food Source**
Allium compounds	Garlic, onion
Anthocyanins	Blue and purple fruits—blueberries, grapes, cherries, raspberries
Carotenoids	Yellow, red, and pink fruits and vegetables; dark green leafy vegetables
Catechins	Green tea
Flavonoids	Most fruits and vegetables
Indoles, isothiocynates	Broccoli, cabbage, cauliflower, radish
Isoflavones	Soy foods
Lignans	Flax seeds, soybeans
Lycopene	Tomato products, watermelon, other pink fruits
Phenolic acids	Berries, grapes, nuts, whole grains

nols is related to their positive influence on heart disease prevention. The phenols are a broad category of antioxidant compounds that work to prevent LDL oxidation. Common phenolic compounds that have been researched fairly extensively include flavonoids and phenolic acids.

Flavonoids became known to the public when research was published reporting that individuals who drink wine may have a decreased risk for heart disease. The flavonoids in wine and grapes started a revolution and much debate about the benefits of wine consumption in combating heart disease. The first link between wine intake and cardiovascular disease became apparent when a French research group[47] found a strong negative correlation between wine intake and death from ischemic heart disease in both men and women from 18 countries.[44] The French have a relatively high consumption of dietary fat and saturated fat, yet a relatively low rate of cardiovascular disease. The increased wine consumption in France may help protect against heart disease, and thus the "French paradox" was born. Some of the reduction in cardiovascular disease may be from the alcohol's ability to increase HDL cholesterol; however, the nonalcohol components of wine, the flavonoids, hold promise as well.

Grape seeds and skins are considered good sources of polyphenolic tannins that provide the astringent taste to wine.[48] The phenolic compounds catechin and anthocyanin are also abundant in grapes.[49] Red wine contains more flavonoids than white wine because the grape skins are incorporated in the fermentation process. The skins and sometimes seeds are used in wine making and in grape juices, making these products high in these phytochemicals. New evidence suggests that nonalcoholic wine and commercial grape juice can provide similar amounts of flavonoids and antioxidant capacity as red wine.[50,51] Because alcohol consumption is generally not recommended as part of an athlete's diet, sparkling grape juice can provide a healthy nonalcoholic alternative.

Teas contain both flavonols and polyphenols, most significantly catechins.[52] Green and black teas both contain these phytochemicals; however, green tea has been found to be more concentrated in polyphenols. This might be related to how the different teas are prepared for consumption. Green tea leaves are steamed and dried, which prevents oxidation of the polyphenols, primarily catechins. Black tea leaves are fermented, which reduces the amount of catechin in black tea compared to green tea.[53] Regardless of the type of tea, the primary antioxidant properties may act in cancer prevention[54,55] and cardiovascular disease protection.[56] Consuming several cups of green or black tea daily will help athletes reap the potential disease prevention benefits of this beverage. The teas can be found in decaffeinated varieties, containing the same beneficial ingredients. The decaffeinated versions are recommended to athletes to help them avoid excessive intake of caffeine.

What are organosulfides?

A growing amount of evidence from epidemiological studies has provided consensus that diets rich in fruits and vegetables are associated with lower risks of developing certain cancers. Several excellent reviews have been published to support this association.[42,43,57] The more difficult determination is what specifically in fruits and vegetables is the protectant. There are many nutrients, fibers, and non-nutrient compounds in fruits and vegetables that may play singular or additive roles in cancer risk reduction. The phytochemicals found in the cruciferous (sometimes called brassica) vegetables and allyl compounds in garlic and onions may play a singular or additive protective role. The cruciferous vegetables contain a variety of organosulfide compounds including glucosinolates, indoles, and isothiocyanates and have long been touted for their anti-cancer properties.[58] Vegetables including broccoli, brussels sprouts, cabbage, rutabaga, and cauliflower are part of the or-

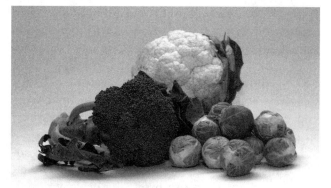

ganosulfide group of phytochemicals. Talalay and Fahey[59] present an excellent review of the role of glucosinolate and isothiocyanate phytochemicals found in cruciferous vegetables in cancer prevention. They cite more than 10 studies and report that "these findings provide additional support for the pivotal role of the glucosinolates and isothiocyanates derived from crucifers in chemoprotection against cancer" (p. 3029S).

Garlic and onions along with leeks, chives, and shallots contain allyl compounds that provide flavor and odor to foods. The allyl compounds in garlic have been researched for many possible health benefits including reducing blood cholesterol levels and cancer risk, and for their antihypertensive potential. A review of more than 20 epidemiological studies suggests that allium vegetables, including onions, may confer a protective effect against cancers of the gastrointestinal tract.[43]

Athletes should include cruciferous vegetables, garlic, onions, and other pungent vegetables in their daily diet to gain the potential health benefits. However, consumption of these vegetables can produce intestinal gas and bloating that may be uncomfortable when training or competing in sport events. Therefore, athletes should avoid high-gas-producing vegetables within several hours before training. Consumption of these vegetables after workouts or competitions is the best practice to avoid uncomfortable gas production while reaping the health benefits.

What is lycopene?

Lycopene is one of the most well studied of the carotenoids and is more widely recognized by the public. Advertisements for vitamin and mineral supplements that "contain lycopene" abound. Lycopene is now added to many vitamin supplements marketed for men because of the strong correlation between ly-

copene intake and prostate health. Lycopene is the most abundant carotenoid in the prostate.[60] In the now classic prospective cohort study of lycopene's effect on the prostate, Giovannucci et al.[61] found that men who consumed at least 10 or more servings of tomato products per week had less than one-half the risk of developing advanced prostate cancer. The proposed mechanism for the reduced cancer risk is the antioxidant property of lycopene.

Tomatoes and tomato products such as ketchup, tomato pastes and sauces, canned tomatoes, and tomato-based products such as enchilada sauce, pizza sauce, picante sauce, and salsa, are good sources of lycopene. Fresh tomatoes appear to have less bioavailable lycopene than processed tomatoes because cooking releases the lycopene stored in the cell walls of fresh tomatoes. Absorption of lycopene is greater with the simultaneous intake of fat. For example, a tomato-based pizza sauce on a pizza with cheese, or an oil and vinegar dressing mixed with canned tomatoes for a salad, will enhance the absorption of lycopene.

Future research may find that lycopene is beneficial in a variety of ways for active individuals. A small study of 20 individuals found that lycopene supplementation of 30 mg per day provided some protection against exercise-induced asthma.[62] There is research, primarily in animal studies, suggesting antioxidant properties of lycopene that may reduce oxidative stress.[63] Research on the effect of lycopene supplementation for providing protection from ultraviolet sunlight has shown some promise,[64,65] which could be significant for athletes who train and compete outdoors. However, many of these studies contained small sample groups, combined other antioxidant supplements with lycopene, and were conducted primarily in animals and not humans. Further research in larger human clinical trials, isolating lycopene, is needed before any definitive answers about lycopene's effects in these areas can be drawn.

How can athletes increase phytochemical consumption through whole foods?

Increasing phytochemical intake means focusing on a plant-based diet. This does not mean that meat needs to be eliminated; it simply means more effort should be spent on trying to incorporate a wide range of fruits, vegetables, and whole grains in the daily diet (see **Training Tables 6.3 through 6.5**). There is still a lot to learn about the actual amount of certain phytochemicals in plants, how they react

Training Table 6.3: Sunshine Broccoli Salad

1 large broccoli head, cut into bite-sized pieces

¼ cup purple onion, chopped

¼ cup sunflower seeds

¼ cup orange juice

8 oz plain or vanilla low-fat yogurt

¼–½ cup raisins

Blend the yogurt and orange juice and set aside. Wash and prepare the broccoli and onion. Mix vegetables and sunflower seeds together in a large bowl. Pour orange juice and yogurt mixture over vegetables and seeds and mix thoroughly. Let salad sit in refrigerator for 2–4 hours before serving, if possible, to blend the flavors. Garnish with or mix in raisins.

Phytochemicals present: Organosulfides

Serving Size: 1¼ cups (Recipe makes four servings)

Calories: 166 kcals

Protein: 6 grams

Carbohydrate: 27 grams

Fat: 5 grams

Training Table 6.4: Salmon Pepper Salad

2 fresh salmon fillets or steaks

1 red bell pepper

2 cups spinach leaves, washed

1 mango or papaya, sliced

2 tbsp fresh lime juice

1 tbsp olive oil

1 clove garlic, crushed

1 tsp dried thyme

Mix lime juice, olive oil, garlic, and thyme together in a small bowl. Rinse and pat dry the salmon steaks. Place steaks in a shallow dish. Pour the lime juice marinade mixture over the salmon; turn to coat. Cover the dish, place it in the refrigerator, and let marinate for at least 10 minutes.

Wash the spinach and spin or pat dry; tear into bite-sized pieces. Wash and core the red pepper; slice into thin strips. Peel the mango or papaya; slice into thin strips or small pieces.

Grill the salmon on an indoor or outdoor grill until fish flakes (approximately 4–6 minutes per side). Arrange salmon on bed of spinach and red pepper. Garnish with mango on top and around the fish. Serve with balsamic vinaigrette salad dressing, if desired.

Phytochemicals present: Lutein, zeaxanthin, and organosulfides; also high in vitamins C and E, and beta-carotene

Serving Size: 3 oz salmon, 2 cups vegetables (Recipe makes two servings)

Calories: 286 kcals

Protein: 19 grams

Carbohydrate: 25 grams

Fat: 13 grams

gaining the performance edge

Phytochemicals are plant-based compounds that appear to have potent antioxidant and anti-cancer effects. Although DRIs have not been established for these substances, athletes can still reap the potential benefits by consuming a variety of fruits, vegetables, and other plant-based foods each day.

in the body, a recommended dietary intake, and their effect on athletic performance. Research on the specific phytochemicals is relatively new, and there are many more different types of phytochemicals than there are vitamins. Establishing DRIs for the various phytochemicals is currently an ongoing process that will take years to decipher; however, that does not diminish the importance of including these essential compounds in an athlete's daily diet.

The following tips will help athletes consume more plant-based foods, thus increasing phytochemical intake:

- Serve hot or cold green tea with meals.
- Keep red or green grapes washed and ready in the refrigerator for snacks.
- Use tomato sauces and pastes and spaghetti sauce as a basis for meals.
- Sprinkle nuts and seeds on salads.
- Use garlic in cooking, dressings, marinades, and sauces.

Training Table 6.5: Berry Soy Smoothie

1 cup frozen blueberries, strawberries, or other berries

1 cup soy milk

½ cup orange juice

4 oz silken tofu

Let berries thaw slightly. Blend all ingredients in blender until smooth. Add enough orange juice and tofu to obtain the desired texture.

Phytochemicals present: Isoflavones, carotenoids, and flavonoids

Serving Size: 3 cups (Recipe makes one serving)

Calories: 295 kcals

Protein: 14 grams

Carbohydrate: 42 grams

Fat: 9 grams

- Prepare side dishes with green leafy vegetables such as kale, spinach, and collards.
- Use soy milk instead of dairy milk on cereal or as a beverage.
- Complement all meals with one or two fruits or vegetables.
- Use whole grain foods more often than processed grains.
- Try a new grain recipe that uses bulgar, barley, or oats.

- Eat fruit for dessert such as a baked apple, chopped melon, or chilled berries.

Athletes should be encouraged to eat a wide variety of foods, including many plant-based items, to assist them in obtaining the energy they need while also consuming valuable nutrient and non-nutrient components in their diet. As research evolves, recommendations similar to the DRIs may be on the horizon for some phytochemicals.

The Box Score

Key Points of Chapter

- Contrary to the body's requirements for carbohydrates, proteins, and fats, the daily dietary requirements for vitamins are very small. However, these micronutrients serve vital functions in the body and thus are essential for survival.

- Vitamins are organic compounds that are essential to at least one vital chemical reaction or process in the human body. In addition, to be considered a vitamin the compound cannot be made by the body itself or cannot be made in sufficient quantities to meet the body's needs. In addition, vitamins contain no calories and are found in very small amounts (i.e., micrograms or milligrams) in the body.

- Vitamin requirements are presented as a collection of dietary values termed the Dietary Reference Intakes (DRIs). The DRI expands on the previously established Recommended Dietary Allowance (RDA) and takes into consideration other dietary quantities such as Estimated Average Requirement (EAR), Adequate Intake (AI), and Tolerable Upper Intake Level (UL). DRIs are continually being reviewed and updated as scientific data become available.

- Vitamins are categorized into two main groups: water soluble and fat soluble. The water-soluble vitamins include the B-complex vitamins, vitamin C, and choline. The fat-soluble vitamins include vitamins A, D, E, and K.

- The B-complex vitamins are actually a group of eight different vitamins. In general, the B vitamins serve as coenzymes in the metabolic pathways, which break down carbohydrates, fats, and proteins for energy. Because they are water soluble, they are not stored in any appreciable amounts and thus present a low risk for toxicity to the body.

- Choline is a vitamin-like compound, but is not considered a B vitamin. Choline is involved in the formation of the neurotransmitter acetylcholine, which is needed for muscle activation. Choline has also been shown to help maintain the structural integrity of cell membranes. The risk for choline deficiency is low; however, toxicity can occur, presenting signs and symptoms of low blood pressure, diarrhea, and a fishy body odor.

- Vitamin C is one of the most recognized vitamins because of its supposed role in enhancing the immune system. It is a strong antioxidant, is critical for the formation of collagen, enhances iron absorption, and aids in the formation of various hormones and neurotransmitters.

- The fat-soluble vitamins are dependent on the presence of dietary fat for intestinal absorption and transport throughout the body. Fat-soluble vitamins can be more toxic to the body than water-soluble vitamins because they are stored in the liver and adipose tissues and can accumulate over time. Caution should be exercised when using supplements containing high doses of these vitamins.

- Vitamin A is associated with the retinoid and carotenoid families of compounds and is important for vision, healthy skin, and cell differentiation. A vitamin A deficiency can result in blindness and hyperkeratosis. Toxicity is rare when the dietary focus is placed on whole foods; however, intake from supplements can quickly reach toxic levels.

- Vitamin D is called the "sunshine vitamin" and is crucial for the maintenance of bone health. Deficiencies are rare as a result of the fortification of milk. Toxicity can result in hypercalcemia and subsequent calcification of various soft tissues throughout the body.

- Vitamin E belongs to the tocopherol and tocotrienol family of compounds and is most recognized for its antioxidant properties. Deficiencies are rare and so is toxicity. However, high levels of vitamin E can have a blood-thinning effect, thereby decreasing blood clotting, which can lead to bruising and other more serious complications.

- Vitamin K is probably the least recognized of the vitamins. The primary role of vitamin K is in blood clotting, but it also plays an important role in bone health. Deficiencies can result in substantial hemorrhaging. Toxicity from food sources is rare.

- Free radicals are highly reactive compounds that can damage cell membranes and other structures, including DNA. They tend to be compounds containing oxygen and can be formed during normal aerobic metabolism. Free radicals can also be introduced into the body from exogenous sources (e.g., pollutants in the air).

- Antioxidants are the body's primary defense against free radicals. They exist in enzymatic and nonenzymatic forms. Vitamins A, C, and E along with other compounds known as phytochemicals serve as the body's nonenzymatic antioxidants. The effectiveness of supplementing the diet with nonenzymatic forms of antioxidants is presently unclear.

- Exercise, particularly aerobic exercise, has been shown to increase free radical production. Although the reasons underlying the free radical increase are not clear, the body's enzymatic antioxidant defense system may up-regulate as an adaptive response to extended training, thus increasing its natural defenses against free radicals. The effect of taking supplements of vitamins A, C, and E and phytochemicals on free radical levels during exercise is presently unclear. For now, making recommendations regarding antioxidant supplementation is not necessary or advisable. The best nutritional advice is to incorporate more antioxidant-containing foods into the daily diet.

- Phytochemicals are biologically active plant chemicals that are not considered nutrients but play a vital role in health. Although there are many different phytochemicals, research has associated three classes as aiding human health: phenolic compounds, organosulfides, and carotenoids.

- Athletes should be encouraged to eat a wide variety of fruits and vegetables to help ensure adequate intake of phytochemicals. Because DRIs have not been established for phytochemicals, the need for supplementation by athletes is currently unknown.

Study Questions

1. What are vitamins and how are they classified? List the specific vitamins that fall under each classification. Which classification of vitamins is potentially more toxic to the body? Explain why.

2. Taken as a group, what major role do the B vitamins play in the body? What implications does this have in regard to athletes and sport performance?

3. List two of the four fat-soluble vitamins and their respective roles/functions for overall health and athletic performance.

4. Should dietary substances that block absorption of fat by the digestive system be used? Defend your answer.

5. What are free radicals? Where do they come from and what effect do they have on the body?

6. What are antioxidants? Which vitamins and related compounds serve as antioxidants in the body? Briefly describe how they work in the body.

7. Should athletes take supplements that boost the body's level of antioxidants? Defend your answer with what is currently known about the substances.

8. What are phytochemicals and where do they come from?

9. What are some of the commonly identified classes of phytochemicals? What roles do they play in the body?

10. What are the current recommendations for the intake of phytochemicals? Should athletes take phytochemical supplements? Defend your answer.

References

1. Schwenk T, Costley C. When food becomes a drug: nonanabolic nutritional supplement use in athletes. *Am J Sports Med*. 2002;30(6):907–916.

2. Institute of Medicine. *Dietary Reference Intakes for Thiamin, Riboflavin, Niacin, Vitamin B_6, Folate, Vitamin B_{12}, Pantothenic Acid, Biotin, and Choline*. Food and Nutrition Board. Washington, DC: National Academies Press; 2000.

3. Van der Beek EJ, van Dokkum W, Schrijver J, et al. Thiamin, riboflavin and vitamins B_6 and C: impact of combined restricted intake on functional performance in man. *Am J Clin Nutr*. 1988;48:1451–1462.

4. Van der Beek EJ, van Dokkum W, Wedel M, Schrijver J, van der Berg H. Thiamin, riboflavin and B_6: impact of restricted intake on physical performance in man. *J Am Coll Nutr*. 1994;13:629–640.

5. Manore M. Effect of physical activity on thiamine, riboflavin and vitamin B_6 requirements. *Am J Clin Nutr*. 2000;72(suppl 2):598S–606S.

6. Suboticanec K, Stavljenic A, Schalch W, Buzina R. Effects of pyridoxine and riboflavin supplementation on physical fitness in young adolescents. *Int J Vitam Nutr Res*. 1990;60:81–88.

7. Winters LR, Yoon JS, Kalkwarf HJ, et al. Riboflavin requirements and exercise adaptation in older women. *Am J Clin Nutr*. 1992;56(3):526–532.

8. Heath E, Wilcox A, Quinn C. Effects of nicotinic acid on respiratory exchange ratio and substrate levels during exercise. *Med Sci Sports Exerc*. 1993;25(9):1018–1023.

9. Jenkins D. Effects of nicotinic acid on carbohydrate and fat metabolism during exercise. *Lancet*. 1965;1:1307–1308.

10. Carlson L, Havel R, Ekelund L, Holmgren A. Effect of nicotinic acid on the turnover rate and oxidation of the free fatty acids of plasma in man during exercise. *Metab Clin Exp*. 1963;12:837–845.

11. Bergstrom J, Hultman E, Jorfeldt L, Pernow B, Wahren J. Effect of nicotinic acid on physical working capacity and on metabolism of muscle glycogen in man. *J Appl Physiol*. 1969;26:170–176.

12. Martineau L, Jacobs I. Free fatty acid availability and temperature regulation in cold water. *J Appl Physiol*. 1989;67:2466–2472.

13. Leklem JE. Vitamin B_6: a status report. *J Nutr*. 1990;120(suppl 11):1503–1507.

14. Coburn SP, Ziegler PJ, Costill DL, et al. Response of vitamin B_6 content of muscle to changes in vitamin B_6 intake in men. *Am J Clin Nutr*. 1991;53(6):1436–1442.

15. Manore MM, Leklem JE, Water MC. Vitamin B_6 metabolism as affected by exercise in trained and untrained women fed diets differing in carbohydrate and vitamin B_6 content. *Am J Clin Nutr*. 1987;46:995–1004.

16. Fogelhom M, Ruokonen I, Laakso JT, Vuorimaa T, Himberg JJ. Lack of association between indices of vitamin B_1, B_2, and B_6 status and exercise-induced blood lactate in young adults. *Int J Sports Nutr*. 1993;3:165–176.

17. Soares MJ, Satyanarayana K, Bamji MS, Jocab CM, Ramana YV, Rao SS. The effect of exercise on the riboflavin status of adult men. *Brit J Nutr*. 1993;69:541–551.

18. Rokitzki L, Sagredos AN, Reuss F, Buchner M, Keul J. Acute changes in vitamin B_6 status in endurance athletes before and after a marathon. *Int J Sport Nutr*. 1994;4(2):154–165.

19. Leonard SW, Leklem JE. Plasma B_6 vitamer changes following a 50-km ultra-marathon. *Int J Sport Nutr Exerc Metab*. 2000;10(3):302–314.

20. Herrmann W. The importance of hyperhomocysteinemia as a risk factor for diseases: an overview. *Clin Chem Lab Med*. 2001;39:666–674.

21. Herrmann M, Schorr H, Obeid R, et al. Homocysteine increases during endurance exercise. *Clin Chem Lab Med*. 2003;41(11):1518–1524.

22. Mock DM. *Present Knowledge in Nutrition*. Washington, DC: International Life Sciences Institute, Nutrition Foundation; 1990.

23. Nice C, Reeves AG, Brinck-Johnsen T, Noll W. The effects of pantothenic acid on human exercise capacity. *J Sports Med Phys Fitness*. 1984;24(1):26–29.

24. Webster MJ. Physiological and performance responses to supplementation with thiamin and pantothenic acid derivatives. *Europ J Appl Physiol*. 1998;77(6):486–491.

25. Hongu N, Sachan DS. Carnitine and choline supplementation with exercise alter carnitine profiles, biochemical markers of fat metabolism and serum leptin concentration in healthy women. *J Nutr*. 2003;133(1):84–89.

26. Sachan DS, Hongu N. Increase in VO_2max and metabolic markers of fat oxidation by caffeine, carnitine and choline supplementation in rats. *J Nutr Biochem*. 2000;11:521–526.

27. Hongu N, Sachan DS. Caffeine, carnitine ad choline supplementation of rats decreases body fat and serum leptin concentration as does exercise. *J Nutr*. 2000;130:152–157.

28. Institute of Medicine. *Dietary Reference Intakes for Vitamin C, Vitamin E, Selenium, and Carotenoids*. Food and Nutrition Board. Washington, DC: National Academies Press; 2000.

29. Rosenblum C. *Sports Nutrition—A Guide for the Professional Working with Active People*. 3rd ed. Chicago, IL: American Dietetic Association; 2000.

30. Institute of Medicine. *Dietary Reference Intakes for Vitamin A, Vitamin K, Arsenic, Boron, Chromium, Copper, Iodine, Iron, Manganese, Molybdenum, Nickel, Silicon, Vanadium and Zinc*. Food and Nutrition Board. Washington, DC: National Academies Press; 2000.

31. Institute of Medicine. *Dietary Reference Intakes for Calcium and Vitamin D*. Food and Nutrition Board. Washington, DC: National Academies Press; 2010.

32. "Special K" takes on new meaning. *Tufts Univ Health Nutr Newsletter*. 1997;15(5):1–7.

33. Alessio HM. Exercise-induced muscle damage. *Med Sci Sports Exerc*. 1993;25:218–224.

34. Clarkson PM. Antioxidants and physical performance. *Clin Rev Food Sci Nutr*. 1995;35:131–141.

35. Kanter M. Free radicals, exercise and antioxidant supplementation. *Proc Nutr Soc*. 1998;57:9–13.

36. Urso ML, Clarkson PM. Oxidative stress, exercise, and antioxidant supplementation. *Toxicol*. 2003;189(1–2):41–54.

37. Jackson MJ. Free radicals in skin and muscle: damaging agents or signals for adaptation? *Proc Nutr Soc*. 1999;58:673–676.

38. Sen CK. Oxidants and antioxidants in exercise. *J Appl Physiol*. 1995;79:675–686.

39. Jenkins RR. Exercise and oxidative stress methodology: a critique. *Am J Clin Nutr*. 2000;72:670S–674S.

40. Steinmetz KA, Potter JD. Vegetables, fruit and cancer II mechanisms. *Cancer Causes Control*. 1991;2:427–442.

41. Block G, Patterson B, Subar A. Fruit, vegetables and cancer prevention: a review of the epidemiological evidence. *Nutr Cancer*. 1992;18:1–29.

42. World Cancer Research Fund and American Institute for Cancer Research. *Food, Nutrition and the Prevention of Cancer: A Global Perspective*. Washington, DC: American Institute for Cancer Research; 1997.

43. Ernst E. Can allium vegetables prevent cancer? *Phytomed*. 1997;4:79–83.

44. Hasler CM. Functional foods: their role in disease prevention and health promotion. *Food Tech*. 1998; 52(11):63–70.

45. Jones CM, Mes P, Myers JR. Characterization and inheritance of the Anthocyanin fruit tomato. *J Heredity*. 2003;94:449–456.

46. Pelletier S, Kundrat S, Hasler CM. Effects of an educational program on intent to consume functional foods. *J Am Diet Assoc*. 2002;102:1297–1300.

47. St. Leger AS, Cochrane AL, Moore F. Factors associated with cardiac mortality in developed countries with particular reference to the consumption of wine. *Lancet*. 1979;1:1017–1020.

48. Yilmaz Y, Toledo RT. Major flavonoids in grape seeds and skins: antioxidant capacity of catechin, epicatechin, and gallic acid. *J Agric Food Chem*. 2004;52(2):255–260.

49. Palma M, Taylor LR. Extraction of polyphenolic compounds from grape seeds with near critical carbon dioxide. *J Chromatogr*. 1999;849:117–124.

50. Day AP, Kemp HJ, Bolton C, Hartog M, Stansbie D. Effects of concentrated red grape juice consumption on serum antioxidant capacity and low-density lipoprotein oxidation. *Ann Nutr Metab*. 1998;41:353–357.

51. Serafini M, Maiani G, Ferro-Luzzi A. Alcohol-free red wine enhances plasma antioxidant capacity in humans. *J Nutr*. 1998;128:1003–1007.

52. Graham HN. Green tea composition, consumption and polyphenol chemistry. *Prev Med*. 1992;21:334–350.

53. Paquay JBG, Guido RMM, Stender G, et al. Protection against nitric oxide toxicity by tea. *J Agric Food Chem*. 2000;48:5768–5772.

54. Clydesdale FM. Tea and health. *Crit Rev Food Sci Nutr*. 1997;36:691–785.

55. Weisburger JH. Tea and health: the underlying mechanisms. *Proc Soc Ep Biol Med*. 1999;220(4):271–275.

56. American Dietetic Association. Position of the American Dietetic Association: functional foods. *J Am Diet Assoc*. 1999;99(10):1278–1285.

57. Institute of Medicine. *Dietary Reference Intakes: A Risk Assessment Model for Establishing Upper Intake Levels for Nutrients*. Food and Nutrition Board. Washington, DC: National Academies Press; 1998.

58. Verhoeven DTH, Goldbohm RA, van Poppel G, Verhagen H. Epidemiological studies on brassica vegetables and cancer risk. *Cancer Epidemiol Biomark Prev*. 1996;5(9):733–748.

59. Talalay P, Fahey JW. Phytochemicals from cruciferous plants protect against cancer by modulating carcinogen metabolism. *J Nutr*. 2001;131:3027S–3033S.

60. Clinton SK, Emenhiser C, Schwartz SJ, et al. Cis-trans lycopene isomers, carotenoids, and retinol in the human prostate. *Cancer Epidemiol Biomark Prev*. 1996;5:823–833.

61. Giovannucci E, Ascherio A, Rimm EB, Stampfer MJ, Colditz GA, Willett WC. Intake of carotenoids and retinol in relation to risk of prostate cancer. *J Natl Cancer Inst*. 1995;87(23):1767–1776.

62. Neuman I, Nahum H, Ben-Amotz A. Reduction of exercise-induced asthma oxidative stress by lycopene, a natural antioxidant. *Allergy*. 2000;55:1184–1189.

63. Porrini M, Riso P. Lymphocyte lycopene concentration and DNA protection from oxidative damage is increased in women after a short period of tomato consumption. *J Nutr*. 2000;130(2):189–192.

64. Greul AK, Grundman JU, Heinrich F, et al. Photoprotection of UV-irradiated human skin: an antioxidative combination of vitamins E and C, carotenoids, selenium and proanthocyanidins. *Skin Pharmacol Appl Skin Physiol*. 2002;15(5):307–315.

65. Heinrich U, Gartner C, Wiebusch M, et al. Supplementation with beta-carotene in similar amount of mixed carotenoids protects humans from UV-induced erythema. *J Nutr*. 2003;133(1):98–101.

Additional Resource

Insel P, Turner RE, Ross D. *Nutrition*. 2nd ed. Sudbury, MA: Jones and Bartlett Publishers; 2004.

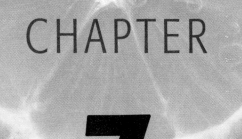

CHAPTER 7

Minerals

Key Questions Addressed

- What's the big deal about minerals?
- What are minerals?
- What are the major minerals?
- What are the trace minerals?

You Are the Nutrition Coach

Anne participates in triathlons. Recently, in a half-Ironman race, she experienced nausea, intestinal cramping, and diarrhea on the run, leading to a poor performance. The entire race took her nearly 6½ hours. During the bike portion, she consumed 100 oz of a relatively new sports beverage that she has been training with this year, as well as two gels. On the run, she consumed sips of the sports beverage provided on the course but switched over to water once she started experiencing the nausea, cramping, and diarrhea. She was frustrated by her performance and wants to ensure that it does not happen again. You ask Anne to bring in the new sports beverage she has been consuming so that you can review the Supplement Facts label. Per 8 oz serving, the following nutrients are provided: 60 calories, 15 g carbohydrates, 0 g protein, 0 g fat, 100 mg sodium, 50 mg calcium, 30 mg magnesium, and 100 mg potassium.

Questions

- What could be a potential cause of Anne's nausea, intestinal cramping, and diarrhea during the race?

- What recommendations would you give to Anne to prevent the symptoms from occurring in future races?

What's the big deal about minerals?

Similar to vitamins, minerals play important roles throughout the body and are considered essential; without minerals, the body could not function. Many minerals are involved in important catalytic reactions (e.g., iron aids in gluconeogenesis) or serve as key structural components of tissues (e.g., calcium provides structure to bones) throughout the body.

The role that minerals play in sport performance has been studied over the years. It is clear that minerals are crucial for a variety of bodily functions, keeping athletes healthy and training strong. Certain athlete populations are more prone to mineral deficiencies, warranting a special focus in the diet. For example, female athletes may be more susceptible to iron deficiencies. Therefore, iron as well as vitamins that enhance iron absorption, such as vitamin C, should receive greater emphasis in their diet. In addition to general health, the intake of several minerals, specifically **electrolytes**, has a great impact on sport performance. Sodium and potassium, the main electrolytes (minerals) lost in sweat, must be replaced on a daily basis as well as during endurance and ultra-endurance sports to optimize performance and prevent medical complications. Other minerals are still under investigation, and their ergogenic effects have yet to be elucidated.

electrolytes Positively or negatively charged ions found throughout the body. The body uses the electrolytes to establish ionically charged gradients across membranes in excitable tissues such as muscle and nerves so that they can generate electrical activity. The most well-known electrolytes are sodium (Na$^+$), potassium (K$^+$), and chloride (Cl$^-$).

What are minerals?

Minerals are unique nutrients in several respects. Unlike carbohydrates, fats, proteins, and vitamins, minerals are not organic molecules. They are basically **inorganic** elements or atoms. Also unlike the macronutrients, minerals contain no calories and, although essential, are needed by the body in very small amounts (i.e., milligrams or micrograms). Furthermore, after ingestion, the structure of minerals is not altered; this is unlike the reaction of macronutrients, which undergo dramatic changes in structure during digestion and utilization by the body. Unlike vitamins, which can be destroyed or altered by exposure to heat, light, alkalinity, or enzymes, minerals remain unaltered. Because of their stability, minerals are unaffected by cooking techniques, digestive processes, and/or exposure to enzymes. In other words, unlike many nutrients, minerals remain unaltered from food source to the human cells.

inorganic A descriptor given to a compound that does not contain carbon atoms in its molecular structure.

However, similar to all nutrients, minerals must be absorbed across the intestinal wall to serve their roles within the body. A variety of factors can affect the bioavailability of minerals. Some minerals are absorbed in proportion to the body's needs. Absorption of other minerals is affected by the fiber content of foods that are ingested simultaneously. High-fiber foods contain compounds that can bind to certain minerals, thus preventing their absorption during passage through the intestines. In some instances, high doses of one mineral, which can occur during supplementation, can cause competition for absorption and thus decrease intestinal uptake of other minerals. Therefore, despite the fact that minerals are needed in limited amounts and are very stable nutrients, athletes cannot afford to be cavalier about their mineral intake, nor can they rely on indiscriminant supplementation to meet their body's mineral requirements.

There are two classifications of minerals: major minerals and trace minerals. The **major minerals** include calcium, phosphorus, magnesium, sodium, chloride, potassium, and sulfur. Minerals are classified as "major" if they are required by the body in amounts greater than 100 milligrams per day. The **trace minerals** include iron, zinc, chromium, fluoride, copper, manganese, iodine, molybdenum, and selenium. Minerals are classified as trace if they are required by the body in quantities less than 100 milligrams per day. Both major and trace minerals are stored in the body; when consumed in excess, stored levels can build and become toxic to the body (e.g., high doses of iron can cause hemachromatosis, a condition discussed later in this chapter). Toxic levels can be achieved through dietary intake, but toxicity is much more likely to be caused by high-dosage supplements.

major minerals The minerals required by the body in amounts greater than 100 milligrams per day. The major minerals include calcium, phosphorus, magnesium, sodium, chloride, potassium, and sulfur.

trace minerals Minerals required by the body in quantities less than 100 milligrams per day. The trace minerals include iron, zinc, chromium, fluoride, copper, manganese, iodine, molybdenum, and selenium.

This chapter discusses the functions, dietary recommendations, effects on energy systems and sport performance, deficiency and toxicity symptoms, food sources, meal-planning tips, and the appropriateness of supplements for athletes in regard to major and trace minerals. Refer to **Table 7.1** for a summary of the DRI values for major and trace minerals.

TABLE 7.1 Dietary Reference Intakes for Major and Trace Minerals

Life Stage Group	Calcium (mg/d)	Phosphorus (mg/d)	Magnesium (mg/d)	Iron (mg/d)	Zinc (mg/d)	Selenium (µg/d)	Iodine (µg/d)	Copper (µg/d)	Manganese (mg/d)	Fluoride (mg/d)	Chromium (µg/d)	Molybdenum (µg/d)
Infants												
0–6 mo	200*	100*	30*	0.27*	2*	15*	110*	200*	0.003*	0.01*	0.2*	2*
7–12 mo	260*	275*	75*	11	3	20*	130*	220*	0.6*	0.5*	5.5*	3*
Children												
1–3 y	700	460	80	7	3	20	90	340	1.2*	0.7*	11*	17
4–8 y	1000	500	130	10	5	30	90	440	1.5*	1*	15*	22
Males												
9–13 y	1300	1250	240	8	8	40	120	700	1.9*	2*	25*	34
14–18 y	1300	1250	410	11	11	55	150	890	2.2*	3*	35*	43
19–30 y	1000	700	400	8	11	55	150	900	2.3*	4*	35*	45
31–50 y	1000	700	420	8	11	55	150	900	2.3*	4*	35*	45
51–70 y	1000	700	420	8	11	55	150	900	2.3*	4*	30*	45
>70 y	1200	700	420	8	11	55	150	900	2.3*	4*	30*	45
Females												
9–13 y	1300	1250	240	8	8	40	120	700	1.6*	2*	21*	34
14–18 y	1300	1250	360	15	9	55	150	890	1.6*	3*	24*	43
19–30 y	1000	700	310	18	8	55	150	900	1.8*	3*	25*	45
31–50 y	1000	700	320	18	8	55	150	900	1.8*	3*	25*	45
51–70 y	1200	700	320	8	8	55	150	900	1.8*	3*	20*	45
>70 y	1200	700	320	8	8	55	150	900	1.8*	3*	20*	45
Pregnancy												
≤18 y	1300	1250	400	27	12	60	220	1000	2.0*	3*	29*	50
19–30 y	1000	700	350	27	11	60	220	1000	2.0*	3*	30*	50
31–50 y	1000	700	360	27	11	60	220	1000	2.0*	3*	30*	50
Lactation												
≤18 y	1300	1250	360	10	13	70	290	1300	2.6*	3*	44*	50
19–30 y	1000	700	310	9	12	70	290	1300	2.6*	3*	45*	50
31–50 y	1000	700	320	9	12	70	290	1300	2.0*	3*	45*	50

This table presents Recommended Dietary Allowances (RDA) and Adequate Intakes (AI). An asterisk (*) indicates AI. RDAs and AIs may both be used as goals for individual intake.

Source: Data from Institute of Medicine's Dietary Reference Intakes for Vitamin A, Vitamin K, Arsenic, Boron, Chromium, Copper, Iodine, Iron, Manganese, Molybdenum, Nickel, Silicon, Vanadium and Zinc. Food and Nutrition Board. Washington, DC: National Academies Press; 2000; Dietary Reference Intakes for Vitamin C, Vitamin E, Selenium, and Carotenoids. Food and Nutrition Board. Washington, DC: National Academies Press; 2000; and Dietary Reference Intakes for Calcium, Phosphorus, Magnesium, Vitamin D, and Fluoride. Food and Nutrition Board. Washington, DC: National Academies Press; 1997. Institute of Medicine. Dietary Reference Intakes for Calcium and Vitamin D. Food and Nutrition Board. Washington, DC: National Academies Press; 2010.

What are the major minerals?

The major minerals are calcium, phosphorus, magnesium, sodium, chloride, potassium, and sulfur. As mentioned earlier, the daily requirements for these minerals exceed 100 milligrams per day. Many of these minerals play a specific role in sport performance such as enhancing the integrity of bones to withstand impact during sports, providing electrolytes lost in sweat, and aiding in the prevention of muscle cramps. This section will review the functions, recommended intakes, signs of deficiency, symptoms of toxicity, food sources, and recommendations for supplementation for each major mineral.

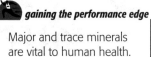

gaining the performance edge

Major and trace minerals are vital to human health. An emphasis should be placed on food sources of minerals, consumed in adequate quantities on a daily basis.

Why is calcium important for athletes?

Calcium is widely recognized as a critical mineral for optimal bone health. However, calcium has many other important roles in the body for health and sport performance that are often unrecognized. An area that is receiving more attention is the fact that many individuals are not meeting their calcium needs as a result of low calcium intake and poor calcium absorption. For those who are low in calcium, deficiency signals generated by the body up-regulate calcium absorption. Diets high in oxalates, fiber, phosphorus, and sodium can negatively affect calcium absorption. Some research has also shown that increased animal protein intake can negatively affect calcium absorption. However, the bottom line is that total calcium intake is the most critical component of the formula for ensuring a healthy body.

What is the RDA/AI for calcium?

The Recommended Dietary Allowance (RDA) for calcium for men ages 19–70 years is 1000 milligrams per day.[1] The RDA for women ages 19–50 years is 1000 milligrams per day. Daily recommendations are increased to 1200 milligrams per day for men older than 70 years and for women older than 50 years. For a complete listing of calcium recommendations across the lifespan, consult Table 7.1.

What are the functions of calcium for health and performance?

Calcium is widely recognized as a bone-strengthening mineral. However, calcium's role in health and performance extends beyond the skeleton:

- *Blood clotting:* Calcium helps to produce fibrin, the protein responsible for the structure of blood clots.
- *Nerve transmission:* Calcium is required for proper nerve function, releasing neurotransmitters that facilitate the perpetuation of nerve signals and activation.
- *Muscle contraction:* Calcium is pumped into and out of muscle cells to initiate both muscle contraction and relaxation in smooth muscle, skeletal muscle, and the heart.
- *Disease prevention and weight management:* Calcium has received more attention recently in the disease prevention arena, specifically in regard to hypertension and colon cancer. The Dietary Approaches to Stop Hypertension (DASH) study developed the DASH diet, which encourages a balanced diet focusing on calcium, magnesium, and potassium because of their role in moderating blood pressure.[3] It has been proposed that a lack of calcium leads to the excessive contraction of smooth muscle, thereby increasing pressure in blood vessels. The DASH diet recommends consuming a minimum of three servings of low-fat dairy products every day. Colon cancer research has focused on the action of calcium combining with bile salts, which are then excreted from the body, thus protecting the cells within the colon from damage. Additional benefits of calcium specific to weight loss are being researched as they relate to increased dairy and calcium intake. Some of this research suggests that the increase in calcium intake aids in body weight and body fat reduction.[4–7] More research is warranted in all of these areas to fully understand the mechanisms involved and the optimal dietary intake guidelines for disease prevention.
- *Bone and tooth formation:* Bone is living tissue, providing a framework for the human body. Bone is composed of two types of cells—osteoblasts (builders) and osteoclasts (destroyers), which are both in constant action. Osteoblasts secrete collagen, and then pull calcium and phosphorus from the blood to form a hardened material that provides the structure of bone. Osteoclasts break down the hardened material, releasing calcium and phosphorus into the blood. During growth and maturation, until peak bone mass is achieved around age 30, the building process dominates over the breakdown process. Throughout adulthood, physical activity levels and diet help to determine whether an individual is in a net state

of building or tearing down. The body adapts to stressors, strengthening in areas that are under stress. Weight-bearing exercises such as walking, running, and weightlifting can create stress that strengthens and builds bone. High calcium intakes help to sustain bone by providing the building blocks for new hardened materials. Calcium is the main component of hydroxyapatite, the solid material of bone. Because calcium is critical for many different functions in the body, if sufficient calcium is not present in the blood, it will be pulled from the reserves located in bone to normalize blood levels. This protective mechanism will ultimately weaken bones if low calcium intake is continued over time.

What are the complications of calcium deficiency?

The body can usually manipulate calcium status by increasing calcium absorption from the intestines or decreasing calcium excretion through the kidneys. Hypocalcemia, or low blood calcium, is uncommon because the body works hard to maintain a constant supply of calcium in the blood. However, in cases of malfunctioning kidneys or other disease states or disorders, it can occur. Signs and symptoms of hypocalcemia include muscle spasms and convulsions. Even though hypocalcemia is rare and occurs mainly in disease states, calcium deficiency in the general population, as well as with athletes, is still one of the most common deficiencies in the United States. The National Osteoporosis Foundation states that more than 18 million people in the United States either have **osteoporosis** or have low bone mass, putting them at high risk for developing osteoporosis in the future (www.nof.org), caused in large part by individuals consuming less than 50% of their calcium requirements daily. Signs and symptoms of calcium deficiency may include impaired muscle contractions and/or muscle cramps; however, these signs are usually rare because the body will pull reserves from bone.

osteoporosis A clinical condition that can result from inadequate calcium intake and is characterized by a significant decrease in bone mass. The result is weak bones that can be easily fractured.

If the body is constantly calcium-challenged, requiring calcium to be withdrawn from the "calcium bank" in the bones, osteoporosis will develop. Osteoporosis, the thinning and weakening of bones, is the most dramatic result of low calcium intake. A strong emphasis needs to be placed on consuming adequate calcium throughout a lifetime, with the younger years being the most influential in creating a high peak bone mass. To prevent low bone density and/or osteoporosis, the Surgeon General reports that diet and physical activity play a significant role.[8] Consuming the recommended daily intake of calcium and vitamin D and achieving at least 30–60 minutes of physical activity per day (including weight-bearing and strength training activities) are lifestyle approaches that can be started at a young age to prevent poor bone health later in life.

Osteoporosis is also one component of the *Female Athlete Triad*, which will be discussed in further detail in Chapter 11 of this text. The triad typically begins with low total calorie intake, which usually equates to low calcium intake, leading to calcium deficiency and low bone density. The lack of sufficient calorie intake on a consistent basis produces hormonal changes resulting in estrogen deficiency. This deficiency, along with other hormonal changes, low calorie intake, and high exercise energy expenditure, can lead to the cessation of menstrual cycles, or amenorrhea. The combination of low calcium intake and amenorrhea contributes to an increased risk for stress fractures, lowered bone mineral density, and potentially osteoporosis.

What are the symptoms of calcium toxicity?

The upper limit (UL) for calcium for men and women ages 19–50 is 2500 milligrams per day.[1] For men and women over the age of 50, the UL decreases to 2000 milligrams per day. Toxicity is typically not a problem with food intake but can be a concern with supplement intake. High calcium intake can impair the absorption of other minerals and in some individuals can contribute to kidney stones. Excess calcium can be deposited in organs and soft tissues and cause altered function. Very high levels of calcium can lead to cardiac arrest and death. Hypercalcemia, or high blood levels of calcium, can be caused by cancer or the overproduction of the parathyroid hormone, often signaled by fatigue, constipation, and loss of appetite.

Which foods are rich in calcium?

Dairy products, including milk, yogurt, cottage cheese, and hard cheeses, are some of the richest sources of calcium. Frozen dairy desserts also have calcium, but are higher in fat and calories than other choices. Many soy alternatives to dairy are fortified with calcium and vitamin D, and in most cases provide equivalent amounts of calcium as their dairy counterparts. Green leafy vegetables are a good source of calcium; however, oxalates present in green vegetables bind to the calcium and prevent some ab-

CALCIUM

Daily Value = 1000 mg
RDA = 1000 mg (males/females age 19–50)
      1200 mg (males 70+/females age 50+)

High: 20% DV or more	Food	Amount	Calcium
	Tofu, calcium processed	85 g (~1/3 cup)	581 mg
	Yogurt, plain, lowfat	225 g (1 8-oz container)	448 mg
	Milk, nonfat	240 ml (1 cup)	352 mg
	Milk, 2% milkfat	240 ml (1 cup)	352 mg
	Milk, 1% milkfat	240 ml (1 cup)	349 mg
	Sesame seeds, whole roasted, toasted	30 g (~1 oz)	297 mg
	Cheese, Swiss	30 g (1 oz)	237 mg
	Sardines, canned	55 g (2 oz)	210 mg
	Cheese, Cheddar	30 g (1 oz)	209 mg
Good: 10-19% DV	Molasses, blackstrap	1 tbsp	172 mg
	Cheese, mozzarella	30 g (1 oz)	151 mg
	Soybeans, cooked	90 g (~1/2 cup)	131 mg
	Collards, cooked	85 g (~1/2 cup)	119 mg
	Salmon, canned, with bones	55 g (2 oz)	117 mg
	Spinach, cooked*	85 g (~1/2 cup)	116 mg
	Turnip greens, cooked	85 g (~1/2 cup)	116 mg
	Black-eyed peas, cooked	90 g (~1/2 cup)	115 mg
	All Bran cereal	30 g (~1/2 cup)	100 mg

*In spinach, oxalate binds calcium and prevents absorption of all but about 5% of the plant's calcium.

Figure 7.1 Food sources of calcium. Calcium is found in milk and other dairy products, certain green leafy vegetables, and canned fish with bones. *Source:* U.S. Department of Agriculture, Agriculture Research Service, 2010. USDA Nutrient Database for Standard Reference, Release 23. Nutrient Data Laboratory Home Page. Available at: http://www.ars.usda.gov/Services/docs.htm?docid=8964. Accessed January 21, 2011.

sorption. Calcium-processed tofu is another option rich in both calcium and plant-based protein. Orange juices, breads, and some cereals are fortified with calcium, and in some cases provide amounts equivalent to that found in milk. Lactose-intolerant individuals can consume lactose-free products, as well as soy or rice products that are fortified, to meet their calcium needs each day. Refer to Figure 7.1 for the calcium content of specific food sources.

What is a suggestion for a calcium-rich meal or snack?

Breakfast: 1½ cups of a layered yogurt parfait including granola and berries (see **Training Table 7.1**) *Total calcium content* = 328 milligrams

Do athletes need calcium supplements?

Calcium supplementation may be indicated for some athletes who are following calorie-restrictive diets. However, the focus should be on calcium-rich foods first. If an athlete is taking calcium supplements, there are a couple things to consider:

- Amounts of calcium greater than 500 milligrams are not well absorbed when consumed at one

time; therefore, it is best to spread supplements throughout the day.

- Calcium is absorbed best when broken down first by stomach acids; calcium supplements should be taken with a small bit of food to stimulate the secretion of digestive juices.
- Calcium tablets should not be taken with other supplements because of nutrient–nutrient interactions; for example, calcium competes closely with iron and zinc, altering the absorption of all nutrients involved and potentially creating other problems.
- Not all supplements are created equal;[9] calcium carbonate supplements tend to yield the highest amount of calcium per tablet but are not as well absorbed as calcium citrate supplements. Avoid calcium supplements that are derived from oyster shells or bone meal because they may be contaminated with lead.

Why is phosphorus important to athletes?

Phosphorus is a mineral that is critical for many functions throughout the body. Because of the phosphorus-rich food supply in the United States, average intakes are well above the RDA, and deficiencies are rare. Unfortunately, Americans' more-than-adequate intake has raised concerns regarding the health complications of excessive phosphorus consumption.

What is the RDA/AI for phosphorus?

The RDA for men and women is 700 milligrams per day.[2]

Training Table 7.1: Poolside Parfait

6 oz low-fat plain yogurt
1/4 cup granola
1/2 cup fresh blueberries, raspberries, or blackberries

In a parfait cup or tall glass, layer 2 oz of yogurt, then 2 tbsp granola and 1/4 cup berries; repeat. Top with remaining yogurt. Chill before serving.

Serving Size: 1½ cups (Recipe makes one serving)

Calories: 290 kcals

Protein: 13 grams

Carbohydrate: 39 grams

Fat: 10 grams

What are the functions of phosphorus for health and performance?

Phosphorus leads to a healthy body in several ways:

- Phosphorus combines with calcium to form hydroxyapatite and calcium phosphate, which provide rigidity to bones and teeth.
- Phosphorus combines with lipids to form phospholipids, which provide integrity to cell membranes.
- Phosphorus activates and deactivates enzymes through phosphorylation.

In regard to athletic performance, phosphorus is a component of adenosine triphosphate (ATP), which provides energy for all forms of cellular function. Phosphorus is also needed for the formation of creatine phosphate (CP). In quick, explosive movements, CP provides an immediate form of energy for cells. During endurance activities, phosphorus buffers acidic end products of energy metabolism, allowing an athlete to sustain his or her effort and delay fatigue. Finally, phosphorus plays a role in energy production by phosphorylating glucose, preparing it to proceed through glycolysis.

What are the complications of phosphorus deficiency?

Because of adequate intake and widespread sources in the American diet, phosphorus deficiencies are rare. Certain disease states, hyperparathyroidism, and taking large doses of antacids (which decrease phosphorus absorption) can contribute to phosphorus deficiencies, producing symptoms such as bone malformation, bone pain, and muscle weakness.

What are the symptoms of phosphorus toxicity?

The upper limit for phosphorus is 4000 milligrams per day for adult men and women.[2] As mentioned previously, phosphorus toxicity is of much greater concern in the United States than is phosphorus deficiency. Americans consume plenty of phosphorus but not enough calcium. This intake imbalance can lead to altered calcium metabolism and an increased risk for osteoporosis.

Which foods are rich in phosphorus?

Phosphorus is found predominantly in animal proteins including meat, fish, eggs, and dairy. Nuts, legumes, and cereals are moderate sources of phos-

PHOSPHORUS

Daily Value = 1000 mg
RDA = 700 mg (males/females)

High: 20% DV or more	Cheese, provolone	85 g (3 oz)	422 mg
	Beef liver, cooked	85 g (3 oz)	355 mg
	Yogurt, plain, nonfat	225 g (8 oz)	353 mg
	Sunflower seeds	30 g (~1 oz)	347 mg
	All Bran cereal	30 g (~1/2 cup)	339 mg
	Milk, 2% milkfat	240 ml (1 cup)	275 mg
	Milk, nonfat	240 ml (1 cup)	275 mg
	Milk, 1% milkfat	240 ml (1 cup)	273 mg
	Herring, cooked	85 g (3 oz)	258 mg
	Beef, ground, extra lean, cooked	85 g (3 oz)	224 mg
Good: 10-19% DV	Chicken, white meat, cooked	85 g (3 oz)	184 mg
	Oysters, cooked	85 g (3 oz)	173 mg
	Lentils, cooked	90 g (~1/2 cup)	162 mg
	Tofu, calcium processed	85 g (~1/3 cup)	162 mg
	Chicken, dark meat, cooked	85 g (~3 oz)	152 mg
	Almonds	30 g (1 oz)	142 mg
	Black beans, cooked	90 g (~1/2 cup)	126 mg
	Soy milk	240 ml (1 cup)	120 mg
	Peanut butter	2 tbsp	106 mg

Figure 7.2 Food sources of phosphorus. Phosphorus is abundant in the U.S. food supply. Meats, legumes, nuts, dairy products, and grains tend to have more phosphorus than fruits and vegetables. Note: The DV for phosphorus is higher than the current RDA of 700 milligrams for males and females age 19 and older.
Source: U.S. Department of Agriculture, Agriculture Research Service, 2010. USDA Nutrient Database for Standard Reference, Release 23. Nutrient Data Laboratory Home Page. Available at: http://www.ars.usda.gov/Services/docs.htm?docid=8964. Accessed January 21, 2011.

phorus; however, these plant foods contain phosphorus in the form of phytic acid, which is not as well absorbed. Refer to **Figure 7.2** for the phosphorus content of specific food sources.

What is a suggestion for a phosphorus-rich meal or snack?

Summer barbeque: Grilled hamburger with cheese, 1 cup of fruit salad, and 1 cup of skim milk
Total phosphorus content = 571 milligrams

Do athletes need phosphorus supplements?

Phosphorus supplements marketed to athletes claim to prevent fatigue as a result of the buffering capacity of phosphorus. Actual research results regarding this claim are equivocal. Studies have explored the effects of sodium phosphate, potassium phosphate, or calcium phosphate on maximal oxygen uptake, anaerobic threshold, and power. Some studies have found an increase in VO$_2$max and ventilatory anaerobic threshold or a decrease in the rating of perceived exertion during submaximal exercise with supplemental phosphates.[10–12] Other investigators report no significant difference with these same parameters as well as power output with phosphate supplements.[13,14] Because a positive result of phosphate supplementation has not been clearly defined, and because long-term excessive intakes of phosphorus can be detrimental to bone health, athletes should focus on dietary intakes of phosphorus to meet daily needs for health and performance.

Why is magnesium important for athletes?

Magnesium is involved in hundreds of enzymatic reactions, bone health, blood clotting, and possibly the regulation of blood pressure. In addition to its many health-related functions, magnesium has recently been investigated for its performance-enhancing effects.[15] Recent magnesium research has focused specifically on its purported ability to prevent muscle cramps. Although its ergogenic effects are still under debate, there is no doubt that adequate daily magnesium intake is critical for overall health.

What is the RDA/AI for magnesium?

The RDA for males 19–30 years old is 400 milligrams per day; for men ages 31–70 years it is 420 milligrams daily.[2] Women require slightly less magnesium. The RDA for females 19–30 years old is 310 milligrams per day; for women ages 31–70 years it is 320 milligrams daily.[2]

What are the functions of magnesium for health and performance?

Magnesium is involved in more than 300 enzyme functions, including DNA and protein synthesis as well as proper blood clotting. Magnesium helps to maintain bone strength through its role in bone metabolism. More recently, magnesium has been highlighted as an aid in the regulation of blood pressure. Research has uncovered that magnesium, potassium, calcium, and protein, as well as the long-time villain sodium, all have an effect on blood pressure. Magnesium has an inverse relationship with blood pressure, with adequate daily intakes protecting an individual from hypertension.

In regard to sports, magnesium plays important roles in bioenergetics. It serves to stabilize the structure of ATP and improves the effectiveness with which the enzyme adenosine triphosphatase acts on ATP and thus releases energy. Magnesium is also involved in glucose and lipid metabolism. It serves as a cofactor for seven key glycolytic enzymes and thus affects both anaerobic and aerobic carbohydrate metabolism. It also plays a role in lipid and protein metabolism. Inside the mitochondria, magnesium is essential for the aerobic production of ATP via the electron transport chain. Finally, during activity, muscles rely on magnesium for proper contraction and relaxation. The important roles that magnesium plays in muscle function and bioenergetics are the driving force behind the development and marketing of sports-related supplements containing magnesium.

What are the complications of magnesium deficiency?

Magnesium deficiency has been shown to cause a variety of problems such as altered cardiovascular function, including hypertension, as well as impaired carbohydrate metabolism.[16,17] Some of the symptoms of magnesium deficiency include loss of appetite, muscle weakness, and nausea. The first signs of a deficiency usually do not surface for several months because a significant amount of magnesium is stored in the bones. If an athlete continues to consume a diet chronically low in magnesium, other symptoms such as muscle cramps, irritability, heart arrhythmias, confusion, and possibly high blood pressure will emerge. If the deficiency is left untreated, death can result.

As mentioned previously, magnesium has been connected to the regulation of blood pressure. Magnesium blocks the stimulating effect of calcium, allowing muscles, particularly in the arterioles, to relax, thereby decreasing blood pressure. Insufficient magnesium intake will allow calcium's contracting effect to dominate, and higher blood pressure will ensue.

Observation of the effect of exercise on magnesium levels in athletes is varied, and study results are equivocal. It has been suggested that prolonged or intense exercise may decrease magnesium levels as a result of increased excretion in sweat and urine as well as increased usage by the cells for energy production. A few studies have shown that levels may drop initially, but rebound to normal levels 2–24 hours postexercise.[18,19] Some researchers have found that the decrease in serum magnesium levels during long-duration exercise contributes to cramping.[20] As a result of this research, products have been developed, suggesting that increasing magnesium intake during prolonged exercise can prevent muscle cramps. However, if athletes are consuming enough calories daily, they typically will consume sufficient amounts of magnesium and therefore do not require extra supplementation during activity. Overall, few studies show a direct link between magnesium deficiency and cramping or impaired performance.[21]

What are the symptoms of magnesium toxicity?

Hypermagnesemia, or high blood levels of magnesium, is uncommon except for those with kidney diseases or malfunction. The signs and symptoms of toxic levels of magnesium include nausea, vomiting, diarrhea, and weakness. The upper limit of 350 milligrams per day refers to the maximum daily dosage of magnesium only from supplements and medicines.[2] There is no evidence of health or performance complications from high magnesium intakes from food sources.

Which foods are rich in magnesium?

Magnesium is widely distributed in foods but is concentrated in plant-based sources. Whole grains, green leafy vegetables, legumes, nuts, and seafood are all good sources of magnesium. Processing causes most of the magnesium to be leached from whole grains; therefore, athletes should incorporate whole, unprocessed grains into meals and snacks. Hard water, with a high mineral content, can also be a significant source of magnesium. Meats and dairy products provide moderate amounts of magnesium. High fiber, phosphorus, and calcium intakes, especially from supplements, can decrease magnesium absorption. If a fiber supplement is prescribed, it should be taken between meals. Refer to Figure 7.3 for the magnesium content of specific food sources.

What is a suggestion for a magnesium-rich meal or snack?

Dinner: Teriyaki tofu stir-fry (see **Training Table 7.2**)
Total magnesium content = 127 milligrams

Do athletes need magnesium supplements?

Recent studies on magnesium supplementation for athletes either are equivocal or show no benefit.[22] Some studies have shown an ergogenic benefit of magnesium potentially enhancing carbohydrate and fatty acid metabolism.[23] A study conducted by Brilla and Haley[24] tested the effects of magnesium supplements on anaerobic performance in young men after a 7-week strength training program. The supplemental group received approximately 500 milligrams of magnesium a day; after the experimental

MAGNESIUM

Daily Value = 400 mg
RDA = 400 mg (males age 19–30) 310 mg (females age 19–30)
420 mg (males age 31–70) 320 mg (females age 31–70)

High: 20% DV or more	All Bran cereal	30 g (1/2 cup)	114 mg
	Sesame seeds	30 g (~1 oz)	107 mg
	Halibut, cooked	85 g (3 oz)	91 mg
	Almonds	30 g (~1 oz)	83 mg
	Oysters, cooked	85 g (3 oz)	81 mg
Good: 10-19% DV	Cashews	30 g (~1/4 cup)	78 mg
	Soybeans, cooked	90 g (1/2 cup)	77 mg
	Spinach, raw	85 g (~3 cups)	67 mg
	Black beans, cooked	90 g (~1/2 cup)	63 mg
	Rice, brown, cooked	140 g (~3/4 cup)	60 mg
	Peanut butter	2 tbsp	56 mg
	Crab, Alaska King, cooked	85 g (3 oz)	54 mg
	Tofu, calcium processed	85 g (~1/3 cup)	49 mg
	Black-eyed peas, cooked	90 g (~1/2 cup)	47 mg
	Yogurt, plain, nonfat	225 g (1 8-oz container)	43 mg
	Whole wheat bread	50 g (2 slices)	43 mg
	Molasses, blackstrap	1 tbsp	43 mg
	Wheat bran flakes cereal	30 g (~3/4 cup)	42 mg

Figure 7.3 Food sources of magnesium. Most of the magnesium in the diet comes from plant foods such as grains, vegetables, and legumes. Note: The DV for magnesium correlates with the current RDA for males ages 19–30. The DV is higher than the current RDA of 310 and 320 milligrams for females ages 19–30 and 31–70, respectively, and lower than the current RDA of 420 milligrams for males 31–70.
Source: U.S. Department of Agriculture, Agriculture Research Service, 2010. USDA Nutrient Database for Standard Reference, Release 23. Nutrient Data Laboratory Home Page. Available at: http://www.ars.usda.gov/Services/docs.htm?docid=8964. Accessed January 21, 2011.

Training Table 7.2: Teriyaki Tofu Stir-Fry

1/3 cup uncooked brown rice

Cooking spray

1 cup broccoli

1/4 cup sliced green or red peppers

1/4 cup sliced red or yellow onions

3 oz teriyaki-marinated tofu

1–2 tbsp teriyaki sauce

Cook rice according to package directions. While the rice is cooking, coat a skillet with cooking spray. Sauté the broccoli, peppers, and onions in the skillet over medium-high heat for 5 minutes. Add the tofu and teriyaki sauce and continue to cook for 3–5 more minutes until the tofu is heated through. Serve over rice.

Serving Size: 3 cups (Recipe makes one serving)

Calories: 432 kcals

Protein: 23 grams

Carbohydrate: 65 grams

Fat: 10 grams

period, peak knee-extension torque increased more in the supplemental group versus placebo. Other studies testing subjects involved in aerobic activities have found no benefit of magnesium supplementation versus controls. Overall, research has found the greatest benefit of supplementation in those who are currently consuming low dietary levels of magnesium.[25] It has been reported that up to half of the athletic population consumes a diet containing less than the current RDA for magnesium.[26] Therefore, similar to all vitamins and minerals, if an athlete is deficient in magnesium, achieving an optimal intake may be helpful in resolving poor performance or deficiency symptoms such as muscle weakness, muscle cramps, and irritability. Athletes should focus on consuming more magnesium-rich foods versus relying on a supplement. The current volume of research is limited, and therefore recommendations for magnesium supplementation for athletes have not been established. If an athlete chooses to take a sport supplement containing magnesium, ensure that the total daily intake remains below the established upper limit by looking closely at the Supplement Facts label for the serving size and magnesium dosage.

Why is sodium important for athletes?

Sodium is a mineral that causes mixed reactions between the health and performance communities. Sodium is often called a demon to health, leading to hypertension and possibly heart disease. In the athletic world, especially for endurance sports, sodium is heralded as a life saver. So, should athletes consume more sodium or less sodium? In general, moderation is the key allowing for flexibility in recommendations based on individual needs.

What is the RDA/AI for sodium?

To function properly, the body requires only approximately 500 milligrams of sodium per day. The most current recommendation sets the AI for sodium at 1500 milligrams per day.[27]

What are the functions of sodium for health and performance?

Sodium is important for maintaining blood pressure, nerve impulse transmission, and muscle contraction. Sodium is most noted for its role in blood pressure. A consistently high intake of sodium has been directly linked to high blood pressure. Approximately one-quarter of American adults and half of those older than age 60 have high blood pressure caused in large part by intakes of sodium in excess of the recommended upper limit.[27] A lower sodium intake

has been the mantra of health professionals for many years, and it will be renewed when statistics become available in upcoming years on Americans' massive sodium consumption as compared to the new stricter DRI guidelines (current AI is 1500 milligrams; previous recommendation was 2400 milligrams).

At the other end of the spectrum, sodium is crowned as a hero for its role during exercise, and its intake is often encouraged. Sodium aids in the absorption of glucose, which makes it a key component of sports beverages designed to provide energy during exercise. Sodium also serves as one of the body's electrolytes. Electrolytes are minerals that become positively or negatively charged ions when dissolved in the fluid medium of the body. They play a role in any physiological function that requires the generation or conduction of electrical signals in the body. An example is the activation of muscle contraction via the spread of electrical activity from the nerves to the muscles. One of the most commonly occurring electrolytes in the body is sodium. The minerals chloride and potassium are other common electrolytes found in the body. Finally, sodium acts in conjunction with the minerals potassium and chloride to create concentration gradients that help maintain proper fluid balance throughout the body. Sodium is lost in sweat during exercise and if the loss is excessive, without replacement, a life-threatening condition called **hyponatremia** can result.

hyponatremia Low blood sodium levels resulting from sodium deficiency and/or the intake of large volumes of water.

What are the complications of sodium deficiency?

Sodium deficiency is not typically a problem on a daily basis because of the checks and balances of hormones regulating uptake and secretion of sodium as well as the high average daily intake. However, short-term sodium deficiency can be an issue for individuals who have prolonged diarrhea or vomiting or who are exercising for a long period of time and have excessive sweat loss. Termed hyponatremia, signs and symptoms of low blood sodium include cramping, nausea, vomiting, dizziness, seizures, coma, and—left untreated—death. Hyponatremia can also be caused by consuming only water, versus sports beverages, during long-duration exercise or by routinely avoiding foods and beverages containing sodium.

What are the symptoms of sodium toxicity?

A rapid intake of large volumes of sodium (e.g., drinking salt water) can cause hypernatremia and hypervolemia—high blood concentrations of sodium and thus high blood volume. This results in swelling and a rise in blood pressure. Most individuals can adequately regulate sodium intake and excretion through the action of aldosterone, the hormone made in the adrenal glands, signaling the kidneys to retain more sodium if intake is low. For those who cannot regulate sodium appropriately, both body fluid volume and blood pressure increase. For these individuals, a reduced-salt diet, below the upper limit of 2300 milligrams per day,[27] can be helpful in regulating blood pressure. It must be noted that sodium is only one player in the game of high blood pressure. Potassium, magnesium, protein, and fiber also have been linked to blood pressure regulation, and therefore intake of all nutrients should be addressed.

Some research also shows that high intakes of sodium may lead to increased calcium excretion, thus contributing to osteoporosis. Similar to blood pressure regulation, osteoporosis risk is increased through deficiencies of some nutrients and excessive intakes of others. Consider the whole picture when evaluating an athlete's risk for osteoporosis to avoid tunnel vision on just one nutrient.

Which foods are rich in sodium?

Sodium is widely distributed in the American diet. Table salt (1 tsp = ~2300 milligrams of sodium), soy sauce, condiments, canned foods, processed foods, fast foods, smoked meats, salted snack foods, and soups are all rich sources of sodium. Most Americans consume well above the upper limit of 2300 milligrams per day, with some intakes reaching into the 8000–11,000 milligrams per day range.[27] Refer to Figure 7.4 for the sodium content of specific food sources.

What is a suggestion for a sodium-rich meal or snack?

Lunch: Grilled cheese sandwich with 1 cup tomato soup
Total sodium content = 1391 milligrams

Do athletes need sodium supplements?

In general, sodium supplements are not required; dietary sources of sodium are more than adequate to cover daily needs as well as losses through sweat.

Food	Serving Size	Sodium (mg)
Cucumber, fresh	1 large (8¼")	6
Dill pickle	1 large (4")	1730
Roast pork	3 oz (85 g)	50
Ham, cured	3 oz (85 g)	1130
Whole wheat bread	1 slice	150
Biscuit from mix	1 (2 oz)	540
Fresh tomato	1 medium	6
Spaghetti sauce, jar	½ cup	515
2% milk	1 cup (240 mL)	115
American cheese	1 oz	420
Baked potato	1 medium	20
Potato chips	1 oz	170

As food becomes more processed, the sodium content increases

Figure 7.4 Sodium content of various foods.
Source: U.S. Department of Agriculture, Agriculture Research Service, 2010. USDA Nutrient Database for Standard Reference, Release 23. Nutrient Data Laboratory Home Page. Available at: http://www.ars.usda.gov/Services/docs.htm?docid=8964. Accessed January 21, 2011.

In activities lasting more than 4 hours, such as long-distance triathlons or adventure racing, sodium supplements may be indicated. Sodium replacement during exercise is covered in detail in Chapter 8 of this text.

Why is chloride important for athletes?

As the major extracellular anion, chloride is primarily involved in fluid balance within the body; however, it is also a key component to many other bodily functions. Chloride (Cl) is widely recognized as the partner to sodium (Na) in salt (NaCl), which in fact is the main source of chloride in the American diet.

What is the RDA/AI for chloride?

The AI for chloride for both men and women is 2300 mg per day.[27]

What are the functions of chloride for health and performance?

Chloride acts as a "disinfectant" to maintain health inside the body. Chloride combined with hydrogen forms hydrochloric acid. In the stomach, hydrochloric acid helps to kill harmful bacteria that have been consumed. White blood cells also use chloride to kill invading bacteria throughout the body. In neurons, the movement of chloride, as well as calcium, sodium, and potassium, allows for the transmission of nerve impulses throughout the body.

In regard to athletes' performance, chloride is one of the extracellular electrolytes that is critical for maintaining fluid balance throughout the body.

What are the complications of chloride deficiency?

Low chloride levels can be caused by frequent vomiting, which removes hydrochloric acid from the stomach. For example, individuals with the eating disorder bulimia can have low chloride levels in the body as a result of frequent vomiting as well as decreased intake. The result is dehydration and metabolic alkalosis, or high blood pH. Even a small rise in blood pH can result in abnormal heart rhythm, decreased blood flow to the brain, and decreased oxygen delivery to various tissues. If left untreated, chloride deficiency can ultimately result in death.

What are the symptoms of chloride toxicity?

For sensitive individuals, high intake of both sodium and chloride may cause hypertension. The upper limit for chloride has been set at 3600 milligrams per day.[27]

Which foods are rich in chloride?

Salt, or sodium chloride (NaCl), is the richest source of chloride in the American diet. Chloride can also be found in small amounts in fruits and vegetables. The dietary sources of sodium shown in Figure 7.4 provide examples of chloride-rich sources of foods as well.

What is a suggestion for a chloride-rich meal or snack?

Dinner: Meatball sub sandwich and a small bag of pretzels
Total chloride content = 3092 milligrams

Do athletes need chloride supplements?

Even though chloride is lost in sweat, athletes generally consume plenty of chloride through a balanced diet. Chloride supplements do not appear to enhance physical performance and therefore are not recommended.

Why is potassium important for athletes?

Potassium is involved in the regulation of many bodily processes, including blood pressure. The most recent dietary recommendations for potassium have increased, creating a large gap between the typical American intake and the recommended values. This gap is caused in large part by the increased consumption of processed foods in the United States, which are generally low in or devoid of potassium. All individuals, including athletes, need to put a stronger emphasis on eating potassium-rich foods on a daily basis.

What is the RDA/AI for potassium?

The most recent recommendation by the Food and Nutrition Board sets the AI for potassium at 4700 milligrams per day for men and women.[27]

What are the functions of potassium for health and performance?

Potassium and sodium perform a balancing act throughout the body. Potassium counteracts the effects of sodium on blood pressure, helping to keep blood pressure low. The interchange and flow of potassium and sodium in and out of cells are responsible for the transmission of nerve impulses and muscle contractions. Potassium is one of the intracellular electrolytes that is critical for fluid balance in the body, especially during exercise. Unfortunately, Americans are not doing a good job of balancing their intake of potassium and sodium. Sodium intakes are too high while potassium intakes are too low, leading to problems such as high blood pressure. Athletes need to make an effort to choose potassium-rich foods while keeping sodium intake under control.

What are the complications of potassium deficiency?

Hypokalemia, or low blood potassium, is caused by frequent vomiting, diarrhea, and use of diuretics, as well as low potassium intake. Athletes with high sweat losses are also at risk for potassium deficiency, which may result in muscle cramps. Common symptoms of potassium deficiency include muscle weakness and loss of appetite. A rapid change in potassium status or long-term low potassium levels can lead to heart arrhythmias.

What are the symptoms of potassium toxicity?

In healthy individuals, kidneys will excrete excess potassium and therefore no upper limit has been set for potassium.[27] However, in those with impaired kidney function, high intake of potassium (combined with low excretion) can lead to hyperkalemia. High potassium levels in the blood over time can lead to a slowing and eventual stopping of the heart.

Which foods are rich in potassium?

Fruits and vegetables are the richest sources of potassium, with potatoes, spinach, and bananas at the top of the list. Meat, milk, coffee, and tea are also significant sources. Food processing tends to remove potassium and add sodium, thereby contributing to the imbalanced intake of these two minerals. Even if potassium is not removed from a food or beverage,

POTASSIUM

Daily Value = 3500 mg
AI = 4700 mg (males/females)

High: 20% DV or more

Good: 10-19% DV

Potato, baked	110 g (1 small)	588 mg
Yogurt, plain, nonfat	225 g (1 8-oz container)	574 mg
Tomato juice	240 ml (1 cup)	556 mg
Clams, cooked	85 g (3 oz)	534 mg
Halibut, cooked	85 g (3 oz)	490 mg
Banana	140 g (1 9" banana)	487 mg
Spinach, raw	85 g (~3 cups)	474 mg
Orange juice, chilled	240 ml (1 cup)	473 mg
Lima beans, cooked	90 g (~1/2 cup)	457 mg
Milk, 1% milkfat	240 ml (1 cup)	443 mg
Baked beans, canned	130 g (~1/2 cup)	385 mg
Cantaloupe	140 g (1/4 medium melon)	374 mg
Acorn squash, cooked	85 g (~1/3 cup)	371 mg
Apricot, fresh	140 g (~ 4 apricots)	363 mg

Figure 7.5 Food sources of potassium. The best food sources of potassium are fresh fruits and vegetables, and certain dairy products and fish. Note: The DV for potassium is lower than the current RDA of 4700 milligrams for males and females age 19 and older.
Source: U.S. Department of Agriculture, Agriculture Research Service, 2010. USDA Nutrient Database for Standard Reference, Release 23. Nutrient Data Laboratory Home Page. Available at: http://www.ars.usda.gov/Services/docs.htm?docid=8964. Accessed January 21, 2011.

the addition of sodium disrupts the ratio of sodium to potassium, leading to potential health and performance complications. Refer to **Figure 7.5** for the potassium content of specific food sources.

What is a suggestion for a potassium-rich meal or snack?
Snack: Summertime Salad (see **Training Table 7.3**)
Total potassium content = 457 milligrams

Do athletes need potassium supplements?
Potassium supplements are not needed and can cause harm in large doses. For athletes, the emphasis should be placed on food sources of potassium because adequate potassium intake is easily attainable through a balanced diet. Large doses of supplemental potassium, at levels of 18,000 milligrams or higher, can disrupt muscle contraction and nerve transmission, ultimately leading to a heart attack.

Why is sulfur important for athletes?
Sulfur is unique because it is considered an essential nutrient, but it does not have an established RDA,

Estimated Average Requirement (EAR), AI, or Tolerable Upper Intake Level (UL).[27] Regardless of the lack of hard numbers, sulfur or sulfate is a nutrient that athletes should consume on a daily basis for proper bodily functioning.

What is the RDA/AI for sulfur?
There is no RDA, EAR, or AI for sulfur because of the fact that it can be obtained from food and water, as well as be derived from specific amino acids in the body.[27]

What are the functions of sulfur for health and performance?
Sulfur is a component of hundreds of compounds in the body. The body synthesizes the majority of these compounds using the sulfur consumed in the diet and from sulfur produced in the body from degradation of the amino acids methionine and cysteine. The most notable sulfur-containing compound in the body is 3-phosphoadenosine-5-phosphosulfate (PAPS). Sulfate derived from methionine and cysteine found in dietary proteins and the cysteine component of glutathione provide sulfate for use in PAPS synthesis.[27] PAPS, in turn, is then used in the biosynthesis of other essential body compounds.[27] Sulfur has also been associated with the growth and development of tissues.

In regard to athletic performance, there is no evidence that the ingestion of excess sulfur is ergogenic.

Training Table 7.3: Summertime Salad

This salad tastes best during the summer months when tomatoes are in season.

1 small tomato, diced
1/4 whole cucumber, diced
1/4 cup red onion, diced
2 tbsp light Italian dressing

Mix together the vegetables and dressing. Chill before serving.

Serving Size: 1 1/2 cups (Recipe makes one serving)

Calories: 95 kcals

Protein: 2 grams

Carbohydrate: 12 grams

Fat: 5 grams

What are the complications of sulfur deficiency?

Deficiencies of sulfur are rare, unless a protein deficiency is also present, which would include a deficiency in methionine and cysteine. Under normal conditions, it appears that adequate sulfur spares cysteine from the synthesis of PAPS, allowing cysteine to instead be used for protein synthesis and growth. When sulfur is present in suboptimal levels, cysteine is required for the production of PAPS, thus sacrificing protein synthesis.

What are the symptoms of sulfur toxicity?

There have been reports of individuals suffering from osmotic diarrhea after consuming large quantities of sulfur.[27] An association has also been suggested between high sulfur intakes and the risk of ulcerative colitis. Unfortunately, at this time there is insufficient evidence to formulate recommendations for sulfur intake, including the establishment of an UL.[27]

Which foods are rich in sulfur?

Sulfur is found in a variety of foods, with the highest concentrations found in some fruits, soy flour, certain breads, and sausages. Juices, beers, wines, and ciders also contain a significant quantity of sulfur. Drinking water is another common source of sulfur; however, quantities can vary dramatically based on the region of the country and the water source.

What is a suggestion for a sulfur-rich meal or snack?

Because no RDA/AI level has been set for sulfur, a "sulfur-rich" meal cannot be recommended. Athletes should include sulfur-containing foods on a daily basis in addition to consuming adequate levels of protein.

Do athletes need sulfur supplements?

Because an insufficient amount of information is available to even draw conclusions on an RDA, EAR, AI, or UL for sulfur, recommending sulfur supplements does not appear to be warranted at this time.

What are the trace minerals?

The trace minerals are equally as important as the major minerals. These minerals are found in smaller amounts in the body than the major minerals and

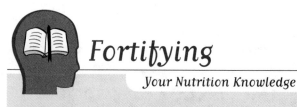

Fortifying
Your Nutrition Knowledge

What Factors Influence Iron Absorption?

The amount of iron absorbed depends on several factors:

1. *Iron status:* The body absorbs iron at the rate needed by the body. If iron stores are low, iron is shuttled into the bloodstream packaged as transferrin (see Figure 7.6), carrying iron to organs and bodily tissues. If iron stores are high, the mineral is stored in the intestinal cells, sloughed off, and excreted when cell life comes to term. Therefore, those with iron-deficiency anemia will absorb iron at a greater rate than those with normal stores.

2. *Gastrointestinal function:* Iron is absorbed in the small intestine, but it must first be prepared for optimal absorption in the stomach. The gastric acids of the stomach help to dissolve iron and convert ferric iron into ferrous iron, which is more readily absorbed through the intestines. Those with altered or malfunctioning gastrointestinal systems, for example, elderly individuals with low production of gastric acid, will have compromised iron absorption.

3. *Type of iron source—heme vs. nonheme:* Heme iron, found mainly in meat/animal products, is most readily absorbed in the body. Nonheme iron, found mainly in plant foods, is absorbed and utilized by the body, but to a lesser degree than heme iron. However, nonheme absorption can be enhanced by consuming vitamin C–rich foods or meat products with nonheme food sources.

4. *Nutrient interactions:* Dietary factors that decrease iron absorption include tannins from tea and coffee, fiber, soy, and high intakes of zinc, calcium, or manganese.

thus are termed *trace* minerals. The trace minerals include iron, zinc, chromium, fluoride, copper, manganese, iodine, molybdenum, and selenium.

Why is iron important for athletes?

Iron is critical for proper health as well as optimal performance. Iron deficiency is one of the most common nutritional deficiencies in the United States and therefore deserves special mention and attention.

What is the RDA/AI for iron?

The RDA for men ages 19–50 years and postmenopausal women is 8 milligrams per day.[28] The RDA for females ages 19–50 years is significantly higher at 18 milligrams per day.[28] The difference is caused by the monthly loss of blood for menstruating women.

What are the functions of iron for health and performance?

Iron is best known for aiding in the formation of compounds essential for transporting and utilizing oxygen; thus, it is critical for aerobic activities and endurance training. Heme is the iron-containing portion of both hemoglobin and myoglobin. Hemoglobin is a protein–iron compound in red blood cells that carries oxygen from the

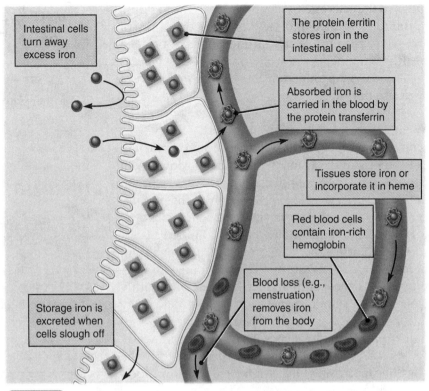

Intestinal cells turn away excess iron

The protein ferritin stores iron in the intestinal cell

Absorbed iron is carried in the blood by the protein transferrin

Tissues store iron or incorporate it in heme

Red blood cells contain iron-rich hemoglobin

Storage iron is excreted when cells slough off

Blood loss (e.g., menstruation) removes iron from the body

Figure 7.6 Iron absorption. The amount of iron absorbed depends on several factors—normal gastrointestinal function, the need for iron, the amount and kind of iron consumed, and dietary factors that enhance or inhibit iron absorption.

Fortifying

Your Nutrition Knowledge

How Is Iron Status Evaluated?

Iron status can be evaluated in several ways. The following blood test parameters are used to measure iron status (see Figure 7.6):

- *Ferritin:* Stores iron within cells; a small amount also circulates in the blood.
- *Serum iron:* Represents the free iron in the blood (small amount) and the iron bound to transferrin.
- *Serum total iron binding capacity (TIBC):* Measures the capacity of transferrin to bind to iron; as iron levels decrease, the binding capacity increases.
- *Hemoglobin:* Measures the iron-containing protein in the blood that is a component of red blood cells.
- *Hematocrit:* Determines the concentration of red blood cells in the blood.
- *Red blood cell count:* Counts the number of red blood cells in the blood, which reflects iron status because of the need for iron to produce red blood cells. The total number of red blood cells is also related to hemoglobin levels.
- *Transferrin saturation:* Transferrin is the transport protein for iron in the blood. The transferrin saturation reflects the percentage of transferrin saturated with iron.

lungs to the cells and tissues of the body. Myoglobin is found in muscle and facilitates the transport of oxygen to the muscle cells. Iron also plays a role in healthy immune function and brain development as well as energy production through its inclusion in various enzymes.

What are the complications of iron deficiency?

Iron deficiency is one of the most common nutrient deficiencies in the United States and worldwide. In contrast to many developing countries, in which iron deficiency affects a large proportion of the population (30–70%), the prevalence of iron deficiency is less than 20% in the industrialized countries of Europe and North America.[29] Iron is lost through skin, hair, sweat, and the intestinal tract. Women lose significantly more iron than men because of monthly iron losses through menstruation. Iron deficiency occurs mainly as a result of poor intake relative to daily needs. Iron deficiency occurs in three stages:

1. *Iron depletion:* Iron stores are depleted from the bone marrow, which is indicated by a low blood ferritin level.

2. *Iron-deficiency erythropoiesis:* Blood results will show a continued decline in serum ferritin and an increase in serum transferrin, while hemoglobin levels remain in the normal range. Athletes will begin to feel the effects of iron deficiency through decreased physical performance results.

3. *Iron-deficiency anemia:* Ferritin and hemoglobin levels are low, resulting in insufficient and/or defective red blood cells. The red blood cells produced are small (microcytic) and pale (hypochromic) in color, and **iron deficiency anemia** is diagnosed. Athletes will complain of cold intolerance, low energy levels, decreased performance, and exercise intolerance. Athletes will also look pale and "sickly."

iron-deficiency anemia A clinical condition commonly resulting from poor iron intake that affects the red blood cells and their ability to transport oxygen.

It is important to realize that there are several types of anemia and it is critical to diagnose the correct one to ensure that individuals receive proper treatment. Refer to **Table 7.2** for an explanation of the anemias that are caused by iron, vitamin B_6, vitamin B_{12}, and folate deficiencies.

Why are athletes at risk for iron-deficiency anemia?

Athletes are at a greater risk than the general population for iron-deficiency anemia. Beard and Tobin

TABLE 7.2	Types of Vitamin and Mineral Deficiency Anemias	
Vitamin/ Mineral	Type of Anemia	Cause of Anemia
Iron	Microcytic, hypochromic anemia	Lack of hemoglobin leads to small red blood cells that are pale in color.
Vitamin B_6	Microcytic, hypochromic anemia	Decreased production of the red blood cell's hemoglobin ring.
Vitamin B_{12}	Pernicious anemia, megaloblastic	Anemia caused by low levels of intrinsic factor, decreasing macrocytic anemia absorption of B_{12} and thus producing altered red blood cells.
Folate	Megaloblastic anemia	Impaired normal red blood cell development and division leads to large, irregular cells.

have reviewed more than two decades of research on iron status and exercise.[30] Their report states that three groups of athletes appear to be at greatest risk for developing altered body iron: female athletes, distance runners, and vegetarian athletes. In fact, similar reports state that as many as 26–60% of female athletes are affected by iron deficiency.[31–34] Due to the large number of athletes at risk, it has been suggested that these groups should pay particular attention to maintaining an adequate consumption of iron in their diets.[30] Although female athletes, distance runners, and vegetarian athletes may be at higher risk, they are not the only athletes at risk. The reasons that any athlete could be at an increased risk for iron deficiency include:

- *Low dietary intakes for both males and females:* Many athletes consume less than their daily requirements for both total calories and iron.

- *Type of food intake:* Vegetarians may be at higher risk if they do not consume enough non-heme sources of iron. Carnivores appear to be at lower risk for deficiency.

- *Increased demand for myoglobin, hemoglobin, and energy-producing enzymes:* Athletes who are training and competing regularly require more oxygen-carrying compounds and more enzymes to produce energy.

- *Type of sport:* Running and other impact sports appear to put athletes at a higher risk than nonimpact sports. Hematuria is the presence of hemoglobin or myoglobin in the urine, caused by a breakdown of red blood cells or hemolysis (releasing of hemoglobin from the kidneys) resulting from repeated impact. Hemolysis has also been observed in weight lifters because of the mechanical stress of lifting heavy weights. Nonimpact sport athletes, such as rowers or cyclists, can also experience hemolysis resulting from loss from the intestinal wall, or in urine or feces due to an irritation caused by equipment and body friction, or the consumption of nonsteroidal anti-inflammatory drugs.

■ *Loss through sweat:* This factor may have a greater impact on the iron status of males because men tend to sweat more than women.

Sports anemia is a unique condition and not a true anemia. With sports anemia, hemoglobin levels are at the low end of the normal range, but other blood parameters test normal. Short-term sports anemia can occur in individuals beginning an exercise program or initiating a period of intense training. To compensate for a sudden shift in duration or intensity of exercise, the athlete's blood volume increases quickly. This rapid change dilutes the blood concentration, which shows up on a blood test as a relatively low level of hemoglobin. After 1 to 2 months of consistent training, blood concentration returns to normal, and the sports anemia is remedied. Long-term sports anemia has been found in highly trained endurance athletes. It is theorized to occur because the red blood cells become very efficient at carrying and releasing oxygen to the tissues and therefore do not require a high level of concentration in the blood.

To prevent iron-deficiency anemia in athletes, the annual development of standard protocols for assessment and treatment of iron deficiency is recommended.[32] Several important steps in the assessment and treatment of iron deficiency anemia are presented in the following Fortifying Your Nutrition Knowledge.

What are the symptoms of iron toxicity?
The upper limit for iron is 45 milligrams per day.[28] Iron toxicity is most common in young children who consume a large number of chewable vitamins/minerals at one time. Toxicity is characterized by nausea, vomiting, diarrhea, rapid heartbeat, and dizziness. If left untreated, toxic levels of iron can lead to death within hours.

For adults, high intakes of iron have other common complications. Excessive iron can cause decreased absorption of other nutrients, such as copper. For those who are genetically predisposed,

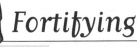

Fortifying
Your Nutrition Knowledge

Dietary Assessment and Treatment of Iron Deficiency

To properly diagnose and treat an athlete, sports dietitians should follow these steps:

1. *Consult with the athlete's physician:* Determine whether the type of anemia is caused by a lack of iron, B₆, folate, or B₁₂ in the diet; the athlete's history of anemia; and the stage of iron-deficiency anemia, if anemia is connected to low iron levels.
2. *Perform a diet analysis:* Review the following: iron intake from foods and supplements, the types of iron sources consumed (heme and/or nonheme), and dietary factors that are enhancing or inhibiting iron absorption at meals and snacks.
3. *Consider the athlete's primary sport and level of training:* Impact vs. nonimpact sport, beginner vs. experienced athlete, and recreational vs. high-volume training regimen.
4. *Inquire about other blood losses:* This could be a result of such causes as a regular blood donation.
5. *Develop a nutritional plan that will increase iron intake and availability, while being sensitive to the athlete's typical dietary patterns:* For example, vegetarians do not have to become carnivores to resolve an iron deficiency. Be sensitive to dietary beliefs and patterns and work within those boundaries, as long as the patterns are not related to disordered eating.

high iron intakes can contribute to a condition termed **hemachromatosis**. This condition causes an accumulation of iron in the liver, which can become toxic and destroy the liver over time. More recent research has shown an increased risk of colon cancer and heart disease with high iron intakes. The theory is that because iron is a pro-oxidant, it may contribute to cell damage, leading to cancerous growths in the colon, or it may accelerate the oxidization of low-density lipoprotein (LDL), leading to atherosclerosis. The exact link or mechanism still needs to be determined by future research.

Which foods are rich in iron?

There are two types of iron: heme and nonheme. Heme iron is found only in animal foods such as beef, poultry, and fish, and boasts a greater bioavailability than nonheme iron, which is primarily found in plant foods such as soy products, dried fruits, legumes, whole grains, fortified cereals, and green leafy vegetables. Nonheme iron's bioavailability can be enhanced when sources are consumed with either a meat product or a vitamin C source. For example, drinking a glass of orange juice, rich in vitamin C, at breakfast will aid in the absorption of the iron from a fortified cereal. Iron absorption can be inhibited by calcium, tannins in tea, phytic acid in grains, or excessive fiber. Therefore, foods rich in these nutrients should be present in small amounts when consuming a good source of iron. Refer to Figure 7.7 for the iron content of specific food sources.

What is a suggestion for an iron-rich meal or snack?

Dinner: 2 cups of meat and bean chili, a whole wheat dinner roll, and 2 cups of spinach salad
Total iron content = 11.3 milligrams

Do athletes need iron supplements?

If an athlete is diagnosed with iron-deficiency anemia, iron supplements are typically suggested, and normalizing iron status will improve performance and endurance. For athletes with normal iron intake and blood levels, iron supplementation will probably not enhance performance and may actually cause harm. "The use of iron supplements must be a judicious choice based on not the likelihood of anemia but, ideally, on hematologic evaluation."[30] Individual iron supplements should be taken only under the care of a physician.

Why is zinc important for athletes?

Zinc is important for every living cell in the body. After ingestion, zinc is transported bound to albumin and is delivered mainly to muscle and bone, with the remainder sent to the liver, kidneys, skin, and other organs. Once at its destination, zinc goes to work to enhance health and athletic performance.

What is the RDA/AI for zinc?

The RDA has been established at 11 milligrams per day for men and 8 milligrams per day for women.[28]

What are the functions of zinc for health and performance?

Zinc is involved in a huge variety of bodily processes and, impressively, is associated with more than 200 enzymatic systems.[35] In addition to its enzymatic role, zinc is critical for optimal health by:

- Playing a role in wound healing, which enhances immune function
- Aiding in the synthesis of RNA and DNA, thus influencing gene expression

IRON

Daily Value = 18 mg
RDA = 8 mg (males and postmenopausal females)
18 mg (females)

High: 20% DV or more

Exceptionally good source		
Clams, cooked	85 g (3 oz)	24.0 mg
Oysters, cooked	85 g (3 oz)	10.0 mg
Corn flakes cereal	30 g (~1 cup)	9.0 mg
Cheerios cereal	30 g (1 cup)	8.1 mg
Beef liver, cooked	85 g (3 oz)	5.6 mg
All Bran cereal	30 g (~1/2 cup)	4.8 mg

Good: 10-19% DV

Lentils, cooked	90 g (~1/2 cup)	3.0 mg
Shrimp, cooked	85 g (3 oz)	2.6 mg
Spinach, raw	90 g (~3 cups)	2.4 mg
Tofu, calcium processed	85 g (~1/3 cup)	2.3 mg
Lima beans, cooked	90 g (~1/2 cup)	2.2 mg
Steak, porterhouse, cooked	85 g (3 oz)	2.2 mg
Sunflower seeds	30 g (~1 oz)	2.0 mg
Turkey, dark meat, cooked	85 g (3 oz)	2.0 mg
Spaghetti, cooked	140 g (~1 cup)	2.0 mg

Figure 7.7 Food sources of iron. Iron is found in red meats, certain seafoods, vegetables, and legumes and is added to enriched grains and breakfast cereals. Note: The DV for iron is higher than the current RDA of 8 milligrams for males age 19 and older and postmenopausal females. *Source:* U.S. Department of Agriculture, Agriculture Research Service, 2010. USDA Nutrient Database for Standard Reference, Release 23. Nutrient Data Laboratory Home Page. Available at: http://www.ars.usda.gov/Services/docs.htm?docid=8964. Accessed January 21, 2011.

- Ensuring the growth and maintenance of various tissues
- Producing hormones
- Synthesizing protein
- Facilitating the proper functioning of the reproductive and gastrointestinal systems
- Maintaining proper brain function

In the area of sport performance, zinc is a component of various enzymes related to carbohydrate, protein, and fat metabolism, especially during exercise. Zinc is a critical nutrient for exercise recovery because of its role in protein synthesis and repair of tissues. Zinc also interacts with insulin and increases the affinity of hemoglobin for oxygen.

What are the complications of zinc deficiency?

Zinc deficiency is not usually an issue for those consuming adequate total calories. Athletes on calorie-restricted diets or poorly planned vegetarian diets may be at increased risk for zinc deficiency resulting from low zinc intake. Increased needs such as during growth and development, malabsorption caused by chronic iron supplementation or high dietary phytate and fiber, and increased losses by means of chronic diarrhea, diabetes, or sweat losses also contribute to low zinc levels. Zinc deficiency can lead to impaired immune function, loss of appetite, diarrhea, dermatitis, and low testosterone levels in men. Similar to iron, if the body detects a low level of zinc, it compensates by increasing the intestinal absorption of the mineral.

Research results are mixed in regard to the acute and chronic effects of exercise on zinc status. The effects vary for high-intensity, short-duration exercise as compared to lower-intensity, long-duration endurance exercise. In addition, the changes in zinc status vary depending on when the tests for zinc levels were performed. For example, immediately after short-duration, high-intensity exercise there is a reported increase in plasma zinc levels that return to baseline levels within 30 minutes after exercise.[36] In regard to endurance training, plasma zinc levels have been reported to remain unchanged in response to chronic training,[37,38] unchanged immediately after an acute bout of endurance exercise,[39] or decreased when measured within minutes or hours postexercise.[40,41] A study of 26 subjects who completed the Houston marathon showed that urinary and serum zinc concentrations measured 15 minutes after the race were unchanged from baseline data taken 2 weeks prior to the marathon.[39] In the studies reporting postexercise zinc decreases, the explanations given include

losses in sweat and urine, increased uptake by the liver and red blood cells, and/or acute inflammation resulting from the exercise. Clearly, controversy exists as to the acute effect of exercise on zinc status. Despite the fact that some studies have reported decreases in plasma zinc levels after endurance-type exercise, the decreases do not appear to lead to long-term zinc deficiencies in endurance athletes, unless athletes are following a calorically restricted diet or are vegetarians.[42,43]

What are the symptoms of zinc toxicity?

The upper limit for zinc is 40 milligrams per day.[28] This level is set based on observed reductions in copper status with intakes of zinc at levels higher than 40 milligrams per day.[28] The body is fairly efficient at excreting excess zinc; therefore, toxicity is rare through a regular diet. However, many athletes are taking zinc supplements in addition to eating zinc-rich foods in their diet. High doses in supplement form can impair iron and copper absorption, which over time may contribute to anemia. Zinc doses of approximately 100 mg per day or greater can increase LDL and decrease high-density lipoprotein (HDL), leading to increased risk for heart disease. More immediate and recognizable signs and symptoms of zinc overload are nausea and vomiting.

Which foods are rich in zinc?

Zinc-rich foods include most animal products, especially beef and other dark meats; fish, with oysters ranking at the top; eggs; whole grains; wheat germ; legumes; and dairy products. Refer to Figure 7.8 for the zinc content of specific food sources.

What is a suggestion for a zinc-rich meal or snack?

Thanksgiving leftovers: A sandwich with 3 oz dark meat turkey and 1 slice of Swiss cheese with ½ cup cranberry sauce and an 8 oz glass of skim milk
Total zinc content = 7.3 milligrams

Do athletes need zinc supplements?

In general, zinc supplements are not essential. Athletes should focus on consuming zinc-rich foods on a daily basis. For individuals who have low dietary intakes and low body stores of zinc, a short-term supplement plan may provide health and performance benefits. For those with adequate intakes and stores, supplementation may have no effect. Research on the effects of zinc supplementation on athletic performance, for those with either low or adequate intakes, is limited and equivocal. Athletes should be encouraged to avoid taking large

ZINC

Daily Value = 15 mg
RDA = 11 mg (males) 8 mg (females)

Exceptionally good source

Oysters, cooked	85 g (3 oz)	154 mg
Wheat bran flakes cereal	30 g (~3/4 cup)	15.8 mg
Crab, Alaska King, cooked	85 g (3 oz)	6.5 mg
Ground beef, extra lean, cooked	85 g (3 oz)	6.0 mg
Beef liver, cooked	85 g (3 oz)	4.5 mg
Turkey, dark meat, cooked	85 g (3 oz)	3.8 mg
Cheerios cereal	30 g (~1 cup)	3.8 mg
Steak, porterhouse, cooked	85 g (3 oz)	3.5 mg
Lobster, cooked	85 g (3 oz)	2.5 mg
Chicken, dark meat, cooked	85 g (3 oz)	2.4 mg
Ham, extra lean, cooked	85 g (3 oz)	2.4 mg
Clams, cooked	85 g (3 oz)	2.3 mg
Yogurt, plain, nonfat	225 g (1 8-oz container)	2.2 mg
All Bran cereal	30 g (~1/2 cup)	1.8 mg
Wheat germ	15 g (1/4 cup)	1.8 mg
Refried beans, canned	130 g (~1/2 cup)	1.5 mg

High: 20% DV or more

Good: 10-19% DV

Figure 7.8 Food sources of zinc. Meats, organ meats, and seafood are the best sources of zinc. Note: The DV for zinc is higher than the current RDA of 11 and 8 milligrams for males and females, respectively, age 19 and older. *Source:* U.S. Department of Agriculture, Agriculture Research Service, 2010. USDA Nutrient Database for Standard Reference, Release 23. Nutrient Data Laboratory Home Page. Available at: http://www.ars.usda.gov/Services/docs.htm?docid=8964. Accessed January 21, 2011.

quantities of supplemental zinc over a long period of time because of toxic effects and mineral–mineral interactions. Zinc supplements are often marketed for common cold prevention and remedy—a claim that is still under investigation. Many zinc supplements recommend a dose that provides several times the RDA. If taken consistently over time, these high dosages can decrease the absorption of iron and copper, leading not only to the toxic effects of zinc, but also to iron and copper deficiency issues.

Why is chromium important for athletes?

Chromium was virtually unnoticed and unheard of by the general population until it was proposed to aid in weight loss. Dietary supplements of chromium then began to fly off the shelves, only to disappoint most consumers, who found that the dream of effortless weight loss was unfulfilled. Chromium is now receiving more attention in the health maintenance and diabetes prevention arenas.

What is the RDA/AI for chromium?

The Adequate Intake level of chromium is 35 micrograms per day for men and 25 micrograms per day for women.[28] As athletes age, the recommendations are lowered.

What are the functions of chromium for health and performance?

The major function of chromium appears to be its ability to enhance the action of insulin. In other words, chromium increases the effects of insulin on the metabolism of carbohydrates, fats, and proteins. Exactly how chromium enhances insulin activity is poorly understood; however, it is does appear that chromium increases the body's tolerance to sugars through its interaction with glucose tolerance factor (GTF). GTF is a molecular complex that strengthens the interaction between insulin and its receptors on the cell membrane.[35] In addition, chromium may increase the number of insulin receptors, thus further increasing insulin sensitivity and improving type 2 diabetes. Because of the relationship between chromium and insulin sensitivity, a deficiency in chromium has been suggested to be a contributing factor in a person's risk for diabetes. Other health-related functions of chromium include a link to blood lipid levels and proper immune function.

What are the complications of chromium deficiency?

Because of its association with insulin, chromium deficiency has been proposed as one cause for high blood glucose, which in the long term may lead to type 2 diabetes. Along with decreased insulin sensitivity and high blood glucose levels, lipid abnormalities can develop. If a chromium deficiency is impairing the action of insulin, the result is altered carbohydrate and protein metabolism. Changes in macronutrient metabolism can ultimately decrease endurance performance as well as the body's ability to build and repair muscle during and after exercise.

What are the symptoms of chromium toxicity?

The absorption rate of chromium is very low. Therefore, toxicity is rare and thus no upper limit has been established.[28] One side effect of chronic high intake of chromium that has been noted is interference with iron and zinc absorption.

Which foods are rich in chromium?

Chromium is found in a unique mix of foods including mushrooms, prunes, nuts, whole grains, brewer's yeast, broccoli, wine, cheese, egg yolks, asparagus, dark chocolate, and some beers. Chromium content in foods is highly variable; therefore, current databases lack thorough information on the quantity of chromium in various dietary sources.[28]

What is a suggestion for a chromium-rich meal or snack?

Dinner: Homemade pasta primavera made with 2 cups of whole wheat pasta and ½ cup each of mushrooms, broccoli, and asparagus in a light tomato sauce sprinkled with 1 tbsp parmesan cheese
Total chromium content = ~35 micrograms

Do athletes need chromium supplements?

Small quantities of chromium have been found to be lost in sweat and urine with strenuous exercise.[44,45] However, for athletes consuming adequate total calories and chromium-rich foods, supplementation is not warranted. Athletes who are following a low-calorie diet for an extended period of time, as is often the case with wrestlers, dancers, runners, or gymnasts, should be monitored for adequate daily chromium intakes. Chromium supplements are often marketed to athletes and touted as a fat burner and muscle builder. Typically the claims focus on chromium's ability to enhance insulin action, which in theory might increase muscle anabolism and improve body composition.

A study of 20 male NCAA wrestlers assessed the use of chromium picolinate or placebo on body composition, weight, and sport performance.[46] Researchers found that 14 weeks of supplementation of chromium picolinate enhanced neither body composition nor performance variables (strength, anaerobic power, or aerobic capacity) as compared to placebo or control subjects. In another report, Vincent reviewed over a decade of human studies researching the effects of chromium picolinate and found that the supplement has not consistently demonstrated effects on the body composition of healthy individuals, even when taken in combination with an exercise program.[47]

Athletes should avoid ingesting too much chromium through supplements. Excessive chromium intake can interfere with iron and zinc absorption, creating deficiency problems.[48] Chromium also competes with iron for binding to transferrin, which could potentially decrease performance because of lower oxygen-carrying capacity.[48] The long-term effects of high doses of chromium supplementation are not fully known at this time. Some research warns that excessive chromium intake over time may cause chromosomal damage, leading to a plethora of health and performance issues.[49] In summary, chro-

mium supplements do not appear to be warranted for health or performance reasons and therefore are not recommended.

Why is fluoride important for athletes?

Fluoride is well-known for its role in the prevention of dental caries. A consistent supply of fluoride was introduced into the U.S. diet when the process of fluoridating water began in the 1940s. Fluoride is well-absorbed and is transported to bones and teeth, which contain most of the body's fluoride. More than 98% of the fluoride in the body is found in the skeleton.[35]

What is the RDA/AI for fluoride?

The Adequate Intake for adults is 4 milligrams a day for men and 3 milligrams a day for women.[1]

What are the functions of fluoride for health and performance?

Fluoride is critical for the mineralization of bones and teeth. Fluoride assists in the deposition of calcium and phosphate in bones and teeth, creating strength and stability. Although not directly involved in energy production or metabolism, fluoride is a key mineral for athletes, considering all sports require a skeleton that is sturdy and enduring. It has also been suggested that fluoride may help strengthen the resistance of interosseous ligaments or muscle tendons during dislocations and sprains and prevent tendonitis in athletes.[35]

What are the complications of fluoride deficiency?

The manifestations of fluoride deficiency are increased dental caries and compromised integrity of bone. Poor denture can lead to a variety of problems in the mouth, which can potentially alter eating patterns or types of foods consumed. Compromised bone integrity can lead to fractures, bone pain, and ultimately decreased performance.

What are the symptoms of fluoride toxicity?

The upper limit established for fluoride is 10 milligrams per day. There is a current debate on whether the U.S. population consumes fluoride in excess of this upper limit on a daily basis. Along with fluoridated water, the use of fluoride toothpaste, floss, mouthwash, and other dental products is common, and thus in theory could lead to overload. **Fluorosis** occurs when too much fluoride is consumed over a period of time, leading to discoloration and pitting of tooth enamel

fluorosis A condition resulting from the overconsumption of fluoride that can lead to pitting and discoloration of the teeth and/or bone and joint problems.

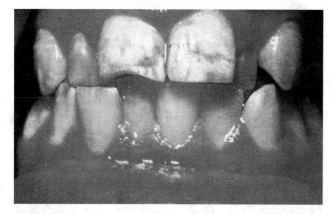

Figure 7.9 Tooth mottling in fluorosis. During tooth development, prolonged excessive fluoride intake can cause fluorosis, which discolors and damages teeth.

(see Figure 7.9), altered bone formation and fractures, chronic gastritis, and weak and stiff joints. Some claim that long-term high doses of fluoride can also contribute to a higher risk for a variety of diseases and poor health.

Which foods are rich in fluoride?

Water is the main source of dietary fluoride in the United States, containing approximately 0.7 to 2 milligrams per liter. Community water suppliers often fluoridate their water to increase the concentration of fluoride in the drinking water. However, not all water in community supplies is fluoridated, and well water varies greatly in fluoride content. Bottled water has varied amounts of fluoride, and often the fluoride content is low.[50] Teas, seafood, and foods that are prepared with water contain appreciable fluoride (see Figure 7.10).

What is a suggestion for a fluoride-rich meal or snack?

Snack: 16 oz hot black tea with a teaspoon of honey
Fluoride content = 1.6 milligrams

Do athletes need fluoride supplements?

Fluoride supplements are generally not recommended. Ingestion of fluoridated water and the topical application of fluoridated toothpaste, floss, and mouthwash are sufficient for protecting the teeth. Fluoride in drinking water is generally adequate for the proper development of bones. Short-term use of fluoride supplements under medical supervision may be appropriate for bone strength-

ening for those who have consistently low fluoride intake. Fluoride supplements are inappropriate for long-term use because of toxic effects and the lack of research data on the safety of long-term use.

Why is copper important for athletes?

Because of the rarity of deficiency complications, copper does not receive much attention. However, it does work "behind the scenes" in conjunction with other minerals to aid in optimal health and performance.

What is the RDA/AI for copper?

The RDA for men and women is 900 micrograms per day.[28]

What are the functions of copper for health and performance?

The health and performance benefits of copper are intertwined. Copper is a component of the enzyme ceruloplasmin, which is involved in iron metabolism. Copper converts ferrous iron to ferric iron, enabling iron to be transported in the blood by transferrin, thus aiding in oxygen metabolism and preventing anemia. Copper is an integral part of a variety of antioxidant enzymes, including superoxide dismutase. This enzyme, as well as other substances with antioxidant properties, helps to protect the body against free radical damage. Lysyl oxidase, another copper-dependent enzyme, is needed for the cross-linking of elastin and collagen, to ensure strength of connec-

Food or Beverage	Fluoride (mcg/100 grams)
Tea, brewed, regular	373
Tea, brewed, decaffeinated	269
Raisins	234
Crab, canned	210
Grape juice, white	210
Wine, white	202
Shrimp, canned	201
Water, bottled, Dannon Fluoride To Go	78
Water, tap, all regions (municipal and well)	71
Water, bottled, Dannon	11

Figure 7.10 Food sources of fluoride. Teas, seafood, and foods that are prepared with water contain appreciable levels of fluoride.
Source: U.S. Department of Agriculture, Agriculture Research Service, 2010. USDA Nutrient Database for Standard Reference, Release 23. Nutrient Data Laboratory Home Page. Available at: http://www.ars.usda.gov/Services/docs.htm?docid=8964. Accessed January 21, 2011.

tive tissues for cardiovascular and respiratory functions, among others.[51] Copper also participates in the electron transport chain. Copper is needed as part of cytochrome c oxidase, the terminal enzyme in electron transport and an important part of energy production.[51]

What are the complications of copper deficiency?

Copper deficiency is rare in the United States. High doses of iron and zinc can interfere with copper absorption and therefore contribute to copper deficiency problems. The signs and symptoms of copper deficiency are anemia, decreased white blood cells, and bone abnormalities. Menkes syndrome is a rare genetic disorder that involves a failure to absorb copper. Instead of being absorbed through the intestinal wall and into the bloodstream, copper accumulates in the intestinal wall and other organs. This buildup of copper can lead to neurological degeneration, abnormal connective tissue development, and low bone mass.

What are the symptoms of copper toxicity?

The upper limit for copper intake is 10,000 micrograms per day.[28] The results of copper overload are gastrointestinal distress and liver damage. Wilson's disease is a genetic disorder characterized by an excessive accumulation of copper, which leads ultimately to anemia, as well as to liver and neurological problems.

Which foods are rich in copper?

Copper is found in organ meats, seafood, nuts, seeds, wheat bran, cereals, whole grains, and cocoa products. Refer to Figure 7.11 for the copper content of specific food sources.

What is a suggestion for a copper-rich meal or snack?

Lunch: 1½ cups clam chowder, 15 wheat crackers, and 1 cup of fruit salad sprinkled with 1 tbsp sunflower seeds
Total copper content: 610 micrograms

Do athletes need copper supplements?

Because most athletes generally consume adequate levels of copper, supplements are not needed or recommended. For example, Gropper et al. studied 70 female collegiate athletes to assess copper intake as

COPPER

Daily Value = 2 mg
RDA = 900 μg (males/females)

Exceptionally good sources

Beef liver, cooked	85 g (3 oz)	12.4 mg
Oysters, cooked	85 g (3 oz)	6.4 mg
Lobster, cooked	85 g (3 oz)	1.6 mg
Crab, Alaska King, cooked	85 g (3 oz)	1.0 mg
Clams, cooked	85 g (3 oz)	0.6 mg
Sunflower seeds	30 g (~1 oz)	0.5 mg
Hazelnuts	30 g (~1 oz)	0.5 mg
Mushrooms, cooked	85 g (~½ cup)	0.4 mg
Tofu, calcium processed	85 g (~⅓ cup)	0.3 mg
Baked beans, canned	130 g (~½ cup)	0.3 mg
Navy beans, cooked	90 g (~½ cup)	0.3 mg
Soy milk	240 ml (1 cup)	0.3 mg
Peanuts	30 g (1 oz)	0.3 mg
All Bran cereal	30 g (~½ cup)	0.2 mg
Refried beans, canned	130 g (~½ cup)	0.2 mg
Cocoa, dry powder	1 tbsp	0.2 mg

High: 20% DV or more

Good: 10-19% DV

Figure 7.11 Food sources of copper. Copper is found in a limited variety of foods. The best sources are seafood, legumes, and nuts. Note: The DV for copper is higher than the current RDA of 900 micrograms for males and females age 19 and older.
Source: U.S. Department of Agriculture, Agriculture Research Service, 2010. USDA Nutrient Database for Standard Reference, Release 23. Nutrient Data Laboratory Home Page. Available at: http://www.ars.usda.gov/Services/docs. htm?docid=8964. Accessed January 21, 2011.

well as ceruloplasmin and serum copper concentrations.[51] The researchers found that copper intake, serum copper, and ceruloplasmin levels were adequate in this population.[51] In addition, high doses of copper can become toxic, leading to side effects such as nausea and vomiting.

Why is manganese important for athletes?

Manganese is not a well-known trace mineral; however, its lack of popularity and recognition is not indicative of its importance to health and performance. Manganese is unique as compared to other minerals in that it can be better absorbed through drinking water and supplements than from whole food products.

What is the RDA/AI for manganese?

The Adequate Intake for manganese is 2.3 milligrams for men and 1.8 milligrams for women daily.[28]

What are the functions of manganese for health and performance?

Manganese activates a variety of health-related enzymes that are involved in skeletal growth, protein and hemoglobin synthesis, metabolism of lipids and carbohydrates, and antioxidant functions. One of these enzymes is superoxide dismutase, which is important for its antioxidant properties. Another enzyme dependent on manganese is glutamic synthetase. Glutathione peroxidase and other antioxidant enzymes such as super-oxide dismutase, catalase, and glutathione reductase function to reduce lipid peroxidation.[23,52] Manganese is also involved in energy metabolism and fat synthesis.

What are the complications of manganese deficiency?

Manganese deficiency leads to poor growth, bone abnormalities, and impaired fat and carbohydrate metabolism. Excessive dietary iron, calcium, and phosphorus inhibit the absorption of manganese. Iron and calcium supplements should be taken between meals to avoid nutrient–nutrient interactions.

What are the symptoms of manganese toxicity?

The upper limit for manganese is 11 milligrams per day.[28] Fatigue and weakness, neurological problems, and mental confusion can all result from large intakes of manganese.

Which foods are rich in manganese?

Whole grains, legumes, green leafy vegetables, tea, and fruit are all good sources of manganese. Refer to Figure 7.12 for the manganese content of specific food sources.

What is a suggestion for a manganese-rich meal or snack?

Dinner: Sweet potato fries (see **Training Table 7.4**)
Total manganese content = 0.85 milligrams

Do athletes need manganese supplements?

Manganese supplements are neither needed nor recommended for athletes. Dietary intake from food sources and daily water intake should be adequate to meet the AI recommended for manganese.

Why is iodine important for athletes?

Iodine has the glory and recognition of being the first vitamin or mineral to be incorporated into a successful fortification program. After more than 75 years, the fortification of salt with iodine is still a success in the prevention of a variety of diseases.

What is the RDA/AI for iodine?

The RDA for iodine is 150 micrograms per day for both men and women.[28]

MANGANESE

Daily Value = 2 mg
AI = 2.3 mg (males) 1.8 mg (females)

Exceptionally good sources

Pineapple, fresh	140 g (~1 cup)	2.3 mg
All Bran cereal	30 g (~1/2 cup)	2.2 mg
Wheat germ	15 g (1/4 cup)	2.0 mg
Hazelnuts	30 g (~1 oz)	1.7 mg
Oatmeal, cooked	1 cup	1.3 mg
Whole wheat bread	50 g (2 slices)	1.2 mg
Blackberries, fresh	140 g (~1 cup)	0.9 mg
Spinach, cooked	85 g (~1/2 cup)	0.8 mg
Lima beans, cooked	90 g (~1/2 cup)	0.7 mg
Soybeans, cooked	90 g (~1/2 cup)	0.7 mg
Tea, brewed	240 ml (1 cup)	0.5 mg
Sweet potato, cooked	110 g (1 small)	0.5 mg
Baked beans, canned	130 g (~1/2 cup)	0.4 mg
Okra, cooked	85 g (~1/2 cup)	0.3 mg
Turnip greens, cooked	85 g (~1/2 cup)	0.3 mg
Beets, cooked	85 g (~1/2 cup)	0.3 mg
Broccoli, cooked	85 g (~1/2 cup)	0.2 mg
Cocoa, dry powder	1 tbsp	0.2 mg

High: 20% DV or more

Good: 10-19% DV

Figure 7.12 Food sources of manganese. Manganese is found mainly in plant foods such as grains, legumes, vegetables, and some fruits. Note: The DV for manganese is lower than the current RDA of 2.3 milligrams for males age 19 and older and higher than the current RDA of 1.8 milligrams for females age 19 and older.
Source: U.S. Department of Agriculture, Agriculture Research Service, 2010. USDA Nutrient Database for Standard Reference, Release 23. Nutrient Data Laboratory Home Page. Available at: http://www.ars.usda.gov/Services/docs.htm?docid=8964. Accessed January 21, 2011.

Training Table 7.4: Sweet Potato Fries

These fries are an excellent side dish for grilled meats and burgers.

1 medium sweet potato
1/2 tbsp olive oil
Ground pepper and garlic salt
Cooking spray

Preheat the oven to 450° F. Wash and cut the sweet potato into 1/4–1/2-in. wedges. Place the potato wedges in a large plastic bag with the 1/2 tbsp olive oil. Add ground pepper and garlic salt to taste. Close the bag and shake to mix the potato, oil, and spices thoroughly. Spray a cookie sheet with cooking spray and spread the potato wedges evenly on the sheet. Bake the potatoes for 20–30 minutes, stirring every 10 minutes to ensure even browning.

Serving Size: 1 potato (Recipe makes one serving)

Calories: 222 kcals

Protein: 4 grams

Carbohydrate: 37 grams

Fat: 7 grams

What are the functions of iodine for health and performance?

The only known role of iodine in humans is to serve as an element essential to the synthesis of hormones secreted by the thyroid gland, namely tetraiodothyronine (thyroxine, or T4) and triiodothyronine (T3). T4 and T3 are involved in the metabolism of all cells of the body during the growth process and in the development of most organs, particularly the brain.[35] Iodine is related to athletic performance through the action of the thyroid hormones, which play a role in protein synthesis in skeletal muscle, energy expenditure, weight control, and body temperature regulation. However, because of the high availability of iodized salt and its use in foods throughout the United States, iodine deficiency is very rare and thus little is known about the impact of iodine on athletic performance.

What are the complications of iodine deficiency?

goiter A clinical condition resulting from iodine deficiency. Goiter causes enlargement of the thyroid gland and results in an observable enlargement of the lower neck.

A lack of dietary iodine can lead to the development of **goiter**, or the enlargement of the thyroid gland. The lack of iodine inhibits the synthesis of the hormones T3 and T4 by the thyroid gland. As a result, the pituitary gland starts producing more thyroid-stimulating hormone in an attempt to initiate the thyroid's production of T3 and T4. The higher blood levels of thyroid-stimulating hormone cause the thyroid gland to grow. In fact, the enlargement of the thyroid can cause a sizeable increase in the outward appearance of the neck. Symptoms of iodine deficiency are similar to symptoms of hypothyroidism, including cold intolerance, weight gain, and decreased body temperature.

What are the symptoms of iodine toxicity?

The upper limit of iodine is 1100 micrograms per day.[28] Excessive iodine intake can also lead to the development of a goiter. Large intakes stimulate the thyroid to produce more hormones, thus stimulating the growth and enlargement of the gland.

Which foods are rich in iodine?

The addition of iodine to salt began in 1924 to increase Americans' intake of this mineral to prevent goiter and other related issues. Iodized salt remains one of the largest sources of dietary iodine in the United

IODINE

Daily Value = 150 µg
RDA = 150 µg (males/females)

Cod, cooked	85 g (3 oz)	99 µg
Corn grits, enriched, cooked	1 cup	68 µg
Milk, 2% milkfat	240 ml (1 cup)	56 µg
Milk, nonfat	240 ml (1 cup)	51 µg
White bread	50 g (~2 slices)	46 µg
Tortilla, flour	55 g	41 µg
Beef liver, cooked	85 g (3 oz)	36 µg
Navy beans, cooked	90 g (~1/2 cup)	35 µg
Shrimp, cooked	85 g (3 oz)	35 µg
Potato, baked	110 g (1 small)	34 µg
Turkey breast, cooked	85 g (3 oz)	34 µg
Whole wheat bread	50 g (~2 slices)	32 µg
Egg, cooked	50 g (1 large)	24 µg
Oatmeal, cooked	1 cup	16 µg

High: 20% DV or more

Good: 10-19% DV

Figure 7.13   Food sources of iodine. Few foods are rich in iodine; it is found mainly in milk, seafood, and some grain products.
Source: U.S. Department of Agriculture, Agriculture Research Service, 2010. USDA Nutrient Database for Standard Reference, Release 23. Nutrient Data Laboratory Home Page. Available at: http://www.ars.usda.gov/Services/docs.htm?docid=8964. Accessed January 21, 2011.

States, although iodine can also be found in seafood, dairy, grains, and cereals. Refer to Figure 7.13 for the iodine content of specific food sources.

What is a suggestion for an iodine-rich meal or snack?

Lunch: A turkey sandwich on whole wheat bread with lettuce and tomato and 1 cup of skim milk
Total iodine content = 105 micrograms

Do athletes need iodine supplements?

Iodine supplements are neither needed nor beneficial for athletes. Food sources are sufficient for meeting daily iodine needs.

Why is molybdenum important for athletes?

Molybdenum is often forgotten when discussing vitamins and minerals because deficiency and toxicity of molybdenum are rare. Regardless of the risk to consume too little or too much, this mineral is an important player in the game of health and performance.

What is the RDA/AI for molybdenum?

The RDA for men and women is 45 micrograms per day.[28]

What are the functions of molybdenum for health and performance?

Molybdenum is an essential trace element needed by virtually all life forms. In humans, molybdenum is known to function as a cofactor for three enzymes.

Two of the enzymes play a role in serving as antioxidants and detoxifying agents in the body. The third enzyme, sulfite oxidase, catalyzes a reaction that is necessary for the metabolism of sulfur-containing amino acids, such as cysteine. Only sulfite oxidase is known to be crucial for human health.[53]

What are the complications of molybdenum deficiency?

Health complications or consequences of low molybdenum intake have not been observed in humans when consuming an adequate diet.[28] The only documented case of acquired molybdenum deficiency occurred in a patient with Crohn's disease on long-term total intravenous nutrition that was not supplemented with molybdenum.[54] Current understanding of the essentiality of molybdenum in humans is based largely on the study of individuals with very rare inborn errors of metabolism and therefore offer little in regard to application for sports nutrition.

What are the symptoms of molybdenum toxicity?

Molybdenum toxicity is rare. The upper limit has been established at 2000 micrograms per day because large quantities can interfere with copper absorption.[28]

Which foods are rich in molybdenum?

Molybdenum is found mainly in plant products such as cereals, whole grains, and legumes. The molybdenum content of plant foods varies depending upon the soil content in which they are grown.[28] Organ meats are the richest source of molybdenum in animal products. Because the methods for analyzing the molybdenum content of foods are not reliable, specific food content information is limited.

What is a suggestion for a molybdenum-rich meal or snack?

Breakfast: 2 cups bran flakes with 12 oz skim milk and a banana
Total molybdenum content = ~17 micrograms

Do athletes need molybdenum supplements?

Molybdenum supplements are neither needed nor beneficial for athletes. Food sources of molybdenum are sufficient, and the usual intake of molybdenum is well above the dietary molybdenum requirement.[28]

Why is selenium important for athletes?

Selenium has only recently received recognition in the nutrition community as an essential nutrient. The connection between human health and selenium intake was made in 1979 after scientists discovered that Keshan disease could be prevented by providing children in China with selenium supplements. Since then, selenium has quickly climbed the ranks of nutritional importance to become a member of the highly regarded antioxidant category of nutrients.

What is the RDA/AI for selenium?

The RDA for selenium is 55 micrograms for both men and women.[55]

What are the functions of selenium for health and performance?

Selenium's role for overall health is closely related to its potential ergogenic effects on athletic performance. Selenium is a component of many bodily proteins, with the selenoproteins being the most notable. Selenocysteine is the selenium form associated with glutathione peroxidase, an antioxidant enzyme that helps to combat free radical damage to cells. Through this breakdown of free radicals, glutathione peroxidase actually helps to spare vitamin E, allowing the vitamin to continue on its free radical scavenger hunt. In other words, selenium and vitamin E work synergistically to quench more free radicals than either nutrient could on its own. Current exercise research has delved into the selenium/antioxidant world, aiming to determine the effects of selenium on exercise-induced free radical formation. For more details about free radicals, antioxidants, and their relationship to exercise performance, refer to the section "What vitamins or compounds have antioxidant properties?" in Chapter 6 of this text.

Selenium-associated enzymes have also been linked to proper thyroid and immune function, as well as to the healthy development of fetuses. Selenium's role in immune function has led to cancer risk reduction claims. In general, selenium research is still in its infancy, with all roles, mechanisms, and health/performance effects still under investigation.

What are the complications of selenium deficiency?

Selenium deficiency is rare in the United States and other industrialized nations because of our geographically diverse food supply. The origin of foods is important because the selenium concentration in soil can vary dramatically around the world. If individuals live in a selenium-deficient area and consume only locally grown foods, a selenium deficiency can result. For example, in areas of China with selenium-poor soil, selenium-deficient residents are more susceptible to a form of viral cardiomyopathy called Keshan disease.

SELENIUM

Daily Value = 70 μg
RDA = 55 μg (males/females)

High: 20% DV or more	Oysters, cooked	85 g (3 oz)	60.9 μg
	Tuna, canned	55 g (2 oz)	44.2 μg
	Lobster, cooked	85 g (3 oz)	36.3 μg
	Pork, loin, cooked, lean only	85 g (~3 oz)	36.0 μg
	Shrimp, cooked	85 g (3 oz)	33.7 μg
	Beef liver, cooked	85 g (3 oz)	30.7 μg
	Spaghetti, cooked	140 g (~1 cup)	29.8 μg
	Whole-wheat bread	50 g (2 slices)	18.3 μg
	Egg, hard cooked	50 g (1 large)	15.4 μg
	Oatmeal, cooked	1 cup	11.9 μg
Good: 10-19% DV	Rice, brown, cooked	140 g (~3/4 cup)	13.7 μg
	Rice, white, enriched, cooked	140 g (~3/4 cup)	10.5 μg
	Cheerios cereal	30 g (1 cup)	10.4 μg
	Cheese, cottage	110 g (~1/2 cup)	9.9 μg
	White bread	50 g (2 slices)	8.7 μg
	Grits, corn, enriched, cooked	1 cup	7.5 μg

Figure 7.14 Food sources of selenium. Selenium is found mainly in meats, organ meats, seafood, and grains. Note: The DV for selenium is higher than the current RDA of 55 micrograms for males and females age 19 and older.
Source: U.S. Department of Agriculture, Agriculture Research Service, 2010. USDA Nutrient Database for Standard Reference, Release 23. Nutrient Data Laboratory Home Page. Available at: http://www.ars.usda.gov/Services/docs.htm?docid=8964. Accessed January 21, 2011.

gaining the performance edge

The trace minerals include iron, zinc, chromium, fluoride, copper, manganese, iodine, molybdenum, and selenium. Each of these minerals plays a specific and important role in overall health and athletic performance. Athletes should strive to consume these nutrients from whole foods first, and rely on supplements only when individually indicated.

Selenium has recently been recognized as an antioxidant mineral, raising questions about the effects of suboptimal intake on cardiovascular parameters and cancer risk. Although it appears that selenium may have a role in these areas, the exact functions, associated mechanisms, and anticipated results of selenium deficiency related to cardiovascular disease and cancer are still under investigation.

What are the symptoms of selenium toxicity?
The upper limit for selenium has been established at 400 micrograms per day.[55] Consumption of selenium in excess of the upper limit can cause brittle hair and nails; if toxic levels continue to be consumed, the loss of hair and nails can occur.

Which foods are rich in selenium?
Selenium is mainly found in animal products, with seafood ranking near the top of the list. Plant foods contain selenium; however, content can vary dramatically based on the selenium concentration of the soil within the region it was grown. Refer to Figure 7.14 for the selenium content of specific food sources.

What is a suggestion for a selenium-rich meal or snack?
Dinner: Shrimp stir-fry with 3 oz of shrimp, 1 cup of mixed vegetables, and 1 cup of cooked brown rice
Total selenium content = 45 micrograms

Do athletes need selenium supplements?
Research on the ergogenic benefits of selenium supplements is still in its infancy. Some research has shown that the antioxidant status of athletes participating in intense training diminishes, leading to the proposal that selenium and other antioxidant supplements may be warranted.[56,57] However, because it is relatively easy to consume adequate amounts of selenium in a well-balanced diet, and because of its toxic effects, selenium supplements are not recommended at this time. Once more information is available, these recommendations may change.

Are other trace minerals important for athletes?
The previous sections have discussed the well-known trace minerals; however, there are a few more that were not discussed. These trace minerals are summarized in **Table 7.3** and **Table 7.4**.

TABLE 7.3	Review of Other Trace Minerals			
Mineral	**RDA/AI for Adults ages 19–50**	**Functions for Health/ Performance**	**Upper Limit**	**Toxicity Complications**
Arsenic	Not determinable	No biological function determined for humans; animal data suggest a requirement.	Not determinable	No adverse effects shown for organic arsenic. Inorganic arsenic known as a toxic substance.
Boron	Not determinable	No biological function determined for humans; animal data suggest a requirement.	20 mg per day	Animal studies reveal reproductive and developmental effects.
Nickel	Not determinable	No biological function determined for humans; animal data suggest a requirement.	1.0 mg per day	Animal studies have observed decreased body weight gain.
Silicon	Not determinable	No biological function determined for humans; animal data suggest it contributes to adverse health effects.	Not determinable	Naturally occurring silicon in foods and water does not appear to be a requirement.
Vanadium	Not determinable	No biological function determined for humans.	1.8 mg per day	Animal studies have observed renal lesions as a result of high intakes.

TABLE 7.4	Food Sources for Other Trace Minerals	
Mineral	**Food Sources**	**Supplements Needed for Athletes?**
Arsenic	Dairy products, meats, fish, grains, and cereals	No. Currently there is no justification for addition of arsenic to the diet.
Boron	Fruit-based beverages, potatoes, legumes, milk, avocados, and peanuts	No. Currently there is no justification for addition of boron to the diet.
Nickel	Nuts, legumes, cereals, sweeteners, and chocolate powders and candies	No. Currently there is no justification for addition of nickel to the diet.
Silicon	Plant-based foods	No. Currently there is no justification for addition of silicon to the diet.
Vanadium	Mushrooms, shellfish, black pepper, parsley, and dill seed	No. Currently there is no justification for addition of vanadium to the diet.

Key Points of Chapter

- Minerals are inorganic nutrients that are essential for normal body functioning.

- Minerals are needed in very small quantities relative to other nutrients because they are structurally very stable and they can be repeatedly used in the body without breakdown. Dietary intake of minerals from foods can lead to a toxic buildup; however, most toxicity is caused by ingesting high-dosage supplements.

- Minerals are classified as either major minerals or trace minerals. Major minerals are those needed by the body in amounts greater than 100 milligrams per day. Trace minerals are those required in daily quantities of less than 100 milligrams.

- Calcium, phosphorus, magnesium, sodium, chloride, potassium, and sulfur constitute the major minerals. The trace minerals include iron, zinc, chromium, fluoride, copper, manganese, iodine, molybdenum, and selenium.

- Calcium is not only required for ensuring healthy, strong bones, but is also important in blood clotting, nerve transmission, and muscle contraction. Adequate intake is approximately 1000 milligrams per day for those 19 to 50 years of age.

- Phosphorus, similar to calcium, is also important for strong bones, and in addition is an integral part of cell membranes and plays a role in enzyme activation. The RDA for phosphorus is 700 milligrams per day, which is easily achieved in the typical American diet.

- Magnesium plays a role in the regulation of blood pressure, is critical for the proper functioning of many cellular enzymes, and is important for bone formation. The RDA for magnesium ranges from 310 to 420 milligrams per day, and supplementation with higher doses has not shown any ergogenic effects in athletes.

- Sodium and potassium are important for maintaining blood pressure, nerve impulse transmission, and muscle contraction. The AI for sodium and potassium is 1500 and 4700 milligrams per day, respectively. Athletes need to make an effort to curb sodium intake and increase potassium consumption to prevent complications such as increases in blood pressure, muscle weakness, and heart arrhythmias.

- Chloride has roles in the body's immune system, digestion of food, and nerve transmission. The AI of 2300 milligrams per day is usually met with diet alone via salted foods.

- Sulfur plays a key role in normal growth and development; however, it does not have an established RDA or AI. Sulfur is found in a variety of foods, and deficiencies are rare.

- The trace mineral iron plays an essential role in the transport and utilization of oxygen throughout the body. Deficiencies do occur in athletes, resulting in anemia; however, universal use of iron supplementation for all athletes is not warranted.

- Zinc is a trace mineral that serves as a cofactor for various enzymes involved in carbohydrate, protein, and fat metabolism during exercise. It also makes an important contribution to recovery because of its role in protein synthesis and repair of tissues. Fortunately, zinc deficiencies are rare in athletes consuming adequate total calories.

- Chromium is a trace mineral touted to increase insulin activity and thus enhance glucose uptake and protein assimilation. As a result, it was speculated that chromium supplementation would increase muscle mass and decrease fat mass. Current research into the effectiveness of chromium supplementation has not supported these claims.

- Fluoride is critical for the mineralization of bones and teeth. Although not directly involved in energy production or metabolism, fluoride is important to athletes, considering all sports require a skeleton and connective tissues that are strong and resilient.

- Copper, iodine, manganese, selenium, and molybdenum are trace minerals in which deficiencies are very rare. Although they play critical roles related to enzyme activity, hormone function, and/or free radical neutralization, their effects on athletic performance are relatively unstudied and/or inconclusive. Supplementation of these trace minerals is not warranted.

- Despite the important roles trace minerals play in the body, the small daily requirements are usually met by the typical American diet. As a result, trace mineral supplementation in excess of that provided by diet alone is not recommended and has not been shown to have any ergogenic effects on athletic performance.

Study Questions

1. What role do minerals play in the body?

2. What are the major minerals? What differentiates a major mineral from a trace mineral?

3. What are some of the common food sources for each of the major minerals?

4. Discuss the various conditions that result as a consequence of deficiencies in the major minerals.

5. Should athletes take supplements containing large doses of the major minerals? Defend your answer based on the benefits versus the risks.

6. What role does the trace mineral iodine play in the body? What condition results from iodine deficiency? Why is this condition very rare in the United States?

7. Besides iodine, list four other trace minerals, discuss their role in the body, and give specific foods that serve as good sources for each.

References

1. Institute of Medicine. *Dietary Reference Intakes for Calcium and Vitamin D.* Food and Nutrition Board. Washington, DC: National Academies Press; 2010.

2. Institute of Medicine. *Dietary Reference Intakes for Calcium, Phosphorus, Magnesium, Vitamin D, and Fluoride.* Food and Nutrition Board. Washington, DC: National Academies Press; 1997.

3. Zemel MB. Dietary patterns and hypertension: The DASH Study. *Nutr Rev.* 1997;55:303–305.

4. Heaney RP, Davies KM, Barger-Lux MJ. Calcium and weight: clinical studies. *J Am Coll Nutr.* 2002;21(2):152S–155S.

5. Teegarden D. Calcium intake and reduction in weight or fat mass. *J Nutr.* 2003;133(1):249S–251S.

6. Parikh SJ, Yanovski JA. Calcium intake and adiposity. *Am J Clin Nutr.* 2003;77(2):281–287.

7. Zemel MB. Role of calcium and dairy products in energy partitioning and weight management. *Am J Clin Nutr.* 2004;79(5):907S–912S.

8. U.S. Department of Health and Human Services. *Bone Health and Osteoporosis: A Report of the Surgeon General.* Rockville, MD: U.S. Department of Health and Human Services, Office of the Surgeon General; 2004.

9. Levenson DI, Bockman RS. A review of calcium preparations. *Nutr Rev.* 1994;52(7):221–232.

10. Goss F, Robertson R, Riechman S, et al. Effect of potassium phosphate supplementation on perceptual and physiological responses to maximal graded exercise. *Int J Sports Nutr Exerc Metabol.* 2001;11(1):53–62.

11. Kreider RB, Miller GW, Williams MH, Somma CT, Nasser T. Effects of phosphate loading on oxygen uptake, ventilatory aerobic threshold and run performance. *Med Sci Sports Exerc.* 1990;22:250–255.

12. Kreider RB, Miller GW, Schenck D, et al. Effects of phosphate loading on metabolic and myocardial responses to maximal and endurance exercise. *Int J Sports Nutr.* 1992;2:20–47.

13. Duffy D, Conlee R. Effects of phosphate loading on leg power and high intensity treadmill exercise. *Med Sci Sports Exerc.* 1986;18:674–677.

14. Bredle D, Stager J, Brechue W, Farber M. Phosphate supplementation, cardiovascular function and exercise performance in humans. *J Appl Physiol.* 1988;65:1821–1826.

15. Golf S, Bohmer D, Nowacki P. *Is Magnesium a Limiting Factor in Competitive Exercise? A Summary of Relevant Scientific Data.* London: John Libbey & Company; 1994.

16. Nadler J, Buchanan T, Natarajan R, Antonipillai I, Bergman R, Rude R. Magnesium deficiency produces insulin resistance and increased thromboxane synthesis. *Hypertens.* 1993;21:1024–1029.

17. Lukaski H, Nielsen F. Dietary magnesium depletion affects metabolic responses during submaximal exercise in postmenopausal women. *J Nutr.* 2002;132(5):930–935.

18. Deuster P, Dolev E, Kyle S, Anderson R. Magnesium homeostasis during high intensity anaerobic exercise. *J Appl Physiol.* 1987;62:545–550.

19. Stendig-Lindberg G, Shapiro Y, Epstein Y. Changes in serum magnesium concentration after strenuous exercise. *J Am Coll Nutr.* 1988;6:35–40.

20. Williamson S, Johnson R, Hudkins P, Strate S. Exertional cramps: a prospective study of biochemical and anthropometric variables in bicycle riders. *Cycling Sc.* 1993;15:20.

21. Clarkson P, Haymes E. Exercise and mineral status of athletes: calcium, magnesium, phosphorus and iron. *Med Sci Sports Exerc.* 1995;27:831–843.

22. Finstad EW, Newhouse IJ, Lukaski HC, McAuliffe JE, Stewart CR. The effect of magnesium supplementation on exercise performance. *Med Sci Sports Exerc.* 2001;33(3):493–498.

23. Clarkson PM. Micronutrients and exercise: anti-oxidants and minerals. *J Sports Sci.* 1995;13:S11–S24.

24. Brilla LR, Haley TF. Effect of magnesium supplementation on strength training in humans. *J Am Coll Nutr.* 1992;11(3):326–329.

25. Lukaski H. Magnesium, zinc and chromium nutriture and physical activity. *Am J Clin Nutr.* 2000;72(2 suppl):585S–593S.

26. Seeling MS. Consequences of magnesium deficiency on the enhancement of stress reactions: preventive and therapeutic implications (a review). *J Am Col Nutr.* 1994;13:492–446.

27. Institute of Medicine. *Dietary Reference Intakes for Water, Potassium, Sodium, Chloride and Sulfate.* Food and Nutrition Board. Washington, DC: National Academies Press; 2004.

28. Institute of Medicine. *Dietary Reference Intakes for Vitamin A, Vitamin K, Arsenic, Boron, Chromium, Copper, Iodine, Iron, Manganese, Molybdenum, Nickel, Silicon, Vanadium and Zinc.* Food and Nutrition Board. Washington, DC: National Academies Press; 2001.

29. World Health Organization. WHO Global Database on Anemia and Iron Deficiency 2000. Available at: http://www.who.int/vmnis/database/anaemia/anaemia_data_status_prevalence/en/index.html. Accessed March 2, 2011

30. Beard J, Tobin B. Iron status and exercise. *Am J Clin Nutr.* 2000;72(2 suppl):594S–597S.

31. Constantini NW, Eliakim A, Zigel L, Yaaron M, Falk B. Iron status of highly active adolescents: evidence of depleted iron stores in gymnasts. *Int J Sports Nutr Exerc Metabol.* 2000;10(1):62–70.

32. Cowell BS, Rosenbloom CA, Skinner R, Summers RH. Policies on screening female athletes for iron deficiency in NCAA division I-A institutions. *Int J Sports Nutr Exerc Metabol*. 2003;13(3):277–285.

33. Malczewska J, Szczepanska B, Stupnicki R, Sendecki W. The assessment of frequency of iron deficiency in athletes from the transferring receptor-ferritin index. *Int J Sports Nutr Exerc Metabol*. 2001;11(1):42–52.

34. Dubnov G, Constantini NW. Prevalence of iron depletion and anemia in top-level basketball players. *Int J Sports Nutr Exerc Metabol*. 2004;14(1):30–37.

35. Speich M, Pineau A, Ballereau F. Minerals, trace elements and related biological variables in athletes and during physical activity. *Clinica Chimica Acta*. 2001;312(1–2): 1–11.

36. Ohno H, Yamashita K, Doi R, Yamamura K, Kondo T, Taniguchi N. Exercise-induced changes in blood zinc and related proteins in humans. *J Appl Physiol*. 1985;58: 1453–1458.

37. Singh A, Evans P, Gallagher KL, Deuster PA. Dietary intakes and biochemical profiles of nutritional status of ultramarathoners. *Med Sci Sports Exerc*. 1993;25: 328–334.

38. Fogelholm GM, Himberg J, Alopaeus K, Gref C, Laakso JT, Mussalo-Rauhamaa H. Dietary and biochemical indices of nutritional status in male athletes and controls. *J Am Coll Nutr*. 1992;11:181–191.

39. Buchman AL, Keen C, Commisso J, et al. The effect of a marathon run on plasma and urine mineral and metal concentrations. *J Am Coll Nutr*. 1998;17(2):124–127.

40. Anderson RA, Polansky MM, Bryden NA. Strenuous running: acute effects on chromium, copper, zinc, and selected clinical variables in urine and serum of male runners. *Biol Trace Element Res*. 1984;6:327–336.

41. Van Rij AM, Hall MT, Dohm GL, Bray J, Pories WJ. Change in zinc metabolism following exercise in human subjects. *Biol Trace Element Res*. 1986;10:99–106.

42. Dressendorfer RH, Sockolov R. Hypozincemia in athletes. *Physician Sports Med*. 1980;8:97–100.

43. Haralambie G. Serum zinc in athletes in training. *Int J Sports Med*. 1981;2:136–138.

44. Anderson RA, Polansky MM, Bryden NA, Roginski EE, Patterson KY, Reamer DC. Effect of exercise (running) on serum glucose, insulin, glucagon, and chromium excretion. *Diabetes*. 1982;31:212–216.

45. Anderson RA, Bryden NA, Polansky MM, Thorp JW. Effects of carbohydrate loading and underwater exercise on circulating cortisol, insulin and urinary losses of chromium and zinc. *Eur J Appl Physiol*. 1991;63:146–150.

46. Walker LS, Bemben MG, Bemben DA, Knehans AW. Chromium picolinate effects on body composition and muscular performance in wrestlers. *Med Sci Sports Exerc*. 1998;30(12):1730–1737.

47. Vincent JB. The potential value and toxicity of chromium picolinate as a nutritional supplement, weight loss agent and muscle development agent. *Sports Med*. 2003; 33(3):213–230.

48. Lukaski HC, Bolonchuk WW, Siders WA, Milne DB. Chromium supplementation and resistance training: effects on body composition, strength and trace element status of men. *Am J Clin Nutr*. 1996;63:954–965.

49. Stearns DM, Belbruno JJ, Wetterhahn KE. A prediction of chromium (III) accumulation in humans from chromium dietary supplements. *FASEB J*. 1995;9:1650–1657.

50. McGuire S. Fluoride content of bottled water. *N Engl J Med*. 1989;321(12):836–837.

51. Gropper SS, Sorrels LM, Blessing D. Copper status of collegiate female athletes involved in different sports. *Int J Sports Nutr Exerc Metabol*. 2003;13(3):343–357.

52. Clarkson PM, Thompson HS. Antioxidants: what role do they play in physical activity and health? *Am J Clin Nutr*. 2000;72(2 suppl):637S–646S.

53. Nielsen FH. Ultratrace minerals. In: Shils M, Olson JA, Shike M, Ross AC, eds. *Nutrition in Health and Disease*. 9th ed. Baltimore, MD: Williams & Wilkins; 1999:283–303.

54. Abumrad NN, Schneider AJ, Steel D, Rogers LS. Amino acid intolerance during prolonged total parenteral nutrition reversed by molybdate therapy. *Am J Clin Nutr*. 1981;34(11):2551–2559.

55. Institute of Medicine. *Dietary Reference Intakes for Vitamin C, Vitamin E, Selenium and Carotenoids*. Food and Nutrition Board. Washington, DC: National Academies Press; 2000.

56. Bloomer RJ, Goldvarb AH, McKenzie MJ, You T, Nguyen L. Effects of antioxidant therapy in women exposed to eccentric exercise. *Int J Sports Nutr Exerc Metabol*. 2004;14:377–388.

57. Subudhi AW, Davis SL, Kipp RW, Askew EW. Antioxidant status and oxidative stress in elite alpine ski racers. *Int J Sports Nutr Exerc Metabol*. 2001;11:32–41.

Additional Resources

Chan S, Gerson B, Subramaniam S. The role of copper, molybdenum, selenium, and zinc in nutrition and health. *Clin Lab Med*. 1998;118(4):673–685.

Dressendorfer RH, Peterson SR, Moss-Lovshin SE, Keen CL. Mineral metabolism in male cyclists during high-intensity endurance training. *Int J Sports Nutr Exerc Metabol*. 2002;12(1):63–72.

Finstad EW, Newhouse IJ, Lukaski HC, McAuliffee JE, Stewart CR. The effects of magnesium supplementation on exercise performance. *Med Sci Sports Exerc*. 2001;33:493–498.

Golf SW, Happel O, Graef V. Plasma aldosterone, cortisol and electrolyte concentrations in physical exercise after magnesium supplementation. *J Clin Biochem*. 1984;22:717–721.

Water

Chad is a collegiate lacrosse player in Arizona. During preseason and in-season training, the team will practice for hours, often in 80–90 degree weather. The coach incorporates fluid breaks during practice; however, he allows the athletes to consume only water. The coach believes that sports beverages hinder performance and therefore forbids the athletes to consume them. The athletes complain of feeling fatigued, lethargic, and light-headed by the end of practices.

Questions

- What are the problems in this scenario?
- What should the athletes do to feel better throughout the duration of their practices?

What's the big deal about water?

Water is arguably the most essential of all the nutrients for athletes despite the fact that it does not provide the body with energy. Death occurs more rapidly in the absence of water than in the absence of any other nutrient. Water restriction can result in death in as little as 3 days. Armed with this knowledge, it doesn't take much imagination to realize the consequences of dehydration on training and/or sport performance.

The phrase "you are what you eat" should be reworded to "you are what you drink." Roughly 55–60% of the average human's body weight is water. Two-thirds of body water is found inside the cells and is referred to as **intracellular water**. Muscle tissue, which is of obvious importance to athletes, is approximately 70% water. This is just another reason why water is so critical to sport performance. The remaining one-third of body water is found outside of cells and is known as **extracellular water**. Most of the extracellular water is found in the spaces between cells, in lymph, and in blood plasma. Intracellular and extracellular water content vary based on several factors:

intracellular water Body water that is found inside the cells. Approximately 66% of the total amount of water in the body is located inside the cells.

extracellular water Body water that is found outside of cells that make up the various tissues of the body. Examples of extracellular water are saliva, blood plasma, lymph, and any other watery fluids found in the body.

- *Protein content of tissues:* Muscle, composed of a large amount of protein, contains a much greater percentage of water than adipose tissue, which is composed of fats. The percentage of total body water can vary tremendously from a lean, muscular athlete with a low body fat composition to an obese, sedentary individual with a high body fat composition.
- *Carbohydrate content of tissues:* Glycogen consists of linked glucose molecules and is stored inside cells along with water. For every gram of glycogen, 3 grams of water are stored. The water released from glycogen breakdown during exercise can be useful for preventing dehydration.
- *Electrolyte concentration within and outside cells:* Intracellular and extracellular minerals such as sodium, chloride, potassium, and calcium affect the flux of fluid into and out of cells.

Large fluctuations in body water storage can contribute to a variety of health concerns as well as poor physical performance in sports. Balancing daily fluid losses with intake is critical in preventing the ill effects of dehydration, as well as overhydration.

What are the functions of water in the body?

As stated earlier, water does not provide the body with energy (i.e., calories) but it is second only to oxygen in regard to its importance for maintaining life (see Figure 8.1). In addition to providing structural integrity to cells, water serves as the body's delivery and waste removal medium. Blood plasma distributes nutrients, hormones, immune cells, and oxygen, just to name a few items, to the billions of cells that make up the tissues of our bodies. In addition, the blood carries away from the cells substances such as carbon dioxide, lactic acid, and ammonia that are formed during the breakdown of nutrients for cellular energy.

The watery environment of the body's tissues serves as a reactive medium. Water is often a product or reactant in many of the chemical reactions that occur in the body. For example, one of the end products of aerobic metabolism is water. Water also serves as the solvent for many essential molecules such as glucose, certain vitamins, minerals, proteins, and enzymes.

Body water also helps in maintaining a stable body temperature. Water has excellent conductive properties and helps move warm temperatures from the core of the body to the periphery. In fact, water conducts heat 26 times faster than air. Body water also serves as the source for sweat that is produced by specialized glands called **sweat glands**. The sweat is

sweat glands Specialized glands located in the deep layer of the skin responsible for the production of sweat and its delivery to the surface of the skin for the purpose of evaporative cooling.

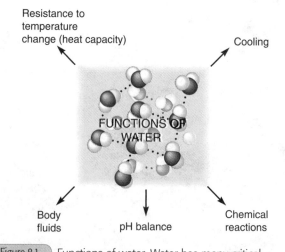

Figure 8.1 Functions of water. Water has many critical functions in the body.

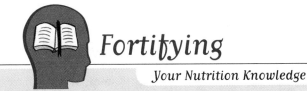

Fortifying

Your Nutrition Knowledge

How Should Athletes Dress for Exercise in the Heat?

When exercising in the heat, it is critical that the clothing worn be functional, not fashionable. The body relies on four processes to cool itself: conduction, convection, radiation, and evaporation. *Conduction* is the transfer of heat from one object to another by direct contact; for example, heat is lost via conduction when a cold water bottle is placed on the skin of the neck. *Convection* is heat loss from the body by the passage of air or fluid molecules over the skin of the body; for example, using a fan to circulate air molecules past the body enhances cooling by convection. *Radiation* is a means of heat loss via electromagnetic waves. Objects that are hotter than their surroundings emit heat waves and thus lose heat. Radiation of heat is how most (~60%) of the body's heat is lost during rest. All three of these mechanisms aid in heat loss as long as the environmental temperatures are below body temperature. Of course, the closer the environment's temperature gets to body temperature, even though it is still below it, the less effective they are at providing cooling. The fourth avenue of heat loss is *evaporation*. It is the process of heat loss via the vaporization of a fluid to a gas, and it is the most important cooling mechanism for the body during exercise. Evaporation of sweat accounts for up to 80% of the body's cooling during exercise or activity. Thus, when thinking about appropriate dress for exercise in the heat, consideration of all of these processes will ensure maximal cooling for the body.

The best clothing for exercise in the heat should be light colored, porous, and constructed of thin material. For example, a cap that is light colored and made of mesh material would be appropriate to wear. It is beneficial to have as much skin exposed to outside air as possible. Some athletes may wet their clothing with water before beginning to exercise.

How Should Athletes Dress for Exercising in the Cold?

When dressing for activity in the cold, the four mechanisms of heat loss must still be considered; however, the goal is to diminish their effectiveness so that the body conserves heat. It is best to dress in multiple layers of thin clothing that cover as much skin as possible. The outside layer should be of a dark color and made of wind-breaking material. The innermost layer should be constructed of absorbent material capable of wicking any sweat away from the surface of the skin. The head and ears should be covered, and a balaclava can be used to cover the face.

When dressing for the cold, it is critical to not overdress. Overdressing will cause excessive sweating, which can soak through all the layers of clothing and thus make a conductive channel for loss of body heat. A simple test to determine the appropriate level of dress for the cold is for an athlete to dress and then step out into the elements. If the athlete is immediately comfortable out in the elements, the athlete is overdressed; if the athlete is slightly chilled and a bit uncomfortable, the level of dress is appropriate. Once exercise has begun, body heat production will increase and the athlete will no longer feel chilled.

directed to the surface of the skin by ducts leading directly from the sweat glands. Once on the surface of the skin, the sweat drop is exposed to the air and can evaporate. It is the evaporation of the sweat that actually provides the cooling effect.

Water also plays a crucial role in maintaining the body's acid–base balance. It serves as the transport medium for protein buffers such as hemoglobin and plays an indirect role in the functioning and formation of the blood's most potent chemical buffer, **sodium bicarbonate**. Under resting conditions when relatively little lactic acid is being produced, the body's pH is slightly alkaline (pH = 7.4).

sodium bicarbonate A chemical compound found in the blood that helps maintain the body's normal acid–base balance. Sodium bicarbonate is considered the blood's most potent chemical buffer.

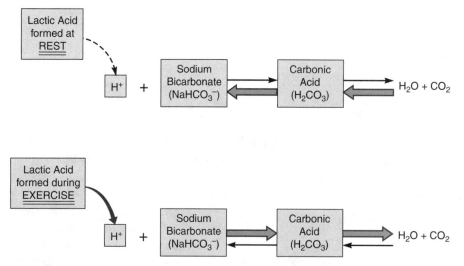

Figure 8.2 The role of water in the sodium bicarbonate buffering system. Water plays a crucial role in maintaining the body's acid–base balance. As depicted, water can either increase or decrease acidity via its relationship to the formation or breakdown of carbonic acid.

electron transport chain (see Figure 2.31). The electron transport chain is the last metabolic pathway associated with the aerobic energy system, and it is here that the hydrogen ions are ultimately transferred to an oxygen atom to form H_2O. In other words, our bodies are constantly producing metabolic water; however, the body does not make enough to satisfy total daily needs.

Is bottled water better than other sources of water?

Bottled water costs more than tap water, but that does not mean that it is superior. Water is water no matter where it comes from. The difference most athletes cite between water sources is the taste, which is determined by what is dissolved in the water. In the case of tap water, the minerals from the ground that leach into the water give it its taste. Each location in the world has its own unique mineral composition, and as a result water can taste very different from location to location. This does not mean that the water itself is more or less effective in hydrating the body; however, it can make a difference in whether athletes drink the water.

Bottled water is usually filtered, and in some instances minerals and/or flavoring have been added back, which enhances only palatability. Of course, savvy marketing would have athletes think that the water is better because it came from natural springs or clear mountain water. On the other hand, athletes should not assume that because the water is bottled it comes from a pristine area. As with food labels, read the water label. Many times the bottled water is coming from the municipal system of a large city, whose water just happens to taste good.

Finally, athletes should not assume that bottled water is safer to drink than tap water. According to the National Resources Defense Council, the Food and Drug Administration's (FDA) rules completely exempt 60–70% of the bottled water sold in the United States from the agency's bottled water standards because the FDA says its rules do not apply to water packaged and sold within the same state. Unfortunately, policing of water regulations within states is underfunded, and one in five states imposes no regulations at all. Even when bottled waters are

Because of the lower hydrogen ion levels (i.e., H+) at rest, water combines with CO_2 to form carbonic acid, which in turn dissociates into sodium bicarbonate and hydrogen ions, thus maintaining resting H+ concentrations (see Figure 8.2). Conversely, intense exercise or sport participation results in the formation of lactic acid, which is buffered by sodium bicarbonate to form carbonic acid. The carbonic acid then dissociates to water and CO_2, which is expelled at the lungs.

Finally, water is critical to the maintenance of blood volume. Adequate blood volume directly affects blood pressure and cardiovascular function. Dehydration, resulting in the loss of as little as 3–5% of body weight, begins to compromise cardiovascular function, which has a direct impact on sport performance, particularly for aerobic sports.

What are the sources of water?

Water is obtained from several different sources. Approximately 80% of daily water needs are supplied in the form of fluids. Less than 20% comes from the water found in fruits, vegetables, and other foods. The remainder is actually formed by the body during normal cellular metabolism. As discussed in Chapter 2 (see Figure 2.23), carbohydrates, fats, and proteins are broken down via the aerobic energy system to form carbon dioxide and water. The water formed during aerobic metabolism is known as "metabolic water." Hydrogen molecules that are part of the chemical structure of carbohydrates, fats, and proteins are basically stripped off and carried to the

covered by the FDA's bottled water standards, those rules are less stringent in many ways than Environmental Protection Agency (EPA) rules that apply to big city tap water. The take-home message is that athletes should not assume that bottled water is better than what comes out of the tap. If athletes do not like the taste of their tap water, many different types of in-home water filtration devices can be purchased, including faucet-mounted filters, pitchers, and even individual water bottles with a filter. These filters will improve the taste of the water and can save the athlete a lot of money.

The exception to this rule pertains to international travel. Each country imposes its own regulations related to water safety. In some instances, bottled water may be safer to consume than tap water. Athletes should investigate the safety of tap water at their destinations before traveling abroad.

What are the ways in which we lose body water?

Body water is lost via urination, defecation, sweating, and insensible processes (see Figure 8.3). Roughly 60% of the body water lost at rest is via formation of urine. However, during exercise in warm environments, sweat formation becomes the primary culprit and can account for up to 90% of water losses. The degree to which sweat formation contributes to water loss is dependent on several factors: the environment (temperature, humidity, and wind velocity), the intensity of the exercise (the metabolic demand and thus the amount of heat generated), the duration of the exercise, and the size of the individual. Water is also lost via a process known as **insensible perspiration**. This is different from the process of sweating. Insensible perspiration is when water from within the body actually seeps through the skin to the skin's surface, where it then evaporates into the air. It is labeled as insensible because, unlike sweat that forms at rates high enough to notice, the water seepage through the skin occurs at a very slow rate, but is ongoing 24 hours a day.

Approximately 15% of the water lost daily is lost by insensible perspiration. Water also is lost during breathing. The air breathed into the body is warmed and humidified by the respiratory passageways that direct the incoming air to the lungs. The drier the air or the greater the volume of air breathed, such

insensible perspiration Loss of water from the body via seepage through tissues and then eventual evaporation into the air. It is labeled as insensible because, unlike sweating, the water loss via seepage through the skin or respiratory passageways occurs relatively slowly and thus goes unnoticed.

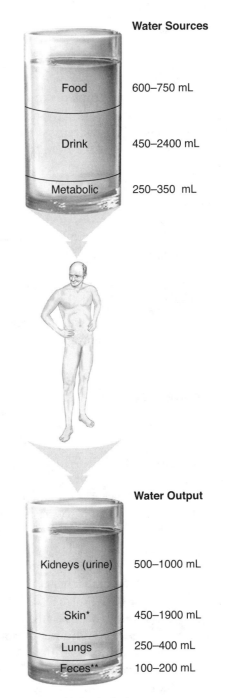

Water Sources

Food	600–750 mL
Drink	450–2400 mL
Metabolic	250–350 mL

Water Output

Kidneys (urine)	500–1000 mL
Skin*	450–1900 mL
Lungs	250–400 mL
Feces**	100–200 mL

* (Insensible and perspiration)
The volume of perspiration is normally about 100 mL per day. In very hot weather or during heavy exercise, a person may lose 1 to 2 liters per hour.

**People with severe diarrhea can lose several liters of water per day in feces.

Figure 8.3 Typical daily fluid intake and output. To maintain fluid balance, your body regulates its fluid intake and output. *Source:* U.S. Department of Agriculture, Agriculture Research Service, 2010. USDA Nutrient Database for Standard Reference, Release 23. Nutrient Data Laboratory Home Page. Available at: http://www.ars.usda.gov/Services/docs.htm?docid=8964. Accessed January 21, 2011.

as during exercise, the greater the loss of body water via this process. Water loss via the respiratory system can be quite significant, particularly in high-altitude sports in cold climates because cold air is very dense and holds little moisture, thus making cold air very dry air. Intense exercise that greatly increases breathing rates in turn increases water loss from the respiratory passageways. The take-home message is that despite the fact that the climate is cold and sweating may not be as great as in warm environments, water intake is still critical to ensure maintenance of hydration levels. The only way to maintain hydration on a daily basis is to ensure that daily water intake is equal to daily water loss. If water intake equals water loss, then **water balance** has been achieved.

> **water balance** Term used to describe the body's state of hydration. If water intake equals water loss, then water balance has been achieved. If water loss exceeds water intake, then negative water balance results. The converse is positive water balance.

What are the consequences of poor water balance?

Failing to maintain water balance can have dire consequences not only in regard to sport performance, but also in regard to survival. With all environmental conditions being the same, a net loss of body water (i.e., poor water balance) can lead to increases in body temperature compared to the hydrated state when performing the same activity (see Figure 8.4). The combination of impaired thermoregulation and environmental heat stress can lead to heat-related disorders such as heat cramps, heat exhaustion, and heat stroke (see **Table 8.1**).

The good news is that heat-related disorders are completely avoidable if commonsense practices regarding heat exposure and hydration are followed. The requirements for maintaining water balance are highly variable among individuals based on size, body composition, activity level, and climate, just to mention a few. If daily water intake is less than daily water loss, the body is in negative balance and **dehydration** will result if water intake is not increased. The opposite scenario, in which the body is in a positive water balance, is referred to as **hyperhydration**.

Being slightly hyperhydrated is preferable to being slightly dehydrated in regard to sport performance. Dehydration leads to a multitude of physiological function

> **dehydration** A condition resulting from a negative water balance (i.e., water loss exceeds water intake).
>
> **hyperhydration** A condition resulting from a positive water balance (i.e., water intake exceeds water loss).

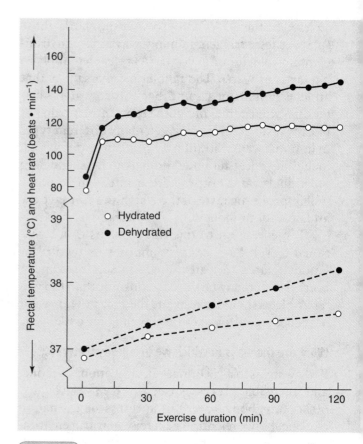

Figure 8.4 Effect of dehydration on heart rate and rectal temperature during exercise of the same intensity. Rectal temperature and heart rate both increase with advancing dehydration.
Source: Brooks GA, Fahey TD, Baldwin K. *Exercise Physiology: Human Bioenergetics and Its Applications.* 4th ed. Boston, MA: McGraw-Hill; 2004. Reproduced with permission of the McGraw-Hill Companies.

changes that are detrimental to training and performance (see Figure 8.5). Dehydration leads to loss of blood volume, which in turn leads to decreases in the amount of blood the heart can pump to the working muscles. Decreased blood flow to muscles means less oxygen is being delivered, and therefore less work can be performed by the muscles. When the aerobic capabilities of muscle to make energy are diminished because of poor delivery of oxygen, the muscles begin to rely more heavily on anaerobic metabolism (refer to Chapter 2). The more the body has to rely on anaerobic metabolism, the quicker lactic acid levels build, the higher the rating of perceived exertion, and the faster fatigue will occur if the athlete does not decrease his or her level of activity. The end result is less-than-optimal sport performance.

Dehydration also leads to extra heat and cardiovascular stress during exercise. As little as a 2–3% decrease in body weight caused by dehydration can result in increases in body temperature and heart

TABLE 8.1 Heat-Related Disorders

Heat-Related Disorder	Degree of Severity	Signs and Symptoms	Corrective Actions
Heat cramps	Least	Muscle cramping	Stretch muscle Moderate activity Provide fluids
Heat exhaustion	Moderate	Profuse sweating Cold, clammy skin Faintness Rapid pulse Hypotension	Cease activity Rest in shade Lie down Consume fluids
Heat stroke	Highest	Lack of sweat Dry, hot skin Muscle incoordination Mental confusion Disorientation	Call for medical help Initiate cooling of body (e.g., fanning, cold towels or ice packs around neck, under arms, and at groin) Immerse or douse with cold water

rate despite the fact that exercise intensity remained the same. The progressive increase in heart rate in the absence of an increase in exercise intensity is known as **cardiac drift**. Cardiac drift occurs because of decreasing blood volume, which in turn requires the heart to pump faster to deliver enough blood to the working muscle (see Figure 8.5). Athletes must understand that intense exercise in hot, humid environments can result in such rapid fluid losses that even increasing fluid intake alone

cardiac drift A progressive increase in heart rate in the absence of an increase in exercise intensity. It is the result of a loss in blood volume.

may not be enough to enable the athlete to prevent dehydration. As a result, athletes must be taught that they may also have to modify their intensity (i.e., pace and/or effort) during competition in hot, humid environments. Failure to do so will lead to progressive dehydration that can eventually lead to cardiovascular collapse, severe heat illness (see Table 8.1), or both. Clearly, maintaining hydration before, during, and after training and/or sport participation is critical.

Is it possible to overhydrate the body?

Although rare, it is possible to consume too much water. The resulting condition is known as **hyponatremia**, more commonly referred to as **water intoxication**. With the advance of extreme endurance sports, hyponatremia has become a more frequent occurrence. "Hypo" refers to low, "na" refers to sodium, and "emia" refers to blood, thus hyponatremia is a condition in which the fluids of the body become very low in sodium content. Sodium is an important electrolyte (refer to Chapter 7) and is critical to normal function of muscle and the nervous system. Symptoms of hyponatremia mimic those of someone who is intoxicated and include muscle

hyponatremia A rare condition resulting from the dilution of sodium levels in the body. Endurance and ultra-endurance athletes who drink copious amounts of water without regard to sodium replacement increase their risk for hyponatremia.

water intoxication A condition resulting from the excessive intake of water. The end result can be a clinical condition known as hyponatremia.

% Body weight loss

0	
1	Thirst
2	Increasing thirst, loss of appetite, discomfort, increasing heart rate
3	Impatience, decreased blood volume
4	Nausea, slowing of physical work
5	Difficulty concentrating, apathy, tingling extremites
6	Increasing body temperature, pulse and respiration rate
7	Stumbling, headache
8	Dizziness, labored breathing
9	Weakness, mental confusion
10	Muscle spasms, indistinct speech
11	Kidney failure, poor circulation
Death	due to decreased blood volume

Figure 8.5 Effects of progressive dehydration.

weakness, muscle incoordination, disorientation, and eventually seizures and coma, if the condition is not recognized and treated.

Endurance and ultra-endurance athletes are at greatest risk for hyponatremia because of their repeated exposure to long training bouts that result in significant fluid loss via sweat. Because sodium and chloride are the main electrolytes lost in sweat, rehydration without replacement of these electrolytes will eventually lead to dilution of their concentrations in the body.[1] One way to prevent hyponatremia is to have athletes ingest sports drinks containing electrolytes, particularly sodium. In regard to nonendurance athletes, hyponatremia is very rare. As a result, the use of electrolyte sports drinks by nonendurance athletes is of lesser importance because of the fact that diet alone in most instances provides enough sodium chloride (i.e., salt) to cover losses in training.

How can hydration status be monitored?

Hydration status can be measured in several ways prior to exercise (see **Table 8.2**). Each method has pros and cons in regard to the ease of administration and related costs. One easy way to monitor whether water balance is being achieved is to monitor body weight. Daily weight fluctuations are caused primarily by changes in water status. As a result, changes in body weight that occur within a 24-hour time frame can give an indication of whether water intake is replenishing daily water loss. For example, if an individual weighs 120 pounds prior to her workout and 118 pounds after the workout, the weight lost during exercise was a result of water loss. The rule of thumb for rehydrating is that 1 pound of weight lost is equal to 2–3 cups (8 oz = 1 cup) of water. An excellent practice for athletes, particularly those in warm climates, is to monitor changes in their pre- and postpractice weights and then follow the rehydrating rule of thumb. If their prepractice weight is not back to the previous day's prepractice weight, then their attempt at rehydrating needs to be increased to prevent progressive dehydration.

Although monitoring body weight is a quick, easy, and inexpensive hydration assessment method, there are several potentially confounding physical and mental issues that need to be considered. Physically, other factors besides water loss during a training session, such as food intake, the time weight

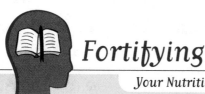

Fortifying
Your Nutrition Knowledge

Teaching Athletes to Self-Monitor Hydration Status

Athletes should be well-versed on the following methods for self-monitoring of daily hydration status:

- *Urine color:* Urine that is clear or the color of pale lemonade indicates positive hydration. Urine the color of apple juice or that is bright yellow or amber in color indicates dehydration. Athletes should monitor urine color throughout the day, not just before or after practice or competition.
- *Urine volume:* Adequately hydrated athletes will need to urinate approximately every 1–2 hours during waking hours. Athletes should notice if they have gone several hours without urinating as a sign that they may be becoming dehydrated. The average daily urine output under normal conditions is approximately 1.5–2.5 liters per day.[28] Athletes, however, will consume more fluids, sweat more, and may have greater urine output. It is not practical to measure urine output; therefore, monitoring the number of times athletes urinate is more practical and helpful to determine hydration status.
- *Daily morning weight:* Athletes may choose to weigh each morning during high heat, humidity, and intense preseason training. A decrease of more than 1% of body weight or more than 1 pound suggests possible dehydration.
- *Weighing-in pre- and postpractice:* Athletes should weigh themselves in light clothing before practice and in the same amount of clothing after practice. Be sure to have athletes remove sweaty T-shirts and towel off before the postpractice weight. Replenish with fluids in the amount of 16–24 ounces for every pound of weight lost.

was taken from last meal, bowel movement patterns, and bladder content at the time of weighing, can affect body weight over the course of 24 hours. As a result, it can be difficult to distinguish which of those factors are contributing to a higher- or lower-than-normal weight, and this can provide confusing or misleading information regarding specific hydration status. Weighing athletes at the same time of day and with an empty bladder can help control for some of these variables and provide a more accurate picture of hydration level.

One mental factor that often is overlooked is the effect of frequent or daily weigh-ins. Requiring an athlete to step on a scale repeatedly in 1 week, especially if in front of other teammates and coaches, can cause the athlete to become excessively focused on weight, which can spiral into distorted eating and body image issues. Because of this risk, other methods of measuring hydration status should be considered for some athletic populations.

One sport that depends heavily on body weight measurements is wrestling. Concern has risen in recent years about unhealthy weight loss practices, including severe dehydration, to cut weight. New guidelines have been instituted through the National Collegiate Athletic Association and the National Federation of State High School Associations to establish a minimum weight for each athlete at the beginning of the competitive season.[2,3] Because it was discovered that wrestlers were arriving at minimum weight testing in a dehydrated state to secure a lower weight minimum, both organizations have included body composition and other hydration tests to be used in conjunction with weigh-ins.

Urine Rating #	Description of Urine Color
1	Urine is clear of color
2	Urine has a very light yellow tint
3	Urine has a light yellow color
4	Urine has a vivid, canary yellow color
5	Urine has a dingy yellow, almost orange color
6	Urine has a medium tan color
7	Urine has a burned orange color
8	Urine has a dark, almost olive-brown color

Figure 8.6 Urine color comparison. Athletes can compare their urine color to the descriptions of urine color in the chart to determine hydration status. The goal for adequate hydration is clear to pale yellow urine (i.e., urine rating 1 or 2). A urine color rating equal to 5 or 6 indicates significant dehydration.
Source: Adapted from Casa DJ, Armstrong LE, Hillman SK, et al. National Athletic Trainers' Association position statement: fluid replacement for athletes. J Athlet Train. 2000;35(2):212–224.

Several other methods of assessing hydration status are related to urine: color, specific gravity, and volume.[4] Urine can be collected in a sample container and compared to a color chart, measured for specific gravity with a refractometer, or evaluated on total volume. Comparing urine color to a chart can be quick and easy but also expensive over time because of the cost of collection containers (see Figure 8.6). Athletes can also subjectively evaluate urine color—typically dark, concentrated urine with a strong smell indicates dehydration. Using a refractometer is simple; however, there are costs associated with purchasing the equipment and issues of ease of portability. Urine volume can be a good indicator of hydration but tends to be cumbersome to collect and measure.

TABLE 8.2 Indexes of Hydration Status

Condition	% Body Weight (BW) Change*	Urine Color**	Urine Specific Gravity
Well-hydrated	+1 to −1	1 or 2	<1.010
Minimal dehydration	−1 to −3	3 or 4	1.010–1.020
Significant dehydration	−3 to −5	5 or 6	1.021–1.030
Serious dehydration	>−5	>6	>1.030

* % BW change = ([postexercise BW − preexercise BW] / preexercise BW) × 100
** See Figure 8.6.

Source: Casa DJ, Armstrong LE, Hillman DK, et al. National Athletic Trainers' Association position statement: fluid replacement for athletes. J Athlet Train. 2000;35(2):212–224. Reprinted with permission.

Each athlete or team needs to determine the most accurate, realistic, convenient, and cost-effective method for measuring hydration status prior to exercise. Any sports requiring weight classes, such as wrestling, are strongly encouraged to measure hydration status in several ways before allowing an athlete to participate in an event. The National Athletic Trainers' Association (NATA) recommends that athletes should be screened for urine specific gravity and urine color at the time of weigh-ins. The upper end of the acceptable range for hydration status is a urine specific gravity of less than or equal to 1.020 or urine color of less than or equal to 4 (see Table 8.2 and Figure 8.6). Body weight changes during and after exercise are also excellent indicators of fluid dynamics and should be included in hydration assessments.

How much fluid do individuals need on a daily basis?

Water is the largest constituent of the human body and is critical for maintaining life, general health, and optimal athletic performance. Proper daily water intake prevents the deleterious effects of dehydration, including metabolic and functional abnormalities. Because water has not been shown to directly prevent chronic diseases, and because of great individual differences in fluid needs based on climate, activity level, and metabolism, an Adequate Intake (AI) has been set for water rather than a Recommended Dietary Allowance (RDA).

What are the current recommendations for daily fluid intake?

The AI for water, published by the Institute of Medicine, reflects the current research and population survey data. For men and women older than age 19, the recommended intake is 3.7 liters and 2.7 liters of water per day, respectively.[5] Refer to **Table 8.3** for the recommendations for younger men and women. These daily quantities reflect total water intake from drinking water as well as from other beverages containing water and from solid foods.

U.S. survey data from the National Health and Nutrition Examination Survey (NHANES) III provide an estimation of the percentage of water required from drinking water and other beverages versus solid food. The results of the survey reveal that fluids provide 81% of total water intake whereas foods contribute 19%. Based on the total water recommendations, men should be consuming approxi-

TABLE 8.3	Dietary Reference Intake Values for Total Water		
Gender and Age Group	AI (L/day) from Foods	AI (L/day) from Beverages	AI (L/day) Total Water
Males, 4–8 years	0.5	1.2	1.7
Males, 9–13 years	0.6	1.8	2.4
Males, 14–18 years	0.7	2.6	3.3
Males, >19 years	0.7	3.0	3.7
Females, 4–8 years	0.5	1.2	1.7
Females, 9–13 years	0.5	1.6	2.1
Females, 14–18 years	0.5	1.8	2.3
Females, >19 years	0.5	2.2	2.7

Source: Institute of Medicine. *Dietary Reference Intakes: Water, Sodium, Chloride, Potassium and Sulfate*. Food and Nutrition Board. Washington, DC: National Academies Press; 2004.

mately 3 liters of fluid (101 oz or ~13 cups) and women should aim for 2.2 liters of fluid (74 oz or ~9 cups) each day. Athletes may need to modify these fluid recommendations to match their individual requirements based on physical activity, environmental conditions during training/competition, and outdoor climate. In general, daily fluid intake driven by thirst can adequately maintain hydration status.

Another method for estimating fluid needs for the average individual under normal circumstances and in moderate environmental conditions relates total energy intake to fluid requirements. It has been estimated that individuals require approximately 1 milliliter of water for every calorie of energy consumed.[6] The average American consumes approximately 2000 calories per day, which equates to 2000 milliliters of fluid. Milliliters are converted to ounces by dividing the number of milliliters by 240 because there are 240 milliliters in 8 ounces of fluid (2000 milliliters ÷ 240 = 8.33 cups of fluid per day). Therefore, the commonly prescribed eight cups (8 oz each) of water per day holds true for the average American.

Determining water needs based on calorie intake can provide a more individualized approach for athletes' daily water needs. Athletes have varied energy intakes based on weight, energy expenditure, and sport performance goals. As energy needs increase and caloric consumption increases, so does the requirement for fluids. For example, according to the calorie and fluid connection, an athlete who consumes 2500 calories per day would need 2.5 liters of fluid per day, but a different athlete who consumes 5000 calories per day would require twice as much fluid daily. Clearly, 5.0 liters of water is more than the values shown in Table 8.3, but athletes in general usually have greater fluid needs. In fact, during intense training of long duration and in high heat and humidity, even the higher water intake recommendation based on the 1 mL per calorie method may be insufficient to maintain water balance. Vigilant assessment of water loss during exercise activities and replacement of these losses at appropriate levels, as described later in this chapter, will help athletes meet their fluid needs for both daily hydration and hydration before, during, and after exercise activities.

Fluid losses can be replenished through drinking water, other beverages containing water, and foods. Water, juices, milk, coffee, tea, and soda all contribute to a person's daily fluid intake. Water is always a good choice because it is calorie-free and inexpensive. Juices and milk contribute not only fluid, but also macronutrients, vitamins, and minerals. They should be consumed in moderation, however, because they can add a significant amount of total calories to the daily diet. Caffeinated coffee and tea will have a slight diuretic effect; therefore, decaffeinated varieties are preferable. Regular sodas are not recommended because of the large quantity of refined sugars they contain. Diet sodas are often considered a better option than regular sodas; however, because of the inconsistent results from research studies on the long-term safety of artificial sweetener consumption, diet sodas should be kept to a minimum.

Solid foods also contribute water to an athlete's total daily fluid intake. Fruits and vegetables contain a large percentage of water, upward of 70–90%. Meats, dairy products, and grain

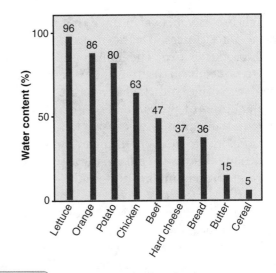

Figure 8.7 Water content of various foods.

products consist of lower percentages of water; however, percentages still range from 30% to 50%. Refer to Figure 8.7 for the water content of various foods. Not only do solid foods directly contribute to water consumption, but the metabolism of foods creates water as a by-product.

Can certain beverages, foods, or medications contribute to fluid losses?

Caffeine and alcohol have been shown to have a diuretic effect, causing the body to excrete fluids in urine. However, the consumption versus loss is not necessarily a 1:1 ratio. For example, humans lose approximately 1 milliliter of water for every milligram of caffeine consumed.[5] One cup (240 mL) of brewed coffee contains an average of 80 mg of caffeine. Consumption of this product would lead to a loss of approximately 80 mL of water, but a gain of 160 mL of water. The fluid loss also tends to be transient in nature, and thus doesn't cause major shifts in fluid balance. Therefore, the Institute of Medicine reports that caffeinated and alcoholic beverages can contribute to an individual's total water intake. For athletes, these beverages should comprise only a small portion of total fluid intake per day because of the damaging physical and mental effects of excess alcohol consumption and the potentially unwanted side effects of large doses of caffeine. However, there appears to be no need to completely eliminate caffeine specifically from the diet. Moderate caffeine intake is unlikely to cause detrimental fluid–electrolyte imbalances, if athletes are eating and drinking normally on a daily basis.[7]

gaining the performance edge

The hydration needs of an athlete can be estimated using the following formula: total calories / 240 = number of cups of fluid needed each day. For example, the number of 8 oz cups of fluid required by an athlete consuming 3000 calories a day can be estimated as follows: 3000 calories / 240 = 12½ cups per day. It is important to remember that fluid losses during exercise must be added to the calculated estimation to cover the hydration needs of athletes.

High-protein diets also have the potential to increase water losses. The normal metabolism of protein produces urea. The human body considers urea a toxic chemical that must be excreted as waste through the urine. Individuals who are consuming large quantities of protein daily, in excess of their daily requirements, may be causing the body to excrete more fluid to flush out the urea. More research is needed in this area to confirm the association between high protein intakes and fluid losses as well as the establishment of any variance to the current daily fluid recommendations for those choosing a high-protein meal plan.

Many prescribed and over-the-counter medications have a diuretic effect on the body. The extent of the diuresis depends on the drug dosage and individual response. Athletes should discuss the side effects of any prescription or over-the-counter drug taken on a routine basis with their physician and adjust their fluid intake accordingly. Coaches need to be aware of the dangers of athletes taking excessively high doses of diuretics without the supervision of a physician. Typically, wrestlers and other athletes attempting to make a weight cut-off, as well as disordered eating athletes, are the individuals taking diuretics. Large doses can cause potassium and other electrolyte disturbances, which can lead to muscle weakness and ultimately cardiac problems.

What are some practical guidelines for consuming fluids on a daily basis?

The goal of daily fluid consumption is to ensure the maintenance of optimal health. To achieve this goal, athletes should consider the following hydration guidelines:

- Each athlete should be aware of his or her individual daily fluid needs and consume fluids accordingly.
- Optimal hydration should stimulate urination approximately every 1–2 hours.
- Urine that is pale or clear in color typically indicates adequate hydration. Athletes need to realize that vitamin and mineral supplementation can create a yellow tint to urine and therefore the color of urine may or may not be an accurate reflection of hydration status.
- Fluids can be obtained from water, milk, juices, coffee, tea, and sports beverages as well as watery foods such as soup, fruits, and vegetables.
- Caffeine should be consumed in moderation. Alcohol consumption should be minimized if not eliminated.

- Athletes should follow a well-balanced diet, including moderate amounts of protein to avoid diuresis as a result of high-protein diets.
- Athletes and coaches should be aware of the diuretic side effects of any medications taken on a regular basis and adjust daily fluid recommendations accordingly.

What is the role of preexercise hydration?

Proper hydration before exercising sets the stage for optimal sport performance. Athletes who avoid fluids intentionally or unintentionally before training sessions or competitive events tend to fatigue quickly, complain of dizziness or faintness, demonstrate a faster rise in core body temperature, have increased heart rates and perceived levels of exertion, and perform suboptimally.[8–10] On the other hand, drinking excessive amounts of fluid prior to exercise can lead to frequent and disruptive urination and possibly hyponatremia. Athletes need to know the benefits of optimal hydration before exercising, accurate measurements of hydration status, and the current guidelines for the quantity, type, and timing of fluid ingestion prior to training sessions and competitive events.

How much fluid should be consumed before exercise?

When establishing a plan for fluid consumption before exercise, consider not only the volume of fluid, but also the timing of ingestion. Generous, but not excessive, amounts of fluids should be consumed in the 24 hours before exercise. Drinking enough fluids to meet daily recommendations will allow an athlete to start an exercise session well hydrated. Fluid intake within the 1 to 2 hours prior to exercise can enhance thermoregulation and lower heart rate during exercise.[9,11] The American College of Sports Medicine (ACSM),[12] the NATA, and the American Dietetic Association (ADA) all recommend the following hydration schedule in the hours immediately prior to exercise:

- Slowly drink approximately 400–600 milliliters (13–20 oz) or the equivalent of about 5–7 mL per kg of body weight at least 4 hours prior to exercise
- If urine is not produced or is dark and highly concentrated, slowly drink more fluid (e.g., ~3–5 mL per kg of body weight) about 2 hours before exercise
- Drink 200–300 milliliters (7–10 oz) in the 10–20 minutes prior to exercise

These volumes of fluid will ensure that athletes are properly hydrated while allowing the kidneys to regulate total body fluid.

What types of fluids should be consumed?

Athletes can choose from a variety of fluids in the hours leading up to a training session or competition, including water, juices, milk, coffee, tea, sports drinks, sodas, and beverages containing glycerol (see Figure 8.8). Each beverage has benefits and drawbacks; therefore, it is critical that athletes experiment with the different choices prior to actual practice or competition to determine their preference and individual tolerance. Water is an appropriate choice, especially if accompanied by a substantial snack or meal. Solid food can provide carbohydrates and electrolytes before exercise whereas water provides fluid without further increasing the concentration or **osmolarity** of the stomach and intestinal contents.

Water is also inexpensive and easy to obtain.

One hundred percent juices provide fluid, carbohydrates, and electrolytes, which are all beneficial prior to exercise, but not without consequences for some athletes. Carbohydrates in juice can help top off glycogen stores for use during exercise. Because juice is a liquid source of carbohydrates, it is digested and absorbed more quickly than are solid foods, making for a speedy delivery of nutrients to the muscles. Potassium, which is found in both fruit and vegetable juices, as well as sodium, found mainly in vegetable juices, are electrolytes that are lost in sweat and therefore beneficial to consume prior to exercise. Seemingly an ideal choice, some athletes swear by juice before training and competitions, whereas others find juices disagreeable to their gastrointestinal systems immediately prior to exercise. The high fructose content of full-strength juices, if consumed immediately before exercise (or within 15–30 minutes) may delay gastric emptying, causing gastrointestinal upset in some athletes. Individual preference and tolerance should guide the choice of whether to include juice in the preexercise hydration plan.

osmolarity Similar to osmolality, it is an indicator of the concentration of dissolved particles per liter of a solvent (mOsm/L). The higher the osmolarity, the greater the tendency to attract water rather than be absorbed.

gaining the performance edge

Water, juice, and milk are excellent choices for preexercise hydration.

Milk provides another seemingly ideal beverage to the lineup of hydration choices. Milk helps athletes meet carbohydrate and protein requirements prior to exercise, in addition to providing fluid. A little protein in the preexercise meal or snack slows the release of nutrients into the bloodstream and thereby allows for a more even supply of energy to the muscles during exercise. Therefore, milk is an excellent preexercise fluid choice; however, many athletes find it difficult to digest, causing stomach upset, bloating, or diarrhea prior to training or competitions. Obviously these effects are undesirable, so milk consumption prior to exercise should be based on individual preference and tolerance.

Coffee and tea are often used as a precompetition beverage because of the claims that caffeine enhances endurance performance. The general consensus in the research is that caffeine does provide an ergogenic benefit by improving endurance time to exhaustion in prolonged events.[13,14] Some of the controversy that exists surrounding caffeine is the balance between an ergogenic benefit and potentially detrimental effects resulting from subsequent dehydration. However, as mentioned earlier in this chapter, the diuretic effects of caffeine do not completely negate the fluid contribution of these beverages. Therefore, coffee and tea do count toward fluid goals prior to exercise. The deciding factor on inclusion of coffee or tea before exercise is an ath-

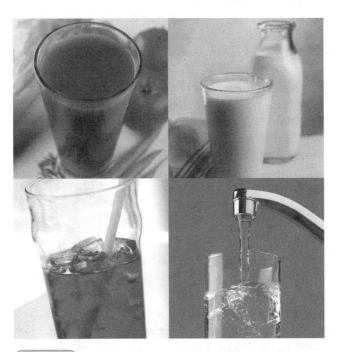

Figure 8.8 Variety of beverages for daily hydration. All beverages consumed count toward daily hydration needs. Limit the use of sodas and other carbonated beverages, which may decrease the effectiveness of overall hydration and nutrition status.

lete's individual tolerance and familiarity with the effects of caffeine. For those who are accustomed to caffeine on a daily basis, coffee or tea should be consumed to avoid headaches or lethargy caused by sudden caffeine withdrawal. For those who do not consume caffeine regularly, coffee and tea should probably be avoided because of the potential side effects of nervousness, tremors, and gastrointestinal distress.

Sports drinks are frequently used by athletes prior to training sessions and competitions. Sports drinks are specifically formulated as a fluid replacement beverage for use during exercise. Athletes should therefore reserve the consumption of these drinks mainly for training sessions and competitions and not necessarily as a refreshment beverage during the day or in the hours leading up to exercise. A small amount of a sports beverage can be appropriately used immediately prior to exercise, with the intention of supplying a small amount of carbohydrates, sodium, and fluids for the initiation of exercise. However, the focus of preexercise fluids should be on more nutritionally concentrated beverages. An additional concern is that, for those embarking on long-duration activities, sports drinks should be consumed during the activity in copious amounts. If sports drinks are consumed before exercise, there is the possibility that the athlete will tire of the flavor of the sports drink before the end of the endurance training session, potentially lowering overall fluid intake and possibly affecting performance.

Sodas are not appropriate for consumption prior to exercise. In general, sodas should be minimized in an athlete's diet because of their large contribution of refined sugars. Besides fluid and simple sugars, sodas are devoid of vitamins and minerals and thus do not have nutritional value. The carbonation in soft drinks tends to cause individuals to drink less because of a feeling of fullness, potentially leading to dehydration at the initiation of exercise. Sodas should not be consumed prior to exercise and in general should be consumed only occasionally.

Methods to enhance preexercise hydration by supersaturating the body with water have been investigated recently. One such method is consuming fluids containing glycerol. The results from well-controlled studies concerning hyperhydration with glycerol have been equivocal.[15–18] Some studies have revealed a thermoregulatory benefit, whereas others have shown no effect. However, it appears that even in cases where glycerol intake has been shown to be positive, the benefits have been somewhat negated when hydration status is maintained during exercise.[19] Therefore, at this time there is not enough evidence to endorse the use of glycerol-containing beverages before exercise. It should also be noted that the side effects of glycerol ingestion include nausea, headaches, and gastrointestinal distress—all of which are undesirable and unfavorable conditions for optimal athletic performance.

What are practical guidelines for consuming fluids before exercise?

The goal of fluid consumption before exercise is to ensure that athletes begin training sessions and competitive events hydrated and fueled to perform at their best and maintain health. To achieve these goals, athletes and coaches should consider the following hydration factors:

- *Drink according to established preexercise hydration guidelines.* Consuming adequate fluids prior to exercise is critical to performance. However, more is not necessarily better.
- *Athletes and coaches should determine a method for assessing hydration status prior to training sessions and competitions to avoid the adverse effects of dehydration.* Urine color, concentration, and odor, as well as body weight, are the most commonly used methods for assessment.
- *Water, juices, and milk are excellent choices for preexercise hydration and can easily be included in the preexercise meal or snack.* Caffeinated coffee and tea should be consumed in moderation. Sodas should be avoided.

What is the role of hydration during exercise?

The goals of hydration during exercise are to maintain plasma volume and electrolyte balance. Through optimal hydration, athletes can avoid abnormal increases in heart rate and core temperature that can potentially lead to health issues, as well as premature fatigue that will zap performance. Both dehydration (insufficient fluids) and water intoxication (excessive fluids) can negatively affect performance.

A water loss of merely 2–3% of total body weight can decrease performance by reducing cardiac output and increasing an athlete's risk for heat

gaining the performance edge

An athlete can drink a variety of fluids prior to competition. However, it is important to experiment with the various drinks to determine taste preference and tolerance before actually using them prior to competition.

gaining the performance edge

Athletes cannot "train" their bodies to increase performance when in a dehydrated state. Proper hydration protocols should be used in all practices and competitions to ensure optimal health and sport performance.

illnesses.[7] Fluid replacement sustains the process of sweating, which cools the body through evaporation. If fluid replacement is suboptimal, blood flow to the skin is decreased, which impairs heat dissipation and elevates body core temperature. Losing 2–3% of total body weight is very common and can happen relatively quickly to athletes during training and competitions. Athletes should note that fluid replacement means *consuming* fluids—not pouring fluids over their heads. Pouring a cold cup of water or ice over the body can provide an immediate sense of relief from the heat but does not elicit the same benefit as consuming the fluids. The most effective way to keep body temperature in check and enhance performance is to actually ingest the cold fluids.

What is the magnitude of water and electrolyte losses during exercise?

Water and electrolyte losses during exercise can vary greatly depending on several factors including body size, exercise intensity, ambient temperature, humidity, clothing choices, and acclimation.[20] For slow-paced, low-intensity efforts conducted in low to moderate temperatures, fluid losses might not exceed 500 mL per hour (~16–20 oz).[21] In hot and humid environments, some athletes can lose up to 2–3 liters of water per hour (~68–102 oz). Considering the size of a 2-liter bottle, consuming upward of one and a half of those bottles during 1 hour of exercise can be daunting! However, each athlete's needs are different, and therefore individual sweat losses should be calculated and hydration protocols developed to replace fluids at a similar rate. Electrolytes lost in sweat include mainly sodium, some potassium, and small amounts of calcium. Sodium losses have been estimated at 50 mmol per liter of sweat, or 1 gram per liter, during exercise, with a range of 20–80 mmol per liter (400–1600 mg per liter). Potassium losses are typically between 4 and 8 mmol per liter (76–152 mg per liter) during exercise.[22] For short-duration activities, normal daily intake of electrolytes may be adequate to replenish losses in sweat. For athletes training and competing for longer durations, at higher intensities, or in hot, humid environments, electrolyte replacement during exercise will be critical for sport performance and prevention of hyponatremia.

As mentioned, individual sweat rates vary dramatically. To prevent dehydration, while also avoiding water intoxication, athletes need to know the current water and electrolyte intake recommendations for during exercise, their individual sweat rates, and how to translate the information into a fluid plan for training sessions and competitions.

How much fluid should be consumed during exercise?

Many national organizations, including the ACSM, NATA, and ADA, have issued position statements regarding their recommendations on the ideal quantity of fluid to ingest during exercise for health and peak performance.[1,4,12,23] The consensus is that athletes should aim for matching their sweat and urine output with fluid consumption to maintain hydration at less than a 2% reduction in body weight. For most individuals, consuming approximately 200–300 milliliters, or 7–10 fluid ounces, every 10–20 minutes during exercise will achieve this goal. However, this recommendation must be confirmed by calculating individual sweat losses through a "sweat trial" to ensure proper hydration based on the factors that contribute to individual variability.

Several studies have revealed no change in performance with varying volumes of fluid ingested during cycling lasting less than 60 minutes in a neutral environment.[24,25] Although consuming fluids may not have a huge impact on short-duration exercise, it does have a large impact on long-duration exercise (~60 minutes), especially in hot, humid environments.[26–28] Any athlete engaging in exercise lasting longer than an hour should measure his or her sweat rate and implement a hydration plan.

How can an athlete calculate his or her individual sweat rate?

Athletes can estimate their individual sweat rate by gathering information from a sweat trial. After collecting the data from the trial, the athlete will be able to estimate his or her individual fluid needs per hour through a series of short calculations. Sweat trials should be performed multiple times during training to provide the most accurate estimation of the quantity of fluid needed on competition day, enabling the athlete to perform at his or her best. Sweat trials should be conducted in several different

gaining the performance edge

Although consuming 200–300 mL of fluid about every 15 minutes will help maintain hydration during exercise for most athletes, sweat trials should be performed to learn individual hydration needs.

environments to gain as much information as possible so that there are no surprises or guesses on competition day. Differences should be compared between indoor and outdoor workouts, summer and winter training sessions, and easy and hard effort days. The data to collect during a sweat trial include the following:

- Body weight (BW), in pounds, before exercise
- BW after exercise (without wearing sweaty clothes)
- Volume of fluid consumed (in ounces) during the workout
- Urine output during exercise
- Total workout/competition time (in hours)[4]

Most of these measurements can be collected easily, with the exception of urine output. To make the calculation more feasible, athletes should exercise for 1–2 hours without urinating, thus negating the need for the urine output data. After collecting the other pieces of data indicated, the sweat rate can be calculated using the following steps:

1. *Determine body weight lost during exercise.* By subtracting the total body weight after exercise from the total body weight before exercise, an athlete can determine the amount of water lost, expressed in pounds:

> BW before exercise – BW after exercise = pounds of water weight lost

2. *Determine the fluid equivalent, in ounces, of the total weight lost during exercise.* Every pound of body weight lost during exercise equals approximately 2–3 cups or 16–24 ounces of fluid (1 cup = 8 oz).[4] The weight loss that occurs during exercise can translate into the number of ounces of fluid the athlete should have consumed, in addition to the fluid actually consumed during the training session or competition, to maintain fluid balance. To determine the number of ounces of fluid lost during exercise, multiply the pounds of water weight lost by 16–24 ounces:

> pounds of water weight lost during exercise × 16–24 oz = number of ounces of additional fluid that should have been consumed to maintain fluid balance during the exercise session

3. *Determine the actual fluid needs of the athlete during an identical workout.* Add the quantity of fluid consumed during the workout to the fluid equivalent of the weight lost during exercise to determine the total actual fluid needs of the athlete:

> ounces of fluid consumed + ounces of additional fluid needed to establish fluid balance = total fluid needs

4. *Determine the number of fluid ounces needed per hour of exercise.* For practical purposes, divide the total fluid needs by the duration of the sweat trial, in hours. This final calculation will provide the athlete with an estimation of his or her hourly fluid needs, which can then be used to plan accordingly for training sessions, and ultimately for competitions of varying lengths.

> total fluid needs / total workout time in hours = fluid ounces per hour of exercise

For example, Alex weighs in before tennis practice at 145 pounds. After 2 hours of playing tennis outdoors on a mild summer day, he weighs in at 143 pounds. During his practice, Alex consumed 20 ounces of fluid. What are Alex's total fluid needs per hour? Following the steps listed previously:

1. Weight loss = 145 lb – 143 lb = 2 lb of water weight loss
2. Additional fluid needed = 2 lb × 16–24 oz = 32–48 oz of additional fluid that should have been consumed to maintain fluid balance during the practice session
3. Total fluid needs = 20 oz + 32–48 oz = 52–68 oz
4. Fluid needs per hour = 52–68 oz / 2 hr of practice = 26–34 oz/hr

From this sweat trial, Alex would estimate his total fluid needs per hour of training or competition to be 26–34 ounces. Therefore, he can plan accordingly for his next practice and bring two 20 oz water bottles filled with a sports drink.

gaining the performance edge

An athlete should not gain weight during an exercise session. Weight gain indicates overhydration and can increase the risk for hyponatremia.

How does the volume of fluid ingested during exercise affect gastric emptying and intestinal absorption?

The goal of determining individual sweat rates is to establish a fluid plan that would closely match fluid intake with fluid losses. This state of fluid balance, or **euhydration**, is not always possible for athletes to achieve. In some cases, athletes' sweat rates exceed maximal gastric emptying rates, which in turn limits the intestinal absorption of fluids. For these athletes, fluid recommendations are set at a volume that matches sweat losses as closely as possible without exceeding gastric emptying rates, thus avoiding stomach cramping and bloating. Using a carbohydrate-containing sports beverage during exercise can enhance absorptive capacity. The section entitled "How much and what types of carbohydrates should be included in a fluid replacement beverage?" later in the chapter describes this in more detail.

However, a majority of athletes are consuming fluids at a rate and volume much lower than their maximal gastric emptying rate. Many athletes consume less than 500 milliliters of fluid per hour during training or competition. For most individuals, gastric emptying rates of 1 liter or more per hour are possible.[20] Therefore, athletes are not reaching their hydration potentials and would benefit from increasing fluid intake during exercise.

By increasing the volume of fluid ingested, athletes will not only more closely match their fluid losses, thus preventing the detrimental effects of dehydration, but also will actually facilitate euhydration by stimulating gastric emptying. Larger volumes in the stomach stimulate the release of fluids into the intestines, leading to a faster delivery of fluids from ingestion to absorption during exercise. If an athlete becomes dehydrated by as little as 2–3% body weight, gastric emptying rates begin to decline, leading to dehydration and often times stomach discomfort.[29]

How does heat acclimatization affect hydration requirements?

Physiological changes occur as an athlete adjusts to warmer environments during exercise. Adjustments are made for both short-term and long-term exposure to heat. An example of a short-term exposure scenario is when athletes are forced to train indoors for several days because of icy winter conditions or heavy snowfall. In this scenario the indoor temperature and humidity are much higher than the athletes are accustomed to. As a result, they sweat more than usual and thus require a short-term adjustment in their hydration requirements. Once the athletes return to the colder outdoor environment, water requirements quickly return to their previous outdoor

training levels. An example of a long-term situation occurs with the change in seasons. As the weather changes from the cool temperatures of spring to the hot, humid conditions of summer, athletes' sweat rates will be altered. Sweat rates will increase initially for 10–14 days. After approximately 2 weeks, an athlete's sweat rate should be reassessed and the hydration plan modified accordingly.

Athletes' hydration status should be monitored closely during acclimatization. Typically, athletes will not replace all lost fluids voluntarily in the heat. As heat acclimatization progresses, voluntary intake usually increases to more closely match losses.[30] One study has reported an opposite trend in fluid intake.[31] Five untrained, unacclimated women performed 3 days of exercise in the heat over a period of 6 weeks. The researcher found that fluid intake decreased, instead of increased, over time. There were several methodological pitfalls to this study, including the lack of sweat volume measurements to compare to intake to evaluate fluid balance. However, the study did confirm previous findings that thirst may not always drive an athlete to drink sufficient amounts of fluids, and thus the recommendation for monitoring hydration status during heat acclimation.

How does altitude affect hydration requirements?

Exposure to high altitude increases the risk for athletes becoming dehydrated. Physiologically, there are several issues that can affect the hydration status of athletes when training or competing at higher altitudes, in particular altitudes above 1.6 kilometers (5280 feet). First, temperatures tend to become progressively colder with increasing altitude (1.8° F for every 500 feet), and colder air is drier air. As altitude increases above 5280 feet, there is less air pressure driving oxygen into the blood. As a result, the body adjusts to the decreased oxygen availability by noticeably increasing breathing rate. The increased volume of dry air coursing through the respiratory passageways, even at rest, leads to increased water loss as the air is humidified on its way to the lungs. When taken in combination, 24-hour exposure to colder, drier air leads to a reduction of body water via dramatic increases in insensible water loss through the skin and respiratory tract. As a result, dehydration can result independent of whether the athlete is training or not. During training, sweat losses are added to the increased water loss via insensible avenues to make fluid turnover even greater. Therefore, athletes need to be particularly conscious about in-

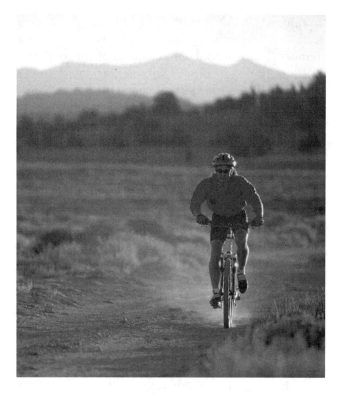

creasing fluid intake at higher altitudes and monitoring urine color and/or body weight fluctuations to help maintain their water balance.

What types of fluids should be consumed during exercise?

The type of fluid consumed during exercise can have a major impact on the hydration status of an athlete. The inclusion of macronutrients, vitamins, and minerals can supply the dietary components to enhance endurance performance and/or muscle building. The temperature of a beverage can affect palatability and digestibility, affecting the volume of fluid an athlete ingests and absorbs. These components and characteristics of fluid replacement beverages have been recognized, studied, and integrated into what most athletes know of as "sports drinks."

How much and what types of carbohydrates should be included in a fluid replacement beverage?

As mentioned previously in Chapter 3, exogenous carbohydrates are extremely beneficial during exercise, especially if the activity is of high intensity or long duration (>45 minutes). In terms of fluids, a carbohydrate-containing beverage has been shown to increase athletic performance versus consuming water alone.[27,32,33] It is recommended that athletes consume 60–66 grams of carbohydrates per hour,

or 1.0–1.1 grams of carbohydrates per minute, during exercise to maintain energy and power output while preventing gastrointestinal upset. Sixty to 66 grams of carbohydrates per hour equate to approximately 1 liter of a 6–8% carbohydrate drink.

Consuming beverages supplying greater than an 8% solution will increase the ingestion of carbohydrates; however, it will also decrease the gastric emptying and intestinal absorption rates.[29,34,35] Higher concentrations in the intestines can cause a reverse osmotic effect, pulling fluids into the intestinal lumen, potentially leading to bloating, cramping, and diarrhea. Therefore, fluids with a higher concentration of carbohydrates, such as fruit juices, sodas, and some sports beverages, are not recommended as the sole beverage during exercise.[4] These fluids can be used appropriately in small amounts during ultra-endurance events when flavor fatigue is of concern. More specific guidelines on alternate fluids for ultra-endurance athletes are discussed in depth in Chapter 12.

The carbohydrate concentration, or % carbohydrate, can be determined by looking at the Nutrition or Supplement Facts label on a product. Look for the number of grams of carbohydrates in 240 milliliters, or 8 ounces, of the product. To determine the carbohydrate concentration, divide the grams of carbohydrates by 240 milliliters, and then multiply the result by 100:

(grams of carbohydrates / 240 milliliters) × 100 = % carbohydrate solution

For example, a sports beverage may have 15 grams of carbohydrates in one 8 oz serving. By using the preceding calculation, it is determined that the sports beverage is a 6% carbohydrate solution:

(15 g of carbohydrates / 240 mL) × 100 = 6% carbohydrate solution

Conversely, a fruit juice might have 35 grams of carbohydrates in one 8 oz serving. The fruit juice is a 15% carbohydrate solution:

(35 g of carbohydrates / 240 mL) × 100 = 15% carbohydrate solution

By using this calculation, athletes can evaluate the appropriateness of new or existing products on the market for use during training sessions or competitions.

The type of carbohydrates in a fluid replacement beverage is also of importance. Glucose, sucrose, and glucose polymers are appropriate types of carbohydrates that digest well for most individuals and are absorbed readily through the intestines. Sports drinks are typically composed of a combination of these sugars. The absorption of carbohydrates is actually maximized when several forms of carbohydrates are used simultaneously, which is the reason why glucose, sucrose, and glucose polymers are included in one product.[36–38] Sources of fructose, such as fruit juice, should be limited because fructose has been shown to increase gastrointestinal distress when consumed during exercise.[36,39] Athletes should note that fructose is sometimes included in small amounts in sports beverages to increase the palatability of the beverage and possibly enhance gastric emptying. A few studies have shown gastric emptying to increase when a beverage contains both glucose and fructose, versus glucose alone.[40] In general, the small amounts of fructose added to some sports beverages can be tolerated without consequence. Each athlete should determine his or her individual preferences and tolerances to evaluate the usage of products that contain fructose.

Taste can affect the amount of fluid consumed during exercise. A flavored beverage has been found to encourage higher fluid consumption during exercise than plain water.[41–43] Some athletes have specific flavor preferences and may consume less total fluid if they are presented with beverages in flavors they dislike. If a team or coaching staff supplies flavored sports drinks to players, providing several different flavors may be helpful to meet specific player preferences. Athletes should be encouraged to try different flavors during their sport activity practices and use the most palatable flavors during competition and training.

Exercise intensity and environmental conditions also dictate what is considered the ideal carbohydrate concentration of a fluid replacement beverage. As the need for fluids during exercise increases, the ideal level of carbohydrate concentration decreases. For example, in hot, humid environments where sweat rates are high

and therefore fluid requirements are great, the level of carbohydrates in a replacement beverage should be below 7% to optimize the rate at which carbohydrates are digested and absorbed. When conditions are mild and the exercise intensity is low, carbohydrate concentrations of greater than 7% may be tolerated.[4] Once again, individual variances will ultimately determine the ideal level of carbohydrate concentration and thus fluid choices.

How much and what types of electrolytes should be included in a fluid replacement beverage?

Sweat is composed mainly of water, along with various electrolytes such as sodium, chloride, potassium, magnesium, and calcium. However, the concentration of electrolytes in sweat can vary greatly based on the rate of sweating, the state of training, and the state of heat acclimatization. Generally speaking, the better the state of conditioning and the more acclimatized the athlete is to hot, humid environments, the lower the concentration of electrolytes found in the sweat. However, considering that sweat rates can be upward of 2–3 liters per hour, the loss of sodium and other electrolytes can be significant. To maintain proper bodily function as well as peak performance, drinks containing electrolytes are appropriate for consumption during exercise, especially prolonged endurance activities. The main electrolytes lost in sweat are sodium and chloride. For exercise durations less than 3–4 hours in length, sodium and chloride replacement does not appear to be physiologically necessary. However, even for short-duration activities, the presence of sodium in a beverage provides an extra bonus in the quest for optimal hydration—sodium typically makes beverages more palatable and stimulates the drive to drink. Therefore, even though the depletion of sodium during short-duration activities does not necessitate concurrent replacement, it can motivate athletes to drink more fluids and thus optimize hydration levels.

There are several situations in which sodium and chloride consumption during exercise is critical. For athletes engaging in exercise sessions lasting longer than four hours, the gradual loss of sodium in sweat over time can lead to depletion and low blood sodium concentrations. Also, within the initial days of heat acclimatization, athletes will lose a larger percentage of sodium in sweat and thus require sodium replacement. In addition to consuming sodium during exercise, athletes acclimatizing to the heat should also consider a temporary increase in their daily intake of sodium, possibly as high as 4–10 grams of sodium per day.[44] This level can be easily consumed by eating salty foods and adding a small amount of table salt to foods during meals. Finally, individuals who are restricting sodium intake or who have not consumed a well-balanced meal prior to exercise should consider choosing a beverage containing sodium during exercise. Therefore, under these conditions, the NATA has recommended adding sodium to fluid replacement beverages in quantities of 0.3 to 0.7 grams per liter. For most athletes the sodium content of sports beverages is sufficient to meet their needs during exercise. However, in some cases additional salt tablets may be indicated. The use of salt tablets is covered in more depth in Chapter 12 of this book.

Other minerals in sweat, though present in small quantities, include potassium, magnesium, calcium, copper, iron, and zinc. These minerals are not universally found in sports beverages but can be found in other sports performance products. Most sports beverages contain a small amount of potassium, which will meet the needs of most athletes during exercise. Potassium tablets should not be taken—excessive amounts of potassium can disrupt the electrical rhythm of the heart. Athletes can easily, and inexpensively, increase their daily food intake of these minerals to compensate for any losses in sweat.

If electrolytes lost in sweat are not replaced, problems can occur. An electrolyte deficiency can occur after one bout of long-duration exercise and/or excessive sweating, or resulting from a low daily intake of electrolytes coupled with consistent depletion of electrolytes through regular physical activity. One of the most common symptoms of electrolyte deficiencies is muscle cramping. Muscle cramps are uncomfortable, distracting, and can halt athletes in their tracks, thus affecting sport performance. In some cases, an electrolyte deficiency not only affects athletic performance but also endangers health. One of the increasingly common health issues associated with electrolyte deficiency is exercise-induced hyponatremia.

Hyponatremia is a disorder of fluid-electrolyte balance that results in abnormally low sodium concentrations (>130–135 mmol/L) in the blood, typically occurring during endurance duration activities lasting longer than four hours. If sustained, hyponatremia can lead to a variety of neurological dysfunctions that, left untreated, can escalate into seizures, coma, and/or death. The signs and symptoms of hyponatremia include headache, nausea, dizziness,

vomiting, or seizures. Hyponatremia can be caused by several factors:

- Drinking too much prior to a workout or event
- Following a salt-free or very low salt diet
- Consuming fluid in excess of individual sweat losses
- Drinking only water, versus a sports beverage containing sodium, during long-duration exercise
- Exercising for greater than four hours
- Taking diuretic medications, typically prescribed for hypertension
- Taking NSAIDs (nonsteroidal anti-inflammatory drugs) such as Advil or Aleve before or during exercise

By following the preexercise hydration guidelines, discovering individual sweat rates, relying on mainly sports beverages during long-duration exercise, and eating sodium in pre- and postexercise meals, a majority of hyponatremia cases can be averted. Special precautions need to be taken for athletes participating in marathons, Ironman distance triathlons, and other ultra-endurance events. These precautions and a greater discussion of hyponatremia can be found in Chapter 12 of this book.

Does the osmolality of the fluid consumed during exercise make a difference?

osmolality An indicator of the concentration of dissolved particles per kilogram of solvent (mOsm/kg). Osmolality affects the movement of water across membranes when the concentrations on either side of the membrane are different. A beverage with a high osmolality tends to draw water to it rather than be absorbed.

The effects of **osmolality** on both gastric emptying and intestinal absorption have been studied. The osmolality of a beverage depends mainly on the carbohydrate and electrolyte content of a product. In general, as osmolality increases, gastric emptying decreases. In recent years, to decrease the osmolality of their products, sports drink manufacturers have started using glucose polymers or maltodextrins, which have less of an effect on osmolality than simple sugars do. Although important, the osmolality of beverages seems to be secondary to other factors in regard to gastric emptying. Gisolfi et al.[45] found that beverages ranging as high as 400 mOsm/kg did not inhibit gastric emptying. Therefore, the osmolality of sports beverages does not appear to be as influential as the volume and calorie content of fluids for gastric emptying.

On the other hand, the osmolality of sports beverages has been shown to greatly affect the intestinal absorption of fluids. Some research has shown that solutions that are hypertonic to plasma (<280 mOsm/kg) stimulate less fluid absorption through the intestines and actually draw water into the intestinal lumen, potentially leading to dehydration and intestinal cramping.[46] Hypotonic and isotonic solutions (<280 mOsm/kg) have been suggested to enhance fluid absorption through the intestinal wall, facilitating hydration.[18,47] However, recent studies have challenged the notion of an upper limit of 280 mOsm/kg for optimal intestinal absorption.[45] More research is needed in this area to determine an ideal osmolality for intestinal absorption at varying levels of exercise intensities. For now, a general recommendation, attempting to optimize both gastric emptying and intestinal absorption, is to choose a fluid replacement beverage with an osmolality close to 280 mOsm/kg. The amount and type of carbohydrates in a beverage have the greatest effect on osmolality; therefore, continuing to use commercially prepared sports drinks of less than or equal to a 6–8% solution (14–18 g carbohydrates/8 oz) is still the best recommendation.

Does the temperature of fluids consumed during exercise matter?

The temperature of fluids consumed during exercise can either encourage or discourage consumption. Most athletes prefer a cool beverage, claiming the lower temperatures make the fluid more appealing and refreshing. Individual preferences vary; however, beverages at 50–59° F are typically recommended.[4]

Should protein be included in fluid replacement beverages?

The inclusion of protein in carbohydrate–electrolyte replacement beverages has recently been explored. The theory is that consuming protein during exercise will increase the body's insulin response to ingested nutrients during exercise, thus sparing glycogen stored in the muscle and liver, in turn enhancing endurance performance. In several studies, the addition of protein to a carbohydrate beverage enhanced the insulin response postexercise.[48–50] It has therefore been theorized that adding protein to a beverage during exercise would have the same effect. However, the results from studies performed during exercise have been inconsistent, with some researchers reporting increased performance without an enhanced insulin response.[51] Therefore, an ergogenic effect may be caused by a mechanism other than insulin. More research is needed in this area to define the advantages of a protein–carbohydrate–electrolyte beverage over a traditional sports drink, as well as the ideal quantity of protein to consume through a beverage during exercise.

For a summary of factors affecting fluid consumption and absorption during exercise, refer to **Table 8.4**.

Why are commercial sports beverages beneficial for athletes?

In the 1960s, the University of Florida Gators were frustrated by the performance of their football team. The players were strong in the first half of a game but faded quickly near the end of the third and beginning of the fourth quarters because of dehydration. Dr. Robert Cade and Dr. Dana Shires developed a beverage that replaced the nutrients lost during exercise and heavy sweating, specifically carbohydrates and electrolytes. Cade and Shires's beverage became known as Gatorade—the original sports beverage. After drinking this new beverage, the athletes felt rejuvenated and therefore played strong throughout their games. The Gators had a record of 7–4 in their first year of drinking Gatorade in 1965 and then improved to a 9–2 record in 1966. Opponents were flabbergasted and intrigued. As the Gators went on to win the Orange Bowl for the first time in their history, the athletes swore that drinking Gatorade was the reason they felt stronger for longer. Although its introduction was not monitored through a controlled study, Gatorade is now one of the most well-researched products in the sports nutrition arena. However, the "ideal" sports beverage for all durations, intensities, and types of sports has not been defined or formulated. To learn more about Gatorade and research on sports beverages, consult the Web site of the Gatorade Sports Science Institute at www.gssiweb.com.

Gatorade currently has many competitors in the sports beverage market, with formulas varying slightly from product to product. The commonality among most sports beverages is the inclusion of fluid, carbohydrates, and electrolytes. The profile of electrolytes, vitamins, and carbohydrate sources as well as the quantity of each of these nutrients create a majority of the differences. Formulas also vary by flavor, sweetness, carbonation, and viscosity in attempts to cater to varying personal preferences. The "optimal" formulation of a sports beverage has

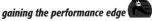

gaining the performance edge

During exercise, drinking chilled fluids is refreshing and may encourage greater fluid consumption.

	TABLE 8.4 Factors Affecting Fluid Consumption and Absorption During Exercise	

Factor	Recommendation	Additional Considerations
Amount of carbohydrate	1.0–1.1 g carbohydrates/minute or 60–66 g carbohydrates/hour	Helps provide energy during exercise.
Carbohydrate concentration	6–8% carbohydrate solution is the best for beverages used during exercise	>8% solution can cause delayed gastric emptying and gastric upset.
Type of carbohydrate	Glucose, sucrose, and glucose polymers	High levels of fructose in sports drinks may cause delayed gastric emptying and gastric upset.
Flavor	Flavored beverages increase fluid intake during exercise versus plain water or unflavored sports beverages	Athletes have varied flavor preferences and should taste test a variety of flavors to find a favorite.
Exercise intensity	8% or lower carbohydrate solution is best tolerated at higher exercise intensity levels	Sports drinks are the recommended beverage for high-intensity exercise.
Environmental conditions	High heat and humidity increase fluid needs; 8% or lower carbohydrate solution is best tolerated in these conditions	More frequent hydration breaks during exercise and competition are needed.
Electrolytes	0.3–0.7 g sodium per liter of fluid consumed	Other electrolytes such as potassium, magnesium, or calcium may be added in small amounts.
Osmolality	~280 mOsm/kg	As osmolality increases, intestinal absorption tends to decrease.
Temperature of the beverage	Cool is best, typically between 50° F and 59° F is best tolerated	Individual preferences will vary.
Protein	No recommendations at this time for the inclusion of protein in sports beverages	More research is needed to fully evaluate the need for protein during exercise.

not necessarily been proven through comparison research; therefore, individual preferences are a major determinant of consumption and thus success with a sports beverage. Overall, the benefit of sports beverages versus water is the inclusion of carbohydrates for sustaining energy levels and electrolytes to prevent conditions such as hyponatremia.

Athletes need to look closely at the Nutrition Facts or Supplement Facts label on beverages to evaluate the type and quantity of carbohydrates, electrolytes, and other nutrients contained in the beverage to determine the appropriateness for their individual sport, the duration of their activities, and individual preferences. The following are some items to look for when reading sports beverage labels:

- *Type of carbohydrate:* Each formula is slightly different. Look for glucose, sucrose, or glucose polymers listed on the ingredients label. Some brands promote their product as a source of "complex carbohydrates," claiming to sustain energy longer. Most of these products use glucose polymers as the carbohydrate source; these are strings of linked glucose molecules versus a

single or "simple" carbohydrate. These products can certainly be beneficial in enhancing performance because they provide carbohydrates, but they may or may not necessarily be more effective than other sports beverages that include a mix of carbohydrate sources. In general, avoid products that contain solely or mainly fructose as the source of carbohydrates. "Natural" sports beverages often contain fructose because fruit juice is used as the sweetening agent versus other sugars. Some athletes may be able to consume fructose without adverse side effects of stomach and intestinal upset and cramping; however, it is better to be safe than sorry and make it a rule to watch out for fructose.

- *Artificial sweeteners:* Some brands of sports beverages include artificial sweeteners. The artificial sweeteners are added to enhance the flavor and palatability of the beverage while keeping the carbohydrate concentration within the guidelines of 6–8%. However, if an athlete is consuming large quantities of fluid during workouts or competitions to match sweat losses, the athlete's intake of artificial sweeteners can rise dramatically with these products. Some athletes experience adverse side effects or possibly allergic reactions to artificial sweeteners. Therefore, products containing artificial sweeteners such as aspartame, saccharin, and acesulfame potassium are not recommended. Look for these sweeteners in the ingredient listing on the label.

- *Stimulants such as caffeine or herbal products:* A newer line of beverages is labeled as "energy" drinks, and these are often marketed for use during exercise. These drinks often contain caffeine and/or a variety of herbal stimulants such as guarana as their major source of "energy." Sugar can be included but is often in concentrations above the recommended 6–8%. Other formulas are sweetened by artificial sweeteners, which provide no carbohydrates. In general, these energy drinks should be avoided during exercise. Look for kola nut, guarana, caffeine, and artificial sweeteners in the ingredients listing.

- *High doses of vitamins and minerals:* To make their formula different, some beverages contain a variety of B vitamins, antioxidant vitamins, or minerals. Sodium, chloride, and potassium are the minerals that are beneficial to include in a sports drink and should be included in sufficient quantities. However, other vitamins or minerals can cause gastrointestinal distress, especially when the beverage is consumed in large quantities to match sweat rates. Look on the Supplement Facts label for the %DV (percent daily value) for each vitamin and mineral in one serving of the product. Multiply the percentage by the number of servings that will be consumed in one exercise session. If the total amount consumed—for nutrients other than carbohydrates, sodium, or potassium—is reaching 200% or more, then reconsider using the product. For example, magnesium is promoted as a mineral that can help prevent cramping. For athletes consuming a well-balanced diet, sufficient daily magnesium can be helpful for the prevention of muscle cramps. However, if an athlete who suffers from muscle cramping chooses a sports beverage containing significant amounts of magnesium, problems can result. As-

suming the athlete will need to drink 4–8 servings of the sports beverage (assuming an 8 oz serving, with the athlete requiring 32–64 oz for a 1–2 hour practice), the total magnesium consumed may exceed the RDA by several times, possibly resulting in gastrointestinal upset and diarrhea—a side effect of excessive intake of magnesium. Therefore, look for the electrolyte basics in a sports beverage—sodium, chloride, and potassium—and avoid products containing large quantities (>10–20% DV in one serving) of other vitamins or minerals.

- *Carbonation:* The vast majority of commercial sports beverages are not carbonated. However, athletes should check the label and avoid carbonated beverages before, during, and immediately after exercise. The effervescent bubbles in these beverages take up space in the stomach, causing a full or bloated feeling. This will decrease the amount of fluid consumed because there is a false sense of fullness. Athletes should limit carbonated beverages as part of their regular fluid intake during the day for the same reason.

- *Specialty formulas:* Sports beverage producers may have an entire line of hydration products. Typically the products will fall into several categories: preexercise, during physical activity, ultra-endurance events, and recovery beverages. The preexercise beverages are generally higher in carbohydrates to help athletes maximize glycogen stores before a training session or competition. These beverages may not be necessary; well-balanced meals and fluids from water, milk, and juice are sufficient for providing carbohydrates and fluids prior to activity. Formulas for during activity focus on carbohydrates and electrolytes. Follow the previously mentioned guidelines when reviewing these products. The endurance formulas are typically higher in sodium and other electrolytes. These beverages can be useful and appropriate for exercise lasting longer than four hours. Evaluate each product for the appropriateness of the types of carbohydrates and quantities of various vitamins and minerals. Recovery beverages generally contain carbohydrates, protein, and antioxidant vitamins and minerals. These beverages can be useful for situations when athletes do not have immediate access to food after exercise. However, if food and beverages are easily accessible, then recovery beverages may not be necessary. For a comparison of sports beverages commonly used during exercise, refer to **Table 8.5**.

What are some practical guidelines for consuming fluids during exercise?

The goal of fluid consumption during exercise is to keep athletes hydrated so that they can perform at their best and maintain health. To achieve these goals, athletes and coaches should consider the following hydration factors:

- *Fluids should be readily available.* Athletes need to take personal responsibility for having fluids on hand at all times during training sessions and competitions. Athletes should have plenty of water bottles to keep in gym bags, in lockers, at home, and in training rooms. Measured water bottles can also help athletes determine whether they are meeting their hydration needs.

- *Fluids should taste good based on personal preference.* If the beverage does not taste good to an athlete, he or she will not drink it. Therefore, allow athletes to choose their fluid replacement beverage, within the guidelines stated in this chapter.

- *Coaches should allow for regular refreshment breaks during training and competitions.* Not only should fluids be on-site and available, but regular breaks should be taken in order for consumption to occur. Breaks will depend on the nature of the sport, such as timeouts in basketball or in between sets in swimming.

Fortifying
Your Nutrition Knowledge

Determine Don's Hydration Needs

Don, an Ironman triathlete, performed a sweat trial to determine his fluid needs per hour. He cycled 50 miles at a 20 mph pace, and then ran 10 miles at a 9-minute-per-mile pace. During the workout, he drank four 24-ounce bottles of a sports beverage on the bike, and then drank another 24 ounces of water during the run. He lost 6 pounds during his workout.

What are Don's fluid needs?

Answer:

- *Determine body weight lost during exercise.* Don lost 6 pounds during his exercise session.
- *Determine the fluid equivalent, in ounces, of the total weight lost during exercise.* Don lost 6 pounds, so 6 lb × 16–24 oz/lb = 96–144 oz.
- *Determine the actual fluid needs of the athlete during an identical workout.* Don consumed 96 ounces on the bike (4 × 24-oz/bottle) plus 24 ounces on the run, for a total of 120 ounces. Adding the fluid consumed during exercise to the fluid equivalent of body weight lost during exercise equals 216–264 oz (120 + [96–144]).
- *Determine the number of fluid ounces needed per hour of exercise.* Don's total fluid needs are 216–264 oz. Because he was on the bike for 2.5 hours (50 miles ÷ 20 mph = 2½ hr) and 1.5 hours on the run (10 miles × 9 min/mile pace = 90 min = 1½ hr), the total exercise time was 4 hours. Dividing the total fluid needs by the total exercise time equals 54–66 oz/hr ([216–264 oz] ÷ 4 hr).
- Don is a "big sweater," losing 54–66 ounces of sweat per hour of exercise. This volume of fluid can be challenging to consume while exercising. Currently, Don is only consuming 30 ounces of fluid per hour (120 oz consumed ÷ 4 hours of exercise = 30 oz/hour). Therefore, Don can start to gradually increase the volume of fluid he ingests each hour during exercise, approaching 54–66 ounces per hour, monitoring for any gastric and/or intestinal discomfort. He may or may not reach the ultimate goal; however, he can strive for it. To maximize the fluid retained, he should focus on the consumption of sports beverages versus solely water.

TABLE 8.5

Sports Beverage Comparison (per 8 oz of product)

Product	Purpose	Quantity of CHO* (grams)	% CHO*	Type of CHO*	Sodium (mg)	K** (mg)	Vitamins and Minerals	Other Ingredients	Comments
	Hydration during short- and long-duration exercise	14–20	6–8%	Glucose, sucrose, and glucose polymers (maltodextrin)	70–200	30–75	If added, only small amounts (0.5–2% of DV) of calcium and magnesium	None	Beverage needs to taste good to encourage consumption. Athletes should be able to consume large quantities of the beverage without risk of reaching toxic levels of any vitamin or mineral.
Accelerade	Hydration during exercise	14	6%	Sucrose, fructose, trehalose (Ascenda)	127	43	67% of DV for vitamin C and E	3.3 grams of protein	Unique product containing protein. Levels of vitamin C and E are too high if consuming large quantities.
All Sport	Hydration during exercise	16	7%	High fructose corn syrup	55	60	40% of DV for vitamin C	None	High fructose corn syrup may cause upset stomach and intestinal cramping.
Carbo-Pro	Hydration during exercise	19	8%	Glucose polymers	0	0	None	None	Neutral flavor may be appealing to athletes who dislike the sweet taste of beverages. Does not contain electrolytes; therefore, it is not appropriate for long-duration activity unless combined with other products.
Gatorade Endurance	Hydration for long-duration events	14	6%	Sucrose, fructose	200	90	Small amounts of calcium and magnesium added	None	Higher sodium and potassium content is beneficial for exercise lasting longer than 3–4 hours. The quantities of calcium and magnesium are kept low and therefore the risk of adverse side effects is also low.
Gatorade Thirst Quencher	Hydration during exercise	14	6%	Sucrose, dextrose	110	30	None	None	The original sports beverage. Contains the basics for replenishment during exercise: carbohydrates, sodium, and potassium.

(continued)

TABLE 8.5　Sports Beverage Comparison (per 8 oz of product) *(Continued)*

Product	Purpose	Quantity of CHO* (grams)	% CHO*	Type of CHO*	Sodium (mg)	K** (mg)	Vitamins and Minerals	Other Ingredients	Comments
Heed	Hydration during exercise	20	8%	Maltodextrin, zylitol, stevia	30	12	Added magnesium, vitamin B$_6$, manganese, and chromium	None	Low sodium and potassium as well as moderately high levels of vitamin B$_6$ and manganese. The sugar alcohol, zylitol, could cause gastric upset.
High 5 Isotonic	Hydration during exercise	19	8%	Maltodextrin, fructose	200	58	None	None	Higher sodium and potassium content is beneficial for exercise lasting longer than 3–4 hours.
Ironman Perform	Hydration during exercise	17	7%	Maltodextrin, dextrose, fructose	190	10	Added magnesium	None	Higher content of sodium versus most sports drinks, but low potassium. Magnesium content is low and should not cause problems for most athletes.
Powerade	Hydration during exercise	19	8%	High fructose corn syrup, maltodextrin	55	30	10% vitamin B$_6$, B$_{12}$, and niacin	None	Low sodium and moderately high levels of vitamins B$_6$, B$_{12}$, and niacin. Some athletes may have problems with the high fructose corn syrup.
Shaklee Performance	Hydration during exercise	25	10%	Maltodextrin, fructose, glucose	130	50	Added calcium, magnesium, and phosphorus	None	Concentration of carbohydrates is high for consumption during exercise. Added minerals are in small quantities and unlikely to cause problems unless very large volumes are consumed at once.

* CHO = Carbohydrate

** K = Potassium

- *Consumption of fluids should begin early in an exercise session.* It takes approximately 10–20 minutes for ingested fluids to reach the bloodstream; by initiating the consumption of fluid replacement beverages early in a training session, athletes can stay ahead of the game in hydration. By consuming fluids gradually during practices and competitions, athletes not only will maintain euhydration to a greater degree, but also will generally tolerate fluids better than in bolus feedings.

- *Use sports beverages for sessions lasting longer than 60–90 minutes.* As the duration of exercise increases, the need for carbohydrate and electrolyte replacement during exercise also escalates. Drinking solely water during long-duration exercise can increase the risk of hyponatremia because of the lack of electrolyte consumption. It should be noted that sports beverages may also enhance performance during slightly shorter duration activities (i.e., 45 to 60 minutes) if they are of high intensity.

- *Consider "hydration training" equal to "physical training" for competition.* Athletes must practice their hydration protocol during training to minimize the risk of gastric and intestinal discomfort during competitions caused by unfamiliar conditions. Hydration training should be considered as seriously as physical training.

What is the role of postexercise hydration?

After exercise, the body is thirsty and hungry for replenishment. Replacing water, as well as electrolytes and carbohydrates lost during exercise, as quickly as possible aids in the recovery of a variety of body processes, including cardiovascular, thermoregulatory, and metabolic activities. Unfortunately, many athletes fail to drink enough to fully restore euhydration and replenish their glycogen and electrolyte stores. Athletes need to be educated on the importance of proper hydration after exercise, current guidelines, and practical tips and hints to put the recommendations into practice.

How much fluid should be consumed?

Ideally, athletes will estimate their sweat losses and then aim to match sweat losses with fluid intake during exercise. However, this situation rarely exists and therefore lost fluids need to be replaced after training sessions or competitions. If pre- and postexercise weight measurements were taken, then the rehy-

dration volume can be calculated. Sweat losses should be matched 100–150% because the kidneys continually produce urine, thus increasing total water excretion.[52] Therefore, for every pound that is lost during exercise, approximately 16–24 ounces of fluid should be consumed. Fluids should be consumed as soon as possible to accelerate recovery, especially if athletes are performing multiple workouts in one day.

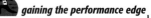

Regardless of whether body weight was measured, athletes should begin hydrating immediately, drinking slowly and consistently. Typically, athletes are encouraged to drink until their urine returns to a clear or pale color. If so, then it is estimated that the athlete will be within 1% of his or her baseline body weight.[53] However, the notion of urine color providing an accurate measure of hydration status has been questioned by some researchers. Kovacs et al.[54] found that urine color, specific electrical conductance, and osmolality were all poor indicators of hydration status in the 6 hours postexercise. More research is needed in this area to fully define the ideal measures of hydration postexercise.

Athletes should be cautioned to avoid drinking very large quantities of water in a short period of time immediately following exercise because this can potentially lead to delayed rehydration or, more seriously, hyponatremia. Large quantities of water are absorbed readily into the bloodstream. The rapid influx of water dilutes the concentration of sodium, causing a decreased plasma osmolality. The body responds to the lower osmolality by increasing urine production and blunting the normal sodium-dependent stimulation of the thirst mechanism. If plain water continues to be consumed, sodium concentrations will continue to plummet, and hyponatremia ensues. Postexercise beverages should ideally contain carbohydrates and electrolytes to replenish stores as well as to assist in optimizing rehydration. Therefore, beverages such as fruit and vegetable juices, milk, soups, or sports drinks are preferred over water after exercise.

What types of fluids should be consumed?

Many athletes' rehydration plans consist of guzzling down plain water. Although water will supply fluid to the body, it may not be the ideal beverage for postexercise replenishment. By consuming

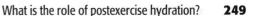

carbohydrates and sodium along with water, euhydration, muscle glycogen, and electrolyte balance can be restored more readily.

As mentioned previously, most athletes do not drink enough fluids voluntarily. Therefore, any method of encouraging fluid consumption after exercise will be beneficial. Part of the concern with consuming only water is that it generally does not stimulate the drive to drink and also can increase urine output, causing both decreased intake and increased losses. The presence of carbohydrates and sodium in either a postexercise beverage or a meal consumed concurrently with water can remedy the situation. Sodium will enhance fluid retention and the drive to drink.[52,55] Carbohydrates can increase the rate of intestinal absorption of both water and sodium.[56–58] Because sodium is lost in sweat and carbohydrate stores are depleted during exercise, it is beneficial to consume these nutrients not only for rehydration purposes but also for electrolyte and glycogen replenishment.

Potassium, another electrolyte lost in sweat, can easily be replaced by consuming whole foods and juices after exercise. In a 2-hour workout session, an average athlete will lose approximately 180 milligrams of potassium. One banana contains ~500 milligrams—more than twice what is lost in 2 hours of exercise. A variety of whole fruits and vegetables and their juices are rich sources of potassium and are ideal to consume after exercise.

Refer to **Table 8.6** for a summary of the daily and exercise-specific fluid recommendations for athletes.

Are supplements beneficial after exercise?

Many fluid replacement products are marketed to athletes to help facilitate hydration while also replacing electrolytes and glycogen stores after exercise. Before reaching for one of these products, athletes should consider the following:

- *How filling is the product?* Many of the products come in a powdered form that is mixed with 8–24 ounces of plain water. If an athlete loses 2 pounds during a workout (the equivalent of 32–48 fluid ounces), but only drinks 8–24

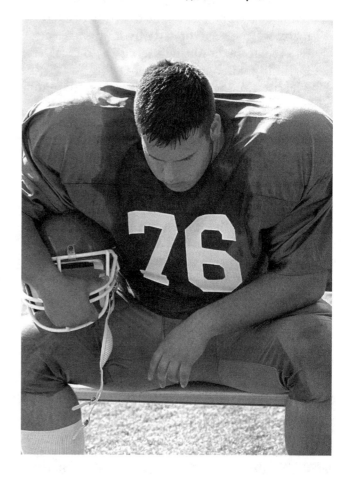

		TABLE 8.6	Daily and Exercise-Specific Fluid Recommendations for Athletes			
	Daily Recommendation	2–4 Hours Prior to Exercise	10–20 Minutes Prior to Exercise	During Exercise	After Exercise
Amount	AI = 3.7 L/day (males); 2.7 L/day females) 1 mL/ calorie consumed	13–20 oz	7–10 oz	7–10 oz every 10–20 minutes	16–24 oz per pound of body weight lost, consumed within 2 hours
Type of Beverage	Water, 100% juices, milk, or other beverages	Water or sports drink; juices or milk if tolerated	Water or sports drink	Sports drink preferable	Water, sports drink, juices, milk, or other beverages

ounces, then he or she is falling short on water replenishment. Recovery products typically contain 120–320 calories and thus can be filling, causing an athlete to voluntarily stop drinking. Although added carbohydrates, sodium, and other nutrients are important to have immediately following exercise, if they prevent an athlete from also consuming the fluid he or she needs, then the supplement should be avoided. If the product tastes good and therefore the athlete drinks more, then the supplement may be beneficial.

- *How much carbohydrate and sodium are present in the supplement?* As mentioned previously, carbohydrates and sodium are beneficial for replenishment and rehydration. However, some products fall short of the recommended doses of each of these nutrients, potentially hindering recovery if no other food or fluid is consumed. Athletes should consume carbohydrates at a rate of 1.2 grams per kilogram of body weight per hour for 3–4 hours postexercise. For every liter of fluid lost in sweat (1 L = 34 oz = ~1.5–2 pounds of weight loss), 300–700 mg of sodium should be consumed after exercise. Based on body weight and sweat losses, athletes should examine the Supplement Facts label on the supplement to determine whether it contains sufficient quantities of carbohydrates and sodium, in addition to fluid.

- *How expensive is the product?* Supplements can cost a fortune! Water, juices, and soups as well as sodium- and carbohydrate-rich foods can deliver equal nutrition, often at a much lower price. However, some athletes prefer using the recovery drink supplements because they require little to no preparation, may not require refrigeration, and can taste good. Athletes should weigh the pros and cons of using a supplement versus "real" food to determine whether it is worth the cost.

- *Are there a lot of "extras" in the supplement?* Some supplements can pack a huge dose of one or several vitamins and minerals in one serving of the product. Keep in mind that the recovery drink is only one item consumed throughout the day. If the supplement, in addition to other foods and beverages, provides mega-doses of nutrients, toxic levels may be reached over time. Look closely at the Supplement Facts label to ensure that none of the nutrients are supplied in doses above 100% DV.

What are some practical guidelines for consuming fluids after exercise?

The goal of fluid consumption after exercise is to restore the body to euhydration status in preparation for the next training or competitive session. To achieve this goal, athletes and coaches should consider the following:

- *Rehydration should begin as soon as possible.* Athletes need to begin drinking water and other fluids within 2 hours of the cessation of activity, but preferably immediately following exercise. Encourage athletes who tend to avoid intake of fluids altogether after exercise to sip on fluids gradually until their stomach is ready to handle more volume.

- *Beverages and/or foods consumed after exercise should contain carbohydrates and sodium.* The addition of these nutrients facilitates fluid absorption and retention while also replacing nutrients lost during exercise. Examples of salty, carbohydrate-rich beverages and foods include vegetable juices, soups, cheeses, luncheon meats, pizza, pretzels, and condiments (such as mustard, ketchup, barbeque sauce, and steak sauce) on sandwiches and burgers.

- *Plan ahead.* Often, athletes will not refuel and rehydrate properly after exercise as a result of limited access to refreshments. Athletes need to take responsibility for ensuring that fluids and foods will be available immediately after exercise to begin the replenishment process. Planning options include packing items before heading to the gym or playing field, purchasing fluids and foods at a nearby grocery or convenience store, and returning home quickly and drinking/eating as soon as possible.

- *Plan for easy-to-prepare snacks and meals.* After hard workouts and competitions, athletes are fatigued and can lack the motivation to prepare a snack or meal in a timely fashion. Athletes should develop a rehydration plan that is easy to follow and easily accessible.

- *Use supplements wisely and sparingly.* Supplements can have a place in an athlete's rehydration plan, if used intelligently. Reserve supplement use for times when other beverages and foods are not available. Read Supplement Facts labels and look for adequate quantities of carbohydrates and sodium and moderate quantities of other vitamins, minerals, and nutrients.

The Box Score

Key Points of Chapter

- Water is arguably the most essential of all the nutrients despite the fact that it does not provide the body with energy. Two-thirds of the body's water is found inside the cells and is referred to as intracellular water. Muscle tissue, which is of obvious importance to athletes, is 70% water. The remaining one-third of the body's water is found outside of cells and is known as extracellular water. Most of the extracellular water is found in the spaces between cells, in lymph, and in blood plasma.

- Water provides structural integrity to cells, serves as the body's delivery and waste removal medium, aids in thermoregulation, helps in maintenance of the acid–base balance, and is critical to the maintenance of blood volume. All of these functions have a direct impact on not only athletic performance but also survival. Dehydration resulting in weight loss of as little as 2–3% of body weight begins to compromise cardiovascular function, which has a direct impact on sport performance.

- Approximately 80% of our daily water needs are supplied in the form of fluids. The remainder (20%) comes from water found in fruits, vegetables, other foods, and metabolic water.

- Water is lost via insensible perspiration, urine, feces, and sweat. The amount lost via sweat is highly variable depending on the environmental conditions as well as the intensity and duration of the exercise training or sport activity. Balancing water intake with water loss is critical for optimal performance, particularly during long-duration activities.

- One easy way to determine the achievement of water balance is to monitor body weight. Daily weight fluctuations are caused primarily by changes in water status.

- Although rare, it is possible to drink too much water, which can result in what is known as "water intoxication." Water intoxication leads to very low blood sodium levels (i.e., hyponatremia), thereby causing muscle weakness, disorientation, and/or coma. Endurance and ultra-endurance athletes are at greatest risk for hyponatremia because of their repeated exposure to long training bouts in which water intake is very high and/or sodium intake inadequate.

- For men and women over age 19, the recommended intake for water is 3.7 liters and 2.7 liters per day, respectively. These daily quantities reflect total water intake from drinking water as well as from other beverages containing water and from solid foods.

- Proper hydration before exercising sets the stage for optimal sports performance. Generous, but not excessive, amounts of fluids should be consumed in the 24 hours before exercise. Drinking enough fluids to meet the daily recommendations will allow an athlete to start an exercise session well-hydrated. Drinking approximately 13–17 oz of fluid 2 hours prior to competition and 7–10 oz of fluid 20 minutes prior will ensure that athletes are properly hydrated.

- The goals of hydration during exercise are to maintain plasma volume and electrolyte balance. Water and electrolyte losses during exercise can vary greatly depending on several factors including body size, exercise intensity, ambient temperature, humidity, clothing choices, and acclimation. For most individuals, consuming approximately 200–300 milliliters, or 7–10 fluid ounces, every 10–20 minutes during exercise will achieve this goal.

- Replacing water, as well as electrolytes and carbohydrates, should begin as quickly as possible after exercise. Two to 3 cups of water or replacement beverage should be consumed for every pound that is lost during exercise.

Study Questions

1. Discuss why the statement "you are what you drink" is appropriate in regard to water's role as a nutrient.

2. What is "water balance"? Which condition, a positive balance or a negative balance, poses the greatest risk to athletes? Defend your answer.

3. Explain why the statement "bottled water is a better source of fluid than tap water" is not necessarily accurate.

4. An athlete concerned about drinking municipal water because of the impurities comes to you to find out where she can buy distilled water. What do you tell the athlete? In other words, what are some of the pros and cons of drinking distilled water?

5. What is the difference between sweat and insensible perspiration? Which is a greater avenue of fluid loss in the athlete?

6. As a dietitian, how can you determine whether your athletes are hydrating well enough during daily training sessions? If they are not taking in enough fluid during training, how do you know how much

to tell them to drink to rehydrate before the next practice?

7. What is the AI for daily fluid intake? What are the body's sources for fluids throughout the day?

8. How much and what types of beverages can be consumed in the hours and minutes leading up to competition? Discuss why fluid intake prior to competition is advantageous.

9. What is a "sweat trial"? What data need to be collected when performing a sweat trial? What are the potential risks associated with not performing a sweat trial on an athlete?

10. What factors can affect how quickly fluids are absorbed by the intestines during training or sport performance?

11. What is hyponatremia? Under what conditions and in which sports might it pose the greatest risk?

12. As a sports nutritionist, what practical guidelines would you give your athletes to help ensure adequate hydration during competition?

13. After competition or training, rehydration is very important. What are the pros and cons of drinking just plain water during recovery?

References

1. Montain SJ, Sawka MN, Wenger CB. Hyponatremia associated with exercise: risk factors and pathogenesis. *Exerc Sport Sci Rev*. 2001;29:113–117.

2. National Collegiate Athletic Association. NCAA Wrestling Rules and Interpretations. Indianapolis, IN: National Collegiate Athletic Association; 2003:WR23–WR34.

3. National Federation of State High School Associations. Wrestling Weight Management Program. Indianapolis, IN: National Federation of State High School Associations; 2001:25–34.

4. Casa DJ, Armstrong LE, Hillman SK, et al. National Athletic Trainers' Association position statement: fluid replacement for athletes. *J Athlet Train*. 2000;35(2):212–224.

5. Institute of Medicine. *Dietary Reference Intakes for Water, Potassium, Sodium, Chloride, and Sulfate*. Food and Nutrition Board. Washington, DC: National Academies Press; 2005.

6. National Research Council. *Recommended Dietary Allowances*. Washington, DC: National Academies Press; 1989.

7. Armstrong LE. Caffeine, body fluid-electrolyte balance, and exercise performance. *Int J Sports Nutr Exerc Metabol*. 2002;12:189–206.

8. Fortney SM, Nadel ER, Wenger CB, Bove JR. Effect of blood volume on sweating rate and body fluids in exercising humans. *J Appl Physiol*. 1981;51:1594–1600.

9. Greenleaf JE, Castle BL. Exercise temperature regulation in man during hypohydration and hyperhydration. *J Appl Physiol*. 1971;30:847–853.

10. Sawka MN, Young AJ, Francesconi RP, Muza SR, Pandolf KB. Thermoregulatory and blood responses during exercise at graded hypohydration levels. *J Appl Physiol*. 1985;59:1394–1401.

11. Moroff SV, Bass DB. Effects of overhydration on man's physiological responses to work in the heat. *J Appl Physiol*. 1965;20:267–270.

12. Sawka MN, Burke LM, Eichner ER, et al. Exercise and fluid replacement. *Med Sci Sports Exerc*. 2007;39(2):377–390.

13. Clarkson PM. Nutritional ergogenic aids: caffeine. *Int J Sports Nutr*. 1993;3:103–111.

14. Dodd SL, Herb RA, Powers SK. Caffeine and exercise performance. *Sports Med*. 1993;15:14–23.

15. Casa DJ, Wingo JE, Knight JC, Dellis WO, Berger EM, McClung JM. Influence of a pre-exercise glycerol hydration beverage on performance and physiological function during mountain bike races in the heat. *J Athlet Train*. 1999;34:S25.

16. Inder WJ, Swanney MP, Donald RA, Prickett TCR, Hellemans J. The effect of glycerol and desmopressin on exercise performance and hydration in triathletes. *Med Sci Sports Exerc*. 1998;30:1263–1269.

17. Kavouras SA, Casa DJ, Herrera JA, et al. Rehydration with glycerol: endocrine, cardiovascular, and thermoregulatory effects during exercise in 37 degrees C. *Med Sci Sports Exerc*. 1998;30(5 suppl):S332.

18. Leiper JB, Maughan RJ. Effect of bicarbonate or base precursor on water and solute absorption from a glucose-electrolyte solution in the human jejunum. *Digestion*. 1988;41(1):39–45.

19. Latzka WA, Sawka MN, Montain SJ, et al. Hyperhydration: thermoregulatory effects during compensable exercise-heat stress. *J App Physiol*. 1997;83:860–866.

20. Convertino VA, Armstrong LA, Coyle EF, et al. Exercise and fluid replacement. *Med Sci Sports Exerc*. 1996;28(1):i–vii.

21. Noakes TD, Adams BA, Myburgh KH, Greef C, Lotz T, Nathan M. The danger of an inadequate water intake during prolonged exercise: a novel concept re-visited. *Eur J Appl Physiol Occup Physiol*. 1988;57(2):210–219.

22. Maughan RJ, Shirreffs SM. Recovery from prolonged exercise: restoration of water and electrolyte balance. *J Sports Sci*. 1997;15:297–303.

23. American Dietetic Association. Position of the American Dietetic Association, Dietitians of Canada, and the American College of Sports Medicine: nutrition and athletic performance. *J Am Dietet Assoc*. 2000;100:1543–1556.

24. Backx K, van Someren KA, Palmer GS. One hour cycling performance is not affected by ingested fluid volume. *Int J Sports Nutr Exerc Metabol*. 2003;13(3):333–342.

25. McConell GK, Stephens TJ, Canny BJ. Fluid ingestion does not influence intense 1-h exercise performance in a mild environment. *Med Sci Sports Exerc*. 1999;31:386–392.

26. Rehrer NJ. Fluid and electrolyte balance in ultra-endurance sport. *Sports Med*. 2001;31(10):701–715.

27. Murray R. Rehydration strategies—balancing substrate, fluid, and electrolyte provision. *Int J Sports Med*. 1998;19:S133–S135.

28. Coombes J, Hamilton K. The effectiveness of commercially available sports drinks. *Sports Med*. 2000;29(3):181–209.

29. Ryan AJ, Lambert GP, Shi X, Chang RT, Summers RW, Gisolfi CV. Effect of hypohydration on gastric emptying and intestinal absorption during exercise. *J Appl Physiol*. 1998;84:1581–1588.

30. Greenleaf JE, Brick PJ, Keil LC, Morse JT. Drinking and water balance during exercise and heat acclimation. *J Appl Physiol*. 1983;54:414.

31. Ormerod JK, Elliott TA, Scheett TP, VanHeest JL, Armstrong LE, Maresh CM. Drinking behavior and perception of thirst in untrained women during 6 weeks of heat acclimation and outdoor training. *Int J Sports Nutr Exerc Metabol*. 2003;13(1):15–28.

32. El-Sayed MS, Balmer J, Rattu AJM. Carbohydrate ingestion improves endurance performance during a 1 h simulated cycling time trial. *J Sports Sci*. 1997;15:223–230.

33. Fritzsche RG, Switzer TW, Hodgkinson BJ, Lee SL, Martin JC, Coyle EF. Water and carbohydrate ingestion during prolonged exercise increase maximal neuromuscular power. *J Appl Physiol*. 2000;88:730–737.

34. Costill DL, Saltin B. Factors limiting gastric emptying during rest and exercise. *J Appl Physiol*. 1974;37:679–683.

35. Bartoli WP, Horn MK, Murray R. Delayed gastric emptying during exercise with repeated ingestion of 8% carbohydrate solution. *Med Sci Sports Exerc*. 1995;27:S13.

36. Hoswill CA. Effective fluid replacement. *Int J Sports Nutr*. 1998;8:175–195.

37. Gisolfi CV. Fluid balance for optimal performance. *Nutr Rev*. 1996;54:S159–S168.

38. Shi X, Summers RW, Schedl HP, Flanagan SW, Chang R, Gisolfi G. Effects of carbohydrate type and concentration and solution osmolality on water absorption. *Med Sci Sports Exerc*. 1995;27:1607–1615.

39. Murray R, Paul GL, Seifert JG, Eddy DE, Halaby GA. The effects of glucose, fructose and sucrose ingestion during exercise. *Med Sci Sports Exerc*. 1989;21:275–282.

40. Neufer PD, Costill DL, Fink WJ. Effects of exercise and carbohydrate composition on gastric emptying. *Med Sci Sports Exerc*. 1986;18(6):658–662.

41. Minehan MR, Riley MD, Burke LM. Effect of flavor and awareness of kilojoule content of drinks on preference and fluid balance in team sports. *Int J Sports Nutr Exerc Metabol*. 2002;12:81–92.

42. Passe DH, Horn M, Murray R. Effect of beverage palatability on voluntary fluid intake during exercise. *Med Sci Sports Exerc*. 1998;30:S156.

43. Rivera-Brown AM, Gutierrez R, Gutierrez JC, Frontera WR, Bar-Or O. Drink composition, voluntary drinking, and fluid balance in exercising, trained, heat-acclimatized boys. *J Appl Physiol*. 86:78–87.

44. Hiller D. Dehydration and hyponatremia during triathlons. *Med Sci Sports Exerc*. 1989;21:S219–S221.

45. Gisolfi CV, Summers RW, Lambert GP, Xia T. Effect of beverage osmolality on intestinal fluid absorption during exercise. *J Appl Physiol*. 1998;85(5):1941–1948.

46. Maughan RJ, Noakes TD. Fluid replacement and exercise stress: a brief review of studies on fluid replacement and some guidelines for athletes. *Sports Med*. 1991;12:16–31.

47. Wapnir RA, Lifshitz F. Osmolality and solute concentration: their relationship with an oral hydration solution effectiveness; an experimental assessment. *Pediatr Res*. 1985;19:894–898.

48. Spiller GA, Jensen CD, Pattison TS, Chick CS, Whittam JH, Scala J. Effect of protein dose on serum glucose and insulin response to sugars. *Am J Clin Nutr*. 1987;46:474–480.

49. VanLoon LJC, Saris WHS, Kruijshoop M, Wagenmakers AJM. Maximizing post-exercise muscle glycogen synthesis: carbohydrate supplementation and the application of amino acid and protein hydrolysate mixtures. *Am J Clin Nutr*. 2000;72:106–111.

50. Zawadzki KM, Yaspelkis BB, Ivy JL. Carbohydrate-protein supplement increase the rate of muscle glycogen storage post-exercise. *J Appl Physiol*. 1992;72:1854–1859.

51. Ivy JL, Res PT, Sprague RC, Widzer MO. Effect of a carbohydrate-protein supplement on endurance performance during exercise of varying intensity. *Int J Sports Nutr Exerc Metabol*. 2003;13(3):382–395.

52. Shirreffs SM, Taylor AJ, Leiper JB, Maughan RJ. Post-exercise rehydration in man: effects of volume consumed and drink sodium content. *Med Sci Sports Exerc*. 1996;28:1260–1271.

53. Armstrong LA, Soto JAH, Hacker FT, Casa DJ, Kavouras SA, Maresh CM. Urinary indices during dehydration, exercise and rehydration. *Int J Sports Nutr*. 1998;8:345–355.

54. Kovacs EMR, Senden JMG, Brouns F. Urine color, osmolality and specific electrical conductance are not accurate measures of hydration status during post-exercise re-hydration. *J Sports Med Phys Fitness*. 1999;39(1):47–53.

55. Wemple RD, Morocco TS, Mack GW. Influence of sodium replacement on fluid ingestion following exercise-induced dehydration. *Int J Sports Nutr*. 1997;7:104–116.

56. Fallowfield JL, Williams C. Carbohydrate intake and recovery from prolonged exercise. *Int J Sports Nutr*. 1993;3:150–164.

57. Maughan RJ, Leiper JB, Shirreffs SM. Rehydration and recovery after exercise. *Sports Sci Exchange*. 1996;9:3.

58. Murray R. The effects of consuming carbohydrate-electrolyte beverages on gastric emptying and fluid absorption during and following exercise. *Sports Med*. 1987;4:322–351.

9

Nutritional Ergogenics

Key Questions Addressed

- What is an ergogenic aid?

- What are dietary supplements?

- What is doping?

- What are some of the commonly encountered doping substances?

- What types of dietary supplements and nutritional ergogenics are commonly used by endurance athletes, strength/power athletes, and team sport athletes?

- Where can information on nutritional ergogenic aids be found?

- What tools are available to research information on ergogenic aids?

You Are the Nutrition Coach

Jason, a 16-year-old high school track athlete, has set a goal to improve his 100- and 200-meter sprint times. He has seen the muscle development evident in elite sprinters and therefore desperately wants to increase his muscle mass, strength, and power. After talking about training regimens, daily nutrition, and supplementation with numerous other athletes at track meets, he has decided to begin taking several supplements to help him reach his goals. His mother is very conscientious about preparing a nourishing supper; however, Jason prepares his own breakfast and lunch, which he admits typically do not consist of quality food choices. Currently he is resistance training two to three times per week and taking the following supplements: "mega" multivitamin/mineral supplement, boron, ornithine and arginine, chromium picolinate, and whey protein.

Question

- What would you suggest to Jason to help him achieve his personal goal of increasing muscle mass to become a stronger, more powerful athlete?

What is an ergogenic aid?

The derivation of the word *ergogenic* gives an indication of its meaning: *Ergo*, which is derived from the Greek word *ergon*, refers to work; *genic* is derived from *genman*, which means to generate or produce. An **ergogenic aid** is anything that enhances a person's ability to perform work or, in the case of athletics, to perform better. The ultimate goal of using ergogenic aids is to gain a competitive edge over the opponent.

ergogenic aid Anything that enhances a person's ability to perform work, or in the case of athletics, to perform better in sport.

Ergogenic aids can take many different forms: physiological, biomechanical, psychological, pharmacological, and nutritional (see **Table 9.1**). Physiological ergogenic aids enhance the functioning of the body's various systems. It is interesting to note that the most often used physiological ergogenic aid is not even thought of as one—it is exercise training. Making a muscle bigger and stronger through strength training improves its ability to generate force and thus enables the athlete to run faster and jump higher. Endurance training causes adaptations by the body that result in greater blood volume, more blood vessels, and a larger, stronger heart. The end result is an enhanced cardiovascular system capable of delivering more blood to working muscles so that faster race paces or longer distances can be maintained.

Biomechanical ergogenic aids enable the athlete to perform better by providing a mechanical advantage. Bigger yet lighter tennis rackets and golf clubs enable athletes to hit balls with less error and more speed. Improved ice skates in which the blade stays on the surface of the ice longer enable speed skaters to provide more thrust and therefore achieve greater speeds. Specially designed running and swim suits decrease wind resistance or drag in the water and thus improve race performances. These are just a few of the innovations in equipment that are designed to improve performance.

Negative thoughts or doubts, lack of mental focus, and physical or emotional inhibitions can all be the nemesis of an athlete. This is where psychological ergogenic aids come into play. Sports psychologists meet with athletes to help them learn mental strategies for overcoming fears and to improve concentration. Visualization is a common psychological ergogenic aid used by athletes. The athlete develops a mental picture of him- or herself performing what he or she is about to do physically. It is not unusual to see divers or gymnasts prior to their competitions with their eyes closed and subtly moving their bodies as they mentally perform a dive or gymnastic routine.

Pharmacological ergogenic aids fall into the category of medicines or drugs. They are chemical substances that were originally designed to treat disease but now are used by healthy athletes with the sole intent of enhancing performance or physical prow-

TABLE 9.1	Types of Ergogenic Aids	
Type of Ergogenic Aid	**Description**	**Examples**
Nutritional	Any supplement, food product, or dietary manipulation that enhances work capacity or athletic performance	Carbohydrate loading; creatine phosphate; amino acid supplementation; vitamin supplementation; glucose polymer drinks; sports gels; carbohydrate-loading drinks; liquid meals
Physiological	Any practice or substance that enhances the functioning of the body's various systems (e.g., cardiovascular, muscular) and thus improves athletic performance	Bicarbonate buffering; any type of physical training (e.g., endurance, strength, plyometric); blood doping via transfusions; the practice of warming up
Psychological	Any practice or treatment that changes mental state and thereby enhances sport performance	Visualization; sessions with a sport psychologist; hypnosis; pep talks; relaxation techniques
Biomechanical	Any device, piece of equipment, or external product that can be used to improve athletic performance during practice or competition	Weight belts; knee wraps; oversize tennis rackets and golf clubs; clap skates; body suits (swimming/track); corked bats
Pharmacological	Any substance or compound classified as a drug or hormonal agent that is used to improve work output and/or sport performance	Hormones (e.g., growth hormone, erythropoetin, anabolic androgenic steroids); amphetamines; caffeine; beta-blockers; ephedrine

ess. For example, amphetamines, painkillers, anabolic steroids, and other synthesized hormones fall under this category of pharmacological ergogenic aids. This category of ergogenic aids is arguably the most dangerous and controversial because misuse can result in serious physical complications or death. Consequently, many of the pharmacological ergogenic aids are banned by sports organizations worldwide.

The main focus of this chapter will be on nutritional ergogenics. Nutritional ergogenic aids are foods, supplements, special diets, and dietary practices that are used by athletes to improve performance. Although for centuries the Chinese have practiced ingesting natural foods or compounds for medicinal and spiritual reasons, it is the ancient Greeks who have been touted as the first to use nutritional ergogenics to gain the "competitive" edge in sports. Today, the sale of substances that fall into the category of nutritional ergogenic aids is a multi-billion-dollar industry. In the following pages, some of the more common dietary supplements and other nutritional ergogenics used by athletes are introduced (see Table 9.1).

What are dietary supplements?

A **dietary supplement**, as defined by the **Dietary Supplement Health and Education Act (DSHEA)** of 1994,[1] is a product (other than tobacco) intended to supplement the diet that contains one or more of the following dietary ingredients:

- Vitamin
- Mineral
- Herb or other botanical
- Amino acid
- Dietary substance to supplement the diet by increasing the total dietary intake
- Concentrate, metabolite, constituent, extract, or a combination of any of the above ingredients

Dietary supplements are not intended to be used as a food or as a sole item of a meal or diet, and these products must be labeled as a dietary supplement. DSHEA broadened the regulatory definition of dietary supplements and altered the federal government's oversight of supplement products. Under DSHEA, the supplement manufacturer is responsible for the safety of the product. However, the supplement manufacturer is not required to test its product for safety, nor does it have to prove that the supplement does what it claims to do.

Since DSHEA there has been increased consumer interest in, use of, and availability of a wide variety of supplements. Dietary supplement use in the United States is a multi-billion-dollar industry. In 2000, 51% of U.S. adults reported taking a multivitamin or mineral supplement in the previous year, and 33.9% of adults in the same survey took a multivitamin and/or mineral supplement daily.[2] In addition, 14.5% of U.S. adults reported using a nonvitamin or mineral supplement within the last year, and 6% used a nonvitamin or mineral supplement daily.[2]

Supplement use among athletes makes up a large percentage of total supplement sales. The sports nutrition product market (including sports bars, drinks, and other supplements) produced more than $25.3 billion in sales according to a 2009 report by the *Nutrition Business Journal*. In a study of NCAA athletes at a Division I university, Froiland et al. reported that 23% of the athletes surveyed regularly (at least five times per week) took a dietary supplement.[3] Thirty-nine percent reported they currently were not taking any supplement; however, all but 6% of the athletes reported using a wide variety of calorie or fluid replacement products. Almost 73% of the athletes reported using energy drinks (e.g., Gatorade, Powerade, All Sport, Red Bull), and 61.4% reported using calorie replacers (e.g., Boost, Slim-Fast type products) and bars (e.g., Personal Edge, PowerBar). Forty-seven percent reported taking a multivitamin. Supplement manufacturers are constantly developing new products and targeting athletes in their marketing strategies because athletes are focused on anything that may be able to improve their sport performance.

Why do athletes use dietary supplements?

Athletes are always looking for an edge over their competitors. Often they turn to dietary supplements that they feel may give them that edge. However, there is no substitute for an appropriately planned training regimen and nutrition schedule. Athletes need to be aware of the safety, efficacy, actions, and laws regarding dietary supplements.

dietary supplement A product (other than tobacco) that is not intended to be used as a food or a sole item of a meal or diet. To be considered a dietary supplement, the product must contain one or more of the following dietary ingredients: vitamin, mineral, herb or other botanical, amino acid, dietary substance to supplement the diet by increasing the total dietary intake, or a concentrate, metabolite, constituent, extract, or combination of any of these ingredients.

Dietary Supplement Health and Education Act (DSHEA) A legislative act passed in 1994 to help regulate the dietary supplement industry. DSHEA broadened the regulatory definition of dietary supplements and altered the federal government's oversight of supplement products.

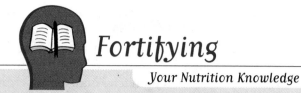

Fortifying
Your Nutrition Knowledge

Removal of Ephedra from the U.S. Market

On February 11, 2004, the Food and Drug Administration (FDA) issued a final ruling that banned the sale of ephedra-containing supplements in the United States.[4] The effective date of the ban was April 12, 2004, giving supplement makers 2 months to pull their supplements containing ephedra or ephedrine alkaloids off the market. This action banning ephedra was the first time the FDA had taken a formal action to halt the sale of a dietary supplement ingredient since the passage of DSHEA in 1994.[5] This final ruling was made after an extensive review of the reports of adverse events, a review of scientific literature on the pharmacology of ephedrine and ephedrine alkaloids, and peer-reviewed scientific literature on the effects of ephedrine alkaloids.

The ephedrine alkaloids, including, among others, ephedrine, pseudoephedrine, norephedrine, methylephedrine, norpseudoephedrine, and methylpseudoephedrine, are chemical stimulants that occur naturally in some botanicals (plants) but can also be synthetically derived. Ma huang, ephedra, Chinese ephedra, and epitonin are several names used for botanical ingredients that are sources of ephedrine alkaloids. The term *ephedrine alkaloids* is used throughout this section and is used by the FDA in the Federal Register final ruling because it is these alkaloids that produce the effects that necessitated the banning of the substances. The commercial common name used for these substances is "ephedra," but ephedrine alkaloids are the actual ingredient source in the dietary supplements. Over the last decade dietary supplements containing ephedrine alkaloids have been labeled and used primarily for weight loss, increased energy, or to enhance athletic performance.[6,7] The following is a time line and explanation of how the FDA came to make its final ruling:

- *October 1995:* The FDA Advisory Committee convened a special working group on products containing ephedrine alkaloids. This group met because the FDA received several reports of adverse events, including deaths related to ephedrine alkaloid use in dietary supplements.

- *August 1996:* A meeting of the Food Advisory Committee (FAC) and the working group was held concerning the potential public health problems associated with the use of dietary supplements containing ephedrine alkaloids. This group recommended good manufacturing practices and warning labels for products containing ephedrine alkaloids.

- *June 1997:* The FDA issued proposed rules on dietary supplements containing ephedrine alkaloids based on the FDA's investigations of reports of serious illnesses and injuries, including a number of deaths, associated with the use of dietary supplements containing ephedrine alkaloids. The proposed rules included:

  - That a dietary supplement is adulterated if it contains 8 milligrams (mg) or more of ephedrine alkaloids per serving or if its labeling suggests or recommends conditions of use that would result in an intake of 8 mg or more in a 6-hour period or a total daily intake of 24 mg or more of ephedrine alkaloids.

  - Dietary supplements containing ephedrine alkaloids must state on the label that the product should not be used for more than 7 days.

  - The use of ephedrine alkaloids in dietary supplements with other ingredients that have a known stimulant effect that may interact with ephedrine alkaloids is prohibited.

  - Labeling claims, such as weight loss or body building, that require long-term intake to achieve the purported effect are prohibited.

- A statement which warns consumers that taking more than the recommended serving may result in serious adverse health effects must accompany products that encourage short-term excessive intake to enhance a purported effect.

  - The labels of all dietary supplements containing ephedrine alkaloids must bear a statement warning consumers not to use the product if they are taking certain drugs.

- *June 4–August 18, 1997:* Open comment period for proposed rules.

- *September 18–December 2, 1997:* Federal Register announced the reopening of the comment period after the correction of inadvertent omissions in the previous administrative record.

- *November 1997:* The Commission on Dietary Supplement Labels (the Commission), an independent agency established by DSHEA, issued its report on ephedrine alkaloids. In the report, the Commission urged the FDA to use its authority under DSHEA to take swift enforcement action to address potential safety issues such as those posed recently by products containing ephedrine alkaloids.

- *September 1998:* The U.S. General Accounting Office (GAO) began a study on the FDA's June 1997 proposal.

- *July 1999:* The GAO concluded that the evidence supported concern that ephedrine alkaloid–containing supplements can cause serious health problems, and it recommended further data collection and review.

- *1999–2003:* Independent reviews of ephedrine alkaloids were under way. Haller and Benowitz[8] reviewed 1997–99 adverse events reports (AERs) and found 31% of events were definitely or probably related to ephedrine alkaloids and another 31% were possibly related; 47% of the definitely or probably related events were cardiovascular events, and 18% were central nervous system events. They determined that ephedrine alkaloids posed a risk to the public. The Council of Responsible Nutrition reviewed 1173 AERs and selected 121 cases to review further.[9] Eight of these resulted in death, and six of the deaths were cardiovascular disease events; of these six, five were males using the supplements as an athletic performance enhancer. Four of these five were concurrently using other performance-enhancing supplements. These researchers could not conclude with certainty that ephedrine alkaloids were the only cause of the events. The RAND Corporation, an independent research organization, was asked by the National Institutes of Health (NIH) to review AERs related to ephedrine alkaloids. Among other findings, the RAND report identified 21 "sentinel events" among the adverse event reports it reviewed, including stroke, heart attack, and death. Sentinel events met the criteria for an AER, had documentation that the person consumed ephedra-containing supplement within 24 hours of the event, and alternative explanations for the event were investigated and excluded with reasonable certainty. The FDA had particular concerns about the effects of ephedra on people engaged in strenuous exercise. Ephedrine produces an adrenaline boost, raising heart rate and blood pressure, and the stimulating effects may produce enough of a boost to mask fatigue even in well-conditioned athletes. RAND concluded that the scientific literature does not support an effect of ephedrine (pharmaceutical) alone on athletic performance, and there were no clinical trials on the effects of dietary supplements containing botanical ephedrine alkaloids on athletic performance.

- *April 2000:* The FDA withdrew parts of the June 1997 proposal. The two parts withdrawn were the proposed finding that a dietary supplement is adulterated if it contains 8 mg or more of ephedrine

(continued)

alkaloids per serving, or if its labeling suggests or recommends conditions of use that would result in the intake of 8 mg or more in a 6-hour period or a total daily intake of 24 mg or more of ephedrine alkaloids. In a separate Federal Register notice, also in April 2000, the FDA announced the availability of additional AERs and related information received after publication of the proposed rule. The additional information included the analyses of these new AERs by experts both inside and outside the agency.

- *April 2001:* The Health and Human Services Office of the Inspector General issued a report entitled "Adverse Event Reporting for Dietary Supplements: An Inadequate Safety Valve" that assessed the effectiveness of the FDA's adverse event reporting system. This report found that adverse event reporting systems typically detect only a small proportion of the events that actually occur after consumption of dietary supplements containing ephedrine alkaloids and that the risks of adverse events increase with strenuous exercise and with the use of other stimulants, including caffeine.

- *March 2003:* The FDA issued a notice for public comment on all additional evidence developed since the publication of the June 1997 proposal. The FDA published a notice making available new information about dietary supplements containing ephedrine alkaloids and requesting public comment on the new information and on regulation of these products.

- In part because of the RAND report, the FDA issued warning letters to 26 firms for making unsubstantiated claims regarding ephedrine alkaloids' effects on enhancing athletic performance. All but one firm complied with the request by either removing the supplement from the market or discontinuing the objectionable athletic performance–enhancing claims.

- *July 2003:* The GAO testified at a House Subcommittee hearing and discussed and updated some of its findings from its prior 1999 report on dietary supplements containing ephedrine alkaloids. This testimony included information that many serious adverse events occurred in relatively young individuals and in those who used the supplements within the recommended dose, frequency, and duration guidelines.

- *February 11, 2004:* The final rule is issued in the Federal Register. The FDA issued a final regulation declaring "dietary supplements containing ephedrine alkaloids to be adulterated under the Food, Drug and Cosmetic Act because they present an unreasonable risk of illness or injury under the conditions of use recommended or suggested in labeling or, if no conditions of use are suggested or recommended in labeling, under ordinary conditions of use. We [FDA] are taking this action based upon the well-known pharmacology of ephedrine alkaloids, the peer-reviewed scientific literature on the effects of ephedrine alkaloids, and the adverse events reported to have occurred in individuals following consumption of dietary supplement containing ephedrine alkaloids."[4]

- This final rule applies to dietary supplements containing ephedrine alkaloids. This final rule does not include OTC or prescription drugs that contain ephedrine alkaloids. The use of ephedrine or pseudoephedrine for the treatment of asthma, colds, allergies, or any other disease is beyond the scope of this final rule.

- *April 12, 2004:* Effective date of the final ruling.

- *May 2004:* Nutraceutical International Corporation sues on grounds that low doses of ephedrine alkaloids have not been proven dangerous.

- *April 2005:* U.S. District Court judge in Utah rules that the FDA failed to prove that ephedrine alkaloids are dangerous in low doses. The judge partially reverses the FDA ban and allows for the sale of ephedrine alkaloid supplements containing <10 mg per daily dose.

- *May 2005:* Low-dose ephedra products return to the market.
- *August 2006:* U.S. Court of Appeals overturns 2005 Utah District Court ruling and upholds the FDA ban of all ephedrine alkaloid products, even those containing low dosages.
- *January 2007:* Nutraceutical International Corporation petitions to challenge the U.S. Court of Appeals ruling in the U.S. Supreme Court.
- *May 2007:* U.S. Supreme Court opts not to hear Nutraceutical's case. The ban of all products containing ephedrine alkaloids is upheld.

Postscript:

Many "ephedra-free" products are now flooding the marketplace. The new "ephedra-free" products, however, often contain stimulant botanical ingredients such as bitter orange (contains synephrine), high amounts of caffeine, kola nut, guarana, and green tea extracts. Safety concerns regarding these stimulant-containing products persist. Athletes need to continue to be aware of the safety and efficacy issues of stimulant-containing supplements.

Athletes consume supplements for a variety of reasons. In the NCAA study previously cited, 43.5% of the athletes surveyed reported taking supplements for their health, 42.5% for improved strength and power, and 42.5% to increase muscle gains.[3] Male athletes tend to choose protein and weight gain products, creatine, and other supplements promoted to help an athlete gain muscle mass and burn fat. Conversely, female athletes are more likely to consume vitamin and mineral supplements, weight loss supplements, and energy enhancers. Some of these supplements may be helpful and even necessary for athletes. For example, calcium and iron dietary supplements may eliminate deficiencies, particularly in females or in athletes who tend to eat fewer calories than their energy demands. In most cases, however, supplements are consumed in the hope of enhancing performance, regardless of the safety or efficacy of the product.

What are the regulations governing dietary supplements?

Supplements are not drugs. Drugs are intended to cure, treat, or prevent disease. Drugs must undergo extensive studies of safety and effectiveness, drug interactions, and dosing effects and must have formal FDA approval prior to marketing the product. On the other hand, dietary supplements do not have to undergo any studies on safety or efficacy prior to entering the market. Supplements are also not food additives, which require testing prior to entering the food marketplace. Dietary supplements containing any new ingredients do not require testing. The manufacturer gathers and interprets safety and efficacy information and then must submit the product and safety information to the FDA 75 days prior to marketing the product. After the 75-day waiting period, the supplement can be placed on the market. However, the FDA does not approve the new ingredient. New supplements that do not contain any new ingredients do not have to submit anything to the FDA prior to marketing the product.

Since 1999, DSHEA has required all supplements to be labeled with all of the product's ingredients and a Supplement Facts panel. The label is very similar in appearance to the Nutrition Facts panel on food labels. Figure 9.1 shows a Supplement Facts panel and ingredient list.

Supplement Facts

Serving Size: 1 Scoop
Servings Per Container: 12

Amount Per Serving		% Daily Value*
Calories	136	
Calories from Fat	18	
Total Fat	2g	
Saturated Fat	1g	
Trans Fat	0g	
Cholesterol	0mg	0%
Sodium	50mg	2%
Potassium	100mg	6%
Calcium	130mg	13%
Carbohydrate	0g	0%
Protein	30g	

Ingredients: whey protein concentrate and isolate, artificial flavors, maltodextrin, acesulfame potassium

Figure 9.1 Supplement Facts panel. Similar to the Nutrition Facts panel on food labels, the Supplement Facts panel required on dietary supplement labels shows the product composition.

Supplement manufacturers cannot make claims that the product can cure or relieve specific health conditions or diseases. They also cannot claim the supplement has pharmacological uses because these claims would then categorize the supplement as a drug, requiring FDA approval. However, similar to food labeling, supplement manufacturers can make structure/function, nutrient content, and health claims. These different types of claims in relation to food-labeling laws have been previously discussed in Chapter 1. The structure/function, nutrient content, and health claims allowed on dietary supplement labels are similar to the food-labeling claims with one big distinction: Food labels are regulated by the FDA and dietary supplement labels are not.

There are regulations limiting the claims allowed on supplement labels. However, the FDA does not regularly monitor these claims. The volume of supplements currently on the market, along with the volume of new ones constantly entering the market, prohibit close monitoring of these claims. The following is an explanation of allowable claims on dietary supplement labels:

- *Nutrient content claims:* Claims on the labels of foods or dietary supplements that characterize the level of a nutrient in that food or supplement can be made if they are in accordance with FDA-authorized regulations. For example, a dietary supplement that states it is a "good source of calcium" must contain at least 10–20% of the daily value for calcium.

- *Health claims:* Health claims are allowed only if scientific evidence or statements from recognized scientific authorities are reviewed by the FDA and meet the standards set for the health claim. This also is similar to making health claims on food labels. For example, a vitamin/mineral supplement that contains 100% of the RDA for folic acid could state a health claim regarding the benefit of folic acid taken during pregnancy in the prevention of neural-tube defects.

- *Structure/function claims:* These claims are not authorized or reviewed by the FDA. Claims about how a supplement affects a function in the body or a structure of the body can be made based on the manufacturer's review and interpretation of the scientific literature. Structure/function claims on labels must be accompanied by a disclaimer such as the following: "This statement has not been evaluated by the Food and Drug Administration. This product is not intended to diagnose, treat, cure, or prevent any disease" (see **Figure 9.2**). Claims such as "glucosamine may strengthen joints" are allowed when accompanied by the disclaimer, but the statement "glucosamine cures arthritis" is not allowed. The manufacturer of a supplement that makes a structure/function claim on the label must notify the FDA no later than 30 days after marketing the product. These structure/function claims on supplement labels fall under a different jurisdiction within FDA than the approved health claims statements allowed on food labels. The food label claims are preapproved by the FDA and only certain claims can be made by law. (See Chapter 1 for more information about these claims.)

It is the structure/function claims that frequently sound too good to be true and often hook athletes into believing they need a particular supplement to gain an edge over the competition. Many sport supplements place structure/function

gaining the performance edge

Nutritional supplements do not require FDA approval, nor do they go through the same rigorous testing and scientific approval process as pharmaceutical drugs. Athletes need to be aware of the possibility that supplements may: (1) contain a banned substance and (2) pose a health risk if consumed in conjunction with other supplements or medications. Athletes should weigh the benefits versus the risks and costs when deciding whether to take a supplement.

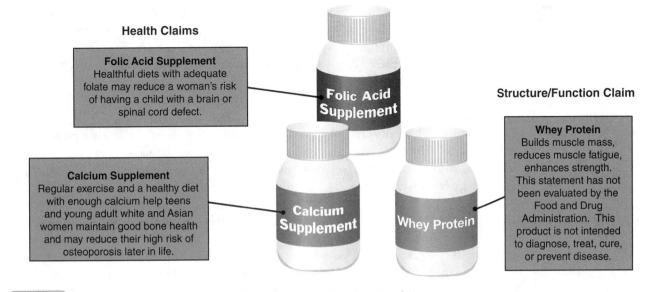

Health Claims

Folic Acid Supplement
Healthful diets with adequate folate may reduce a woman's risk of having a child with a brain or spinal cord defect.

Calcium Supplement
Regular exercise and a healthy diet with enough calcium help teens and young adult white and Asian women maintain good bone health and may reduce their high risk of osteoporosis later in life.

Structure/Function Claim

Whey Protein
Builds muscle mass, reduces muscle fatigue, enhances strength. This statement has not been evaluated by the Food and Drug Administration. This product is not intended to diagnose, treat, cure, or prevent disease.

Folic Acid Supplement

Calcium Supplement

Whey Protein

Figure 9.2 Examples of supplement labels with health and structure/function claims.

claims on their labels to entice athletes to buy their products.

In addition, DSHEA states that the supplement label must list all ingredients, including the active ingredients. However, product testing and regulation are not required as part of DSHEA *before* a supplement is marketed or while on the market. The manufacturer is responsible for the labeling and safety of the product; however, because companies do not have to prove their products' safety, efficacy, or accuracy of ingredients before hitting the market, the product could contain any or none of the ingredients listed. Some supplements could contain ingredients that are not listed on the label as well. This can be important for athletes in sports that perform drug testing. Athletes have had winning performances challenged and awards withdrawn because of inadvertent consumption of a seemingly benign dietary supplement that contained a banned substance. Athletes must understand that manufacturers can mislead consumers by omitting ingredients on the label, putting ingredients on the label that are not actually in the product, or falsely claiming a structure/function application, and because of poor regulatory oversight may never have had action taken against them.

The **Federal Trade Commission (FTC)** regulates the advertising of dietary supplements. It is the responsibility of the FTC to ensure truth in advertising on supplement labels, in print advertising, and in commercials. The mission of the FTC is to prevent unfair competition and to protect consumers from unfair or deceptive practices in the marketplace. The agency encourages self-monitoring by the supplement industry and intervenes when deceptive or unsafe advertising occurs. Advertisements that make false claims or fail to use appropriate structure or function disclaimer statements are subject to action by the FTC. The FTC can take action against the manufacturer for providing false or misleading claims or if the product claims safety in the absence of evidence of safety. For example, over the past few years the FTC has sent letters to various weight loss supplement makers requesting they discontinue claims about fantastic amounts of weight loss or misleading information about the scientific research behind specific weight-loss claims.

A few of the common marketing ploys manufacturers use to entice athletes to purchase their products include:

- Product endorsement by a well-known professional athlete.
- Testimonials from other supplement users claiming amazing results. These spokespeople are often very fit and athletic looking, adding to the mystique and "credibility" of the product.
- Claiming "scientific research," but studies are not published in scientific journals or unpublished research is cited.

Federal Trade Commission (FTC) A government agency whose mission is to ensure truth in advertising on supplement labels, in print advertising, and in commercials, thereby preventing unfair competition and protecting consumers from unfair or deceptive practices in the marketplace.

- False label or health claims. If the FTC learns of these claims and finds them to be false, the FTC can take action against the supplement manufacturer.

Many supplements are marketed to athletes as fat burners, muscle builders, and energy enhancers. Some of these products are effective, but others are not. For example, creatine has shown promise as a muscle-building sport supplement. Many controlled studies have been performed on creatine's effects on weight gain and increased muscle mass and have been published in peer-reviewed scientific journals. Sports drinks, containing electrolytes and carbohydrates, have significant scientific backing for ergogenic effects on endurance training. Although these two examples have been well researched, the majority of sports ergogenic supplements that arrive on the market each year do so with minimal or no testing at all. Some supplements have had minimal testing on animals or in vitro but no human testing. Still others take already published research and misapply it to new supplements. These loose applications may include scientific-sounding jargon that promises quick results with minimal or no side effects.

Are some supplements better or safer than others?

Differences in plant species, growing practices, soil content, harvesting, the part of the plant used (leaf, seed, stem, fruit), and storage practices all can influence the content of a dietary supplement and therefore the effect of the product on the consumer. Because supplements do not require proof of testing and the contents of a product are not always consistent,[10] two bottles of an identically packaged supplement made by the same manufacturer can vary greatly and thus alter the effect on the body. This can happen if a different plant species is used, if the supplier provides a different plant product with or without the manufacturer's knowledge, and if the manufacturer does not use quality control measures during the production of the supplement.[11,12] Some manufacturers voluntarily use quality control measures, however, and can verify the content of their products.

Good manufacturing practices (GMPs) for pharmaceuticals have been in place for many years and are administered by the FDA. GMP means that the drug was manufactured and packaged with established quality control measures. This includes controls in personnel, facilities design and cleanliness, equipment, testing, storage, production and process controls, yield, packaging, and shipping. Essentially, all areas from the supply of ingredients used to the actual manufacturing and packaging, labeling, and distribution of pharmaceuticals must follow established good manufacturing practices.

Good manufacturing practice guidelines are currently being developed to help ensure that safety and quality control measures are used during the production of dietary supplements. Many supplements are prepared in quality-controlled environments where contamination from other substances is not likely. However, other supplement makers may use poor manufacturing practices; use the same equipment to prepare or package different products, which can lead to contamination of supplements; and do not use quality control measures for ingredients, storage, and packaging.[10,13]

Standards published by the **United States Pharmacopeia (USP)** provide a set of guidelines for the quality, purity, manufacturing practices, and ingredients in supplement products. The USP has been in existence since 1820 and is a not-for-profit organization dedicated to setting public standards for the quality of health care products. In 2003, the USP developed a program to verify the quality standards it publishes for dietary supplements. The USP-verified mark is used only on supplements that have been through the extensive verification process required by the USP (see Figure 9.3). To obtain the USP-verified mark, the USP will test the listed ingredients and verify the ingredients and amounts listed, test for contaminants, test that the supplement will break down and release ingredients in the body, and ensure that the product was manufactured using good manufacturing processes.

Manufacturers voluntarily choose to participate in the USP program to test and verify their dietary supplements. Athletes who purchase dietary supple-

good manufacturing practices (GMPs) A set of quality control measures adopted by the United States Pharmacopeia that establishes guidelines for personnel, facilities design and cleanliness, equipment, testing, storage, production and process controls, yield, packaging, and shipping of products.

United States Pharmacopeia (USP) A not-for-profit organization that establishes and verifies standards for the quality, purity, manufacturing practices, and ingredients in supplement products.

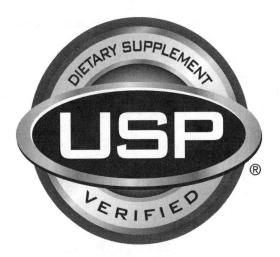

Figure 9.3 U.S. Pharmacopeia verification mark. Dietary supplements can earn the USP verification mark through a comprehensive testing and evaluation process.
Reprinted with permission from The United States Pharmacopeial Convention, 12601 Twinbrook Parkway, Rockville, MD 20852.

ments with the USP-verified symbol on the label may be getting a higher-quality product than those without the seal. Information on the products that have undergone the USP-verified process is available on the USP Web site (see Table 9.10 later in this chapter).

Choosing a supplement manufactured by a well-known company may provide for a better product. The manufacturing and labeling used by larger, established companies will likely have better standards such as an accurate listing of all the ingredients in the product and the dosage levels of all active ingredients. Some pharmaceutical manufacturers also make dietary supplements. The standards in place that these companies must use to have their drugs approved may also be used when they develop dietary supplements. Although it is not guaranteed that supplement makers that also make pharmaceuticals will have better quality dietary supplements, it is one more thing athletes can look for when making supplement choices.

There is no question that some dietary supplements, especially certain vitamins and minerals, offer potential health benefits. However, most dietary supplements marketed to athletes for increased sport performance have not had vast amounts of scientific research to back the products' claims. Athletes also need to realize that the supplements they are taking, knowingly or unknowingly, may contain banned substances that can have serious ethical and physical consequences.

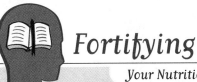

Fortifying
Your Nutrition Knowledge

Questions Athletes Should Consider When Deciding Whether to Purchase a Dietary Supplement

Athletes should consider the following questions when considering the use of a dietary supplement:

- *Is there scientific research that supports the reported claims?* Quality research that supports efficacy of the product should include well-controlled reproducible studies that have been published in scientific and peer-reviewed publications.
- *Is the supplement safe?* Scientific research may be able to help determine safety as well as efficacy of the supplement. Look for the USP-verified and U.S. Pharmacopeia symbols on the supplement label. Check the product out by using some of the resources listed in Table 9.10 later in this chapter.
- *How much does the supplement cost?* Decisions about cost should consider cost versus proposed benefit. If the benefit appears to be proven and the athlete can afford the product, then purchase may be worthwhile. However, athletes should always focus first on obtaining foods that are healthful and training appropriately to meet sport performance goals.
- *Is the supplement just a gimmick packaged with a great advertising message?* If it sounds too good to be true, it probably is. Testimonials by famous athletes or bulked-up and fit-appearing athletes should not take the place of searching for actual research on the safety and efficacy of the supplement.
- *Does the product contain a banned substance?* Look on the ingredient list to determine what substances are found within the product. Use the resources in Table 9.10 to help make reasonable assessments about the products. Even if an athlete's sport does not engage in drug testing, banned substances are those that can cause potential harm to athletes.

What is doping?

Doping is the practice of enhancing performance through the use of foreign substances or other artificial means. According to the **World Anti-Doping Agency (WADA)**, the word *doping* was originally derived from the Dutch word *dop*, which was the name of an alcoholic drink made from grape skins. The drink was used by Zulu warriors to enhance their physical prowess in battle. However, it wasn't until the turn of the 20th century that the word *doping* began to be used regularly and referred to the drugging of racehorses. Doping has become an epidemic in sports and presents risks not only to the health of athletes, but also to the basic tenet of fair play in competition.

Athletes, and the general public, must understand that DSHEA significantly reduced the regulation of supplements and broadened the category to include herbals and botanical products. In short, according to DSHEA, the FDA has the power to oversee the supplement industry but cannot investigate a supplement unless a safety problem has been reported. The bottom line is that the vast majority of supplements sold to the general public have not been tested for effectiveness or safety.

Despite this fact, the sale of dietary supplements is a multi-billion-dollar industry. Sports nutrition professionals and the athletes they counsel must be knowledgeable about the ingredients found in any dietary supplements because they may contain substances banned by the International Olympic Committee (IOC) (see **Table 9.2**) and other govern-

doping The practice of enhancing performance through the use of foreign substances or other artificial means.

World Anti-Doping Agency (WADA) An international, nongovernmental organization whose mission is to foster a doping-free culture in sports. WADA was established in 1999 and is headquartered in Montreal, Canada.

TABLE 9.2	World Anti-Doping Code–2010 Prohibited Substances List	
Prohibited Substance Category	**Name of Substances**	**Actions**
Stimulants**	Adrafinil, adrenaline, amfepramone, amiphenazole, amphetamine, amphetaminil, benfluorex, benzphetamine, benzylpiperazine, bromantan, cathine, clobenzorex, cocaine, cropropamide, crotetamide, dimethylamphetamine, ephedrine, etamivan, etilamphetamine, etilefrine, famprofazone, fenbutrazate, fencamfamin, fencamine, fenetylline, fenfluramine, fenproporex, furfenorex, heptaminol, isometheptene, levmethamfetamine, meclofenoxate, mefenorex, mephentermine, mesocarb, methamphetamine, p-methamphetamine, methylenedioxyamphetamine, methylenedioxymethamphetamine, methylhexaneamine (dimethylpentylamine), methylephedrine, methylphenidate, modafinil, nikethamide, norfenefrine, norfenfluramine, octopamine, oxilofrine, parahydroxyamphetamine, pemoline, pentetrazol, phendimetrazine, phenmetrazine, phenpromethamine, phentermine, 4-phenylpiracetam (carphedon), prenylamine, prolintane, propylhexedrine, pseudoephedrine, selegiline, sibutramine, strychnine, tuaminoheptane, and other substances with similar chemical structure or similar biological effects	Stimulate the sympathetic nervous system: enhance mental alertness, increase concentration, decrease mental fatigue, delay onset of physical fatigue
Narcotics**	Buprenorphine, dextromoramide, diamorphine (heroin), fentanyl and its derivatives, hydromorphone, methadone, morphine, oxycodone, oxymorphone, pentazocine, pethidine	Mask perception of pain and exertion
Cannabinoids**	Natural or synthetic Δ9-tetrahydrocannabinol (THC) and THC-like cannabinoids (e.g., hashish, marijuana, HU-210)	Act on central nervous system, mode of action not clearly understood
Anabolic agents*	1-androstendiol, 1-androstendione, bolandiol, bolasterone, boldenone, boldione, calusterone, clostebol, danazol, dehydrochloromethyltestosterone, desoxymethyltesterone, drostanolone, ethylestrenol, fluoxymesterone, formebolone, furazabol, gestrinone, 4-hydroxytestosterone, mestanolone, mesterolone, metenolone, methandienone, methandriol, methyldienolone, methyl-1-testosterone,	Mimic actions of testosterone; build tissue, especially muscle; enhance recovery

Prohibited Substance Category	Name of Substances	Actions
Anabolic agents* (continued)	methasterone, methyltrienolone, methyltestosterone, metribolone, methylnortestosterone, mibolerone, nandrolone, 19-norandrostenedione, norboletone, norclostebol, norethandrolone, oxabolone, oxandrolone, oxymesterone, oxymetholone, prostanozol, quinbolone, stanozolol, stenbolone, 1-testosterone, tetrahydrogestrinone, trenbolone, androstenediol, androstenedione, prasterone (dehydroepiandrosterone (DHEA)), dihydrotestosterone, testosterone (includes isomers and its metabolites), clenbuterol, selective androgen receptor modulators (SARMs), tibolone, zeranol, zilpaterol, and other substances with similar chemical structure or similar biological effects	
Peptide hormones, growth factors, and related substances*	Erythropoiesis-stimulating agents (e.g., erythropoietin (EPO), darbepoetin (dEPO), methoxy-polyethylene-glycol-epoetin beta (CERA), hematide), chorionic gonadotrophin (CG) and luteinizing hormone (LH) in males, insulins, growth hormone (hGH), insulin-like growth factor (IGF-1), mechano growth factors (MGFs), platelet-derived growth factor (PDGF), fibroblast growth factors (FGFs), vascular-endothelial growth factor (VEGF), hepatocyte growth factor (HGF), platelet-derived preparations (e.g., platelet-rich plasma, blood spinning), corticotrophins, and other substances with similar chemical structure or similar biological effects	Enhance actions of existing hormones by increasing concentrations in the body
Beta-2 agonists*	All beta-2 agonists, including their D- and L-isomers, are prohibited. Their use requires a Therapeutic Use Exemption. Exceptions include salbutamol and salmeterol by inhalation only to prevent and/or treat asthma and exercise-induced asthma.	Block binding of sympathetic hormones, thus producing a calming effect
Hormone antagonists and modulators*	Aromatase inhibitors including but not limited to aminogluthetimide, anastrozole, androsta-1,4,6-triene-3,17-dione (androstatrienedione), 4-androstene-3,6,17 trione (6-oxo), exemestane, formestane, letrozole,and testolactone.	Block conversion of testosterone to estrogen plus diminish effects of estrogen in the body
	Selective estrogen receptor modulators (SERMs) including but not limited to: raloxifene, tamoxifen, and toremifene.	
	Other anti-estrogenic substances including but not limited to: clomiphene, cyclofenil, and fulvestrant.	
	Agents modifying myostatin functions including but not limited to: myostatin inhibitors.	
Diuretics and other masking agents*	Masking agents are prohibited. They include: diuretics, probenecid, plasma expanders (e.g., glycerol; intravenous administration of albumin, dextran, hydroxyethyl starch, and mannitol) and other substances with similar biological effects.	Impair excretion or change blood or urine measures to conceal use of other substances
	Diuretics include: acetazolamide, amiloride, bumetanide, canrenone, chlortha-lidone, etacrynic acid, furosemide, indapamide, metolazone, spironolac-tone, thiazides (e.g., bendroflumethiazide, chlorothiazide, hydrochlorothiazide), and triamterene, and other substances with a similar chemical structure or similar biological effects (except drosperinone, pama-brom and topical dorzolamide and brinzolamide, which are not prohibited).	
Glucocorticosteroids**	Glucocorticosteroids are prohibited when administered orally, rectally, intravenously, or intramuscularly. Their use requires a Therapeutic Use Exception. Dermatological preparations are not prohibited.	Delay fatigue via increased fat mobilization and utilization
Beta blockers**	Beta blockers include, but are not limited to, the following: acebutolol, alprenolol, atenolol, betaxolol, bisoprolol, bunolol, carteolol, carvedilol, celiprolol, esmolol, labetalol, levobunolol, metipranolol, metoprolol, nadolol, oxprenolol, pindolol, propranolol, sotalol, timolol.	Mute the effects of the sympathetic hormones and thereby decrease heart rate

* Prohibited from use at all times.

** Prohibited from use only during competition.

ing sports organizations. Failure to pay attention to supplement ingredients could lead to positive testing for doping and implementation of associated punitive sanctioning.

An additional concern for athletes centers on the purity of the dietary supplement and the possibility of **inadvertent doping**. Inadvertent doping results when an athlete is taking a dietary supplement that, unbeknownst to him or her, can result in a positive test for doping. Inadvertent doping can occur in the following ways:

inadvertent doping A situation resulting from an athlete ingesting a dietary supplement that unbeknownst to him or her can result in a positive test for a banned substance.

- The ingredient was listed on the food label but the athlete did not know it was on the banned list or that the ingredient could cause a positive test.
- The supplement label lists all of the ingredients, but the names given are not recognized as being related to banned substances. For example, Ma Huang herbal products may be listed on the ingredients list, but athletes may not know that it contains ephedrine, which is banned.
- The supplement manufacturer may not declare a banned substance in its ingredient list. In some cases the ingredient may be included but deliberately not listed, or the banned substance was added inadvertently by the manufacturer as a by-product of other ingredients, or via contamination in the production process.

Although the FDA has established guidelines for good manufacturing practices and accurate labeling of supplements, there has been little enforcement. In short, this means that the quality control of supplement manufacturing is left to the supplement companies. Unfortunately, several studies have revealed evidence of deceptive and inaccurate labeling practices.[10–13]

Inadvertent doping does not exempt athletes from punishment and embarrassment if they test positive for a banned substance. Sports nutrition professionals must be knowledgeable about not only the list of banned substances, but also herbal substances that are related to or may be converted to banned substances within the body.

What are some of the commonly encountered doping substances?

Doping substances used by athletes range from natural herbals to chemically engineered compounds,

and literally are too numerous for discussion within the confines of this chapter. A visit to the local nutrition/health food store will quickly leave a lasting impression of the number of dietary supplements available to athletes. A discussion of each nutritional ergogenic is beyond the scope of this book, so rather than being discussed individually, the substances will be divided into functional groups as delineated by Antonio and Stout.[14] In the following sections each group is briefly discussed, and the more commonly encountered supplements within each group are listed in Tables 9.3 to 9.9. In the tables, the "Claimed Actions" column describes the touted benefits of the nutritional aid. These are merely claims from manufacturers or proposed actions, not the actual results of research. The "Human Research" column indicates whether any human studies have been done and published on the product. A "yes" in this column does not mean the product works, it merely means published human studies using the product exist. The "Potential" column gives an indication as to whether the nutritional aid has some merit for use based on findings from currently available research data. The "Comment/Concerns" column provides other pertinent information on the nutritional aid. The following functional groups of nutritional ergogenics are covered:

- Anabolics
- Prohormones and hormone releasers
- Fat reducers
- Anticatabolics
- Vitamins and minerals

Which nutritional ergogenic aids are commonly used as anabolic agents, prohormones, and hormone releasers?

An **anabolic agent** is a substance that enhances the body's ability to build tissue. In regard to sports, anabolic agents are typically those that lead to an increase in muscle mass by promoting protein synthesis (see **Table 9.3**). The word *anabolic* is usually associated with anabolic steroids, which technically are synthetic hormones that play a similar role to that of testosterone. Because anabolic steroids are synthetic hormones and are not considered dietary supplements, they will not be covered in this chapter. However, there are several compounds classified as dietary supplements that are touted to increase the body's levels of anabolic hormones. These supplements are known as

anabolic agent A substance that enhances the body's ability to build tissue. In regard to sports, anabolic agents are typically those that lead to an increase in muscle mass by promoting protein synthesis.

TABLE 9.3	Anabolic Nutritional Ergogenics				
Supplements (other names)	Claimed Actions	Human Research	Potential	Comments/Concerns
Beta-hydroxy-beta-methyl-butyrate (HMB)	Prevents protein breakdown and enhances synthesis, increases strength, improves body composition	Yes	Moderate-high	Long-term effects unknown. Benefits appear to decline with continued use.
Chromium picolinate	Enhances action of insulin; increases muscle mass	Yes	Low	Sufficient amounts can be consumed in the daily diet.
Conjugated linoleic acid (CLA)	Increases response to tissue growth factors, hormones, and cell messengers; increases muscle mass	Yes	Low	Animal studies suggest it is safe; long-term effects unknown.
Creatine monohydrate	Increases anaerobic output (strength/power) in events lasting 6 seconds to 4 minutes	Yes	Moderate-high	Long-term effects (>5 years) are still unknown.
Octacosanol	Improves neural functioning, thus increasing ability to utilize muscle and intensify training	Yes	Low	Has been used in foods since 1950; appears safe.
Protein powder/bars	Increases strength, aids in muscle growth and development	Yes	Low-moderate	Effective only for athletes who are protein deficient. Watch for other added ingredients.
Vanadyl sulfate	Enhances/mimics effects of growth factors in muscle	Yes	Low	Animal studies demonstrate severe side effects; human effects less clear.

prohormone A molecule or substance that can be readily converted to a biologically active hormone.

hormone releaser A substance or substances that stimulate an increased quantity and/or frequency of release of hormones within the body.

prohormones and hormone releasers.

Prohormones are precursor substances that can be readily converted to biologically active hormones by the body. Marketers of prohormones promote their products based on the theory that the fewer the enzymatic steps the prohormone has to go through to become biologically active (i.e., the closer in structure it is to the "real thing"), the greater its effectiveness as an ergogenic aid. Although this is not the case, millions of dollars have been spent on substances touted to be close relatives to actual hormones in the body. Androstenedione, commonly referred to as "Andro," is probably the most well known of the prohormones and requires only one enzymatic step to be converted to testosterone.

Unlike prohormones, which are converted by the body into the targeted hormone, hormone re-

leasers are substances that stimulate an increased quantity or frequency of release of the specific hormone within the body, thus increasing physiologic levels. Clonidine is one such hormone releaser that has been touted to increase growth hormone levels in the body. Some of the more commonly encountered nutritional ergogenics classified as anabolic agents, prohormones, or hormone releasers are the following:

- Androstenedione (Andro)
- Beta-hydroxy-beta-methylbutyrate (HMB)
- Boron
- Clonidine
- Conjugated linoleic acid (CLA)
- Creatine monohydrate (creatine)
- Vanadium (vanadyl sulfate)

These substances as well as other anabolic, prohormone, or hormone releaser supplements frequently encountered are summarized in Table 9.3 and **Table 9.4**.

TABLE 9.4 Prohormones and Hormone Releasers

Supplements (other names)	Claimed Actions	Human Research	Potential	Comments/Concerns
Andro supplements (androstenedione, androstenediol, 19-nor-4-androstenedione; 19-nor-4-androstenediol)	Increases testosterone levels	Yes	Low	May decrease muscle mass and increase estradiol levels.
Arginine and ornithine supplementation	Increases growth hormone production	Yes	Low	No research supports that amino acids increase growth hormone levels.
Boron	Increases plasma testosterone	Yes	Low	No research support for effectiveness; can be toxic.
Clonidine	Increases growth hormone production	Yes	Low	No research supporting claims.
Dehydroepiandrosterone (DHEA)	Increases testosterone levels, decreases fat and builds muscle	Yes	Low-moderate	Research does not support claims; may decrease HDL levels and insulin sensitivity; female athletes may experience increases in androgen levels.
Tribulus terrestris	Increases body's production of testosterone	Yes	Low	Promoted as safe alternative to steroids, but can be toxic.

Which nutritional ergogenic aids are commonly used to reduce fat mass?

At first glance one may wonder how a compound that decreases body fat would be considered an ergogenic aid. However, for some athletes fat is considered dead weight and, therefore, supplements that lead to decreases in body fat could enhance performance by making the athlete lighter. Some of these nutritional agents increase the body's ability to mobilize and utilize fats for energy. Others decrease appetite, which lowers daily caloric intake and causes the body to turn to fat stores for energy, while still others block the absorption of ingested fats. Regardless of the mode of action, this category of dietary supplements is sought after by endurance athletes, athletes in appearance sports, athletes participating in weight-tiered sports, and the general public. Some of the more commonly encountered fat reduction nutritional aids are as follows:

- Caffeine
- Chitosan
- Chromium
- Dehydroepiandrosterone (DHEA)
- Ephedrine
- L-carnitine
- Yohimbe

Refer to **Table 9.5** for a summary of these dietary supplements.

Which nutritional ergogenic aids are commonly used as anticatabolics?

Anticatabolics are nutritional compounds that decrease the breakdown of body tissues. Body tissues, and in particular proteins, are in a constant state of turnover, so the idea behind anticatabolics is to slow protein degradation. If protein degradation is decreased and protein synthesis is maintained, the end result would be an accumulation of protein (in the case of athletes, increased muscle mass). Body builders,

anticatabolic A nutritional compound that slows the breakdown processes in the body (catabolism), thus tilting the metabolic balance toward increased tissue building (anabolism).

TABLE 9.5 Fat Reducers

Supplements (other names)	Claimed Actions	Human Research	Potential	Comments/Concerns
Caffeine	Stimulates central nervous system, increases lipolysis	Yes	Moderate-High	Elevates blood pressure and heart rate; can cause loose bowels and gastric upset.
Chitosan	Decreases amount of dietary fat absorbed across intestinal lining during digestion	Limited	Moderate	Can cause diarrhea; decreases absorption of fat-soluble vitamins.
Chromium	Enhances the actions of insulin; increases muscle mass, thus increasing metabolic rate	Yes	Low	Kidney failure and muscle wasting have been reported at high doses.
Dehydroepiandrosterone (DHEA)	Increases testosterone levels and thus muscle mass, which increases metabolic rate	Yes	Low	In women, can increase testosterone level and increase risk for heart disease.
Ephedrine	Increases lipolysis and resting metabolic rate, suppresses hunger	Yes	High	No longer sold over the counter because of reported adverse side effects.
L-carnitine	Assists in transfer of fats into the mitochondria, thereby increasing fat oxidation	No	Low	Appears to be safe but lack of research support raises questions about use; avoid D-carnitine supplements, as they may be toxic.
Yohimbe	Blocks receptors that inhibit lipolysis, thereby increasing fat loss	Yes	High	Side effects include anxiety, nausea, tremors; purity of supplements is a concern.

power lifters, Olympic weight lifters, and throwing athletes in field events all could potentially benefit from anticatabolics. Anticatabolic dietary supplements include:

- Alpha-ketoglutarate
- Branched chain amino acids
- Casein protein
- Glutamine
- Leucine
- Whey protein

These anticatabolics are summarized in **Table 9.6**.

Which vitamins and minerals are commonly used as nutritional ergogenic aids?

The micronutrients (i.e., vitamins and minerals) and their function within the body are discussed in detail in Chapters 6 and 7. These nutrients serve key roles in body functions critical to sport performance and thus supplement manufacturers have

had little trouble selling their products by touting their potential benefits. However, because the body can reuse vitamins and minerals as they serve in their various roles, our physiologic need for daily intake is very small. This is the reason vitamins and minerals are classified as "micronutrients." The majority of research investigating vitamins and minerals indicates that unless the athlete is deficient, supplementation beyond the RDA has no effect on sport performance. In other words, under most circumstances the small daily requirement for vitamins and minerals is usually more than met by a well-balanced diet. Just to make sure that adequate intakes are met, many sports nutrition professionals recommend taking a good quality multivitamin/mineral as an "insurance policy," but warn that megadosing on any one vitamin or mineral in hopes of an ergogenic effect is neither warranted nor recommended.

TABLE 9.6   Anticatabolic Nutritional Ergogenic Aids

Supplements (other names)	Claimed Actions	Human Research	Potential	Comments/Concerns
Alpha-ketoglutarate	Spares glutamine, thus sparing muscle tissue, which is the biggest source of glutamine	Yes	Moderate-high	Long-term safety is unknown, but limited evidence indicates it is well tolerated.
Branched chain amino acids (BCAA)	Increases availability of valine, leucine, and isoleucine for various functions, thereby sparing muscle tissue, which is the usual source	Yes	Moderate-high	Appears to be safe.
Casein protein	Source of essential amino acids, which decreases muscle protein degradation and stimulates protein synthesis	Yes	Moderate-high	Potential for allergic reactions but rare; can increase cholesterol levels.
Glutamine	Increases availability of glutamine, which is used in energy metabolism in the kidneys, gut, liver, and cells of the immune system, thus sparing muscle	Yes	High	High doses are required but seems to be safe; long-term effects unknown.
Leucine	Spares muscle by increasing availability of leucine, which is used by various tissues for energy	Yes	Moderate	Appears to be safe.
Whey protein	Source of essential amino acids, which decreases muscle protein degradation and stimulates protein synthesis	Yes	High	Potential for allergic reactions but rare; no serious side effects have been reported even with high doses.

What types of dietary supplements and nutritional ergogenics are commonly used by endurance athletes, strength/ power athletes, and team sport athletes?

Athletes are keenly attuned to the physical, nutritional, and energetic requirements necessary for optimal performance in their sport. Many athletes self-identify areas that they believe to be weak and then seek products that will address their shortcomings. Shrewd marketers take advantage by using key words or phrases (e.g., increased power, improved endurance) that draw attention to their product and entice the athlete to "give the product a go." The following paragraphs identify some of the dietary supplements and nutritional ergogenics used by various types of athletes in hopes of enhancing their sport performance.

Because of the nature of endurance sports, any supplement promoting an enhancement of energy, muscular endurance, cardiorespiratory capacity, or recovery between workouts, as well as decreased body fat, has great appeal to the endurance athlete. **Table 9.7** lists a variety of products commonly used by endurance athletes. The list ranges from supplements that are highly effective and researched (e.g., sports beverages) to those that appear to be minimally effective and not well documented (e.g., L-carnitine). An athlete's individual decision to experiment with a particular supplement should occur only after careful consideration of the potential benefits and risks.

Strength/power athletes are attracted to supplements or ergogenic aids promoting an enhancement of strength, power, anaerobic metabolism, and muscle mass. **Table 9.8** lists a variety of ergogenic aids commonly used by strength/power athletes. The list

TABLE 9.7 Common Nutritional Ergogenics Used by Endurance Athletes

Supplements (other names)	Claimed Action	Human Research	Potential	Banned	Comments/Concerns
Branched chain amino acids (BCAA)	Essential amino acids that are touted to enhance endurance performance	Yes	Low	No	BCAAs are supplied by whole foods, which also provide other nutrients.
Caffeine (kola nut, guarana)	Enhances performance by increasing serum FFA/use of muscle triglycerides, sparing muscle glycogen	Yes	Moderate	No	Elevates heart rate and blood pressure; can cause irritability, nervousness, and gastrointestinal distress.
Coenzyme Q_{10} (ubiquinone or CoQ_{10})	Enhances function of electron transport chain; increases endurance performance	Yes	Low for athletes	No	Potential for cell damage when consumed in large amounts and exercising intensely.
Energy bars	Provides energy for prolonged endurance performance	Yes	High	No	Should not be used as a meal replacement.
Energy gels	Quick supply of carbohydrates during endurance exercise	Yes	High	No	Consume with 8–12 oz of fluid; may be better tolerated taken in small amounts.
Ginseng	Increases stamina; ability to adapt to training stressors; enhances immune function	Yes	Low	No	Ginseng content in supplements can vary greatly; may increase blood pressure.
Glycerol	Energy source during exercise; promotes hyperhydration status before endurance exercise	Yes	Low-moderate	Yes	USOC/IOC bans use. May cause gastrointestinal upset and cramping.
L-carnitine	Fat transporter within cells; increases endurance performance	Yes	Low	No	Avoid D-carnitine supplements, as they may be toxic and can deplete L-carnitine.
Medium-chain triglycerides (MCT)	Quickly metabolize fatty acids that spare glycogen and thus delay fatigue	Yes	Low	No	May cause gastrointestinal upset and cramping.
Multivitamin/mineral	Supply essential vitamins and minerals to endurance athletes for optimal health and performance	Yes	Moderate	No	Look for supplements containing no more than 100–200% of the Daily Value.
Pyruvate	Accelerates Krebs cycle; enhances use of glucose; greater fat loss; increases glycogen storage	Yes	Low-moderate	No	Limited research available on ergogenic effects and side effects of long-term use.
Sodium bicarbonate	Buffers lactic acid, thereby delaying the onset of fatigue	Yes	Low	No	May cause nausea, diarrhea, irritability, and/or muscle spasms.
Sodium/electrolyte tablets	Prevents hyponatremia by supplying sodium during exercise and other electrolytes as buffers	Yes	High	No	Avoid supplements using mainly sodium bicarbonate; can cause diarrhea/cramping.
Sports beverages	Enhances endurance performance and delays fatigue by supplying fluid, carbohydrates, and electrolytes	Yes	High	No	Practice during training to avoid gastrointestinal distress during competitions.

TABLE 9.8

Common Nutritional Ergogenics Used by Strength/Power Athletes

Supplements (other names)	Claimed Action	Human Research	Potential	Banned	Comments/Concerns
Anabolic androgenic steroids	Increases muscle mass and strength	Yes	High	Yes	Harmful side effects: abnormal growth, liver and heart disease, stroke, and aggression.
Beta-hydroxy-beta-methyl butyrate (HMB)	Prevents protein breakdown and enhances synthesis; increases strength; improves body composition	Yes	Moderate-high	No	Long-term effects unknown. Benefits appear to decline with continued use.
Chromium	Increases muscle mass, decreases fat mass, improves blood glucose and lipid levels	Yes	Low	No	Sufficient amounts can be consumed in the daily diet.
Conjugated linoleic acid (CLA)	Increases production of growth hormone, weight loss, fat loss, increases muscle mass	Some	Low	No	Most research showing benefits was conducted on animals. Watch for gastric/intestinal distress.
Creatine monohydrate	Increases anaerobic output (strength/power) in events lasting 6 seconds to 4 minutes	Yes	Moderate-high	No	Long-term effects (>5 years) are still unknown.
Human growth hormone	Increases muscle mass, strength, and power; decreases fat mass	Yes	High	Yes	Causes pathological enlargement of organs and increases risk of chronic disease.
Medium-chain triglycerides (MCT)	Increases energy and muscle mass; decreases fat mass	Yes	Low	No	Side effects often experienced are intestinal cramping and diarrhea.
Multivitamin/mineral	Supplies essential vitamins and minerals to athletes for optimal health and performance	Yes	Moderate	No	Look for supplements containing no more than 100–200% of the Daily Value.
Protein powder/bars	Increases strength; aids in muscle growth and development	Yes	Low-moderate	No	Effective only for athletes who are protein deficient. Watch for other added ingredients.

ranges from ergogenic aids that are highly effective but also possess severe side effects (e.g., steroids) to those that are minimally effective and relatively safe (e.g., chromium). Some of these supplements are illegal and/or banned by sports agencies and should obviously be avoided. Others may offer potential benefits but should be evaluated on an individual basis.

Many nutritional ergogenics used by team sport athletes overlap those of the endurance and/or strength/power athletes. In other words, each athlete uses supplements that he or she feels will help meet the physical or energy requirements of the position the athlete plays. For example, the typical power, contact team sport athletes are likely to take the same supplements as strength/power athletes, namely those designed to increase muscle mass, improve speed, or enhance strength. Baseball, hockey, football, and basketball players commonly report using creatine. They

also are more likely to try hormone releasers, prohormones, and/or anabolic steroids. Volleyball, soccer, and field hockey athletes tend to seek out different supplements. These athletes are more interested in maintaining or losing weight, keeping energy levels high, and taking supplements that will not increase weight but will increase power. The nature of their sport is less dependent on size and brute strength and more dependent on agility, quickness, and muscular endurance. Supplements that team sport athletes often report using are listed in **Table 9.9**.

Regardless of the demands of a particular sport, there are nutritional ergogenic aids available that claim to enhance performance. Although some supplements/nutritional ergogenics do have potential, it must be understood that research evidence on most is far from conclusive. In addition, even fewer nutritional aids have been evaluated in regard to

TABLE 9.9

Common Nutritional Ergogenics Used by Team Sport Athletes

Supplements (other names)	Claimed Action	Human Research	Potential	Banned	Comments/Concerns
Androstenedione	Increases testosterone; increases muscle mass, strength, and power	Yes	Low	Yes	Research does not support claims; may increase estrogens in body.
Beta-hydroxy-beta-methyl-butyrate (HMB)	Anticatabolic; spares muscle mass; increases muscle mass and strength	Yes	Moderate-high	No	Possible effect in the untrained; benefits appear to decline with continued use.
Branched chain amino acids (BCAA)	Increases muscle endurance; serves as an anticatabolic	Yes	Moderate	No	No consistent support of endurance effects but some potential as an anticatabolic.
Caffeine	Boosts metabolism; increases free fatty acid levels in blood; enhances endurance performance	Yes	High	No	Can cause gastric upset and nervous irritability.
Creatine monohydrate	Increases anaerobic power; increases strength	Yes	High	No	Research supports claims; may cause diarrhea and muscle cramping; long-term effects unknown.
Dehydroepi-androsterone (DHEA)	Prohormone; increases testosterone levels; decreases fat; builds muscle mass, strength, and power	Yes	Low-moderate	Yes	Research does not support claims in young trained athletes; female athletes may experience increased androgen levels and decreased HDL levels and insulin sensitivity.
Ephedrine (Ma Huang/ephedra)	Increases metabolism; suppresses hunger; decreases body fat	Yes	High	Yes	No longer sold over the counter due to reported adverse side effects.
Inosine	Enhances ATP levels, thereby increasing anaerobic power	Yes	Low	No	Supplementation can elevate uric acid levels and thus cause gout.
Ornithine and arginine	Increase release of growth hormone; increases muscle mass	Yes	Low	No	No research supports that amino acids increase growth hormone levels.

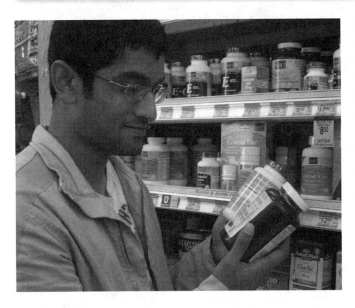

long-term use and associated side effects. Nutrition professionals need to be able to provide athletes with up-to-date information so that they can make educated decisions regarding the use of nutritional ergogenics based on grounded information and not on manufacturers' claims.

Where can information on nutritional ergogenic aids be found?

Table 9.10 provides a listing of several different resources that supply information on dietary supplements. Some of the Internet sources provide information about banned substances, and others are designed to help consumers make informed choices about supplement use. Athletes in sports in which drug testing is likely

TABLE 9.10 Dietary Supplements Resource List

Source	Location	Information
Web Sites		
National Collegiate Athletics Association	www.ncaa.org/wps/portal/ncaahome?WCM_GLOBAL_CONTEXT=/ncaa/ncaa/academics+and+athletes/personal+welfare	Find specific supplements, list of NCAA banned substances, nutrition information, and videos for athlete education
FDA, CFSAN (Center for Food Safety and Applied Nutrition)	www.fda.gov/Food/DietarySupplements/default.htm	Information on legislation of dietary supplements, warning letters, industry regulations
American College of Sports Medicine	www.acsm.org	Online articles from Medicine & Science in Sports and Exercise; ACSM position statements
International Bibliographic Information on Dietary Supplements (IBIDS) Database	http://ods.od.nih.gov/Health_Information/IBIDS.aspx	Can search for information on specific supplements and supplement safety and find research articles
National Institutes of Health, Office of Dietary Supplements	http://health.nih.gov	Dietary supplements fact sheets, health information related to supplements, IBIDS database (International Bibliographic Information on Dietary Supplements)
Food and Nutrition Information Center	http://fnic.nal.usda.gov/nal_display/index.php?info_center=4&tax_level=1	Credible information on dietary supplements, herbs, and botanicals; can search for specific supplements
Consumer Labs	www.consumerlab.com	Product reviews of many supplements, sports bars, and sports drinks
Supplement Watch, Inc.	www.supplementwatch.com	Scientific reviews of research related to supplements; provides a rating system for any supplements it has reviewed and comprehensive and up-to-date information concerning dietary supplements
U.S. Pharmacopeia	www.usp.org/USPVerified	Lists dietary supplements that have the USP-verified seal; provides information on selecting supplements
MedWatch	www.fda.gov/Safety/MedWatch/HowToReport/ucm053074.htm	Consumers or medical professionals can report adverse events suspected to be related to supplement use
National Center for Complementary and Alternative Medicine	http://nccam.nih.gov	Information on various dietary supplements and other alternative medicines
World Anti-Doping Agency	www.wada-ama.org	Provides lists of banned ergogenic aids and other information to athletes and the public
United States Anti-Doping Agency	www.usantidoping.org	Provides lists of banned ergogenic aids and other information to athletes and the public
Natural Medicines Comprehensive Database	www.naturaldatabase.com	Provides reliable information on natural medicines, herbal, and nonherbal supplements
PubMed	www.ncbi.nlm.nih.gov/pubmed	A free service of the U.S. National Library of Medicine that enables searches on life science topics such as nutritional ergogenic aids
Publications		
Ergogenics Edge, by Melvin Williams[15]	www.humankinetics.com	Good review of many dietary supplements and other methods of doping
Sports Supplements, by Jose Antonio and Jeffrey Stout[14]	www.lww.com	Reviews sports supplements as they are marketed for different exercises and activities; some discussion of ethics, credibility of science related to supplements

Sports nutrition professionals working with athletes need to determine what, if any, supplements are being taken. This inquiry should include current and past dietary supplement use and why the athletes are taking the supplements.

should be aware that many dietary supplements that do not carry the USP-verified seal could contain banned substances, even if the label does not list the ingredient. Using the list of resources will help athletes make informed choices about which supplements to use, appropriate supplement doses, potential side effects, and purported benefits of taking dietary supplements.

The best sports nutrition professionals are well versed in the vast array of dietary supplements that athletes commonly use. Athletic trainers working predominantly with strength athletes should become very familiar with the supplements marketed toward muscle gain and fat loss. Similarly, nutrition professionals working with female athletes will find it helpful to become familiar with common weight loss, energy, fat burning, and vitamin/mineral supplements. Athletes appreciate being educated about the pros and cons of using supplements, including the risks of positive drug testing and the cost of these supplements. Well-balanced nutrition is often much less expensive than consuming dietary supplements regularly. Sports nutrition professionals should not advocate a universal "supplements should never be taken" policy. Those who do will often lose credibility with athletes. Certain dietary supplements may have significant benefits for some athletes. Sports nutrition professionals should work with athletes to help them make informed decisions about supplement use by helping them understand the safety, efficacy, and economics of taking dietary supplements for improved sport performance.

What tools are available to research information on ergogenic aids?

New dietary products and supplements are appearing on store shelves faster than research can keep up. As noted earlier, most of these nutritional products have not been tested for effectiveness or safety. Unless the manufacturer sponsors placebo-controlled studies, which is very rare, or the ergogenic aid garners the attention of sports organizations or the FDA, experimental testing is unlikely. As a result, ineffective products continue to sell until word of mouth from one user to another eventually kills the demand. Unfortunately, that can take years. In the meantime, bogus products continue to defraud athletes and the general public.

Sports nutrition professionals must be aware of the various research tools available to help them gain as much information as possible, when available, on nutritional products. Sports nutrition professionals are often the first line of defense in protecting athletes and the public from ineffective and potentially unsafe nutrition products. Learning as much as possible about the product and its ingredients is vital so that the sports nutrition professional can educate athletes about the product. Many times, merely instructing someone not to use a product is not an effective deterrent. However, explaining in layperson's terms what the product contains and what is known about the main ingredients, and offering supportive research evidence, will provide logic for the recommendation.

When investigating a dietary supplement, the anti-doping agencies should be consulted. WADA and the **United States AntiDoping Agency (USADA)** were created in 1999 with the sole intent of educating athletes about supplements and other ergogenic aids. Their Web sites (found in Table 9.10) provide a wealth of information on banned substances, the latest information releases on various aids, and contact information for questions.

One of the best ways to determine whether any peer-reviewed research has been conducted on a specific product is to use the Internet to tie into the library site of an area university or college. University libraries often provide access to several research journal databases that will allow individuals to search for a specific product or ingredients. Some of the more common databases that include journals covering research in the area of sports nutrition are **Medline**, **CINAHL**, and **SportDiscus**. If nothing can be found using the research databases, then

United States Anti-Doping Agency (USADA) A national-level, nongovernmental organization that serves as an extension of the World Anti-Doping Agency. Its mission is to educate athletes about doping, reinforce the ideal of fair play, and sanction those who cheat.

Medline The U.S. National Library of Medicine's premier bibliographic database that provides information from the following fields: medicine, nursing, dentistry, veterinary medicine, allied health, and preclinical sciences.

CINAHL The acronym used for the Cumulative Index to Nursing & Allied Health, which is a reference database that provides authoritative coverage of the literature related to nursing and allied health.

SportDiscus A reference database of citations, books, conference proceedings, dissertations, reports, monographs, journals, magazines, and newsletters covering information in the following areas: sports medicine, exercise physiology, biomechanics, psychology, training techniques, coaching, physical education, physical fitness, active living, recreation, history, facilities, and equipment.

using a database covering the popular media, magazines, journals, and newsletters such as EBSCOhost may provide an informational article on the product. Often an expert will be cited, or unpublished studies involving the product will be mentioned. Usually a quick search on Google can provide contact information for the experts or investigators mentioned in the article. An email or phone call to these contacts can be a goldmine of information.

The Web sites of other professional organizations such as the American College of Sports Medicine (www.acsm.org), the National Strength and Conditioning Association (www.nsca-lift.org), and the International Society of Sports Nutrition (www.sportsnutritionsociety.org) can also be consulted. Occasionally, information in the form of position statements, pronouncements, or press releases can be found on specific nutritional ergogenics.

The Box Score

Key Points of Chapter

- An ergogenic aid is anything that enhances a person's ability to perform work. Ergogenic aids can take many different forms: physiological, biomechanical, psychological, pharmacological, and nutritional.

- According to DSHEA, to be categorized as a dietary supplement a substance should not be intended to be used as a food or sole item of a meal and must contain one or more of the following dietary ingredients: vitamin, mineral, herb or other botanical, amino acid, dietary substance to supplement the diet, or concentrate, metabolite, constituent, extract, or combination of any of the above ingredients.

- Dietary supplements do not require FDA approval and do not go through the same rigorous testing and scientific approval process as pharmaceutical drugs. Athletes need to be aware of the possibility that the supplement they take could contain a banned substance or could pose a health risk if consumed in conjunction with other supplements or medications.

- Good manufacturing practice guidelines are being developed to help ensure that safety and quality control measures are used during the production of dietary supplements. However, supplement makers are not required to follow these practices. As a result, athletes should purchase products displaying the USP seal, which ensures product quality.

- Doping is the practice of enhancing performance through the use of foreign substances or other artificial means. Doping is banned in most sport competitions. Unfortunately, doping has become an epidemic in sports, which presents risks not only to the health of athletes, but also to the basic tenet of fair play in competition.

- Endurance athletes should fully evaluate any supplement before purchasing and ingesting it. Some products are well researched and highly beneficial, whereas others are expensive, ineffective, and potentially harmful.

- Numerous nutritional ergogenic aids are being used by strength and power athletes. Unfortunately, few of these products have been proven to be effective, and most that have are banned from use by sports organizations.

- Use of nutritional ergogenic aids in team sports is as varied as the physical demands of the different positions. Nutritional ergogenic aids that boost muscle building, enhance strength/power, and delay fatigue are prevalent. Athletes must be educated as to the risks and benefits of each as well as to whether their use is banned. Failure to do so can have ramifications affecting the entire team.

- One of the best ways to determine whether any peer-reviewed research has been conducted on a nutritional ergogenic aid is to tie into a university or college library Web site and search one of several literature databases. Some of the more common databases that include journals covering research in the areas of sport nutrition are Medline, CINAHL, and SportDiscus.

- Other excellent sources of information are the World Anti-Doping Agency (WADA) and the United States Anti-Doping Agency (USADA), which provide a wealth of information on banned substances, the latest information releases on various nutritional aids, and contact information for questions.

Study Questions

1. Define "ergogenic aid" and discuss the various types of ergogenic aids. What are some examples of each type?

2. What does the acronym DSHEA stand for? What are the ramifications of DSHEA in regard to the use and safety of certain ergogenic aids?

3. What tools does a sports nutrition professional have available to research information about old or new nutritional supplements and other ergogenic aids?

4. Discuss why the statement "Buyer beware" is appropriate, particularly for athletes.

5. What roles do the FDA and FTC have in regard to dealing with dietary supplements?

6. List four nutritional ergogenics that might be encountered when working with endurance athletes.

7. List two nutritional ergogenic aid categories that strength athletes are likely to use or to have questions about.

8. What is the most common nutritional ergogenic used by team sport athletes? Discuss the need for and effectiveness of this type of supplement for team sports and other athletes.

9. What is the difference between nutritional supplements that are classified as "anabolic" versus "anticatabolic"?

10. What is the "placebo effect," and why is it important that research involving ergogenic aids controls for it?

11. Define "doping." What world organization was formed in 1999 to prevent it?

12. What is CINAHL, and how might a sports nutrition professional use it?

13. An athlete asks you about a nutritional supplement with which you are not familiar. How would you research the supplement to become well versed in its purported actions, side effects, legality for sport, and so on?

References

1. 103rd Congress. Public Law 103-417. Dietary Supplements Health and Education Act of 1994.

2. Millen AE, Dodd KW, Subar AF. Use of vitamin, mineral, non-vitamin, and non-mineral supplements in the United States: the 1987, 1992, and 2000 National Health Interview Survey results. *J Am Diet Assoc*. 2004;104(6):942–950.

3. Froiland K, Koszewski W, Hingst J, Kopecky L. Nutritional supplement use among college athletes and their sources of information. *Int J Sport Nutr Exerc Metabol*. 2004;14(1):104–120.

4. Food and Drug Administration. Final rule declaring dietary supplements containing ephedrine alkaloids adulterated because they present an unreasonable risk. *Federal Register*. 2004;69:6787–6854.

5. Rados C. Ephedra ban: no shortage of reasons. *FDA Consum Mag*. 2004;38(2):6–7.

6. Agency for Healthcare Research and Quality. Ephedra and ephedrine for weight loss and athletic performance enhancement: clinical efficacy and side effects. File inventory, Evidence Report/Technology Assessment Number 76; AHRQ Publication No. 03-E022; 2003.

7. Soni MG, Carabin IG, Griffiths JC, Burdock GA. Safety of ephedra: lessons learned. *Toxicol Lett*. 2004; 150:97–110.

8. Haller CA, Benowitz NL. Adverse cardiovascular and central nervous system events associated with dietary supplements containing ephedra alkaloids. *N Engl J Med*. 2000;343:1833–1838.

9. Council for Responsible Nutrition. *Safety Assessment and Determination of a Tolerable Upper Limit for Ephedra*. Mississauga, Ontario: Cantox Health Sciences International; 2000:1–169.

10. Gurley BJ, Wang P, Gardner SF. Ephedrine-type alkaloid content of nutritional supplements containing Ephedra sinics (Ma Huang) as determined by high performance liquid chromatography. *J Pharm Sci*. 1998;87: 1547–1553.

11. Hahm H, Kujawa J, Ausberger L. Comparison of melatonin products against USP's nutritional supplements standards and other criteria. *J Am Pharm Assoc*. 1999;39:27–31.

12. Parasrampuria J, Schwartz K, Petesch R. Quality control of dehydroepiandrosterone dietary supplements products. *JAMA*. 1998;280:1565.

13. Catlin DH, Leder BZ, Ahrens B, et al. Trace contamination of over-the-counter androstenedione and positive urine test results for a nandrolone metabolite. *JAMA*. 2000;284:2618–2621.

14. Antonio J, Stout JR. *Sports Supplements*. Philadelphia, PA: Lippincott Williams & Wilkins; 2001.

15. Williams MH. *The Ergogenics Edge: Pushing the Limits of Sports Performance*. Champaign, IL: Human Kinetics; 1998.

CHAPTER

10

Nutrition Consultation with Athletes

Key Questions Addressed

- Why is nutrition consultation and communication with athletes important?

- How much do athletes know about sports nutrition?

- Who provides nutrition assessment and education to athletes?

- How does the consultation process with athletes begin?

- What is a diet history?

- How are food records analyzed?

- What are the steps for the initial consultation with the athlete?

- What are the steps for a follow-up consultation with the athlete?

- What should walk-in or short sessions with athletes involve?

- Are there any concerns about the confidentiality of the health, nutrition, and exercise information provided by the athlete?

You Are the Nutrition Coach

Jennifer is a freshman and plays shortstop on her college softball team. Her coach thinks that she has the skill to be a starter her sophomore year. She is thin and has a hard time hitting home runs, despite consistently hitting over .325 for the past three seasons of play in high school. She and her coach feel that if she were to gain some muscle mass and strength, her home-run hitting would improve, thus securing the starting position next year. Jennifer agrees but is also concerned about gaining too much weight. She decides to consult with the sports dietitian at her college to develop a plan to gain muscle mass and a small amount of weight.

Questions

- What information would you like to have Jennifer bring to the first consultation session?

- How do you determine whether Jennifer is ready to make the changes in dietary intake needed to produce weight gain?

- What type of follow-up and continued nutrition consultation would you recommend for Jennifer?

Why is nutrition consultation and communication with athletes important?

Athletes need coaches to help them train to succeed in their sport. They need athletic trainers to help them prevent and rehabilitate injuries that may occur during sport activities. Athletes are not expected to know how to prevent injuries or train appropriately on their own. However, it is often assumed that athletes know about nutrition and know how to eat for improved sport performance. Similar to working with a coach or trainer to improve sport-specific skills, gaining education or seeking consultation about nutrition can help improve athletes' sport performance. Unfortunately, many athletes have had limited nutrition education, gaining no further knowledge than the information presented during K–12 classes. Some athletes are fortunate enough to have coaches or parents who are knowledgeable about good nutrition and how it affects sport performance. Often, access to a sports dietitian with expertise specifically in sports nutrition is limited. However, for all athletes, acquiring the knowledge and skills that support good nutrition behaviors can help individuals meet their sport-specific goals.

The role of sports nutrition in improving sport performance has been well documented. The well-hydrated and well-nourished athlete who pays attention to dietary intake before, during, and after workouts/competitions can gain a competitive edge over opponents. Therefore, empowering athletes with nutrition education is essential to any individual or team athlete. Educational opportunities can be provided in team sessions, in individual consultations, on the playing field, and by giving athletes information about credible sports nutrition resources.

Written educational materials designed specifically for a particular sports team or athlete can be valuable resources initially and for future reference. Communicating messages appropriately that meet the athlete's needs, goals, and lifestyle will help the athlete be successful in making dietary changes. Regardless of the format of the communication, it is important that athletes receive accurate and timely nutrition information to improve their sport performance.

This chapter reviews why athletes need nutrition education, who should provide nutrition assessments and educational sessions, common information-gathering methods, consultation, and sport-specific nutrition planning. Information about and examples of nutrition analysis, the recording of dietary history, how to provide successful individual consultations, and how to develop interviewing skills is provided. An example consultation using an athlete case study near the end of the chapter can help the learner piece all of the communication concepts together.

How much do athletes know about sports nutrition?

Athletes who train, compete, and socialize together often obtain their nutrition information from each other. They also get nutrition information from coaches, trainers, and college courses. However, many athletes lack accurate and up-to-date knowledge of the nutrition practices that can enhance sport performance. Most athletes are aware of general nutrition concepts for overall health, but struggle with sport nutrition specifics.

A study conducted by Jonnalagadda et al.[1] on the dietary practices, nutrition education, and attitudes of freshman football players at an NCAA Division I school reported the following:

- Sixty-one percent of these athletes believed that protein is the main source of energy for working muscles.
- Seventy-one percent disagreed that sports drinks are better than water for replacing fluid losses.
- Sixty-five percent believed that vitamin and mineral supplements increased energy levels.

Another study of 330 athletes in various sports in Division I schools found that athletes had poor knowledge of the recommended percentage of total calories for the macronutrients.[2] Only 29% identified the correct carbohydrate intake, 11.8% the correct fat intake, and just 3% knew the correct protein intake. A more recent study of the dietary practices of NCAA Division I football players in-

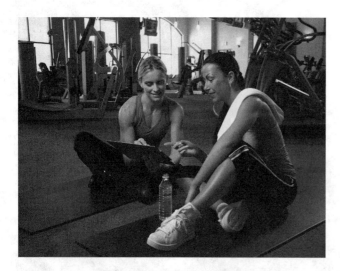

dicated that nutritional knowledge is still poor.[3] In regard to hydration, Nichols et al. reported that athletes had adequate general knowledge but lacked information on appropriate behaviors for consuming sports drinks.[4]

The study of 330 Division I athletes also surveyed athletes to determine whether and where athletes received sports nutrition information.[2] They found that 55% had received nutrition information or counseling in their college careers (60% of the women and 49.5% of the men). Most of the information was distributed by the strength and conditioning coaches (21.9%), athletic trainers (19.0%), or university classes (12.5%), and 10% of the education was provided by dietitians. Similarly, Burns et al. report that athletes in several different sports at eight NCAA Division I universities received their nutrition information primarily from athletic trainers (39.8%) and strength coaches (23.7%).[5] Coaches, athletic trainers, dietitians, and others working closely with athletes all should work together to provide accurate nutrition information to athletes.

A study of a Division I hockey team revealed that many hockey players obtain their information from their peers.[6] In this study, the freshman players observed the dietary intake of and comments from the older players on the team and subsequently modeled their eating style after these more experienced players. Fortunately, the older players in this study chose lower-fat, more nutrient-dense foods. Even though these older players did not have formal nutrition education, they passed healthful eating and nutrition information on to the younger players. This modeling behavior worked well in this instance because the older players made food choices that benefited their health and sport performance. However, if misinformation is passed along by more senior members of the team, the entire team could be making food choices that are not optimal for sport performance. Some form of traditional education about sports nutrition practices led by knowledgeable staff, followed with peer team support and well-respected role models, will help provide accurate information to sports teams and individual athletes.

Who provides nutrition assessment and education to athletes?

Athletes can benefit from nutrition education from a variety of sports professionals. Coaches have a significant influence on athletes and can affect their knowledge of nutrition and encourage healthy nutri-

tion behaviors. Athletic trainers often have the most contact with athletes, especially an athlete who is injured or needs regular taping, ice, or other daily treatments pre- and postpractice. Strength and conditioning coaches also have regular contact with athletes and work with them to improve sport performance with proper training regimens. Registered and licensed dietitians (RDs and LDs) can provide an in-depth assessment of an athlete's current nutrition status; calculate specific calorie, macronutrient, and micronutrient goals; aid in meal planning/cooking tips; generate proper hydration schedules; and address specific health-related nutrition questions/concerns, thus making RDs and LDs valuable resources for athletes. The involvement of an RD or LD is also essential to the athlete with medical complications such as diabetes, anemia, weight control issues, or an eating disorder.

All of these professionals can and should provide basic nutrition information to athletes; however, the extent to which information and recommendations are disseminated will vary based on each person's qualifications. Coaches, athletic trainers, and strength/conditioning coaches typically have a high credibility rating with athletes, making them valuable nutrition educators for players. However, most coaches, athletic trainers, and strength/conditioning coaches do not have a college degree in dietetics or nutrition certifications and therefore are qualified to educate athletes only on information that is considered "public domain." There is a plethora of public domain information available that is provided by government agencies and research organizations geared for sports professionals working on improving the nutrition status of athletes. Examples of public domain information include the following:

- MyPlate Food Guidance System—both print and online information
- Dietary Guidelines for Americans
- Information in position papers published by major nutrition and sport organizations such as the American College of Sports Medicine, National Athletic Trainers Association, and American Dietetic Association
- Nutrition information found in textbooks and scientific peer-reviewed journals
- Food and nutrition information found on product labels, Web sites, and printed brochures

The key for any individual working with athletes, regardless of licensure and registration, is to provide nutrition education to athletes using accurate, scientifically based information. Instances where individuals can cross legal and ethical boundaries are when nutrition assessment and subsequent nutrition therapy, particularly medical nutrition therapy, are provided without a license. Chapter 16 provides additional information about this topic.

However, some cases are best handled and required by law to be provided by licensed and registered dietitians. Licensure laws for dietitians exist in 35 states and Puerto Rico.[7] An additional 12 states have less strict certification laws. The number of states that have licensure laws will change as new legislation is passed at the state level. These laws provide legal definitions of what type of nutrition assessment and education can be conducted by non-licensed professionals and what cannot be provided unless the individual is licensed. Most licensure laws for dietitians are similar to other allied health professionals such as athletic trainers, physical therapists, pharmacists, and nurses. The purpose of licensure is to help the public find qualified and trained professionals who have completed minimum education requirements, maintain their education in a timely manner, and have passed an exam that verifies a high level of knowledge and proficiency in their profession. Licensure protects the public against fraudulent practices and also allows the state to have regulatory authority over these professions.

In states where licensure is mandated for dietitians, the term *dietitian* and/or *nutritionist* may be licensed. That means that only a registered dietitian who meets the qualifications set by the state to obtain a license can use the term *dietitian* or *nutritionist* in his or her title or practice. The states also legislate what types of assessments or education can be offered by licensed dietitians only. In most cases, licensed, registered dietitians are the only professionals allowed to provide nutrition assessments and medical nutrition therapy to individuals. This means that licensed and registered dietitians are the only professionals allowed to provide athletes with a full assessment of their dietary intake, medical nutrition needs, and individual recommendations based on those assessments. In cases when athletes need this type of assessment, licensed and registered dietitians should be consulted.

In this chapter, the majority of information related to nutrition consultations with athletes is provided as examples of a registered and/or licensed dietitian performing the assessment. Certainly many additional sports professionals will consult with athletes about their nutrition needs and provide some education regarding nutrition and sport performance.

The information in this chapter will be valuable for individuals interested in obtaining the registered dietitian credential as well as for other professionals working with athletes in primary roles that are not in the nutrition field but relate to the overall health and physical performance of athletes.

How does the consultation process with athletes begin?

Ideally, the athlete will document his or her personal health history and dietary intake information prior to the first nutrition education session. The information gathered should include basic demographics, including contact information, a health history questionnaire, a list of current medications and supplements, a food record, and a training or exercise log. If this information is collected and reviewed prior to the first visit, it can be evaluated more thoroughly, and specific suggestions could be generated during the first visit with the athlete. Each of these pieces of information adds value to the assessment and consultation process; collectively they provide sports nutrition professionals with the information needed to develop a sound nutrition plan for the athlete.

What is a diet history?

A **diet history** is the most comprehensive form of dietary intake data collection. It is an interview process that reviews recorded dietary intake, eating behaviors, recent and long-term habits of food consumption, and exercise patterns. A skilled and trained interviewer is needed to take the diet history. Most dietitians use a form of diet history interview in every individual assessment with a new client. This process is time-consuming but well worth the effort.

diet history The most comprehensive form of dietary intake data collection. It involves an interview process that reviews recorded dietary intake, eating behaviors, recent and long-term habits of food consumption, and exercise patterns. A skilled and trained interviewer is needed to take the diet history.

A direct interviewing process can help the dietitian take a diet history relatively quickly. In this process, a combination of open-ended and closed questions can pace the interview within the time allotted for the session. Using an initial health history questionnaire and any food records completed, a set of clarifying questions can be formulated prior to the first visit. If the questionnaire and food records are brought in on the day of the visit, the dietitian can quickly scan the information and ask questions in the order of the questionnaire and food record. The questions and format will vary for each athlete. Most sessions are time-limited and the information must be obtained as quickly and efficiently as possible to allow for education, meal planning, and goal setting.

Assessing dietary adequacy should include assessment not only of food intake data, but also biochemical and anthropometric parameters. Height, weight, body composition, and body mass index should be compared to appropriate standards. Laboratory assessments such as hemoglobin, albumin, electrolytes, and any clinical diagnoses should also be considered when making a complete dietary assessment. Clinical observations of the athlete's skin, hair, and nails can provide information necessary to make accurate assessments of usual dietary intake and adequacy. Dietary adequacy should be assessed and diet plans formulated based on the totality of the evidence, not on dietary intake data alone.[8] Information about and examples of tools used in the diet history are described in the following sections in this chapter.

What is a health history questionnaire?

health history questionnaire A survey that includes a variety of questions about current health, past medical history, and other daily health and wellness topics. The information collected in the health history questionnaire about chronic diseases, current or past injuries, surgeries, and regular medications help nutrition professionals make a thorough assessment of the athlete's needs and subsequently develop a sound nutritional program.

The **health history questionnaire** asks a variety of questions about current health, past medical history, and daily health and wellness topics. These may have implications for nutrition care and should be addressed as part of the sports nutrition consultation. It is often assumed that athletes are healthy and are not likely to have medical conditions. However, many high-level athletes and recreational athletes do have underlying medical issues that may affect nutrition status and thus dietary recommendations. Information about chronic diseases, current or past injuries, surgeries, and regular medications helps nutrition professionals make a thorough assessment of the athlete's needs and subsequently develop appropriate nutrition recommendations. A sample health and nutrition history questionnaire is shown in Figure 10.1.

In addition to information about current medical conditions, information about family history of major chronic illnesses should also be obtained. Nutrition professionals need to look at the athlete as a whole and make the best nutrition recommendations possible for the athlete's health and sport performance. This may include providing assessment and education on medical nutrition topics when the need arises. For example, a college athlete states on his health history that he has no chronic illnesses but has a paternal and maternal history of diabetes. Nutrition education for this athlete should focus on the athlete's goals for sport performance, as well as on information about diabetes prevention.

A listing of medications is also valuable information to obtain from athletes. Some medications may have drug–nutrient interactions. Others may need to be taken with food or on an empty stomach. This may affect the timing of meals and snacks, thus affecting pre- and postexercise food intake. Reviewing current medications can also provide the dietitian with insight about medical conditions that the athlete may have forgotten to disclose. For example, a diuretic on the athlete's medication list could suggest that he or she has hypertension or some other cardiac condition. Inquiring about the reasons for taking the diuretic and how often it is used will clarify the effects the medication may have on hydration status and medical nutrition management of the athlete. Athletic trainers and coaches working daily with athletes also need to be aware of medications in case of emergencies. These professionals play a pivotal role in helping athletes maintain their medication regimen and monitoring the effects of these medications on sport performance. In addition, athletic trainers, coaches, and the team physician should be aware of the list of banned substances for athletes that may be present in various medications.

Additional health and wellness information gathered in a health history questionnaire provides more information about the nutrient needs of the athlete. Routine questions about smoking habits and consumption of alcohol should be included on the health history questionnaire. Athletes are less likely to smoke, but if they do, smoking may increase the need for some nutrients such as vitamin C. Alcohol consumption can add extra calories with little nutrient value and may play a role in the discussion about meeting the athlete's goals. Information about current exercise can be requested on a health history questionnaire or within a more detailed exercise log.

Many athletes seek the assistance of a dietitian because they want to change their weight or body composition. Some may desire weight gain, whereas others desire weight loss. Others may just want to

Health and Nutrition History Questionnaire

The following information is confidential and will not be disclosed to anyone outside of this organization.

Name:_____ Date:_____ Home Phone #:_____

Address:_____ Alt. Phone #:_____

Email address:_____

Birth Date:_____ Height:_____ Weight:_____

Medical History

Indicate if you currently have or ever had any of the following:

Condition			Explanation:_____
Asthma	❏ yes	❏ no	_____
Anemia	❏ yes	❏ no	_____
Cancer	❏ yes	❏ no	_____
Diabetes	❏ yes	❏ no	_____
High blood pressure	❏ yes	❏ no	_____
High cholesterol	❏ yes	❏ no	_____
Heart disease	❏ yes	❏ no	_____
Heart attack	❏ yes	❏ no	_____
Heart surgery	❏ yes	❏ no	_____
Kidney disease	❏ yes	❏ no	_____
Osteoporosis	❏ yes	❏ no	_____
Stomach/GI disorder	❏ yes	❏ no	_____
Stress fracture	❏ yes	❏ no	_____
Other_____	❏ yes	❏ no	_____

Do you have a family history of any of the above? ❏ Y ❏ N   If yes, please explain:

_____

_____

Please list any medications you are currently taking and the reason for taking them:

_____

_____

Do you take vitamin or mineral supplements? ❏ Y ❏ N   If so, list the type and amounts: _____

_____

Do you take any supplements to try to boost athletic performance or increase energy (e.g., protein supplements, ginseng, green tea, chromium picolinate)? ❏ Y ❏ N   If so, list the type and amounts: _____

_____

Do you smoke? ❏ Y ❏ N   If so, how much?_____

Are you currently engaging in an exercise program? ❏ yes ❏ no   If so, please list:

Type of Exercise: Frequency: (times/week)_____ Length of Session: (minutes/hours)_____ Intensity: (light, mod, hard)_____

Do you consider yourself overweight? ❏ yes ❏ no   Would you like to lose weight? ❏ yes ❏ no

Have you ever been on a diet for weight loss? ❏ yes ❏ no   If so, please explain:
(i.e., when did you diet/join weight loss program, type of program, how much weight lost/regained)

_____

_____

Have you ever purposefully restricted food intake and obtained what you or others felt was an extremely low or unhealthy weight? ❏ Y ❏ N
If yes, please explain:

_____

_____

Have you ever thrown up, used laxatives, fasted or exercised for extremely long periods to try to lose weight? ❏ Y ❏ N   If yes, please explain:

_____

Please circle the typical meals and snacks that you consume on an average day:

Breakfast   Snack   Lunch   Snack   Dinner   Snack   Other

Figure 10.1   Sample health and nutrition history questionnaire. Taking a health and nutrition history in the first meeting with athletes helps the dietitian determine any health concerns that should be addressed when developing the nutrition plan.
Adapted from the National Institute for Fitness and Sport, www.nifs.org.

alter their body fat percentage without a change in weight. Therefore, obtaining information on their current height, weight, and body composition; how the athlete feels about their current weight; and whether or not the desired weight loss is appropriate. If an athlete states he considers himself overweight, but the anthropometric measurements suggest otherwise, the dietitian knows to proceed with caution. Athletes that are overly concerned about their weight may be at risk for developing eating disorders, or eating behaviors that inhibit optimal sport performance. Information about past and current dieting and weight loss practices also can be useful in the initial consultation session.

Why is an inquiry about supplement use important?

Many athletes use one or more dietary supplements on a regular basis. There are two main issues to explore regarding an athlete's use of supplements. First, a listing of all supplements currently being used helps determine safety and efficacy for the athlete. As discussed in Chapter 9, some supplements may not be safe for regular consumption, may not be proven effective, or could be banned by several sports organizations. Sports nutrition professionals need to know which supplements might fall into these categories and share that information with the athletes. The second question about supplements is to determine why the athlete is taking each of the supplements. This can provide clues about the goals of the athlete and his or her drive to achieve these goals. If the athlete is taking three different weight-gainer and protein supplements several times each day, this is a significant clue that the athlete has a strong desire to build muscle mass. In addition, there may be myths about certain supplements that need to be addressed with individual athletes. Taking a thorough history of past and present supplement use will help guide the discussion and education necessary to help the athlete remain safe when consuming supplements.

Many athletes take a multivitamin and mineral supplement, or single vitamins or minerals. Specifically asking about vitamin and mineral supplement use may be necessary because many athletes and the general population often do not recognize vitamins and minerals as supplements. Although taking a multivitamin/mineral supplement in most cases is appropriate and for some athletes beneficial, taking mega-doses of single vitamins or minerals may not be safe. Follow-up questions to clarify the daily doses of vitamins and minerals along with a review of food records will help determine whether these supplements are necessary and safe, and whether doses can be decreased or should be discontinued.

What type of food intake information should be obtained from the athlete?

Any type of direct food recording provides valuable information for the initial consultation. Reviewing the types and amounts of food usually consumed, when and where meals are consumed, and how they are prepared provides a wealth of information to begin the evaluation of current intake. This information will be used to formulate a nutrition plan for the athlete. There is a variety of methods for collecting food intake data. The most common is direct recording of food intake using a **food record**. The athlete is asked to keep a 1-, 3-, or 7-day food record of all foods and beverages consumed in the designated time period. Documentation of intake throughout the day should be recorded as soon as possible after consumption to obtain the most accurate information. The recall method requires the athlete to remember all foods and beverages consumed in a distinct period of time, usually within the past day. This **24-hour dietary recall** can be obtained in the first session if food records are not available. Another tool is a **food frequency questionnaire** that asks the athlete to record how often common foods are eaten on a daily, weekly, monthly, or even yearly basis. All of these tools can be helpful to the dietitian and may be used separately or collectively to obtain substantial information about the athlete's food intake. Each of these methods has advantages and disadvantages.[9,10] The three methods are described in more detail in the following sections.

> **food record** The most common method for collecting food intake data. It requires the direct recording of all food and beverage intake over a 1-, 3-, or 7-day period. Documentation of intake should occur at the time of consumption or as soon as possible afterward to obtain the most accurate information.
>
> **24-hour dietary recall** A method of collecting food intake information that requires the athlete to remember all foods and beverages consumed within the past day (i.e., 24 hours). Although not the most accurate way of collecting food intake information, it can provide an idea of an athlete's nutritional intake in the first consultation session if other types of food records are not available.
>
> **food frequency questionnaire** A nutritional analysis survey tool that asks an athlete or client to record how often common foods are eaten on a daily, weekly, monthly, or even yearly basis.

How are food records used in nutrition consultation?

The first step for nutritional assessment of the athlete is to gather accurate information about food intake. The nutrition plan developed later in the consultation will be based partly on this initial information. The goal of any food recording is to gain specific information about foods consumed by the athlete. A food record kept prior to the first visit decreases the reliance on memory to determine recent food intake.

The number of days an athlete should keep a food record depends on several variables. Many athletes will not take the time or see the need for recording food intake. A 1-day food record gives a snapshot view of only 1 day of eating patterns. The athlete is asked to write down foods eaten in a "typical" day. The athlete has to determine which day is typical. This could be a weekday when practices are intense, a school day, or a weekend day. Although this 1-day record provides some dietary intake information, additional recorded days will provide better information about usual dietary intake.

A 3-day food record provides more information about foods eaten and consumption pattern differences throughout a week than a 1-day record, but is not as time-intensive as a 7-day log. A 3-day food record is most useful when two weekdays and one weekend day are recorded. Often individuals eat differently on weekdays than on the weekends. Training schedules, access to meals, and time for meal preparation may vary on different days of the week. In general, a 3-day food record will provide an estimate of nutrient intake that can be used to develop a nutrition plan. This may not be an accurate reflection of long-term nutrient intake, but it does provide a reliable assessment of short-term patterns that are valuable for conducting an intake evaluation and subsequent meal plans.

A sample completed food record is shown in Figure 10.2 . To help cue the athlete to record a thorough and accurate food log, sections for the date, time of meals/snacks, amount and type of food consumed, feelings or emotions about food, and location should be included on the recording form. Instructions on how to complete the food record should be included for the athlete, such as a sample 1-day record with examples of the amount of detail requested when recording dietary intake. Instructions on determining the amount of each food eaten, specific brands chosen, restaurant names if dining out, and where the food was eaten are necessary for cueing the athlete. If possible, the dietitian should review the recording process on the phone, or have the information available in detail on a Web page that the athlete can access. This will help ensure the most accurate food recording prior to the first session.

Obtaining a complete and accurate food record from an athlete can be a challenge. Athletes who are not accustomed to keeping a food journal may forget to record every food eaten each day. Even the most conscientious athletes may forget to write down a snack or beverage consumed. The accuracy of the food record is questionable in many cases. Several studies have documented a high incidence of underreporting of food intake.[11,12] A number of studies also have reported variations in nutrient intake based on the day of the week[13,14] or appetite fluctuations, especially related to physical activity or menstrual cycle changes.[15,16]

Many factors affect day-to-day variations in dietary intake.[9] Some athletes will eat the same thing for breakfast and lunch every day of the week, and only have variety with the evening meal and snacks. Other athletes have wide variations in meal intake daily. The day of the week is almost certain to affect intake based on individual training and competition schedules. Food intake during the competitive season versus the off-season may influence dietary differences. The season of the year could also have an effect. Less food may be consumed in hot, humid months and more during cold winter months. Athletes may have changes in appetite based on their training schedule. During intense training, athletes may not eat as much as in less intense training times. Therefore, a food record ideally covers at least 3 days, combining weekdays and weekends, as well as capturing heavy and light training days.

How is a 24-hour dietary recall used in a nutrition consultation?

Even when documented food records are obtained from the athlete, a 24-hour dietary recall can be a valuable tool. The purpose of the dietary recall is to get a complete and detailed picture of what the athlete consumed over the last 24 hours. In many cases, asking the athlete for a recall of a "typical" day of food intake will also provide information to help with the evaluation of an athlete's usual intake. The athlete can document all foods eaten in the past 24 hours on a blank 1-day food record. This organizes the information, making review and evaluation easy. The dietitian can then prompt the athlete by asking

gaining the performance edge

Completing food records provides substantial information for the assessment of the athlete's dietary intake. A 3-day food record is recommended when assessing dietary intake. It provides enough information to learn about typical intake patterns without being time-intensive for busy athletes.

Please complete the three days of food intake using the attached blank forms. The three-day food record is designed to give an accurate description of your typical diet. Record two weekdays and one weekend day. Please eat your typical diet on the days you record. Because the information will be used to plan appropriate dietary changes, it is important that you not change your usual eating pattern. Be as accurate as possible, recording all foods, beverages, and snacks consumed. Provide as much detail as possible on the record including the brand name of foods, restaurants, food preparation method, portion size, and type of food such as fat-free, sugar substitute, high-protein, reduced calorie. Record any comments about where you ate or how you felt when you ate in the location/feelings section. A sample of a one-day food record is listed below to help you complete your three days.

| 1 cup fluid = 8 oz | 1 pint = 16 oz = 2 cups | 3 oz meat = size of deck of cards |
| 3 tsp = 1 tbsp | 4 tbsp = ¼ cup | 1 oz cheese = size of three dice |

Date:_____

Time	Food/Beverage	Amount	Location/Feelings
5:30 AM	Granola bar	1 bar	Hurrying to practice
	Gatorade	1 24-oz bottle	
8:30 AM	Cereal (corn flakes)	2 cups	Home
	Milk, 1%	2 cups	
	Cranberry juice cocktail	1 cup	
	Toast, whole grain	2 slices	
	Peanut butter	2 tbsp	
	Jam	2 tbsp	
1:00 PM	Wrap Sandwich: chicken, cheese,	1 large	Panera Bread Co.
	vegetables, lite ranch dressing, wheat wrap	4 oz chicken	Large pita, lettuce, tomato, sprouts
		2 slices cheese	
		3 tbsp dressing	
	Lemonade	24 oz	
	Side salad, mostly romaine lettuce	1 cup	
	Lite vinaigrette salad dressing	1 tbsp	
6:00 PM	Hamburger patty, 93% lean	4 oz	Home, hungry after practice
	Ketchup, mustard, pickle relish	1 tbsp each	
	Wheat bun	1 large	
	Baby carrots, steamed	1.5 cups	
	Potato chips	~20 chips	
	Water	12 oz	
9:00 PM	Milk, 1%	1 cup	Stressed about doing homework
	Peanut butter cookies	2 large, homemade	

Figure 10.2 Sample 1-day food record. Completing a 1-, 3-, or 7-day food record provides information on specific foods athletes eat each day.

questions about specific types of foods or beverages consumed, condiments on food, and clarification of portion sizes. Using food models can visually aid individuals in correctly estimating the portion size of foods/beverages consumed. Clarifying questions such as "Did you have anything to drink with that meal?" or "Did you put anything on your sandwich in addition to the turkey and cheese?" prompt the athlete to be more specific about all foods consumed. A 24-hour recall is not going to provide a truly accurate picture of what an athlete eats on a regular basis, but it does provide information about general eating habits.

How is a food frequency questionnaire used in a nutrition consultation?

Food frequency questionnaires (FFQs) look at intake over a longer period of time than food records and dietary recalls. The FFQ puts foods into broad categories and asks the client to record intake over time. For example, a FFQ may ask, "How often do you consume dairy products?" The responses may be daily, weekly, or monthly, and the athlete is asked to write in the number of servings typically consumed in those three time periods. A sample portion of a food frequency questionnaire is shown in Figure 10.3 . Many FFQs have been developed to as-

Food Frequency Questionnaire

Instructions:
1. Answer each question as best as you can.
2. Use a no. 2 pencil and put an X in the box that corresponds with your answer.
3. Follow instructions for each question.

1. In the last 12 months, how often did you eat cold cereal?
   - ❏ Never (Go to question 4)
   - ❏ 1 time per month
   - ❏ 2–3 times per month
   - ❏ 1 time per week
   - ❏ 2–3 times per week
   - ❏ 1 time per day
   - ❏ 2 or more times per day

2. When you ate cereal, what type of cereal did you choose most often?
   - ❏ Oatmeal
   - ❏ Whole grain
   - ❏ Whole grain with dried fruit
   - ❏ Granola-type cereal
   - ❏ Sugar sweetened

3. When you eat cereal, what is the typical serving size you consume in one sitting?
   - ❏ Less than ½ cup
   - ❏ ½ cup
   - ❏ ¾ cup
   - ❏ 1 cup
   - ❏ 1–1½ cups
   - ❏ More than 1½ cups

4. In the last 12 months, how often did you drink 100% fruit juice?
   - ❏ Never
   - ❏ 1 time per month
   - ❏ 2–3 times per month
   - ❏ 1 time per week
   - ❏ 2–3 times per week
   - ❏ 1 time per day
   - ❏ 2 or more times per day

Figure 10.3 Sample food frequency questionnaire. A food frequency questionnaire captures long-term dietary patterns of intake.

sess a specific population's intake of a certain type of food or designed by organizations for research purposes, such as the National Cancer Institute Diet History Questionnaire.[17] Other FFQs provide a more general view of dietary intake and are best for the information needed to assess athletes' usual intake over time. When selecting a food frequency questionnaire, consider an instrument that is already validated, provides information on either a group or an individual's needs, and is appropriate for the population being assessed.[18] Food frequency questionnaires provide information about long-term dietary patterns, which is an advantage as compared to food record data. However, assessing FFQs is time-consuming, the FFQs can be costly to administer and evaluate, and they may not provide information specific to the athletic population. If the athlete has time to complete food records and an FFQ, and the dietitian has time to evaluate both tools, using them in combination is valuable. With less available time, food record data is more beneficial in assessing an athlete's dietary intake.

How is an exercise/training log used in a nutrition consultation?

Documentation of how much exercise is completed daily and weekly is essential to any sports dietitian's assessment and nutritional plan.[19] The training log is a valuable tool in determining energy expenditure and thus energy needs. It also provides information on the time spent training and competing that may influence food preparation and consumption patterns. Information about the type, duration, and intensity of training provides an even more accurate picture of caloric expenditure.

A sample exercise log is shown in Figure 10.4 . As with food records, a specific form requesting information regarding daily/weekly exercise and a sample of how the log should be completed will help athletes complete the record in the detail desired. Detailed energy expenditure logs that record all activity within a 24-hour period are available; however, these are extremely cumbersome to complete with accuracy and are very time-consuming. An exercise log that reveals actual duration, intensity, and type of exercise provides adequate information for developing a nutrition plan that includes nutrition needs for energy expenditure.

Which clinical assessments should be conducted in the initial consultation session?

Access to laboratory data and other medical documen-

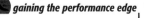
gaining the performance edge

The initial information gathering for the first session can be extensive or minimal. The amount of time available prior to the first visit and the athlete's interest in and ability to keep food records and to complete an exercise log will all be factors the dietitian will consider when asking the athlete to complete information before the first visit.

Exercise Log

Complete the exercise log for each day of the week. Please write down the type of Activities (A), Duration (D) in minutes, and the Intensity level (I) of the exercise. For example: Running, 75 minutes, at 80% of race pace or Weight training, 45 minutes, light day.

Week		Sunday	Monday	Tuesday	Wednesday	Thursday	Friday	Saturday
1	A							
	D							
	I							
2	A							
	D							
	I							
3	A							
	D							
	I							
4	A							
	D							
	I							

Comments/Goals:

Figure 10.4 Sample exercise log. Keeping track of the time, amount, and intensity level of exercise helps determine energy expenditure.

tation is extremely helpful when consulting with athletes who present with various medical conditions. Nutrition consultations requiring the interpretations of laboratory assessments are regarded as medical nutrition therapy and should be completed by registered and licensed dietitians. Laboratory assessment can help to determine an athlete's nutrition status, which will affect the development of a nutrition plan. For example, female athletes, especially long-distance runners, have a tendency to develop iron deficiency during their training and competitive careers. Athletes' laboratory reports of total iron, hemoglobin, serum ferritin, and hematocrit levels can help the dietitian evaluate iron status and thus provide education on ways to improve dietary iron intake if needed. Common laboratory reports often requested by dietitians include electrolyte levels, albumin, pre-albumin, total protein, and potentially any clinical laboratory report related to a current disease condition. Dietitians will need detailed glu-

cose monitoring values for athletes with diabetes and lipid levels for athletes with known heart disease or dyslipidemias.

Other health/sports professionals may use laboratory or diagnostic data to evaluate and educate athletes regarding nutrition status. For example, athletic trainers may request radiology reports for athletes with potential stress fractures and MRI reports for any soft or hard tissue injuries. When stress fractures are determined, the athletic trainer and physician may discuss medical as well as nutritional treatment to help the athlete heal. This is an opportunity to talk with the athlete about regular calcium and vitamin D intake, and decide whether supplementation would be a helpful adjunct to treatment. The dietitian, physician, and athletic trainers or physical therapists work together as a team to develop the best nutrition and health care plan for the athlete based in part on the clinical medical information available.

How are food records analyzed?

Once the data are collected from the athlete, clarification of the food record will help ensure that the most accurate information is obtained for analysis. In the initial consultation, clarifying questions can be asked to help learn more about actual food intake. Often the food consumption information is incomplete. The most frequently *omitted* items on a food record include:

- Actual portion sizes
- Condiments used
- Restaurant or name brand of item
- Method of food preparation
- Beverages consumed with meals or snacks
- Snacks between meals

A sample food record with clarifying questions is shown in (Figure 10.5). Clarification questions such as those listed in Figure 10.5 help jog the athlete's memory without making judgments about the foods eaten, or trying to lead the athlete to add or omit foods during the discussion. The question "What else did you eat at lunch on Wednesday?" might sound judgmental to the athlete. The athlete may feel that the dietitian does not believe the information provided on Wednesday's food record. Asking, "Did you have any juice with breakfast?" could lead the athlete to say yes if he or she feels that is the answer the dietitian wants to hear. Asking the question "Did you have something to drink with breakfast?" helps clarify the meal without suggesting a particular beverage or making any judgments about the intake.

Information from the food record is most often entered into a nutrient analysis computer program. Many software databases are available to calculate the content of the diet to estimate macronutrient and micronutrient values. Books of nutrient composition tables are also available to research a specific food item that may not be available in nutrient databases. Some nutrient analysis products are available on the Internet and offer free access to any user. All of these programs perform the mathematical calcula-

Food Record and Clarifying Questions

Food	Amount	Location/Comments	Clarifying Question
Breakfast:			
Juice	1 cup		What type of juice did you have?
Eggs	2	Fried	
Toast	2 slices	Whole grain	Did you put anything on your toast?
Grapes	1 big bunch		How much is a "big bunch" of grapes?
Lunch:		At Wendy's	
Chicken sandwich	1 whole		How was the chicken cooked—grilled, baked or fried?
Frosty	Small size		
Side salad	1 small	Just vegetables, no meat or cheese	Did you put any dressing on the salad? Were there croutons on the salad?
Snack:			
Granola bar	1 bar	Nature Valley	Did you have one bar out of the two-pack portion, or did you eat both bars? Did you have anything to drink with the granola bar?
Dinner:		At home	
Frozen vegetable Lasagna	1 single serving		Could you estimate the size of the container of lasagna?
Milk	2 glasses		What size glass of milk? What type of milk did you drink?
Ice cream	1 bowl	Chocolate	How big was the bowl? Was it ice cream, frozen yogurt, etc?
			Did you eat or drink anything after your evening meal?

Figure 10.5 Sample food record and clarifying questions. Food recording provides valuable information when developing nutrition plans for athletes. The accuracy of the recording process can be improved by providing a sample record and asking clarifying questions about the foods eaten during the consultation.

tions and comparisons to the food database, saving significant time.

Table 10.1 provides a list of software, Web sites, and books that provide nutrient analysis information. Most computerized nutrient analysis packages come with a standard nutrient database loaded on the software's CD-ROM or DVD. Occasionally, the purchaser has the option of selecting which database to include in the software package. The database is used to compare the food data input from the dietary records to estimate nutrient intake. The most common database used in software packages is the U.S. Department of Agriculture (USDA) Database for Standard Reference. This database is appropriate for the analysis of diets of people in the United States and reflects typical foods consumed. It is regularly updated with new foods and uses the most current Dietary Reference Intake (DRI) tables. The database used is important when selecting software or Web sites to assess the nutrient content of food record data. The database should be updated regularly, and updates should be included in any software package contract. The nutrient information is only as good as the database used to calculate the nutrient composition. The U.S. food supply is highly fortified and also contains highly processed foods. This may be very different in other countries. So, using an appropriate database matched for the athlete's typical intake will provide a more accurate reflection of nutrient intake.

New food products enter the food market daily, and no one database can keep up with the changing food market. Sports nutrition products are increasing in popularity and new sports drinks, bars, supplements, and foods are marketed regularly to athletes. Many of these items are not in standard databases. These foods could make up a substantial portion of an athlete's intake and need to be accounted for in the nutrient analysis. Many software and Web analysis databases allow the user to add new foods to their own nutrient analysis database. Information from the food label can be added to the database for each new item. Not all micronutrients are required to be listed on the supplement label, so many of them will not be available for the data analysis. There will, however, be calorie, macronutrient, cholesterol, and fiber information on the label

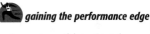

gaining the performance edge

Assessing athletes' intake using computer analysis provides detailed information about the various nutrients consumed in the diet. Athletes tend to consume sports foods and beverages that typically are not included in standard nutrient databases. Software purchased to analyze the diets of athletes should include the option of adding these foods to the database to produce an accurate dietary analysis for all foods and beverages consumed.

TABLE 10.1	Resources for Dietary Analysis	
Resource	**Contact Information**	**Comments**
Nutrition analysis tool	nat.illinois.edu/mainnat.html	Web-based analysis tool, free to all Internet users. Will save personal data and allows users to add more days; includes an energy calculator.
USDA Database for Standard	www.ars.usda.gov/main/site_main.htm?modecode=12-35-45-00	Large database of foods consumed in the United States; Reference updated regularly; often the database used for computerized nutrient analysis software
Nutritionist Pro	1-800-709-2799 www.nutritionistpro.com	Accurate, up-to-date food and nutrient data for complete analysis on over 35,000 foods and ingredients, including brand-name, fast foods, ethnic foods, and enteral products.
Fit Day	www.fitday.com	Web-based analysis tool, free to all Internet users but requires setting up a free user account.
NutriBase	www.dietsoftware.com	Commercially available nutrition analysis program for professional or personal use
MyPlate	www.choosemyplate.gov	Web-based analysis tool, free to all Internet users.
Bowes and Church's Food Values of Portions Commonly Used. 19th ed.	Lippincott Williams and Wilkins Publishers www.lww.com	Well-organized book of many common foods listed in standard portion sizes. Includes brand names and some restaurant items. Gives macro- and micronutrient values. Excellent for determining nutrient content of a specific food.

of sports-related or other foods that are not in the database. When working with athletes, nutrition professionals should be prepared to add new foods to the nutrient analysis database to provide the most accurate nutrient analysis.

How do you compare dietary intake to nutrition recommendations?

There are many ways that an athlete's diet can be compared to national standards to help determine nutritional adequacy. Three common ways are to compare intake to the DRIs, to the MyPlate food guidance system, or to the Dietary Guidelines for Americans. In addition, published data on nutrition intake specific to athletes can be used to compare the intake of similar athletes. There are advantages and disadvantages to all of these methods of assessment, and several can be used in conjunction to provide the best assessment of dietary intake.

How can the DRIs be used to assess athletes' nutritional adequacy?

Most frequently, the dietary information obtained from the dietary assessment is compared to the DRI standards. The DRIs include Recommended Dietary Allowance (RDA), Adequate Intake (AI), Estimated Average Requirement (EAR), and Tolerable Upper Intake Level (UL), as previously described in this text. Most computerized dietary analysis software uses the RDA or AI data for comparing intake to dietary standards. If the RDA or AI of the athlete's intake is met, the dietitian can determine with confidence that the athlete is consuming adequate amounts of the nutrient. When a UL is available, the dietitian should compare that number to each nutrient and determine whether too much of any nutrient is being consumed. Using the appropriate DRI values that are available for each nutrient and comparing these to the established RDA or AI are essential to any accurate dietary intake assessment.

How can the MyPlate food guidance system be used to assess athletes' nutritional adequacy?

A quick and easy way to assess overall adequacy of dietary records is to use the MyPlate food guidance system. This can be an excellent, easy guide to help the dietitian and athlete compare the number of servings from each food group consumed to the number recommended. If an athlete is consuming the minimum number of servings in all of the food groups on the plate, there is relatively good assurance that the dietary intake will meet minimum recommendations for most nutrients. This does not ensure that

an athlete will obtain adequate calories, but may help determine generally healthful food intake with adequate micronutrients. The MyPlate system is an excellent tool for any professional trying to quickly assess an athlete's dietary intake. However, it is not the best tool for a detailed analysis of current dietary intake.

Table 10.2 provides a sample comparison of an athlete's 1-day food intake to the recommended servings from MyPlate. In the example, the athlete's intake meets or exceeds the minimum number of daily servings for all MyPlate categories, based on a 2200 calorie per day meal plan. Although meeting the minimum number of servings will provide adequate vitamins and minerals, it may not be enough total calories to meet the athlete's energy requirements. Additional assessment of energy intake is discussed later in this section.

Can the Dietary Guidelines for Americans be used to assess athletes' nutritional adequacy?

The Dietary Guidelines for Americans are a set of general goals for food intake and dietary comparison developed by the USDA and the Department of Health and Human Services (HHS). They are intended to help educate Americans about healthful food consumption patterns to reduce the development of chronic diseases such as hypertension, diabetes, cardiovascular disease, obesity, and alcoholism. These are very general guidelines for the average American and are tools that all individuals can use to decipher how their diets match up to healthy guidelines. However, athletes expend more energy and may need or tolerate higher levels of some of the nutrients than the guidelines suggest as an average intake for Americans. This public domain information is valuable for anyone working with athletes on a nutrition plan for general health. For a review of the Dietary Guidelines for Americans, refer to Chapter 1 of this book. Although useful, comparing athletes' intakes to the Dietary Guidelines alone is the least useful method for helping to determine the best nutrition plan for individual athletes.

How is energy intake assessed?

Energy intake can be determined by using food record analysis data. The total calories consumed for each day or series of days is listed on the food record analysis report. This information can then be compared to the athlete's estimated energy needs. In most cases, estimating athletes' energy needs is done using one of several prediction equations (see Chapter 11 for example equations and calculations). One

1-Day Food Intake	MyPlate Categories					
	Grains	Fruit	Vegetables	Protein Foods	Dairy/ Alternative	Oils/Empty Calories
Puffed oat cereal, 2 cups	1.5 oz					
Milk, skim, 1 cup					1 cup	
Raisins, ½ cup		1 cup				
Eggs, poached, 2				2 oz		
Apple juice, 12 oz		1½ cups				
Cereal bar	1 oz					
Pita bread sandwich:						
Whole grain pita, 1 whole	2.5 oz					
Roast beef, 3 oz				3 oz		
Tomato, lettuce, cucumber, green pepper			½ cup			
Potato chips, 1 oz						2 tsp oils
Iced tea, 16 oz, unsweetened						
Vegetable juice, 12 oz			1½ cups			
Fruit and yogurt smoothie, small		1 cup			1 cup	
Cashews and almonds, ⅓ cup				1 oz		
Veggie burger, 1			2 oz			
Bun, 1	2 oz					
Steamed broccoli and carrots, 1 cup			1 cup			
Milk shake, chocolate, 12 oz					1½ cups	2 tsp oils, plus discretionary sugar calories
Daily Total:	**7 oz**	**3.5 cups**	**3 cups**	**6 oz**	**3.5 cups**	**4 tsp oils + some sugars**

of the equations is listed in **Table 10.3**, where resting energy expenditure (REE) indicates the basic energy needs of the body, and this number is multiplied by an activity factor that reflects the energetic demands of the sport and/or level of training. The dietitian can calculate energy needs for individual athletes by using the athlete's body weight and gender and age category and selecting an appropriate activity factor. Activity factors are on the low end for athletes training for less time and at lower intensity levels, and are on the high end if they are highly competitive, training hard for many hours each day.

The dietitian should then compare the estimated energy expenditure to the dietary intake. In some cases, dietary intake may be below recommended energy needs based on the energy expenditure calculations. If this is the case, the athlete and dietitian can discuss ways to increase calorie intake. When energy intake is higher than calculated energy expenditure, additional discussion about weight changes may be helpful. If the athlete has not lost or gained weight recently and his or her diet has been consistent over time, then the dietary energy intake is probably meeting energy demands. The goals of the athlete must be considered when determining the appropriateness of energy intake versus energy expenditure. If the athlete desires weight loss, then a calorie deficit is appropriate. When the athlete wants to gain weight, then additional calorie consumption above calculated energy needs should be encouraged. (Figure 10.6) provides an example of a dietary analysis report of an athlete's 1-day food record. Note that the calories, macronutrients, and micronutrients are displayed in absolute numbers (e.g., grams, milligrams) as well as a percentage of the established dietary recommendations.

TABLE 10.3	Resting Energy Expenditure (REE) Calculations and Activity Factors		
Gender and Age (years)	Equation (BW in kilograms)		Activity Factor
Males, 10–18 years	REE = (17.5 × BW) + 651		1.6–2.4
Males, 18–30 years	REE = (15.3 × BW) + 679		1.6–2.4
Males, 30–60 years	REE = (11.6 × BW) + 879		1.6–2.4
Females, 10–18 years	REE = (12.2 × BW) + 749		1.6–2.4
Females, 18–30 years	REE = (14.7 × BW) + 496		1.6–2.4
Females, 30–60 years	REE = (8.7 × BW) + 829		1.6–2.4

BW, body weight.

Source: World Health Organization. Energy and Protein Requirements, Report of a Joint FAO/WHO/UNU Expert Consultation. Technical Report Series 724. Geneva, Switzerland: World Health Organization; 1985:206.

Dietary Analysis Printout

Nutrient	Total	Recommendation (Rec.)	% Rec
Calories	2278.51	2200*	103.57
Pro (g)	73.76	48	153.67
Fat (g)	68.12	73.33	92.9
Carb (g)	353.24		—
Fiber (g)	22.31	30	74.37
Cal (mg)	698.43	1000	69.84
Iron (mg)	31.37	10	313.7
Na (mg)	4363.33	2400	181.81
Pot (mg)	2887.23		—
Phos (mg)	1171.30	700	167.33
Ash (g)	15.34	330	4.65
vitA (IU)	7991.13	4000	199.78
vitC (mg)	216.32	75	288.43
Thia (mg)	2.79	1.1	253.64
Ribo (mg)	2.36	1.1	214.55
Nia (mg)	35.14	14	251
Sat Fat (g)	13.47	24.44	55.11
Mono Fat (g)	21.21	24.44	86.78
Poly Fat (g)	10.47	24.44	42.84
Chol (mg)	66.62	300	22.21

Analysis completed using the Nutrition Analysis Tool; http://nat.crgq.com/[20]

*Note: The 2200 calorie recommendation is based on the computer analysis tool used in this example and is not necessarily appropriate for calorie comparison for athletes. Using dietary analysis software helps nutrition professionals assess dietary intake, but additional assessments of nutrition adequacy for specific athletes must be made. Carbohydrate recommendations are not listed because the reference amount is difficult to determine for whole populations.

Figure 10.6   Dietary analysis report. Many computer programs are available that provide detailed dietary analyses of food records.

If calorie intake needs to be altered, the absolute value and/or the relative contribution of the macronutrients as compared to total calories may require adjustment. Carbohydrate intake should be assessed first because it is the macronutrient that should be consumed in the highest percentage of calories for the athlete's diet.[20] Whether working with a team sport, strength, or endurance training athlete, carbohydrates are going to be used as fuel during exercise. The recommended range of intake of carbohydrates for athletes is 5–10 g/kg body weight. The lower end of the range is adequate for athletes performing mainly strength-training exercises and short duration competition, the high end of the range is for endurance athletes, and the middle range is appropriate for team sport athletes. Information from the analysis of the grams of carbohydrate intake should be compared with the calculated needs and adjusted to meet the athlete's requirements.

Protein intake is assessed after carbohydrate intake and needs are established. Protein intake should be compared to overall calorie intake as well as to fat and carbohydrate intake to provide a well-rounded picture of the athlete's diet. The recommended range of protein intake for athletes is 1.2–2.0 g/kg body weight. The low to middle end of the range is adequate for the endurance and many team sport athletes. The middle to higher end of the range is appropriate for strength and power athletes who engage primarily in anaerobic exercise. Comparing protein intake from dietary assessment data to the protein range appropriate for athletes will help the dietitian determine the optimal protein needs for the individual athlete and adjust the dietary intake recommendations accordingly.

Fat is the last macronutrient to be compared to overall calorie intake and to have its levels assessed. Once the carbohydrate and protein needs are established, the rest of the calories should be derived from fat intake. A minimum of 20% of calories should come from fat in the athlete's diet, especially for athletes performing long-duration, low to moderate intensity workouts.[21,22] A range of 20–35% of calories consumed as fat is safe and adequate for most athletes. This range allows for plenty of flexibility in

gaining the performance edge

Comparing an athlete's dietary intake to estimated calorie and macronutrient requirements as well as to established RDAs or AIs provides information on the adequacy of his or her daily diet. Using this information in combination with other dietary assessment methods can help the dietitian accurately assess dietary intake and the athlete's needs.

fat intake based on the other macronutrient needs for each athlete.

How is vitamin and mineral intake assessed?

Most computer programs compare the vitamin and mineral intake to the RDA/ AI values. This provides information on how an athlete's vitamin and mineral intake compares to the recommendations for the general population. The RDA and AI are designed to prevent nutrient deficiencies for men and women in various age categories and are not targeted specifically for physical activity needs. For example, the calcium recommendation for a 30-year-old female athlete is 1000 mg and for a 15-year-old female is 1300 mg, regardless of activity level. Similarly, a female athlete in childbearing years may have higher iron needs than a male athlete or a female athlete who is postmenopausal.

There are no specifically designed standards for vitamin and mineral intakes of athletes. When assessing an athlete's vitamin and mineral intake, use the correct gender and age categories. There are research studies, many listed throughout this book, that have assessed both intake and nutrient needs of athletes. Some comparison to these studies may be appropriate. However, comparisons to these studies should be made only when the athlete is in the same gender and age group and has an equivalent exercise level as the subjects in the published study.

What are the steps for the initial consultation with the athlete?

The initial consultation with an athlete is designed to gather information, assess dietary intake, develop goals, provide nutrition education based on these goals, and develop a nutritional plan. A review of why the athlete has sought nutrition education and what goal(s) he or she has regarding nutrition and sport performance is the first step in the consultation process. Information from food and exercise records are then assessed and compared to appropriate standards. Education on ways to improve intake is completed and goals are set to help monitor progress. This process is completed in the general

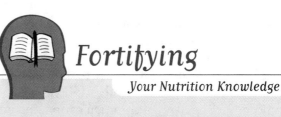

Fortifying
Your Nutrition Knowledge

Steps for the Initial Consultation Interview

Not every initial consultation with an athlete will follow these particular steps in order. The dietitian must be flexible in gathering information and providing education based on the athlete's needs and goals. The following steps will help guide dietitians in providing an efficient and effective consultation with an athlete:

- Establish rapport.
- Clarify athlete's reasons for nutrition consultation.
- Complete the nutrition assessment (anthropometrics, food record analysis, exercise assessment).
- Assess readiness for change.
- Determine nutrition goals.
- Provide education related to goals.
- Summarize and set follow-up visit date and time.

format listed in the following **Fortifying Your Nutrition Knowledge**. However, each initial consultation will be different from the next. The dietitian must remain flexible in the consultation session and be willing to complete these steps in a different order based on how the interview progresses.

Establish rapport

The key to any good interview is establishing rapport early in the session. Coaches, strength and conditioning staff, and athletic trainers may already have established rapport with the athlete. A consultant dietitian may not have, and might need to spend more time initially on rapport building. Addressing the athlete by name and asking a few general questions about the sport, the athlete's position on the team, or his or her specialty in the sport can set the athlete at ease with the process of the interview. When a dietitian knows about the sport and can converse about the type of play, positions, and typical workouts and competitions, the athlete feels that he or she is understood. This helps establish a personal relationship with the athlete in a supportive environment.

Projecting a positive demeanor and body language helps put the athlete at ease. Communication experts and social scientists believe that the image a person projects accounts for more than half of the total message conveyed to another individual at a first meeting.[23] Nonverbal communication, including tone of voice, eye contact, facial expressions, posture, and physical environment, contributes to the ability to communicate with clients. A simple nod and cordial greeting can set the stage for effective communication. Conversely, a sour facial expression, lack of eye contact, and a physical barrier such as a desk between the client and interviewer can immediately put the athlete on the defensive.

The setup of the physical space where the consultation occurs can be arranged to help the athlete feel at ease. Sitting behind a desk while the athlete is in a chair on the other side of the desk places the consultant in a position of power over the athlete. A better situation is to sit next to the athlete, with a table or part of a desk nearby on which to place papers or educational materials. There should be a comfortable distance between the athlete and the nutrition educator. Sometimes, education and assessment are conducted on the playing field or in the athletic training room. Providing a comfortable environment that is quiet and conducive to communication can be achieved in even the most cramped or open spaces. Simply paying attention to the details of the environment and creating a comfortable, nonthreatening space between the athlete and the professional can provide an excellent opportunity for communication.

Clarifying reasons for consultation

After establishing rapport, clarification of the purpose of the visit and the athlete's goals will define what type of additional information the dietitian needs to elicit from the athlete. Asking specific questions about the athlete's goals will help clarify what is necessary to improve nutrition, weight, and health or sport performance status. It also helps the dietitian to determine the nutrition plan and education required to assist the athlete. Some questions to determine the nutrition goals of the athlete may include:

- What would you like to improve regarding your daily diet?
- What has motivated you to seek nutrition advice?
- How do you feel about your current body weight and/or body composition?

- Do you want to change your weight or body composition?
- What are your sport performance goals?
- How do you think nutrition can help you achieve these goals?

Once the athlete verbalizes initial reasons for requesting the consultation and specific nutrition/performance-related goals, the nutrition assessment part of the consultation can take place.

Nutrition assessment

The majority of this section regarding the assessment stage provides a case study example of how a dietitian can interact with an athlete. The concepts in this section can be applied by all health professionals working with athletes to improve their nutrition; however, the actual assessment and nutrition plan development in this section are examples of nutrition assessment and nutrition therapy, and thus should be conducted by a registered and/or licensed dietitian.

Jennifer's Case Study Jennifer is a freshman and plays shortstop on her college softball team. Her coach thinks that she has the skill to be a starter her sophomore year. She is thin and has a hard time hitting home runs, despite consistently hitting over .325 for the past three seasons of play in high school. She and her coach feel that if she were to gain some muscle mass and strength, her home-run hitting would improve, thus securing the starting position next year. Jennifer agrees, and she has started to eat more calories in an attempt to gain weight but is also concerned about gaining too much body fat. She is fast around the bases and her defensive quickness is a huge asset to her team. She decides to consult with the sports dietitian at her college to develop a plan to gain muscle mass and a small amount of weight.

Specific Information from Jennifer's Initial Diet History

Height: 5′9″

Weight: 142 lbs

Body Mass Index: 21

Body Fat: 18%

Usual Body Weight: 140–144 lbs

Recent Weight Change: None

Jennifer's 1-day food record is shown in Figure 10.7 .

Jennifer works out with the softball team 6 days per week. This includes playing time at practices, three aerobic conditioning sessions per week, and morning strength training three times per week. She burns a

One Day of Jennifer's Food Intake Record

Time	Food	Amount	Location/Feelings
8:00 AM	Cheerios cereal	2 cups	Home, tired
	Milk, 1 %	1 cup	
	Bagel, plain	½	
	Peanut butter	1 tbsp	
	Orange juice	1 cup	
12:30 PM	Turkey sandwich	2 oz	Home from class
	Whole wheat bread	2 slices	
	Lite mayo	1 tbsp	
	Lemonade	12 oz	
	Sugar cookies	2	
6:30 PM	Spaghetti	2 cups	Home from practice
	Spaghetti sauce, premade in a jar	1 cup	
	Salad (lettuce, tomato, pepper, cucumber)	2 cups	
	Lite ranch dressing	2 tbsp	
	Garlic bread	1 slice	
	Gatorade	16 oz	
9:30 PM	Graham crackers	2	Studying, bored
	Apple	1	

Nutritive Analysis of Selected Nutrients from Jennifer's One-Day Food Record

Nutrient	Total	Comparison to Jennifer's needs
Calories	2278	Meets calculated needs for weight maintenance
Protein (gm)	73 (13% of total calories)	Should increase protein for goal of muscle mass gain
Fat (gm)	68 (27% of total calories)	Meets needs; may increase to meet total calorie goals
Carbohydrate (gm)	350 (61% of total calories)	Adequate for athletic needs
Calcium (mg)	698	Below recommended daily intake of 1000 mg
Iron (mg)	31	Meets recommended needs
Vitamin C (mg)	216	Meets recommended needs

Figure 10.7   Jennifer's 1-day food record. This 1-day food record was analyzed by a computerized dietary analysis program. An abbreviated summary of the analysis highlights the categories in which Jennifer is either meeting her needs or falling short of recommendations.

lot of energy in these workouts and gets very hungry after practice. She has started to increase her food intake but does not like many meat foods and is concerned she may not be getting enough protein in her diet.

In the first appointment, Jennifer shares her concern about wanting more power and strength but without losing speed. After analyzing her food record and assessing current intake, the dietitian works to develop goals and objectives to achieve muscle mass gains. Jennifer states that her outcome goal is to add approximately 5 pounds of muscle mass in the next 3 months.

Three short-term process-oriented goals were developed to help her achieve her long-term goal of gain-

ing muscle mass. First, she needs to eat an additional 300–500 calories daily for weight gain. Second, she should include a minimum of two servings of high-quality protein daily to allow for protein to be used for development of additional muscle mass. Third, because her calcium intake was low, she needs to consume a minimum of two milk/alternative servings per day. Jennifer will measure her progress toward these goals by keeping a food record for 3 days each week for the next 2 weeks. She will weigh herself once per week, and body composition analysis will be performed once each month for the next 3 months.

Education is provided to help Jennifer meet her goals. The dietitian gives Jennifer handouts on ways to increase calorie intake with nutrient-dense foods, including meat, beans, and other protein foods. Information about grocery shopping and meal and snack selection as well as foods to choose that are higher in calcium is also provided.

At the end of the first consultation, the dietitian summarizes the goals developed and the education related to achieving those goals. She asks Jennifer to restate the goals and how she plans to take action to meet the goals. Jennifer verbalizes a list of foods she is prepared to purchase the next time she goes grocery shopping.

The dietitian offers to meet with Jennifer again in the future to provide support and additional education, and to monitor progress toward her goals. Jennifer decides she would like to meet again in approximately 2 weeks. She plans to bring her food records to the follow-up consultation as well as a list of additional questions or concerns that may arise over the next 2 weeks. They mutually decide on a date and time, and the consultation is ended.

Anthropometric data

An important part of developing a nutrition plan for athletes is to analyze their current nutrition intake and compare it to weight and/or body composition data. Weight and body composition data may not be readily available except in terms of a stated height and weight. In an office setting, the dietitian can measure the athlete's height and weight in the first visit to establish an accurate measurement rather than relying on stated information. Body mass index (BMI) can be calculated from height and weight; however, body composition must be measured through specific assessment tools.

Dietitians are sometimes trained in body composition assessment and can perform these measurements. In an office or field setting, skinfold calipers or a bioelectrical impedence analyzer is the easiest way to measure body composition. If a dietitian has access to and is trained in using more elaborate and accurate body composition analysis tools such as the BOD POD or underwater weighing, these methods are preferred (see Chapter 11 for more details). Often athletic trainers or strength and conditioning coaches are skilled in body composition techniques. This is an excellent opportunity for dietitians and other staff to collaborate in assessing body composition and developing a plan for improvement if needed. Comparing body weight over time is necessary to determine whether energy intake is appropriate. Asking probing questions about weight changes, training

status, energy level fluctuations, fatigue, or a drop in performance at different times during the training and competitive season will help the dietitian and the athlete determine whether intake is consistently adequate to meet weight and training goals.

Jennifer's Case Study Jennifer's BMI is 21 and she appears slight of build with good muscular definition. Her BMI of 21 is in the normal healthy range (BMI healthy range = 18.5–24.9; see Chapter 11 for more details); however, considering her musculature and high level of activity, an increase in BMI is appropriate to meet her goal. Assessment of body composition is indicated in Jennifer's case. Her body fat percentage was measured at 18%, which is considered within the healthy range for athletic women (see Chapter 11 for more details). Since Jennifer has not gained or lost more than 5 pounds in the last 3 years, she is eating an appropriate number of calories per day for weight maintenance. To gain weight, she will need to add 300 to 500 calories per day.

Reviewing and analyzing the food record

Ideally, the food record is obtained and analyzed before the athlete arrives at the initial assessment appointment. The dietitian can also ask questions about usual intake to determine whether the foods listed on the food record are typical of the athlete's intake. If food record data are not provided in advance, the dietitian can elicit a 24-hour recall or have the athlete complete a brief 1-day food record at the very beginning of the consultation. This is an opportunity to start immediately interviewing the athlete and clarifying dietary intake information.

Once information from the food record or 24-hour recall is clarified, analysis of the information should be completed (covered in detail earlier in this chapter). This analysis can be done using computer software or by the dietitian comparing the information and making judgments based on clinical knowledge and sport nutrition practice. Most often a combination of comparing foods consumed to set guidelines such as MyPlate, assessing food purchasing/preparation practices and the time available for meal preparation and consumption, and simply assessing the quality and quantity of food consumed will all be a part of this analysis. The anthropometric, dietary, and exercise assessments will be used in conjunction to determine whether energy needs are appropriate and will aid in creation of the athlete's nutrition plan.

Jennifer's Case Study One day of Jennifer's 3-day food record is listed in Figure 10.7. Jennifer's food record contains only one serving from the milk/alternative group. Clarifying whether this is a typical amount of dairy product consumption daily will help in assessing calcium and protein intake. For example, Jennifer may state that she rarely has more than one serving of milk each day, mainly on her cereal in the morning. The dietitian should then further clarify whether this is a food preference or a lactose intolerance problem.

Overall, Jennifer's dietary intake is adequate in energy to meet her estimated needs to maintain weight (approximately 2300 calories daily). To gain weight she will need to add calories to her regular dietary intake. Her protein intake is 1.1 g/kg and 13% of her total caloric intake. Although 13% is within the normal range of protein intake for athletes, 1.1 g/kg is on the low end of normal. To increase muscle mass and weight, some of the additional calories she needs to consume should come from additional protein sources. Jennifer's intake of vitamins and minerals exceeded the RDAs/AIs except that for calcium. Her calcium intake was less than half of the recommended AI, and this needs much improvement.

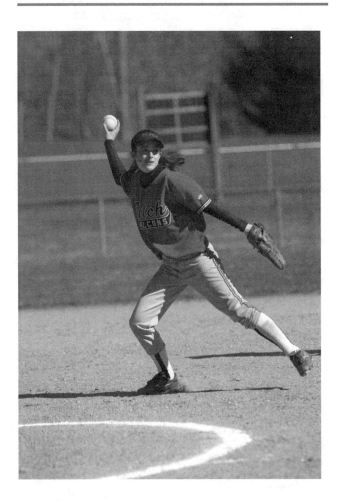

Exercise assessment

A review of when and how often the athlete exercises will provide information on energy expenditure. A quick exercise recall or review of an exercise log provides information on the duration, intensity, and frequency of exercise sessions. Additional questions should be asked about overall activity level that does not include exercise sessions. For example, a college athlete who drives to all classes will have a lower energy expenditure than one who walks to all classes on campus. Information about exercise and activity habits is then compared to information obtained from dietary records and the assessment of nutrient intake to determine whether calorie intake should be increased, decreased, or maintained at the current level.

Jennifer's Case Study Determining overall energy expenditure is necessary, especially in Jennifer's case because her goal is to gain weight and muscle mass. Jennifer is a very active athlete on and off the field. She usually walks to classes and drives only to off-campus activities. She exercises 6 days per week with the softball team at afternoon practices. They have additional strength-training sessions three mornings each week. When comparing her activity level to her energy intake, and knowing that her weight has been stable for 3 years, the dietitian determines that she is consuming enough calories to meet but not exceed her energy needs.

Assess readiness to change

Assessing readiness to make nutrition and behavior changes is an important part of any initial consultation. There is a variety of methods to assess readiness for change. Whichever method is chosen, it is essential to determine whether the athlete realizes the need to make nutrition changes and is ready to take action. Only an athlete with some level of readiness will be able to make the changes needed to meet goals.

The **Transtheoretical Model**, developed by Prochaska and DiClemente, is a research-based model that approaches behavior change as a process versus a distinct event.[24] The process involves a progression through a series of six stages that ultimately leads to permanent lifestyle behavior change. Each of these stages

Transtheoretical Model A conceptual model of how humans go about changing their behaviors. It involves six stages, each of which represents a different mind-set toward change. Knowing which change stage an athlete or client is in can be helpful in developing strategies for altering their health or nutrition behaviors.

can be applied to helping athletes change their eating patterns to improve overall health and maximize athletic potential. The following overview of the Transtheoretical Model briefly describes the six stages of behavior change and how each stage can apply to working with athletes on changing nutrition habits. The final part of each section highlights tips for how to help athletes move progressively from stage to stage.

Stage 1: Precontemplation

An athlete is in the precontemplation stage if he or she states no intention of making a change in the foreseeable future (within the next 6 months). Most of the athletes in this stage are merely uninformed or unknowledgeable of the reasons why making dietary changes can influence their overall health and athletic performance. Unfortunately, these athletes are generally categorized as resistant to change and unmotivated, which may cause them to receive little attention from coaches, athletic trainers, or dietitians. Providing a clear explanation of why dietary changes are needed and the personal benefits they will realize by making positive behavior changes is essential in this stage. Educating athletes about the importance of proper dietary habits in relation to their sport will help them move from the precontemplation stage to the next stage, contemplation.

Stage 2: Contemplation

An athlete is in the contemplation stage if he or she has stated the intention to make a specific dietary change within the next 6 months. Athletes in this stage are fully aware of the benefits of making dietary changes, but also are acutely aware of the disadvantages of changing. Athletes in this stage know they should make a change, but the barriers to achieving their goal overshadow their ability to move forward. For many athletes, the acknowledgment that their season is quickly approaching causes them to initiate some action to improve their dietary habits. Dietitians can help athletes move out of this stage and into the preparation stage by discussing the pros and cons of changing versus not changing their dietary habits and the resulting effects on their athletic performance.

Stage 3: Preparation

An athlete is in the preparation stage if he or she has stated an intention to change within the next month. These athletes have taken steps to prepare for change (e.g., they have scheduled an appointment to see a registered dietitian or bought a new healthy eating cookbook). Once they have reached this stage, the athletes are ready for traditional behavior change programs/services.

As a dietitian, this is an exciting and important stage—athletes are ready for change and open to professional guidance. It is critical not to overwhelm a person in this stage with too much information. Providing information on ways to change dietary patterns, intake, and behaviors while emphasizing how these changes will benefit the athlete is the best educational method in this stage. Identifying one or two small changes to focus on will build the athlete's confidence in his or her ability to make more changes and therefore will help move the athlete toward the action stage.

Stage 4: Action

An athlete is in the action stage if he or she has made specific, overt modifications in dietary habits within the last 6 months. The changes made must be significant enough to improve athletic performance or reduce the risk of disease. These athletes are not only ready for professional guidance, but also are actively putting the professional recommendations into practice. Athletes in this phase are hungry for examples of easy ways to make healthy eating a reality.

Individualization is a key component in this phase. The calculation of individual energy and macronutrient requirements, the development of an individualized daily meal plan and exercise hydration schedule, and the provision of quick, easy recipes are popular topics often requested by clients. Athletes want to know not only why they need to make a change, but also how they can make the change so that implementation happens with ease. Athletes require consistent guidance by dietitians, who can provide the practical tools they need to continue making positive dietary changes over several months to reach the next stage, maintenance.

Stage 5: Maintenance

Athletes in the maintenance stage are actively working on preventing a relapse. This phase consists mainly of working on self-efficacy and the confidence that they will not resort to old habits—a process that can last from 6 months up to several years. Encouragement should be provided to make the changes fit into the athlete's lifestyle. It should be noted that "relapse" is often thought to be an actual stage. However, in the Transtheoretical Model, relapse is not a distinct stage; it is instead a backward step to an earlier stage. If an athlete has progressed to the action or maintenance stage, he or she generally will not relapse all the way back to precontemplation. The backward step usually falls somewhere between contemplation and preparing for taking another action. This stage does not necessarily involve "change," but it can involve finding alternatives or additional ways to meet their goals.

Stage 6: Termination

Athletes who have reached the termination stage have zero temptation of ever returning to old habits. These individuals have established such a solid plan that no emotional state, situation, or environment will cause them to resort to old habits. There is controversy regarding whether most individuals ever reach this stage. It appears that most people will remain in the maintenance stage for a lifetime—constantly working to adjust, adapt, and learn how to keep on track with healthy eating patterns. Reaching termination is possible; however, dietitians should realize that it is rare for individuals to fully reach termination. Therefore, athletes should be supplied with a constant stream of tools and resources to keep them at least in the maintenance stage, with termination as an ultimate goal.

Jennifer's Case Study Jennifer is in the action stage. She asked for the nutrition consultation because she realizes she needs guidance to improve her nutrition. She has already started to make some small changes to improve her nutrition intake for muscle mass gains by eating more at some of her meals. Additional education and tips for improving calorie and nutrient intake should help her continue taking action to complete the nutrition changes recommended.

Determine nutrition goals

Athletes should set both short- and long-term nutrition and/or weight goals. Athletes generally have a long-term goal in mind such as to gain muscle or lose body fat. This long-term goal is the final outcome the athlete would like to achieve and is also referred to as the **outcome-oriented goal**. Outcome-oriented goals help guide the athlete and dietitian to develop a nutrition plan, revise the plan as needed, and

outcome-oriented goal The final outcome or end result that an athlete would like to achieve as a result of changing dietary habits. For example, a slightly overfat athlete may have an outcome-oriented goal of losing 3 pounds of body fat in 6 weeks. Outcome-oriented goals help guide the athlete and dietitian to develop a nutrition plan, revise the plan as needed, and continue behavior change toward meeting the desired end result.

continue behavior change to meet these goals. An outcome-oriented goal will be measured throughout the educational process to determine the effectiveness of the nutrition plan and the implementation of the plan by the athlete. However, this long-term goal is difficult to reach quickly, and therefore several short-term goals may be necessary to help guide the athlete to the final outcome.

A short-term or **process-oriented goal** is designed to help the athlete achieve the outcome desired but with small steps. Process-oriented goals may also be considered objectives. These goals help provide interim steps and ways of measuring success before the final outcome goal is achieved. Short-term goals must be made difficult enough to be challenging, but also be attainable in a short period of time. If goals are developed in this manner, success is seen in small steps, and progress toward the final goal is defined by the success of the short-term goals.

Helping athletes set realistic, achievable goals is an important part of the nutrition consultation. Both the athlete and the dietitian should mutually decide upon goals. If goals are set too high, or if expectations for how quickly goals should be met are too aggressive, then meeting the goals will be difficult. The athlete can help determine how many goals and what goals to start with based on his or her motivation and lifestyle. In general, a maximum of three process-oriented goals should be agreed upon initially. Nutrition professionals can gauge how many goals to suggest based on assessment of readiness to change as well as the interaction in the initial and follow-up sessions. Once short-term goals are developed, the athlete and dietitian should develop a plan for measuring and monitoring progress toward goal achievement. The challenge with nutrition goal setting is to develop goals that encourage small changes in gradual, manageable, and measurable steps to reach the ultimate (outcome) goal.

gaining the performance edge

By understanding the stages of change, a dietitian can be more effective in counseling, educating, and motivating athletes to make healthy dietary changes by catering to their individual needs and preparedness for change.

process-oriented goal An achievement based on following or complying with procedures designed to cause a specific outcome. Process-oriented goals are focused on the steps required to reach the desired outcome and not so much on the final outcome itself. For example, an athlete wishing to lose weight may formulate a process-oriented goal of training 30 minutes longer 4 days of the week. The end result is to lose weight, but the goal is to meet the additional exercise requirements.

Jennifer's Case Study The dietitian recognizes that to gain weight and muscle mass (Jennifer's long-term, outcome-oriented goal) Jennifer will need to increase total calories and protein in her diet. Intake of other nutrients is adequate except for calcium. Because calcium is essential to bone health, improving calcium intake is another goal the dietitian shares with Jennifer. They discuss how the long-term goal can be achieved and together they decide on the following short-term (process-oriented) goals:

- *Goal 1:* Eat an additional 300–500 calories per day, focusing on nutrient-dense foods.
- *Goal 2:* Eat a minimum of two servings in the protein foods group each day.
- *Goal 3:* Consume at least two servings of dairy products each day.

Each of the short-term goals is focused on the ultimate goal of gradual muscle gain without excessive weight gain. Jennifer is already in the action stage of change and is likely to succeed with three goals because her motivation level is high.

To determine progress toward these three goals, Jennifer will keep food records for at least 3 days of each week for the next 2 weeks. To assess the overall outcome goal, an accurate height, weight, and body composition analysis is performed in the initial appointment. These measures can be repeated at 1-month intervals to assess changes in body weight and composition. Jennifer is asked to weigh herself only once a week, at the same time each week, to help her avoid becoming overly concerned about her weight. This will allow a monitoring process and feedback mechanism for her as well as for the dietitian.

Education related to goals

Education about healthful eating is likely to be done throughout the initial consultation process. There may be moments in the conversation at the beginning of the session when education is provided. If athletes share information that they have learned that appears to be inaccurate, the dietitian can clarify that information and provide accurate information at that time. Near the end of the session, specific education should take place that will help the athlete achieve his or her goals.

Dietitians should have a variety of sample meal patterns ready in handout form to avoid the time-consuming process of developing the plan in the first session. Having sample plans available in a variety of calorie levels, for vegetarian and nonvegetarian patterns, and for different age levels that can be adapted for different athletes is extremely valuable for dietitians and their athletes. Adjustments to these sample patterns can be made quickly based on specific short-term and long-term goals.

Jennifer's Case Study For Jennifer's first goal, she is provided with a handout describing healthy weight gain for athletes that includes nutrient- and calorie-dense foods. This handout provides examples of 300–500 calorie snacks and ideas for higher calorie beverages to consume with meals and snacks. Encouraging Jennifer to consume nutrient-dense foods to increase calories rather than consuming high-fat, high-sugar snacks helps her increase nutrient intake. Providing a handout about grocery shopping that includes tips on purchasing a variety of protein foods including vegetarian, meat, and dairy sources will help her purchase the necessary protein foods, increasing the likelihood of regular consumption. By focusing on obtaining extra calories from protein-rich foods and dairy, she is learning how to increase her total calorie intake, while focusing on her other two goals of increasing protein and dairy in her diet.

Because Jennifer is not a consistent meat eater, she needs some information on nonmeat protein sources to meet her second goal. Using the MyPlate food guidance system is a simple way to show her how to incorporate both nonmeat and meat sources of protein into her daily diet.

To meet her third goal, Jennifer needs to consistently consume two dairy/alternative servings daily. The MyPlate food guidance system recommendation for dairy/alternative intake is actually two to three servings per day. However, because Jennifer is currently consuming only one dairy/alternative serving daily, and has expressed difficulty with dairy food consumption, setting a goal of increasing to two servings of dairy daily is more realistic for her than aiming for three servings. A list of dairy foods and beverages, and creative ways to consume more dairy, will help her meet this goal. For example, she currently consumes milk only on cereal. The dietitian could suggest milk as a beverage to consume at her evening meal. Or, if the taste of milk is unappealing, then alternate dairy sources such as soy milk, grain milks, dairy or nondairy cheese or yogurt, and foods made with these items could help her meet this goal.

A sample meal plan for Jennifer is shown in **Training Table 10.1**. The changes in the revised meal plan are based on her food preferences gleaned from the consultation.

Training Table 10.1: Jennifer's Sample Meal Plan

Jennifer's Initial 1-Day Food Intake	Jennifer's Revised Meal Plan
Cheerios cereal	Cheerios cereal
Milk, 1%	Milk, 1%
Bagel, plain	Bagel, plain
Peanut butter	Peanut butter
Orange juice	Calcium-fortified orange juice
	Banana
Turkey sandwich	Turkey sandwich
Whole wheat bread	Whole wheat bread
Turkey, 3 oz	Turkey, 3 oz
Lite mayo	Lite mayo
Sugar cookies	Sugar cookies
Lemonade	Lemonade
	Apple
Spaghetti	Spaghetti
Spaghetti sauce, premade in a jar	Spaghetti sauce, premade in a jar plus 3 oz lean ground beef
Salad (lettuce, tomato, pepper, cucumber)	Salad (lettuce, tomato, pepper, cucumber)
Lite ranch dressing	Lite ranch dressing
Garlic bread	Garlic bread
Gatorade	Gatorade
Graham crackers	Graham crackers
Apple	Hot chocolate made with milk
Total Calories: 2304	Total Calories: 2726
Total Carbohydrate: 350 (61%)	Total Carbohydrate: 399 (59%)
Total Protein: 73 g (13%)	Total Protein: 98 g (14%)
Total Fat: 68 g (27%)	Total Fat: 82 g (27%)
Total Calcium: 698 mg	Total Calcium: 1076 mg

Summary and closing

As the initial consultation process comes to an end, a summary of the goals and meal-planning ideas, education provided, and questions from the athlete will provide a framework for further sessions. The athlete should be given an opportunity to ask for clarification or information on additional topics not covered in the session. The athlete should be asked to state, in his or her own words, how the suggested changes will be made based on the information provided. This helps the athlete understand the goals and how to implement them after leaving the consultation. If the athlete is unsure of how to put the nutrition information into practice, a review of the goals and education methods should be done prior to the athlete's departure.

It is helpful to provide the athlete with a brief written list of the main objectives of the nutrition plan and how the plan can be implemented. This can be written on the back of an educational handout or on a separate form that the dietitian creates. These goals and the educational plan to achieve them can be shared with other sports professionals if the athlete gives permission to do so. This improves continuity of care and helps the athlete and the rest of the professionals work together toward a common goal. At the closing of the interview, plans for follow-up appointments should be discussed.

Jennifer's Case Study The dietitian summarizes Jennifer's three goals and asks how Jennifer plans to implement the dietary changes. Jennifer appears to understand the goals and how to add calories to her diet. She verbalizes protein sources she is going to purchase when she goes grocery shopping. She verbalizes concern about increasing dairy products, but states she is going to try to purchase more dairy foods as well. Jennifer states she would like to meet again in 2 or 3 weeks. The appointment is set and appropriate closing comments are shared.

What are the steps for a follow-up consultation with the athlete?

Providing the athlete with an opportunity to meet with the dietitian after the initial assessment allows the athlete to attempt some of the changes recommended and then review these changes. This process is critical to the athlete's continued success in accomplishing established short-term and long-term goals. Making permanent dietary changes can be more challenging than most athletes initially perceive. Athletes need guidance along the way to help them meet their goals and provide a continued resource for education, goal revision, and ultimate success in behavior change. Accountability to someone else for making recommended changes is also a motivating factor in making and keeping follow-up appointments.

Follow-up visits may be more frequent for athletes with many changes to make and less frequent for others. In some cases, a one-time visit is enough to help the athlete move toward healthier eating for optimal sport performance. In most cases, at least one follow-up visit is recommended. Athletes who present with eating disorders or disturbed eating patterns will likely need several follow-up sessions. Athletes presenting with weight concerns, trying to either gain weight or lose weight, or those with medical conditions will likely require a series of sessions.

The process for a follow-up appointment is similar to the initial consultation but is usually much shorter. Typical follow-up sessions are scheduled for approximately half the amount of time as for an initial consult. Less time is needed for the rapport-building part of the session because the athlete and dietitian already know each other. The beginning of the follow-up visit often consists of a quick review of goals and a review of any food records. A comparison of the record to the stated goals helps provide input to the athlete about progress made.

Assessment of how the athlete is feeling, energy levels, and any subjective information about sport performance should be discussed. Often the subjective information is the first progress an athlete notices. The scale or body composition assessments may not reveal a change in body weight or body composition, but the athlete might recognize feeling better, or having more energy during practice and competitions. Eliciting this subjective information is a skill all dietitians working with athletes need because it can be a strong motivating factor in continuing the dietary changes that influence the attainment of short- and long-term goals. Assessing weight, body composition, and any laboratory or clinical assessments may also occur during the follow-up visit.

Based on all of the information obtained in the follow-up session, revision of short-term and long-term goals can take place. If the athlete has mastered one or more process-oriented goals, then adding another goal may be indicated. If the athlete is having difficulty meeting some short-term goals, then revision of goals may be necessary.

The final step in the follow-up process is to determine whether additional appointments are indicated. Determining this may depend on the time the athlete has to keep appointments, finances for appointments if nutrition consultations are not covered by the team

or by insurance, and the need for additional sessions. Telephone consults may be an easy alternative to having face-to-face contact. Brief consultations and questions may be handled through email; however, nothing confidential should be shared through email. The dietitian and athlete together can determine the best follow-up plan for the athlete. Developing a plan for follow-up or deciding to terminate additional appointments should be clear to both the athlete and the dietitian in the closing of the appointment.

Jennifer's Case Study Jennifer returns after 2 weeks for a follow-up visit. She has brought in food records for 5 of the past 14 days since the last visit. Upon review of the records, the dietitian sees that Jennifer is meeting two of her three goals consistently. Her calorie intake is excellent and she is consistently consuming two or even three high-quality protein sources each day. However, dairy intake is still averaging only one serving per day. The dietitian reviews dairy intake with Jennifer to determine why this is a difficult goal to meet. Jennifer states that she just does not like the taste of milk and yogurt. The dietitian provides a handout with dairy and nondairy sources of calcium to Jennifer. Calcium-fortified orange juice, instant oatmeal, and hot chocolate made with milk are options that Jennifer states she will try to incorporate into her diet for the next 2 weeks. They set another follow-up appointment date for 2 weeks later and continue with the three original goals set. At the upcoming follow-up appointment, weight and body composition assessments will be made to determine progress toward the long-term weight and muscle-gain goals.

What should walk-in or short sessions with athletes involve?

Often a dietitian will meet with many athletes on a walk-in or first-come, first-served basis. In these brief sessions, completed food records and health history questionnaires are generally not available. These sessions, however, can be valuable for the athlete despite the short time and limited availability of prior information. This may be the only opportunity for an athlete to speak with a nutrition professional, so making the most out of the short time can significantly help the athlete.

An excellent opportunity for brief sessions occurs after a group nutrition session with a team. Athletes may be encouraged to ask questions after the group session is over. In this case, the athlete often has one specific question that can be answered relatively easily. The dietitian should be prepared for a variety of questions from the athletes. These may include questions about popular sports supplements or dietary regimens seen in the media, clinical questions related to health conditions, and questions about specific nutrients in foods or how to obtain certain nutrients from different foods. Answering questions and having a variety of written materials on hand for more detailed information provides a valuable service to several athletes in a short period of time.

Other settings in which brief consults with athletes can occur include health and wellness fairs, sports competitions, or booths at conferences. All of these settings are excellent opportunities to present accurate and helpful nutrition information to interested and engaged athletes. Providing general sports nutrition information at the table or booth for athletes to read later is often the best way to provide information in these settings. Providing a list of Web sites with credible information on a variety of sports nutrition topics will be helpful for the busy athlete who may choose not to stop and talk at the table but is willing to pick up a flyer. A typical sports nutrition table display should include:

- An attractive table cover and information about what professional or company is sponsoring the display.
- Short, one-page flyers on sports nutrition topics including hydration, energy needs, carbohydrates, proteins, fats, pre- and postexercise eating guidelines, and additional resources such as reputable Web sites, books, and cookbooks. If the display is at a particular sporting event (e.g., a marathon), then nutrition and hydration information specific to the sport should be displayed.
- Interactive displays that attract attention and aid with education are desirable. Displays could include food models, samples of sports gels or bars, different options for water bottles to use during exercise, and short quizzes.
- Information about services offered and how to make appointments, including business cards, should be made available on the table.

In many sports medicine clinics or physicians' offices, a dietitian may be available on an as-needed basis after seeing the athletic trainer, physical therapist, or sports medicine physician. In these cases, a shortened nutrition questionnaire that the athlete can complete in just a few minutes will help guide the individual session. The questionnaire can be similar to the one presented in Figure 10.1, but with much less detail. Demographic information, reason for the visit, anthropometric data, and brief questions about how often an athlete eats, where meals are consumed, and dietary supplements used should be included in the brief questionnaire. This will help guide the session to meet the athlete's needs while providing critical initial information to the dietitian.

A brief diet history and 24-hour dietary recall can be done for walk-in sessions with athletes. Information about type, duration, and intensity of exercise can also be quickly obtained. An experienced dietitian can review all of this information quickly to get a basic idea of the athlete's current nutrient and energy intake and make assessments about changes needed. Because time is limited, only one goal may be developed to help the athlete improve nutrition intake. The dietitian and the athlete can mutually decide on the most important aspect of dietary change and develop a nutrition plan to meet that goal. Additional appointments can be made to follow up with the athlete. These appointments can include more time to allow for a better assessment and for education, goal setting, and nutrition plan development.

Are there any concerns about the confidentiality of the health, nutrition, and exercise information provided by the athlete?

Any health and medical information is considered confidential. Privacy acts that safeguard medical information obtained from the patient verbally or during medical treatment are in place throughout the United States. The Health Insurance Portability and Accountability Act of 1996 (HIPAA) is designed to protect insurance coverage for workers and their dependents if they lose or change jobs. It also addresses the security and privacy of health data and addresses issues to improve the efficiency and effectiveness of the nation's health care system by encouraging electronic data interchange in health care.[25] This act requires any health care provider and all health care organizations to inform patients about their rights to privacy. In some settings, dietitians, athletic trainers, physical therapists, and team physicians may have to comply with HIPAA privacy standards. All traditional hospitals and clinics that require fees for service and/or bill insurance companies or Medicare/Medicaid must comply with HIPAA.[25] Some private consultants, such as dietitians in private practice, may also fall under HIPAA regulations. The Department of Health and Human Services (HHS) administers HIPAA, and the Centers for Medicare and Medicaid Services (CMS) agency within HHS is responsible for implementing some provisions of HIPAA. For more information on health information privacy and HIPAA regulations, consult www.hhs.gov/ocr/privacy/hipaa/understanding/index.html. Even if the HIPAA regulations do not apply in some athletic settings, confidentiality of information should be strictly maintained.

Nutritional assessment information, including analyses of food records, health history information, and nutritional plans developed, should be kept confidential. Ensuring the privacy of this information is essential to building and maintaining the trust of the athlete-dietitian relationship. Information should not be shared with other athletes, teammates, coach-

---

Consent for Disclosure of Confidential Medical Information Form

Health Care Agency
Address
Phone/fax

I, _____ authorize _____ to
   (patient/athlete name)   (agency/institution name)

Disclose to: _____
              (Medical facility, person, parent)
              _____
                          (Address)
              _____
              _____
                      (Phone and fax)

The following information:
_____
_____
_____

(Should list specific information such as nutrition intake, concerns with nutrient density, eating behaviors, any information that the agency/person being given the information will need to help the athlete.)

Method of Disclosure:
_____

(Verbal only—phone or in person, fax, mailed medical record copy)

_____ _____ _____
Patient/Athlete Name (printed)   Identifying number   Date of Birth

Patient/Athlete's Rights:*
Each institution will have specific patient rights and provisions of the consent for disclosure. Typical provisions include:
• The right to know what information is being disclosed
• The right to revoke the consent for disclosure at any time
• If consent is revoked by the patient, the following consequences (if any) may
  occur _____
*Note—each medical institution, athletic agency, or sports medicine clinic will have their own patient rights and provisions for disclosure. These should be described in the consent for disclosure form in writing.

Consent is valid until: _____
                                  (date)

Patient/Athlete Signature: _____   Date: _____

Figure 10.8 Sample medical information disclosure form. Medical information is considered protected information under HIPAA. Written permission to disclose medical information must be obtained prior to sharing the information with any medical personnel or other individuals.

ing staff, or the media. Care should be taken to avoid casual conversations that seem harmless but if overheard could be misconstrued as sharing of confidential information. If the athlete gives permission to release the information to a coach, parent, spouse, or any other individual, then this information can be exchanged. However, in the absence of permission, no information should be given to anyone but the athlete, even when asked directly. Most health care organizations and many athletic departments also have strict confidentiality policies regarding release of medical information to persons or organizations outside the providing organization. Permission to disclose medical information is best given in written form, thus providing the athlete with a clear understanding of what information can be disclosed, and to whom. A sample medical information disclosure form is shown in Figure 10.8. The form clearly stipulates what information is going to be released, to whom, and in what format (verbal, written, medical record documents). The form must have the athlete/patient signature and should have a date when permission to release the information will expire.

The issue of confidentiality and permission to disclose information may seem excessively cautious, especially as it relates to nutrition information; however, to develop a good working relationship with athletes, trust is critical. Athletes may share sensitive information in individual consultations that they have never shared with other people. This is often the case for athletes with eating disorders or weight concerns. Athletes seeking help for eating disorders may be less likely to return for follow-up visits if they are afraid that their coaches, parents, or teammates will learn about their personal eating behaviors. Maintaining confidentiality is designed to protect the athlete and to protect the dietitian as well.

The Box Score

Key Points of Chapter

- Nutrition consultation and communication help athletes acquire the knowledge and skills necessary to foster healthy dietary behaviors that will help them achieve their sport-specific goals.

- Nutrition assessments of athletes should be completed by a registered and/or licensed dietitian. Dietitians have the education and experience to assess dietary intake, analyze medical information, and develop specific nutrition plans for athletes. Other sports professionals such as coaches and athletic trainers can support athletes' nutrition knowledge and behavior changes by using nutrition information from public domain sources regularly when working with athletes.

- Assessing the needs of the athlete is the first step in effective nutrition consultation. The more information the dietitian can gather about the athlete's goals, health history, training regimens, medications, and dietary practices, the more effective the first nutrition consulting session will be.

- The diet history is the most comprehensive form of dietary intake data collection and involves an interview process that reviews food intake records, eating behaviors, recent and long-term eating habits, and exercise patterns. The process is very time-consuming but provides a wealth of information that can help the dietitian design an individualized diet plan for the athlete.

- Health history questionnaires are valuable tools for gathering information about an athlete's current health and medications, past medical history, and other health-related behaviors.

- Obtaining information about food intake is done using a variety of tools. The most common food intake tool is the food record. Food intakes can be recorded for 1-, 3-, or 7-day periods. Other food intake assessment methods include the 24-hour food recall, food frequency questionnaires, and diet histories.

- Documentation of how much training or exercise the athlete is currently performing is essential to any sports dietitian's assessment and dietary plan.

- Food records must be as detailed and accurate as possible if they are to be effective tools. Commonly omitted pieces of information such as portion sizes, use of condiments, food brands, names of restaurants, method of food preparation, beverage use, and snacks can severely limit a food record's accuracy. To obtain this information the dietitian needs to be armed with the appropriate clarification questions.

- The initial consultation with athletes includes many steps to gather information, make a nutrition assessment, and develop a nutritional plan that meets the athlete's needs. These steps include rapport building, clarifying reasons for the consultation, nutrition assessment, assessing readiness to change, goal setting, education, and summarizing.

- When assessing an athlete's readiness to change his or her dietary habits, the six stages of behavior change presented in the Transtheoretical Model need to be considered. The six stages are precontemplation, contemplation, preparation, action, maintenance, and termination. The stage the athlete is in dictates which tools or motivational strategies can be used to help the athlete change his or her nutritional behaviors.

- Follow-up consultations with athletes are required to review how the imposed changes are working, to address any problems encountered, to answer questions, and to foster a sense of accountability on the part of the athlete. Follow-up visits may be more frequent for athletes with many goals/objectives, and less frequent for others.

- Walk-in sessions are often very brief consulting sessions that are done without the dietitian being armed with previous health and dietary information about the athlete. These sessions are more athlete-directed and consist of the dietitian answering an athlete's questions. Despite their brevity, walk-in sessions can still be very educational and may lead to the athlete desiring a more complete consultation.

- Any health or medical information is considered strictly confidential and is protected by the Health Insurance Portability and Accountability Act (HIPAA). Even if the HIPAA regulations do not apply to some of the information collected, confidentiality of information should be maintained.

Study Questions

1. What information should the sports dietitian obtain from the athlete prior to the first nutrition counseling session?

2. What information can be gleaned from a health history questionnaire? Why does a sports dietitian working with athletes need this information?

3. Besides information provided in a health history questionnaire, what other information is important for the dietitian to obtain?

4. What tools can be used to obtain information about an athlete's diet? What are the pros and cons of each?

5. Food records must be complete to get an accurate representation of an athlete's diet. What information about food intake is usually missing or not clearly identified in most food records?

6. Once dietary information has been collected from an athlete, what standards, tools, and/or dietary measures can be used by the dietitian to assess that athlete's diet? What are the advantages and disadvantages of each?

7. What are the basic steps required for conducting an effective initial dietary consultation? Is it necessary for the steps to be completed in a specific sequence? Defend your answer.

8. What is the purpose of a follow-up visit? What should be discussed in the follow-up session?

9. How do walk-in dietary consult sessions differ from the typical planned consultation? What can and cannot be accomplished in these short sessions?

10. What does HIPAA stand for? How does HIPAA affect sports dietitians and their handling of the information gathered during counseling?

References

1. Jonnalagadda S, Rosenblum C, Skinner R. Dietary practices, attitudes, and physiological status of collegiate freshman football players. *J Strength Cond Res*. 2001;15(4):507–513.

2. Jacobson B, Sobonya C, Ransone J. Nutrition practices and knowledge of college varsity athletes: a follow-up. *J Strength Cond Res*. 2001;15(1):63–68.

3. Cole CR, Salvaterra GF, Davis JE, Borja ME, Powell LM, Dubbs EC, Bordi PL. Evaluation of dietary practices of National Collegiate Athletic Association division I football players. *J Strength Con Res*. 2005;19(3):490–494.

4. Nichols PE, Jonnalagadda SS, Rosenbloom CA, Trinkaus M. Knowledge, attitudes, and behaviors regarding hydration and fluid replacement of collegiate athletes. *Int J Sport Nutr Exerc Metab*. 2005;15(5):515–527.

5. Burns RD, Schiller MR, Merrick MA, Wolf KN. Intercollegiate student athlete use of nutritional supplements and the role of athletic trainers and dietitians in nutrition counseling. *J Am Diet Assoc*. 2004;104(2):246–249.

6. Smart L, Bisogni CA. Personal food systems of male college hockey players. *Appetite*. 2001;37:57–70.

7. American Dietetic Association. Advocacy and the Profession, Licensure and Certification. Available at: www.eatright.org/ada/files/licensure_laws1.pdf. Accessed June 25, 2007.

8. Institute of Medicine. *Dietary Reference Intakes: Applications in Dietary Assessment*. Washington, DC: National Academies Press; 2000.

9. Beaton GH, Milner J, Corey P, et al. Sources of variance in 24-hour dietary recall data: implications for nutrition study design and interpretation. *Am J Clin Nutr*. 1979;32:2546–2559.

10. Driskell JA, Wolinsky I. *Nutritional Assessment of Athletes*. Boca Raton, FL: CRC Press; 2002.

11. Lichtman SW, Pisarska K, Berman ER, et al. Discrepancy between self-reported and actual caloric intake and exercise in obese subjects. *N Engl J Med*. 1992;327:1893–1898.

12. Mertz W, Tsui JC, Judd JT, et al. What are people really eating? The relation between energy intake derived from estimated diet records and intake determined to maintain body weight. *Am J Clin Nutr*. 1991;54:291–295.

13. Tarasuk V, Beaton GH. The nature and individuality of within-subject variation in energy intake. *Am J Clin Nutr*. 1991;54:464–470.

14. Van Staveren WA, Hautvast JG, Katan MB, Van Montfort MA, Van Oosten-Van Der Goes HG. Dietary fiber consumption in an adult Dutch population. *J Am Diet Assoc*. 1982;80:324–330.

15. Barr SI, Janelle KC, Prior JC. Energy intakes are higher during the luteal phase of ovulatory menstrual cycles. *Am J Clin Nutr*. 1995;61:39–43.

16. Tarasuk V, Beaton GH. Menstrual cycle patterns in energy and macronutrient intake. *Am J Clin Nutr*. 1991;53:442–447.

17. National Cancer Institute, Division of Cancer Control and Population Sciences. Diet History Questionnaire. Available at: riskfactor.cancer.gov/DHQ. Accessed June 20, 2007.

18. Subar AF. Developing dietary assessment tools. *J Am Diet Assoc*. 2004;104(5):769–770.

19. Clark KS. Sports nutrition counseling: documentation of performance. *Top Clin Nutr*. 1999;14(2):34–40.

20. Maughan RJ, Greenhaff PL, Leiper JB, Ball D, Lambert CP, Gleeson M. Diet composition and the performance of high-intensity exercise. *J Sports Sci*. 1997;15(3):265–275.

21. Bloch TD, Wheeler KB. Dietary examples: a practical approach to feeding athletes. *Clin Sports Med*. 1999;18:703–711.

22. Kleiner SM. Eating for peak performance. *Physician Sportsmedicine*. 1997;25(10):123.

23. Holli BB, Calabrese RJ. *Communication and Education Skills: The Dietitian's Guide*. 2nd ed. Philadelphia, PA: Lea & Febiger; 1991.

24. Prochaska JO, Norcross JC, DiClemente CC. *Changing for Good*. New York, NY: Avon Books; 1994.

25. Centers for Medicare and Medicaid Services. The Health Insurance Portability and Accountability Act of 1996 (HIPAA). Baltimore, MD. Available at: www.cms.hhs.gov/hipaa. Accessed August 20, 2004.

Key Questions Addressed

- What are the common weight management concerns for athletes?
- What are the prevalence and significance of overweight and obesity?
- What methods are used to determine weight status?
- Why is body composition important?
- What are the components of energy intake and energy expenditure?
- What methods do athletes use to lose weight?
- What are the weight loss issues for athletes in weight classification sports?
- What happens when weight loss efforts develop into disordered eating patterns?
- How can athletes gain weight healthfully?

You Are the Nutrition Coach

Ian is an 18-year-old gymnast training at a private gym with many other male and female gymnasts. He is competing at an advanced level and is likely to make the next Olympic team. Lately he has been finding some of his balance and strength moves on the rings and parallel bars more difficult. He has gone through a bit of a growth spurt and gained approximately 5 pounds over the last year. He suspects the weight gain is causing his performance difficulties. He decides to try a weight loss program that will help him lose weight before his next big competition in 6 weeks. He is not sure how many calories to consume and therefore arbitrarily decides to eat 1500 calories per day.

Questions

- Which assessments are required to determine whether Ian needs to lose weight?

- What type of diet and exercise plan would you recommend for Ian?

- What additional concerns do you have for Ian's health and sport performance?

What are the common weight management concerns for athletes?

Almost all athletes are looking for ways to improve sport performance. To gain a performance edge on their competitors, athletes may try to lose weight, gain weight, or modify their body composition. Overall health is also a concern for most athletes; weight modifications may be necessary in some cases if the athlete presents with risk factors such as prehypertension, insulin resistance or prediabetes glucose levels, or lipid abnormalities.

A common reason athletes strive to lose weight is aesthetics. Athletes have similar concerns as the general population about weight and body composition. They are concerned about their appearance and try to meet the ideals of cultural norms. Athletes often perceive additional pressure to maintain or achieve an ideal weight to enhance, improve, or sustain optimal sport performance.

Performance may improve following weight loss in some athletes. For example, a few pounds lost, especially as body fat, may improve speed. If an athlete has less body weight to carry but maintains the same muscle mass and power, speed may improve. Agility may increase as well for similar reasons. Less body fat may help the athlete jump higher or plant and turn with greater speed. Therefore, in some cases, weight loss may improve sport performance. In other cases, attempting to make these changes may lead to an obsession about weight or body composition and result in disordered eating.

Some sports have weight classifications requiring athletes to compete in a specific weight category. These athletes must "make weight" before each event or they will not be able to compete in the event. This places extra pressure on athletes to lose or maintain their body weight, which often involves altering their daily diet, sometimes in a dramatic fashion.

Many athletes want to gain weight or increase lean muscle mass to improve sport performance. As the strength-to-weight ratio increases, more power per pound can be produced and potentially an athlete can increase speed, decrease time over long distances, and produce more power in explosive sports. Increasing lean mass or overall weight requires nutrition and exercise changes to enhance the ability of the body to develop and maintain additional body mass.

This chapter discusses the various weight management concerns of athletes and ways athletes can alter body weight if needed. The chapter begins with an introduction of the prevalence and health consequences of overweight and obesity concerns and assessment of weight and body composition. A discussion of energy balance, including intake, needs, and expenditure in athletes and the general population, provides the background necessary for the reader when the topics of weight loss and weight gain in athletes are discussed. A section on issues pertaining to weight-classified sports and eating disorders in athletes is also included in this chapter.

What are the prevalence and significance of overweight and obesity?

There has been a significant rise in the incidence of overweight and obesity based on data from the National Health and Nutrition Examination Survey (NHANES).[1,2] Figure 11.1 shows the alarming trends in the rise of overweight and obesity in adults in the United States from 1960 to 2008.[1] Overweight and obesity are determined in these data sets using body mass index (BMI) measurements. A BMI of 18.5–24.9 is considered normal weight, ≥ 25 is considered overweight, and ≥ 30 is considered obese. The NHANES data show that 68% of adult Americans are overweight or obese, with 33.8% of these being obese.[1] Overweight and obesity in children and adolescents ages 2–19 has also been on the rise, with approximately 16.9% of this age population being obese.[2] The causes of overweight and obesity and this trend toward increases in the numbers of overweight and obese children and adults are complex and include many factors. Environmental factors such as lack of exercise and higher caloric consumption as well as sociocultural, behavioral, hormonal, metabolic, genetic, psychological, and physiological factors all contribute to this growing trend in overweight in the United States.

The prevalence of overweight and obesity in athletes in most competitive

> **body mass index (BMI)** An indicator of nutritional status that is derived from height and weight measurements. Body mass index has also been used to provide a rough estimate of body composition even though the index does not account for the weight contributions from fat and muscle.

> **gaining the performance edge**
>
> Overweight and obesity affect nearly two-thirds of the adult American population. Athletes have a much lower prevalence of overweight than the general population. However, athletes participating in some power sports and sports in which a greater body mass is beneficial (e.g., football, heavyweight wrestling, some field events) have a higher incidence of overweight or obesity.

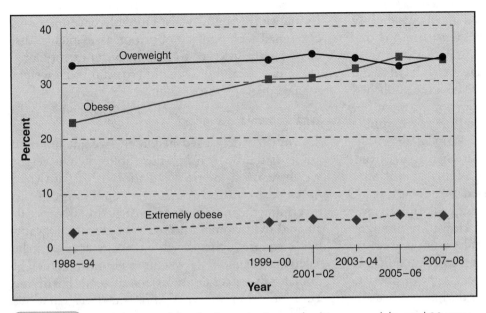

Figure 11.1 Trends in overweight, obesity, and extreme obesity among adults aged 20 years and over: United States, 1988–2008.
Notes: Age-adjusted by the direct method to the year 2000 U.S. Census Bureau estimates, using the age groups 20–39, 40–59, and 60 years and over. Pregnant females were excluded. Overweight is defined as a BMI greater than 25 but less than 30; obesity is defined as BMI ≥ 30; extreme obesity is defined as BMI ≥ 40.
Source: Centers for Disease Control and Prevention, National Center for Health Statistics. National Health and Nutrition Examination Survey III 1988–1994, 1999–2000, 2001–2002, 2003–2004, 2005–2006, and 2007–2008.

What are the main health consequences and health risks of overweight and obesity?

The health consequences associated with obesity as a risk factor carry with them significant morbidity and mortality in adults and health problems in children and adolescents. Some of the major health conditions associated with obesity include hypertension, type 2 diabetes, coronary heart disease, stroke, osteoarthritis, respiratory problems, and some types of cancer. There are additional psychological, emotional, and social costs to obese individuals as well. Obese athletes are at risk for developing these health consequences as well. Despite their high activity levels, which offer some preventive effects, obese athletes can develop obesity-related conditions, and professionals working with them should provide screening and education for the athlete just as they would the general population.

Body mass index and mortality rates have a strong correlation. Individuals in the underweight (<18.5 BMI) and obese (≥30 BMI) categories have increased mortality relative to individuals in the normal weight category.[4] There is relatively low risk in the 18.5–24.9 and even the 25–29.9 BMI categories when there is an absence of concurrent comorbid conditions. Obesity is generally defined as an excess of body fat accumulation. It is the excess adipose tissue that is the cause of the comorbid conditions, not necessarily the excess weight.[5] A person's absolute risk status is based not only on the BMI classification, but also on **waist circumference** measurements, existing disease conditions, and summation of other obesity-associated diseases. Increased risk is found in individuals with cardiovascular disease risk factors and other obesity-associated risk factors such as osteoarthritis, physical inactivity, hypertension, and gynecological abnormalities. Very high absolute risk status would include individuals

> **waist circumference** A measure of abdominal girth taken at the narrowest part of the waist as viewed from the front.

sports is relatively low. However, in some sports, such as football, heavyweight wrestling, and boxing, the prevalence of overweight and obesity may be high. As an example, for the past decade there has been a perception that bigger is better in almost all positions in football. Indeed, players are bigger than in years past. This may or may not pose additional health risks to the athlete. If the majority of the weight gain is fat-free mass, then the increase in disease risk is negligible. A study of Division I football players to determine body mass and body composition found the mean BMI of all positions was 29.4 ± 0.6%.[3] Body fat percentages ranged from 15.2% to 25.4%. Quarterbacks, defensive and offensive backs, and receivers were the leanest and weighed less, whereas the linemen were the heaviest and had the highest body fat percentages. Prevalence data presented earlier provide a background on the significant problem of overweight and obesity of the U.S. population. Though the NHANES data are reflective of the U.S. population as a whole, not an athletic population, the trends toward overweight and obesity in the general population are likely to affect the health and performance of athletes, particularly young athletes in the future.

with high BMI that already have an existing disease such as coronary heart disease, atherosclerotic disease, diabetes, or sleep apnea.

The National Institutes of Health (NIH) and the National Heart, Lung, and Blood Institute published practical guidelines for identification, evaluation, and treatment of overweight and obesity in adults in 2000.[6] This guide includes a treatment algorithm that helps the client and practitioner assess overweight and obesity as well as associated educational tools and treatment options based on the assessment. The treatment algorithm was designed primarily for use in a clinical medical setting. However, this algorithm can be applied to the athletic population to assess and help prevent or treat medical conditions that may be associated with overweight or obesity. The initial assessment can occur during a preseason physical or at other times throughout the athletic season when need arises. The main steps in assessing, preventing, and treating overweight and obesity, adapting the algorithm for use with athletes, are the following:

1. Measure height, weight, waist circumference, and body composition.
2. Calculate BMI.
3. Determine whether BMI, waist circumference, and body composition are within normal ranges for the athlete.
4. Assess health parameters (such as cholesterol and blood pressure).
5. If within normal limits, encourage weight maintenance.
6. If above normal limits, determine athlete's interest in and ability to attempt weight loss; provide education and monitoring of behaviors.
7. Follow up assessments and provide education regularly to determine progress toward goals.

The treatment algorithm is focused on disease risk factors and prevention of disease complications related to obesity. A discussion of BMI and waist circumference measures and their relevance to health and sport performance are presented in the next section.

What methods are used to determine weight status?

The two most commonly used ways to assess weight status are BMI and waist circumference. Both of these measures are used to determine health and health risk and can be used as a starting point when determining a weight that is best for athletic per-

formance. BMI and waist circumference measures combined with body composition assessments (discussed in the next section) offer sport nutrition professionals helpful information to establish a weight management plan for athletes.

What is body mass index?

The most widely used height for weight index in adults is the BMI. It is a measure of height versus weight using a metric calculation. BMI data were obtained from large general population groups to determine the midpoint range of health. BMI is calculated by dividing a person's weight in kilograms by the square of their height in meters. It can also be calculated using body weight in pounds and height in inches (versus kilograms and meters). **Fortifying Your Nutrition Knowledge** presents the calculations for both methods.

Table 11.1 outlines the recommended classifications for BMI adopted by the National Institutes of Health Expert Panel on the Identification, Evaluation, and Treatment of Overweight and Obesity in Adults.[7] The BMI is not gender-specific and therefore is appropriate for all men and nonpregnant women of all race and ethnic groups. A BMI of 18.5 to 24.9 is considered normal or healthy for the average pop-

Fortifying

Your Nutrition Knowledge

Calculating Body Mass Index

Metric Calculation Equation:
    Weight in kilograms ÷ (Height in meters)^2
Height: 74 inches
Weight: 195 pounds
Convert inches to meters:
    74 inches × 2.54 cm/inch = 188 cm = 1.88 meters
Convert pounds to kilograms:
    195 lbs ÷ 2.2 = 88.6 kg
    88.6 kg ÷ (1.88 meters)^2 = 25.1 BMI
Nonmetric Calculation Equation:
    (Weight in pounds ÷ {Height in inches}^{2}) × 703
Height: 74 inches
Weight: 195 pounds
    (195 ÷ {74 inches}^{2}) × 703 = .0356 × 703 = 25.1 BMI

TABLE 11.1	Body Mass Index Classifications
BMI (kg/m²)	**Classification**
<18.5	Underweight
18.5–24.9	Normal weight
25.0–29.9	Overweight
30.0–34.9	Obesity class I
35.0–39.9	Obesity class II
≥40	Obesity class III (extreme obesity)

ulation, 25 to 29.9 is considered overweight, greater than or equal to 30 is considered obese, and greater than or equal to 40 is considered extreme obesity. The BMI should be used to classify overweight and obesity and to estimate relative risk for disease compared to normal weight. Nomogram charts with calculated BMIs for various heights and weights are widely available. This makes BMI an easy and available tool for both health professionals and the public to use to assess their weight and health status.

Body mass index correlates well with body fatness.[8,9] There is evidence to support the use of BMI in risk assessment because it provides a more accurate measure of total body fat than does the assessment of weight alone.[7,10] However, BMI has some limitations when applied to athletes. Individuals with higher muscle mass (like most athletes) may have a BMI above 24.9 because muscle tissue is denser than fat tissue, weighing more when compared with an equal volume of fat tissue, leading to a higher body weight and BMI. Although total body weight in these athletes may be higher, they may be very lean and thus have a lower health risk despite being in the overweight BMI category. Athletes can use BMI for a general idea about their weight status, but body composition measures (lean muscle to fat ratio) will provide a better understanding of their overall health status as well as their sport performance needs. BMI can be used as a basic screening tool for athletes. It is a quick and easy way to assess weight; however, it is only one part of a comprehensive assessment to help an athlete determine the best weight for both health and sport performance.

What can measures of body fat distribution tell us?

Body mass index can be used to predict potential health risks. Other measures of risk assessment also can be employed to obtain a clearer picture of health.

Waist circumference measures the degree of weight distribution around the waist. Fat located in the abdominal area is associated with a greater health risk than fat in the gluteal-femoral region. A waist circumference over 40 inches (>102 cm) in men and over 35 inches in women (>88 cm) is considered high, placing individuals at greater risk for disease.

Waist circumference is measured using a flexible tape at the narrowest part of the waist as viewed from the front while the person is standing. The measure is best conducted against bare skin or tight-fitting clothing. The tape should be snug but not compress the skin, and should be parallel to the ground all the way around the waist. For individuals who do not have an obvious narrow part of the waist on visual inspection, it is best to measure the waist at the midpoint between the iliac crest and the lower rib. Waist circumference can be an independent predictor of disease risk. However, often waist circumference and BMI are used together to estimate risk status. A high waist circumference measure when BMI is between 25 and 34.9 is associated with an increased disease risk for type 2 diabetes, dyslipidemia, hypertension, and cardiovascular disease.[11,12] **Table 11.2** presents the relative risk of waist circumference combined with BMI levels. At a BMI ≥35, waist circumference measurements have little added predictive power over BMI alone, and it may not be necessary to measure waist circumference in this case. Measuring waist circumference is part of the evaluation guidelines from the NIH and is preferred over waist-to-hip ratio measurement for assessing overweight and obesity. Although waist circumference measures are primarily used to determine health risk, athletes, especially those in heavyweight sports, should have a waist circumference measure as part of an annual sport physical.

Waist-to-hip ratio (WHR) is another fat distribution measure that compares abdominal circumference to hip girth. It gives an indication as to where fat deposition is occurring (i.e., upper body versus lower body). For example, individuals with fat deposition that occurs primarily in the hips are described as having a pear shape (see Figure 11.2). The opposite fat deposition pattern results in a body shape resembling an apple. To determine WHR, the waist measurement is taken as described above for the waist circumference. The hip measurement is taken around the hips and over the buttocks wherever the greatest girth is found. Once

waist-to-hip ratio A comparison of waist girth to hip girth that gives an indication of fat deposition patterns in the body.

TABLE 11.2 Classification of Overweight and Obesity by BMI and Waist Circumference, and Associated Disease Risk*

Underweight, Normal, Overweight, Obesity, and Extreme Obesity	BMI (kg/m²)	Obesity Class	Men ≤ 102 cm (≤40 in) Women ≤ 88 cm (≤35 in)	Men > 102 cm (>40 in) Women > 88 cm (>35 in)
Underweight	<18.5	—	—	—
Normal+	18.5–24.9	—	—	—
Overweight	25.0–29.9	—	Increased	High
Obesity	30.0–34.9	I	High	Very high
	35.0–39.9	II	Very high	Very high
Extreme obesity	≥40	III	Extremely high	Extremely high

* Disease risk for type 2 diabetes, hypertension, and CVD.

+ Increased waist circumference can also be a marker for increased risk, even in persons of normal weight.

Source: National Heart, Lung, and Blood Institute, National Institutes of Health, U.S. Department of Health and Human Services. Clinical Guidelines on the Identification, Evaluation, and Treatment of Overweight and Obesity in Adults, Evidence Report, 1998. NIH Publication No. 98-4083.

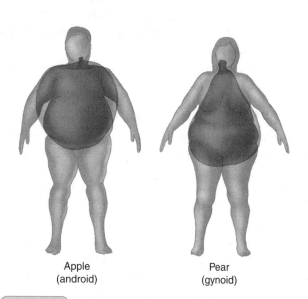

Apple (android)   Pear (gynoid)

Figure 11.2 Apple vs. pear shape. Android and gynoid fat distribution patterns. Individuals exhibiting android fat distribution have high waist-to-hip ratios and are at greater risk for cardiovascular disease.

eas are simple, noninvasive, and inexpensive ways to determine appropriate weight and the health risk status of individuals. However, these measures do not provide specific information about the actual quantity of body fat, muscle mass, and other components in the body that make up total body mass. Determining actual body fat, muscle mass, and bone mineral mass percentages (body composition) helps further determine health status and, for athletes, is an excellent way to determine whether weight is optimal for sport performance.

gaining the performance edge

Height, weight, and waist circumference measures are fast, easy, inexpensive, and noninvasive tools that every health care provider should use. Calculating BMI or using a nomogram with BMI levels for various heights and weights is simple and gives reliable information quickly about the patient. Waist-only and waist-to-hip circumference measures can give additional information to help assess health risk as well as body fat distribution.

the measurements are taken, the WHR is calculated by dividing the waist girth by the hip girth. Females and males with WHRs >0.80 and >0.91, respectively, run a higher risk for cardiovascular disease, diabetes, hypertension, and certain cancers.[13] A low-risk WHR value is <0.73 and <0.85 in women and men, respectively.[13]

Why is body composition important?

Measures of height versus weight and measures of distribution of body fatness in the waist and hip ar-

What makes up the composition of the body?

The body is made up of a variety of tissues and substances that contribute to total body mass. **Fat mass (FM)** is the weight of body fat. Body fat is made up of about 10% water and 90% adipose tissue. **Essential body fat** is the fat associated with the internal organs, central nervous system, and bone marrow. Without fat in these areas, the body can-

fat mass (FM) The portion of body composition that is fat. Fat mass includes both fat stored in the fat cells and essential body fat.

essential body fat Fats found within the body that are essential to the normal structure and function of the body.

nonessential body fat Fat found in adipose tissue. Nonessential body fat is also called "storage fat."

fat-free mass (FFM) The weight of all body substances except fat. Fat-free mass is primarily made up of organ weight and the skeletal muscles, including minerals, protein, and water.

lean body mass (LBM) The portion of a body's makeup that consists of fat-free mass plus the essential fats that comprise those tissues.

bone mineral mass (BMM) The weight of the mineral content of bone.

percent body fat (PBF) The amount of fat mass found on the body expressed as a percentage of total body weight.

not function properly. In females, some essential body fat is also associated with mammary glands and in the pelvic region. The essential body fat percentage or the minimum level of body fat compatible with health in men is approximately 3–5% and in women is approximately 12–14%.[14] **Nonessential body fat** is found in adipose tissue.

Fat-free mass (FFM) is the weight of all body components except fat and is primarily made up of the skeletal muscles, including minerals, protein, and water, as well as organ weight. The term FFM often is interchanged with **lean body mass (LBM)**; however, LBM includes essential fat and FFM does not. Approximately 70% of the FFM is made up of water. **Bone mineral mass (BMM)** is the weight of the mineral content of bone based on estimations of bone density. Bone consists of approximately 50% water and 50% minerals and protein. Total bone weight is approximately 12–15% of total body weight, but only 3–4% of this is minerals.

Percent body fat (%BF) is the percentage of total body weight that is fat mass. The %BF is the number that most athletes and their coaches and trainers use to determine whether the athlete is at an optimal body composition. This combined with BMI will give a better picture of overall health and ability to perform in the sport.

The World Health Organization (WHO) and the NIH have not yet determined body composition recommendations for the average population. These organizations have not made these recommendations primarily because there are many techniques used to determine body composition, thereby making it difficult to compare results and make recommendations. In addition, some methods are costly, are time-consuming, may lack reliability, and are not readily available to the public or the average medical provider. As previously discussed, BMI and waist circumference measures are available, easy, and inexpensive, making these assessments appropriate for the general population. For athletes, body composition remains the preferred assessment (versus BMI and waist circumference) because it is a better

method for determining the quantities of both FFM and FM.

Body composition varies greatly between individuals. It is influenced by a myriad of factors including genetics, gender, age, disease, diet, and activity level. Young individuals tend to have higher resting metabolic rates, are more active, and as a result are lean. As puberty approaches, the males begin to build more muscle mass and the females more fat mass because of increasing sex hormone levels. In adulthood, job and family responsibilities tend to replace regular exercise, sports participation, or recreational activities, and the result over time is muscle mass decreases and fat mass increases. In older individuals, the continued decreased activity level and onset of certain chronic diseases such as osteoarthritis can compound muscle loss and fat accumulation. For these reasons and based on genetics and response to training, athletes in the same sport and with the same training regimen will have varied body composition measures.

What are the methods for measuring body composition?

Body composition can be measured in a variety of ways. Some methods are quick and relatively inexpensive to complete, whereas others are time-consuming, highly technical, and costly. The accuracy of the various body composition measurements is also highly variable. In fact, even the most accurate techniques have measurement errors in the 2–3% range. This section addresses the commonly used body composition measurement tools used in the field and laboratory, which include underwater weighing (UWW), air displacement plethysmography, bioelectrical impedence analysis, skinfold measurement, dual-energy X-ray absorptiometry (DEXA), and others.

The gold standard (or criterion) methods of determining body composition are underwater weighing (i.e., densitometry) and DEXA. These techniques are considered accurate, and their validity and reliability have been established in the research literature. UWW and DEXA are used to help validate other methods of body composition.

Underwater weighing

Underwater weighing or hydrostatic weighing is an assessment of body composition based on the determination of body density

underwater weighing The gold standard of body composition determination that involves weighing a person while he or she is totally immersed in water.

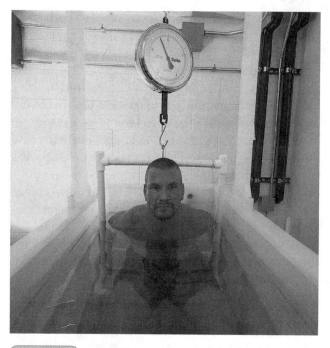

Figure 11.3 Underwater weighing. During underwater weighing, the subject must exhale completely, submerge without taking a breath, and remain motionless until the water is still and the scale is steady.

or densitometry. To determine the density of the body, the athlete is first weighed on land and is then submerged in a tank of water to determine his or her underwater weight (see Figure 11.3). The basic premise of this technique is that fat-free mass sinks and fat floats; therefore, the more the body weighs in the water, the less fat within the body. Because air in the lungs will also make a person float when submerged in water, the volume of air in the lungs at the time of weighing has to be determined and its effects factored out. After accurate measures of body weight in air and water have been determined, Archimedes' principle is used to determine body volume. Archimedes' principle states that the difference between the weight in air and the weight in water equals the weight of the volume of water displaced by the person's body:

$$\text{Mass}_{(\text{water displaced by body volume})} = \text{Body weight}_{(\text{in air})} - \text{Body weight}_{(\text{in water})}$$

Because the density of water is a known physical property, body volume can be calculated using the following formula for density:

$$\text{Density}_{(\text{water})} = \text{Mass}_{(\text{water})} / \text{Volume}_{(\text{water})}$$

When the density formula is rearranged to solve for the volume of water, it becomes:

$$\text{Volume}_{(\text{water})} = \text{Mass}_{(\text{water})} / \text{Density}_{(\text{water})}$$

Once the volume of water is calculated, it can be plugged into the following formula for determining density of the body:

$$\text{Density}_{(\text{body})} = \text{Mass}_{(\text{body})} / \text{Volume}_{(\text{body})}$$

The mass of the body equals the body weight in air, and the volume of body is equal to the volume of water, which was calculated above. Once the density of the body is calculated, it is converted to percent body fat based on data from laboratory studies that have measured the densities of various tissues of the body. The various tissues of the body have densities ranging from 0.9 g/mL to 1.1 g/mL. In short, the higher the body density, the more fat-free mass and the leaner the athlete is.

Most of the error associated with this method arises from the assumptions made when converting body density to percent body fat. Although fat density from one person to the next is fairly consistent, assumptions about fat-free mass can decrease accuracy. The problem is that it is assumed that all of the component tissues making up fat-free mass exist in the same percentages and make up the same percentage of FFM from person to person. This assumption is flawed because, for example, an osteoporotic female would have less dense bones than normal and her skeletal weight would therefore make up a lower percentage of her FFM than assumed. Fortunately, the induced error is relatively small under most circumstances, which is why underwater weighing is still considered the standard for body composition assessment. In addition, researchers have developed conversion equations for various subpopulations to account for known differences in FFM to increase the accuracy of this technique. Under ideal measurement conditions and applying the appropriate conversion formula, the standard error of measurement is approximately ±2.5%.[13]

The disadvantages of underwater weighing are that it has to be conducted in a laboratory because the water tank is not mobile; the protocol is fairly complex, so obtaining all the data needed requires some technical expertise; and many people do not like getting into a small tank of deep water, much less totally submerging themselves for several seconds while their underwater weight is measured. Finally, the test requires the person being measured to follow some very specific directions that some populations, especially children, can find difficult.

Air displacement plethysmography

A newer method of body composition analysis that is similar to UWW but enables determination of body volume based on air displacement rather than water is **air displacement plethysmography**. Just as in UWW, once body volume is known, the density of the body can be calculated and used to determine percent body fat. The commercially available machine that uses air displacement plethysmography is called the BOD POD. The BOD POD is an egg-shaped container in which the person sits (see Figure 11.4). Inside the container are two air chambers (one where the subject sits and another located behind the person) separated by a wall with a moving diaphragm. Once the person is seated inside the front chamber, the diaphragm between the chambers is used to produce pressure fluctuations in the chambers. Difference in the pressures between the two chambers is used to calculate volume in the

air displacement plethysmography A technique that measures the volume of air displaced by an object or body. In body composition assessment, air displacement plethysmography is used to determine the volume of the body so that the density of the body can be determined.

front chamber, which in turn can be used to calculate the person's body volume.

The accuracy of air displacement plethysmography is similar to underwater weighing. It is prone to many of the same assumption errors as UWW because once body density is calculated, assumptions have to be made to convert to percent body fat. The advantages to this method over UWW are that subject participation in the measurement is minimal, the subjects stay dry, and the fear of going underwater is removed. It is relatively simple to use and obtaining the measurement is quick. Also, the BOD POD is easier to maintain than the water tank used for UWW and is smaller, lighter, and more portable. The disadvantage is that the BOD POD is expensive and well above the budget of many facilities.

Dual-energy X-ray absorptiometry

Dual-energy X-ray absorptiometry has been used for measuring bone mineral density for research and health assessment for many years. It is commonly used to assess risk for osteoporosis and

dual-energy X-ray absorptiometry (DEXA) A method of body composition assessment that involves scanning the body using radiography technology to distinguish between fat and lean body tissue.

can measure bone mineral density (BMD) by region in the body. In addition to assessing BMD, DEXA also can be used for body composition determination. During assessment the individual is placed in a supine position on a table in the DEXA machine, and the DEXA scanner passes over the entire length of the body (see Figure 11.5). Just as with any X-ray technology, the various body tissues absorb or reflect the X-rays to varying degrees, allowing for differen-

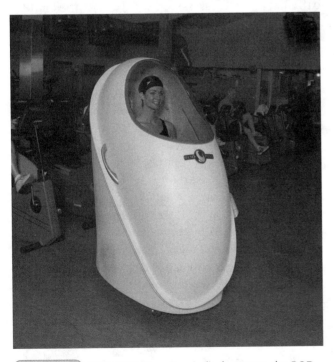

Figure 11.4 BOD POD. By using air displacement, the BOD POD provides an alternative to underwater weighing that is easier, cheaper, and of similar accuracy.

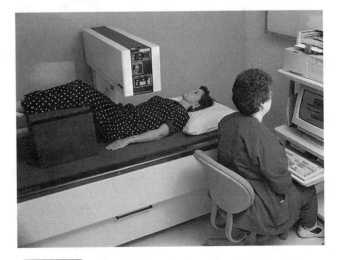

Figure 11.5 DEXA (dual-energy X-ray absorptiometry). The two-dimensional image produced from a DEXA scan can be used to assess body composition.

tiation between tissue types. The X-ray information is analyzed by computer software that differentiates between the various tissue types and calculates body fat percentage. Unlike UWW and the BOD POD, which are based on a two-component model of body composition (FM and FFM), the DEXA provides a three-component look at body composition (FM, bone mass, and lean body mass). Most studies have concluded that DEXA is accurate and correlates well with results from UWW.[15,16]

DEXA's advantages are that it is the only method that provides regional as well as whole body composition measures; it requires minimal cooperation from the participant, thus expanding its use to all ages and levels of health; it is easy to operate; and it is relatively fast (it takes 15 to 20 minutes). The limiting factors in using DEXA are that the machine is large, costly, and not mobile. As a result, these machines are usually found only in research institutions or clinical settings.

Bioelectrical impedance analysis

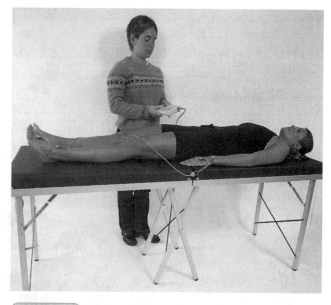

Figure 11.6 Bioelectrical impedance analysis (BIA). The measured resistance to a small electrical current passed through the body is used to estimate body composition.

bioelectrical impedance analysis (BIA) A body composition assessment technique that measures the resistance to flow of an insensible electric current through the body; percent body fat is then calculated from these impedance measurements.

Bioelectrical impedance analysis (BIA) has become a popular way to assess body composition. A variety of BIA machines are available to the general population for home use, and more sophisticated machines are available for clinical and research settings. During BIA in a lab, the person lies flat on a nonconducting surface. Electrodes are placed on two different parts of the body, usually one on the foot and one on the hand on the same side of the body (see Figure 11.6). An insensible electrical current is passed between the electrodes, and the resistance to the flow of the electricity is measured. Because the physical properties of fat make it an insulator, the greater the resistance to flow (i.e., impedance) of the electric current, the higher the percent body fat. Computer software then uses prediction equations based on gender and age to convert the impedance measures to percent body fat.

The accuracy of BIA depends on which prediction equations are used and whether certain premeasurement conditions are met. Of particular concern are any preassessment activities that might affect hydration level.[17] An athlete who is overhydrated prior to BIA assessment is likely to have a higher calculated body fat percentage, and a dehydrated athlete is likely to have a lower calculated body fat percentage than if the measures were taken in a normal hydrated state.[17] To obtain accurate measures, subjects should avoid alcohol consumption within 48 hours of testing; avoid moderate or vigorous physical activity within 12 hours of assessment; abstain from eating within 4 hours of the test; avoid ingestion of any substances that have diuretic effects, including caffeine, prior to assessment; and empty the bladder immediately before the test. When the appropriate prediction equation is applied and measurement conditions are met, the standard of error for BIA can be fairly small (±5%).[18]

The handheld or foot bathroom scale types of BIA do not provide as accurate of a measure as the typical laboratory devices. However, they can be used in combination with body weight to assess changes in mass over time. Athletes making dietary and exercise changes to alter body composition (either to gain FFM or to lose FM) may use these scales as an adjunct to weight measures alone. They can plot changes in %BF and weight over time to determine the trend in changes in these two parameters. For better success with assessing trends in using the handheld or foot scales, measurements should be done weekly on the same day and at the same time of day, before exercise and with the same average amount of hydration.

Skinfold assessment

Body composition can be estimated by measuring subcutaneous fat. The thickness of the layer of fat

skinfold calipers An instrument used to measure the thickness of skinfolds in millimeters.

directly underneath the skin is measured using **skinfold calipers**. During skinfold measurement, the tester pinches a fold of skin between the thumb and index finger. While holding the fold, the thickness of the fold is measured by placing the skinfold calipers perpendicular to and about a half an inch below the pinching fingers. The spring tension in the caliper jaws slightly presses in on the fold, and the skinfold thickness is measured in millimeters. (Figure 11.7) shows the skinfold calipers being used to measure the thickness of the triceps skinfold. Measurements are taken at several anatomical locations on the body. **Table 11.3** lists the common skinfold sites and their anatomical locations.

After the skinfold measurements are taken, prediction equations can be applied to determine the overall percentage of body fat. The accuracy of skinfold assessment depends on many factors. First, not all fat is deposited under the skin. In fact, up to 50% or more of the body's fat can be found in areas other than subcutaneously. As a result, an assumption has to be made that subcutaneous fat levels are accurate indicators of overall body fat. Many formulas have been used to improve the accuracy of subcutaneous measures as they relate to total body fat. In addition, technical errors in the skinfold measurement can decrease accuracy. Learning to take skinfold measurements requires proper instruction, education, and substantial practice. Pinching poorly shaped skinfolds, taking measurements at the wrong locations, placing the calipers incorrectly on the fold, and so on can all affect measurement accuracy. For example, if the caliper is left on the site too long (>4 seconds) before taking the measurement, the caliper jaws, which are spring-loaded, will continue to compress the underlying fat, thereby reducing the measurement at that site. If experienced testers follow the standardized measurement techniques and apply the correct prediction equations, then skinfold assessment can accurately predict %BF to within 3–4% of UWW.[19]

As has been discussed, many methods can be used to assess body composition in athletes. Selection of the method used will depend on what equipment and staff are available and its cost. Regardless of the method selected, the athlete should use the same body composition method in subsequent reevaluations. This reduces data variability caused by methodological differences between body composition protocols and makes it easier to follow actual changes that may be occurring in body composition over time. Generally, a lowered body fat percentage and higher lean mass are optimal for athletes. However, the ideal body composition for each athlete can be very different. Therefore, coaches and nutrition professionals should be careful not to set a single body composition level that an entire

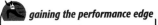

gaining the performance edge

Monitoring body composition in athletes provides a standard of measure that more accurately reflects body fatness than BMI or waist circumference measures. Periodic assessment of body composition, using the same mode of testing and following standardized protocols, will provide an ongoing way for athletes to assess their body composition over the course of a season and thus help them evaluate whether weight loss or gain is needed.

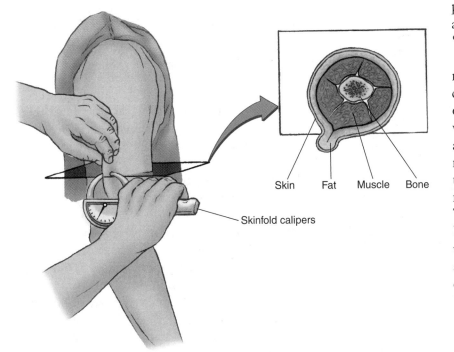
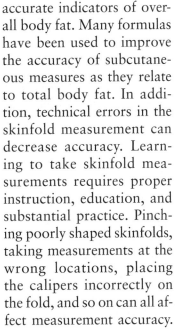

Skin Fat Muscle Bone

Skinfold calipers

Figure 11.7 Skinfold measurements. A significant amount of the body's fat stores lies just beneath the skin, so when done correctly, skinfold measurements can provide an indication of body fatness. An inexperienced or careless measurer, however, can easily make large errors. Skinfold measurements usually work better for monitoring malnutrition than for identifying overweight and obesity. They also are widely used in large population studies.

TABLE 11.3	Common Sites for Skinfold Measurements	
Name of Skinfold Site	Direction of Fold	Anatomical Location
Abdominal	Vertical	2 centimeters to the right of the umbilicus
Biceps	Vertical	Anterior midline of upper arm over the mid-belly of bicep muscle, 1 centimeter above the level of the triceps skinfold
Triceps	Vertical	Posterior midline of upper arm halfway between acromion process and olecranon process
Chest or pectoral	Diagonal	Men: half the distance between anterior axillary fold and nipple
		Women: one-third the distance between anterior axillary fold and nipple
Medial calf	Vertical	Midline of the medial aspect of calf muscle at the level of greatest girth
Midaxillary	Vertical	Midaxillary line at the level of the xiphoid process of sternum
Subscapular	Diagonal	1 to 2 centimeters below inferior angle of scapula
Suprailiac	Diagonal	Anterior axillary line just superior to iliac crest
Thigh	Vertical	Anterior midline of thigh halfway between inguinal crease and proximal edge of patella

Source: American College of Sport Medicine. Physical fitness testing and interpretation. In: Franklin BA, Whaley MH, Howley ET, eds. *ACSM's Guidelines for Exercise Testing and Prescription*. 6th ed. Philadelphia, PA: Lippincott Williams & Wilkins; 2000.

team or group of athletes should attain. Rather, body composition levels should be developed based on the individual athlete, their genetics, the physical demands of their sport, their performance goals, and their overall health.

How does body composition affect sport performance?

There are basic body composition levels identified for health of the general population but no set standards or ideals for athletes in specific sports or athletes as a group. When considering weight management and body composition issues, each athlete and his or her support staff must look at both the actual value of body fatness and lean body mass and determine whether changes in weight or body composition are warranted for that *individual athlete*. Assessment data can be compared to any published data for the specific sport, and additional considerations of the athlete's current sport performance, goals, diet, exercise patterns, and health should be made to determine whether body composition is in the ideal range.

Although the WHO and NIH have yet to set body composition standards for the general population, others have suggested healthy body fat ranges of 10–20% for men and 20–30% for women.[20] These general recommendations may not reflect sport performance norms for athletes. Athletes often assume there is an ideal weight or body composition that

is best for their sport and thus for them personally. Suggesting ideal body composition or body fat percentages by sport assumes that there is a known optimal combination of fat mass and fat-free mass that is best for sport performance in a particular sport or activity. However, "ideal" is difficult to define from athlete to athlete because there are so many individual considerations that contribute to body composition. Genetics, natural physique differences, and muscle and fat distribution are just a few things to consider. Sport performance is determined by a myriad of factors, only one of which is the makeup of FM and FFM in athletes.

The body composition levels required for maintaining health tend to be more lenient than those required for optimal performance in many sports. Therefore, body composition recommendations for athletes have been determined by taking the average body weights and fat percentages from large groups of elite athletes in various sports. Manore and Thompson did an extensive review of body fat percentages in male and female athletes in a large variety of sports.[21] Their report found variations in the ranges of body fat percentage in athletes within the same sport and of the same gender. These body fat percentages ranged from approximately 5–19% for male athletes and 7–20% for female athletes. These levels, and those from other research studies of body composition in athletes, can be healthy for some athletes but also could be quite low for other athletes and should not necessarily be considered ideal for a specific sport.

Different sports have different typical body composition levels. For example, sports such as gymnastics, track, and others in which the athlete must work against his or her own body weight to perform in competition tend to benefit from low body fat percentages. In these sports, excess body fat merely weighs the athlete down and does not provide any benefit in regard to force or energy production. In other words, fat weight in these athletes is considered "dead weight." At the other extreme are athletes performing in events where weight may be advantageous. For example, football linemen and sumo wrestlers benefit from the extra fat weight. Increased body weight in these athletes improves their stability, helps them to hold their ground, and/or helps them move lighter opponents out of the way. Another example where fat can be beneficial is for an athlete participating in long-distance cold water swimming; increased levels of body fat help the athlete float, decreasing drag and providing thermal insulation from the cold water. In these cases, excess body fat can enhance sport performance but is not good for cardiovascular health.[22]

There are many sports that fall somewhere in between the extremes in regard to body fat requirements. In some sports, body height is more important than body fat (e.g., basketball). In other sports, moderate levels of body fat can be beneficial as long as it is not at the expense of speed (e.g., rugby, hockey). Despite the fact that body fat levels vary from sport to sport, with all other sport-related requirements (e.g., skills, height) being equal, *excess* body fat is generally a disadvantage for athletes.

Many athletes closely monitor their body weight as if it is a good indicator of fat levels or body composition. Nothing could be further from the truth. Two athletes can weigh the same on a scale and even be the exact same height but have vastly different FM and FFM percentages. As a result, athletes who train regularly should not only track body weight but also have body composition measured routinely, especially if they are planning to either increase or decrease weight. Assessing body composition along with body weight can help the athlete determine which component of body mass is changing and thus whether the program is working. For example, if an athlete loses body weight, it could be resulting from either a decrease in muscle mass or a decrease in body fat. A decrease in muscle mass is not ben-

TABLE 11.4	Considerations and Information Needed when Setting Body Weight or Body Composition Goals for Athletes

1. The goal is to find the weight that is best for the athlete, not necessarily the lowest possible weight.
2. Assess genetics, resting metabolic rate (RMR), body composition, and activity level.
3. Calculate BMI.
4. Measure waist circumference.
5. Measure body composition.
6. Assess current eating habits.
7. Determine changes in dietary intake and exercise patterns that may naturally produce weight and body composition changes.
8. Assess training regimen—strength, cardiovascular, stretching, time, and intensity.
9. Review data on typical body composition for sport and assess whether this is reasonable for the athlete.
10. Determine whether modifying body composition or weight poses a risk (e.g., for injury, for an eating disorder) to the athlete.
11. Assess the athlete's attitude toward nutrition and behavior change.

eficial because of its negative impact on metabolism, strength, and power, thus indicating a change is needed in either the athlete's training regimen or his or her daily diet. Alternatively, an athlete aiming to lose weight on a particular diet and exercise program may not see a change in total body weight as measured by a scale. The failure to see a body weight loss does not necessarily mean the program is not working because muscle mass could have increased and balanced out any weight loss caused by decreased fat levels. Obviously, tracking changes in body composition over time is preferable and more informative than monitoring changes in body weight alone. **Table 11.4** provides a list of considerations and information that should be collected to help determine an optimal body weight and body composition for individual athletes and their sport.

What are the components of energy intake and energy expenditure?

An individual is in **energy balance** when energy intake is equal to energy expenditure. When an individual is in energy balance, weight remains stable. **Positive energy**

energy balance A state in which energy intake is equal to energy expenditure.

positive energy balance A state in which the total daily calories consumed are greater than the total daily calories expended. A positive energy balance will result in weight gain.

negative energy balance A state in which the total daily calories consumed are less than the total daily calories expended. A negative energy balance will result in weight loss.

balance occurs when energy intake is greater than energy expenditure, leading to weight gain. **Negative energy balance** is the opposite—when energy expenditure is greater than energy intake, causing weight loss. Maintaining energy balance is essential for the maintenance of lean tissue mass, immune and reproductive function, and optimal athletic performance.[23] When trying to lose weight, athletes must achieve negative energy balance. However, the right balance must be struck, where the calorie intake deficit or the increase in energy expenditure through training is not so great that it compromises sport performance. This section will cover energy balance, including assessing energy expenditure as well as the multiple components of energy intake and energy expenditure.

What influences energy intake?

Energy intake is simply calories consumed in the form of the macronutrients (carbohydrates, fats, and proteins) and alcohol. As discussed in earlier chapters, carbohydrates and proteins contain 4 kcal/gram and fats contain 9 kcal/gram. Alcohol contains 7 kcal/gram but does not provide any appreciable nutrients, vitamins, or minerals. Energy intake is usually higher in athletes versus nonathletes because of their higher energy expenditures. Food records, 24-hour dietary recalls, and dietary history interviews (see Chapter 10) are used to determine an athlete's energy intake.

Physiological, environmental, social, and emotional factors all regulate food consumption. These include both internal and external cues for eating. Internally, hunger and satiation provide signals for intake (see Figure 11.8). External factors include environmental stimuli such as smell, sight, and taste of food as well as the influence of the eating environment.

Internally, **hunger** prompts eating through physical cues such as gurgling or growling of the stomach. These are physiological signs that the body is depleted of energy and needs fuel. **Satiation** is the feeling of fullness that accompanies food intake and signals the

hunger A physical cue such as gurgling or growling of the stomach that prompts an individual to eat.

satiation The feeling of fullness that accompanies food intake and signals the time to end a meal.

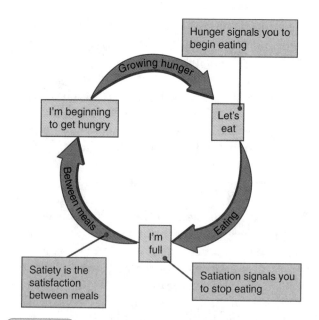

Figure 11.8 Hunger, satiation, and satiety. Hunger helps initiate eating. Satiation brings eating to a halt. Satiety is the state of nonhunger that determines the amount of time until eating begins again.

time to end a meal. **Satiety** refers to the feeling of fullness that maintains after a meal and helps determine the intervals between meals. The composition of the diet can influence hunger, satiation, and satiety. Protein has an increased satiety effect compared to fat and carbohydrates. The fiber content of a meal or food can enhance satiety by slowing gastric emptying. Total energy content can affect satiation and satiety as well. Energy-dense diets (those high in fat and low in fiber) tend to delay satiation and may encourage overeating. When any type of food is eaten, the stomach and intestines become enlarged and distended; this internal action has a satiation effect.

Appetite often is confused with hunger and therefore a distinction between the two is important in discussions of dietary intake and attempts to lose weight. Appetite is a psychological or emotional desire for food, whereas hunger is driven by a physiological need or drive for food. A number of factors stimulate appetite. External factors such as the smell of fresh baked bread or the anticipation of the taste of a favorite dessert can stimulate appetite. Social influences such as the time of day, social circumstances, and social events all affect appetite. Cultural influences of family and friends, foods that have special

satiety The feeling of fullness that maintains after a meal and helps determine intervals between meals.

appetite A psychological or emotional desire for food.

meaning, and traditions around food all can influence the desire to eat regardless of physiological hunger. Stress or other emotions can also encourage or discourage food intake that is not related to a physiological need for food.

What are the components of energy expenditure?

Three main components make up the total amount of energy expended each day. These components include the resting metabolic rate (RMR), the thermic effect of food (TEF), and the thermic effect of activity (TEA). Our body expends energy to maintain basic physiological functions (e.g., circulation, respiration, cellular functions), to allow for muscular activity, to process nutrients consumed, and to a lesser degree to help with temperature control. Energy expenditure increases during physical trauma, growth periods, fevers, and in extreme hot or cold environments and during exercise. Figure 11.9 illustrates the primary components of energy expenditure.

What is resting metabolic rate?

Figure 11.9 demonstrates that the largest portion of calorie expenditure is attributable to fueling basic physiologic functions. The body is constantly building and tearing down cells to continue functions for life. This portion of total energy expenditure is termed basal metabolic rate (BMR) or resting metabolic rate (RMR). RMR and BMR are often used interchangeably. However, RMR is usually slightly higher than BMR because RMR is assessed several hours after a meal or physical activity and BMR is assessed while the individual is in a totally rested state (no exercise for 12–18 hours and after an overnight sleep). RMR reflects a more practical measure. The functions included in RMR are the respiratory process, circulation, heartbeat, muscle functions, nervous functions, temperature regulation, and all of the organ functions that are very metabolically active. It is estimated that 60–75% of the total energy expenditure daily is RMR.[24]

Many factors can influence RMR. Individuals with higher body weight or larger surface area have a higher RMR. Those with increased lean body mass have a higher RMR because muscle tissue is more metabolically active than fat tissue. Caffeine intake and smoking increase RMR, as does hot or

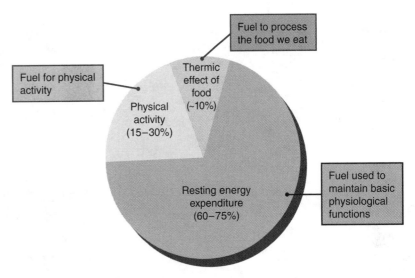

Figure 11.9 Major components of energy expenditure. The majority of daily energy expenditure is used to maintain physiological functions. Energy expended by athletes during physical activity and exercise is significant and could equal or exceed the energy needed for maintaining resting energy expenditure. The thermic effect of food is the energy required to digest, absorb, transport, metabolize, and store food.

cold ambient temperature. Rapid growth and some medical conditions can increase or decrease RMR. Each individual's RMR remains relatively consistent over time, but significant differences in RMR can be found when comparing different individuals.

There are several ways to assess actual total daily energy expenditure. Many are used in research or hospital settings and are available only to research participants or hospitalized patients. These measures include direct calorimetry using a whole body calorimeter; indirect calorimetry, which measures oxygen consumed and carbon dioxide produced; and doubly labeled water that measures isotope excretion rates. These methods are costly to administer and not widely available to the public. Because these methods are not quick and easy to use in the athletic training room, on the field, or in a sports professional's office, other methods to estimate energy expenditure must be used.

Regression or prediction equations are the most commonly used practical method to help determine energy expenditure and thus energy requirements. **Table 11.5** presents four calculation methods that can be applied in clinical and training settings to provide an estimation of daily energy requirements. One consideration when using prediction equations to estimate energy needs of athletes is how the equations were developed. Most prediction equations used the general population, both obese and nonobese, and

TABLE
11.5
Calculating Energy Needs

Harris-Benedict Equation Method

Adult Males

Resting energy expenditure = 66.5 + 13.7 (Weight in kg)
    + 5.0 (Height in cm) − 6.8 (Age)

Adult Females

Resting energy expenditure = 655 + 9.6 (Weight in kg)
    + 1.8 (Height in cm) − 4.7 (Age)

Source: Harris J, Benedict F. *A Biometric Study of Basal Metabolism in Man.* Washington, DC: Carnegie Institute of Washington; 1919.

Dietary Reference Intakes (DRI) Method: Estimated Energy Requirements for Adults

Males

662 − 9.53 (age) + PA × (15.91 × [weight in kg]
    + 539.6 × [height in meters])
PA (physical activity):
    1.0 Sedentary
    1.11 Low active
    1.25 Active
    1.48 Very active

Females

354 − 6.91(age) + PA × (9.36 × [weight in kg]
    + 726 × [height in meters])
PA (physical activity):
    1.0 Sedentary
    1.12 Low active
    1.27 Active
    1.45 Very active

Source: Institute of Medicine. *Dietary Reference Intakes for Energy, Carbohydrate, Fiber, Fatty Acids, Cholesterol, Protein, and Amino Acids (Macronutrients).* Food and Nutrition Board. Washington, DC: National Academies Press; 2005.

Resting Energy Expenditure (REE) Calculations and Activity Factors

Gender and Age (years)	Equation (BW in kilograms)	Activity Factor
Males, 10–18 years old	REE = (17.5 × BW) + 651	1.6–2.4
Males, 19–30 years old	REE = (15.3 × BW) + 679	1.6–2.4
Males, 31–60 years old	REE = (11.6 × BW) + 879	1.6–2.4
Females, 10–18 years old	REE = (12.2 × BW) + 749	1.6–2.4
Females, 19–30 years old	REE = (14.7 × BW) + 496	1.6–2.4
Females, 31–60 years old	REE = (8.7 × BW) + 829	1.6–2.4

Source: World Health Organization. Energy and Protein Requirements. Report of a Joint FAO/WHO/UNU Expert Consultation. Technical Report Series 724. Geneva, Switzerland: World Health Organization; 1985.

Cunningham Equation

Males and Females

RMR = 500 + 22 FFM (kg)

Source: Cunningham JJ. A reanalysis of the factors influencing basal metabolic rate in normal adults. *Am J Clin Nutr.* 1980;33:2372–2374.

did not use athletes in their studies that resulted in the development of the equations. Each equation can be applied to athletes, but the sports nutrition professional must be aware that these are prediction equations, meaning just that—they predict or estimate energy expenditure. Practitioners working with athletes should use their clinical and sport knowledge and expertise along with the equations to determine baseline energy needs for athletes.[25] Here is an example of how two different equations applied to the same athlete produce different results:

Male athlete, 180 lb, 5′11″, 24 years old, high-intensity training 1–1.5 hours/day

WHO equation:

REE = 15.3 × 81.8 + 679 = **1930**

Harris-Benedict equation:

REE = 66.5 + (13.7 × 81.8) + (5 × 180.3)
− (6.8 × 24) = **2251**

The WHO and Harris-Benedict equations predict *resting* energy expenditure for 24 hours. To arrive at estimates of 24-hour total energy expenditure, the REE must be multiplied by an activity factor to account for the thermic effect of exercise or activity.[26] Activity factors range from 1.2 if confined to bed rest, low activity 1.3, average activity 1.5–1.75, and highly active 2.0.[27] The WHO equation listed in Table 11.5 uses activity factors of 1.6–2.4, which may be a better estimate of the thermic effect of activity for athletes.

To complete the example for the 180 lb male athlete with high-intensity training, an activity factor of 2.0 is applied:

WHO equation:

$$REE = 1930 \times 2.0 = 3860$$

Harris-Benedict equation:

$$REE = 2251 \times 2.0 = 4502$$

Both equations are applied correctly but result in more than a 600-calorie estimate difference. This is a good example of why sports nutrition professionals must use their expertise and experience in figuring athletes' needs. Providing a range of calories, calculating two or three different ways, and using clinical judgment based on the diet and exercise information from the athlete can help determine the best calorie-level range for each individual athlete.

What is the thermic effect of activity?

In the average population, RMR is the highest percentage of total daily energy expenditure. In athletes, the energy expended through exercise can actually meet or exceed estimated RMR rates. The **thermic effect of activity (TEA)** includes the energy costs for skeletal muscle contraction and relaxation as well as the costs to maintain posture and position. **Table 11.6** lists the energy costs of various daily and sport activities. For example, a male triathlete weighing 60 kilograms who bikes for 4

thermic effect of activity (TEA) The amount of energy required to meet the energy demands of any physical activity.

TABLE 11.6	Energy Expenditure of Sport Activities							
				Kcal/hr at Different Body Weights				
Description	Kcal/hr/kg	Kcal/hr/lb	50 kg 110 lb	57 kg 125 lb	68 kg 150 lb	80 kg 175 lb	91 kg 200 lb
Aerobics							
light	3.0	1.36	150	170	205	239	273
moderate	5.0	2.27	250	284	341	398	455
heavy	8.0	3.64	400	455	545	636	727
Bicycling							
leisurely < 10 mph	4.0	1.82	200	227	273	318	364
light 10–11.9 mph	6.0	2.73	300	341	409	477	545
moderate 12–13.9 mph	8.0	3.64	400	455	545	636	727
fast 14–15.9 mph	10.0	4.55	500	568	682	795	909
racing 16–19 mph	12.0	5.45	600	682	818	955	1091
BMX or mountain	8.5	3.86	425	483	580	676	773
Daily activities							
sleeping	1.2	0.55	60	68	82	95	109
studying, reading, writing	1.8	0.82	90	102	123	143	164
cooking, food preparation	2.5	1.14	125	142	170	199	227
Home activities							
house painting, outside	4.0	1.82	200	227	273	318	364
general gardening	5.0	2.27	250	284	341	398	455
shoveling snow	6.0	2.73	300	341	409	477	545
Running							
jogging	7.0	3.18	350	398	477	557	636

(continued)

TABLE 11.6

Energy Expenditure of Sport Activities *(Continued)*

Description	Kcal/hr/kg	Kcal/hr/lb	Kcal/hr at Different Body Weights				
			50 kg 110 lb	57 kg 125 lb	68 kg 150 lb	80 kg 175 lb	91 kg 200 lb
running 5 mph	8.0	3.64	400	455	545	636	727
running 6 mph	10.0	4.55	500	568	682	795	909
running 7 mph	11.5	5.23	575	653	784	915	1045
running 8 mph	13.5	6.14	675	767	920	1074	1227
running 9 mph	15.0	6.82	750	852	1023	1193	1364
running 10 mph	16.0	7.27	800	909	1091	1273	1455
Sports							
Frisbee, ultimate	3.5	1.59	175	199	239	278	318
hacky sack	4.0	1.82	200	227	273	318	364
wind surfing	4.2	1.91	210	239	286	334	382
golf	4.5	2.05	225	256	307	358	409
skateboarding	5.0	2.27	250	284	341	398	455
rollerblading	7.0	3.18	350	398	477	557	636
soccer	7.0	3.18	350	398	477	557	636
field hockey	8.0	3.64	400	455	545	636	727
swimming, slow to moderate laps	8.0	3.64	400	455	545	636	727
skiing downhill, moderate effort	6.0	2.73	300	341	409	477	545
skiing cross country, moderate effort	8.0	3.64	400	455	545	636	727
tennis, doubles	6.0	2.73	300	341	409	477	545
tennis, singles	8.0	3.64	400	455	545	636	727
Walking							
strolling < 2 mph, level	2.0	0.91	100	114	136	159	182
moderate pace ~3 mph, level	3.5	1.59	175	199	239	278	318
brisk pace ~3.5 mph, level	4.0	1.82	200	227	273	318	364
very brisk pace ~4.5 mph, level	4.5	2.05	225	256	307	358	409
moderate pace ~3 mph, uphill	6.0	2.73	300	341	409	477	545

Source: Adapted from Nieman DC. *Exercise Testing and Prescription*. 4th ed. Mountain View, CA: Mayfield Publishing; 1999.

hours (average speed 18 mph) and runs (7:30 minute per mile) for 1 hour could expend 3690 calories during one training day.

What is the thermic effect of food?

thermic effect of food (TEF) The increase in energy expenditure associated with food consumption.

The **thermic effect of food (TEF)** is the increase in energy expenditure associated with food consumption. The digestion and absorption processes of food intake require energy, as does the metabolism and eventual storage of nutrients throughout the body. The TEF is estimated to account for approximately 10% of total daily energy expenditure when a mixed diet is consumed.[28] For example, an athlete who consumes 3000 calories per day will expend approximately 300 calories (10% TEF) to metabolize the food. Simply eating calories contributes to the daily total energy expenditure.

Variance in the type of macronutrient consumption may affect TEF. Protein and carbohydrates have slightly higher TEF because they require more calories to be converted into storage forms

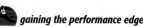

gaining the performance edge

Athletes may have a high total energy expenditure because of a higher RMR and the high energy costs of training. RMR is increased in most athletes because they have higher levels of lean body mass, which is highly metabolically active tissue. The energy costs of training and daily activity (TEA) could be as high or even higher than RMR, resulting in very high total energy expenditure daily.

(i.e., fat and glycogen) than fat. Conversely, fat consumed in the diet takes little energy to digest and then store as fat in the body. It appears that consuming a diet that contains a higher percentage of carbohydrates and protein and a lower percentage of fat may be beneficial in producing weight loss. However, regardless of the TEF, the most important reason that reducing intake of dietary fat can produce a calorie deficit resulting in weight loss is because fat is more calorically dense than carbohydrates or protein.

What methods do athletes use to lose weight?

Weight loss methods for athletes contain similar components as weight loss plans for nonathletes. There must be a calorie deficit through reduced calorie intake, increased exercise, or a combination of both. Weight loss should occur slowly, at a rate of approximately 1 to 2 pounds per week and should include goal setting and a monitoring system to encourage continued progress toward the weight and fat loss goals. Weight loss programs specific to competitive athletes should maintain a good balance of macronutrients for sport training (emphasizing adequate carbohydrate for glycogen use and replenishment and protein for lean tissue maintenance) and contain adequate energy and nutrients to continue to train and improve sport performance. If weight loss (fat loss) is desired, it should start early, before the athlete starts the competitive season.[23]

This section of the chapter covers calculating calorie needs, calorie deficit, macronutrient composition, meal planning, exercise, goal setting, and monitoring to help athletes lose weight.

How are weight and body composition goals for athletes determined?

After it has been determined that weight or body fat loss is indicated for an athlete, a goal weight or body fat percentage should be determined. Sports nutrition professionals should help athletes avoid choosing an arbitrary goal weight and use individual weight and body composition data to determine the best weight and body composition for each athlete individually.

Body mass index can be used initially to determine weight goals. In using a BMI nomogram or Web calculator, athletes plug their height and weight in the chart to determine current BMI. Next, they can choose a weight on the chart that is one or more

points below their current BMI, or one that may correspond with a BMI in the normal range. The choice of a BMI goal weight depends greatly on current BMI, level of overweight or obesity, weight history and/or history of recent weight gain, level of exercise, and commitment to a long-term weight management plan. The weight goal chosen also should fall within the general guideline of not losing more than 1 to 2 pounds per week and, as discussed earlier in the chapter, should fall within the goal of a 5–10% loss of current body weight.

In many instances, athletes should use weight and body composition data to determine appropriate weight (fat) loss goals. Athletes attempting to lose weight should have both BMI and body composition measured before starting a weight loss program. Once %BF is determined, a calculation can be completed to determine optimal body weight based on desired body fat level. For example, a 20-year-old college male middle-distance runner had a BOD POD measurement of 11% body fat. He is 5′10″ and weighs 160 pounds (BMI = 23). Typically, college middle-distance runners have 6–9% BF. He and his sports dietitian determine that 8% body fat is a good goal for him based on his BMI and current percentage of body fat. His weight loss goal can be calculated using the following formulas:

> FM = %BF × Body weight (lbs or kg)
>
> FFM = Body weight − FM
>
> Desired body weight = FFM ÷ (1 − [desired %BF])
>
> Calculate FM: 0.11 × 160 = 17.6
>
> Calculate FFM: 160 − 17.6 = 142.4
>
> *Desired Body Weight:* 142.4 ÷ (1 − 0.08) = 154.8

This example shows that a modest weight loss of approximately 5 pounds (primarily fat loss) could be enough for this athlete to achieve a 3% drop in his body fat percentage and a reduction to a BMI of 22. Once the goal weight and body composition are determined, athletes in consult with their sports dietitian need to determine energy intake that will produce this loss.

How are energy needs for weight loss determined?

To lose weight, energy expenditure must be greater than energy intake. When exercise and activity are equal to energy intake, weight maintenance occurs. If dietary intake is greater than energy expenditure, weight gain occurs. To achieve negative energy balance for weight loss, athletes can decrease food intake, modify exercise and activity levels, or both, creating a total energy deficit.

The first step in helping athletes lose weight is to calculate an athlete's estimated calorie needs using one of the equations listed in Table 11.5. This establishes an estimate of the athlete's baseline energy expenditure and a starting point for determining the number of calories the athlete should reduce to produce weight loss. Once this baseline is established, calorie intake recommendations should decrease this number by 250–1000 calories per day. This general guideline allows for a modest change in energy intake that will most likely not affect daily energy levels or the athlete's ability to recover from workouts. This large range of 250–1000 calories allows the athlete and the sports nutrition professional to have flexibility in calorie reduction levels based on the athlete's weight, current dietary intake, and goal rate of weight loss. Athletes must be reminded not to dramatically decrease calorie intake because it can negatively affect sport performance. The calorie recommendations for weight loss should always be compared to actual current intake and evaluated for necessary adjustments. For example, an athlete's total energy needs may be calculated at 3500 calories, which would translate into a weight loss recommendation of about 3000 calories per day. However, if the athlete is currently consuming 4000 calories, then suggesting a decrease in caloric intake merely to the originally calculated 3500 estimate may initiate some weight loss and appear less drastic to the athlete.

Combining a dietary reduction in calories with increased caloric expenditure is most likely to produce weight loss results for athletes. Obtaining a daily 500–1000 calorie deficit by changing only diet or exercise by itself may be challenging. Cutting calories too low often leads to hunger and discomfort. Most athletes cannot tolerate being hungry and thus have trouble adhering to the strict weight loss diet. In addition, very low calorie diets can result in the body going into a protective mode, thus lowering basal metabolic rate making further weight loss and long-term weight management difficult. Conversely, creating the calorie deficit solely from physical activity and exercise can lead to overtraining and injury. A combination of a 250–500 calorie dietary reduction and a 250–500 calorie deficit produced from increased exercise and physical activity can produce a weight loss of approximately 1–2 pounds per week.

What dietary changes are necessary for athletes to lose weight?

Dietary changes to reduce caloric intake are necessary for athletes to lose weight. Athletes need to concentrate on matching the macronutrient intake recommended for weight loss to that required for continuing sport activities. Portion control, regardless of macronutrient composition of the diet, is important in helping athletes reduce calories. Eating regular meals to avoid becoming ravenous as well as proper meal planning also play an important role in any healthful weight reduction nutrition plan for athletes.

How does the macronutrient composition of the diet affect weight loss for athletes?

When weight loss diets are objectively studied, it appears that regardless of macronutrient composition, if calories are reduced, then weight loss occurs. Macronutrient intake in athletes is of great importance in regard to sport performance. As previously discussed in Chapters 3, 4, and 5, carbohydrates, fat, and protein all perform essential functions within the body related to overall health, energy production, and sport performance. Therefore, when modifying an athlete's total daily intake, consider the relative importance of the various macronutrients.

Carbohydrates are the primary macronutrient that athletes need to perform well in sport and exercise activities. Carbohydrates are essential fuel for the working muscles during exercise and are valuable to muscles after exercise to replenish muscle glycogen stores. Many popular diets recommend severe restriction in carbohydrates, including those foods that contain valuable nutrients (fruits, vegetables, whole grain breads, milk, and yogurt); these plans are recipes for performance disaster, often depleting an athlete's body of carbohydrates as well as essential vitamins and minerals. It can be beneficial to reduce some carbohydrates in the diet if the sources of carbohydrates do not provide nutritional value; for example, reducing foods that contain high amounts of added sugars (candy, cookies, soda, etc.) will reduce overall calories consumed without reducing the nutrient density in the athlete's diet. Substituting higher-fiber foods such as grains, fruits, and vegetables for some of these calorie-dense foods can increase feelings of fullness and satiety so that athletes may consume fewer calories throughout the day.

Protein is important in any athlete's diet for maintaining muscle mass, building and repairing tissues, and providing satiety. Consuming adequate

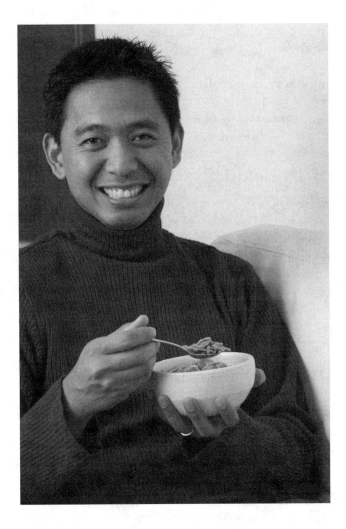

amounts of protein to maintain these functions is critical, especially when athletes are making lifestyle changes for weight loss. Maintenance of muscle mass can help keep the resting metabolic rate elevated, aiding in the weight loss effort and improving the likelihood of weight loss maintenance. Athletes who consume at least the minimum amount of protein recommended for their sport activities should obtain enough protein to maintain protein's necessary functions in the body. Protein intakes at the high end of the recommended ranges may be appropriate for some athletes to produce better satiety levels. Athletes should be encouraged to choose lean, low-fat protein sources that will contribute fewer total calories than high-fat options.

Fat is an essential component of a healthful athlete's diet; however, intake should be moderated while trying to lose weight. Fat contains more than twice the amount of calories per gram as carbohydrates or protein. Therefore, a reduction in fat can help produce a calorie deficit for weight loss because it is more calorie-dense. It should be emphasized that athletes are not encouraged to eliminate fat from the diet; a modest decrease in total fat intake to a level of approximately 20% of total calories will allow for the consumption of essential fatty acids without the contribution of excessive calories.

A weight loss plan that produces a reduction in calories, regardless of the macronutrient composition, should lead to weight loss. For all athletes, the macronutrient composition of the reduced-calorie diet should match their individual needs to produce weight loss while maintaining quality sport performance. Athletes should be educated on the detrimental effects of some popular diet plans that dramatically decrease or eliminate certain macronutrients, while encouraging the excessive intake of other macronutrients. For athletes aiming to lose weight, balance, variety, and moderation should remain the mantras of healthy eating, to ensure that all nutrient needs are being met.

How does portion control affect weight loss?

No matter the composition of the diet, portion sizes of foods consumed have an effect on calorie consumption and thus weight management. A small reduction in the size of portions eaten at each meal or snack can produce a calorie deficit for weight loss. This deficit can occur even without any change in the types of foods eaten. The MyPlate food guidance system and food labels can help individuals determine the serving size of different foods.

The standard serving sizes for the MyPlate food guidance system and the range of servings per day are found in Chapter 1 of this text. Food labels are required to list the nutrient information in one serving of the food and also to identify how many servings are contained in the entire package. Athletes may assume that the food contained in one package is one serving size, but that may not be the case. A discussion of how athletes can use the food label to aid in meal planning also is covered in Chapter 1.

Because serving sizes in restaurants and in food packages have become enormous, individuals mistakenly assume that one item or one meal served is a "normal" serving size. For example, a serving size from the MyPlate food guidance system for a bagel is ½ of a 2 oz bagel. A 2 oz bagel (2 servings of grains) contains approximately 150 calories. A 6 oz plain bagel, typical of many gourmet bagel and coffee shops, counts as 6 servings of grains and contains approximately 450 calories. This phenomenon of large servings of carbohydrate-rich foods has mistakenly led people to believe that carbohydrates cause

Training Table 11.1: Portion Control Tips

- Choose low-calorie, nutrient-dense foods such as vegetables, fruits, and whole grains.
- Serve smaller portions than usual on meal and snack plates.
- Purchase preportioned meals, entrée, and snacks and read labels to determine how many servings are in each package. Purchase more economical sizes of foods and package them into single serving sizes immediately once home from the grocery store.
- Use the MyPlate food guidance system serving sizes as a guide for portions consumed.
- Weigh or measure cooked food for a week to gain an understanding of appropriate serving sizes.
- At restaurants, plan ahead to take home leftovers. Remove bread and chips from the table and focus on enjoying the meal. Ask the wait staff to bring a take-out box when the entrée is served. Place half of the meal into the take-out box before starting the meal.
- Order off the appetizer or lunch menu. Many appetizers when combined with a salad or soup can make a meal.

weight gain. In actuality, it is the large number of calories consumed, which is often underestimated, that is contributing to weight gain. In the example of the 2 and 6 oz bagels, the larger bagel has an additional 300 calories! Therefore, a reduction in portions, regardless of the food item, can produce the necessary calorie deficit for weight loss. The portion control tips shown in **Training Table 11.1** can help athletes reduce total calorie intake.

How can athletes plan meals to meet weight loss and body composition goals?

If possible, athletes should attempt initial dietary changes for weight loss in the off-season. This allows the athlete to focus on moderating eating behaviors without the concern of how these changes might affect sport performance. Off-season modifications also allow time for the dietary changes to become a habit that the athlete can then follow throughout the season.

The emphasis of dietary changes should be on how athletes can decrease calorie intake without compromising sport performance. Meal skipping to reduce calories is not recommended because the lack of fuel prior to or after training can decrease exercise performance. However, consuming smaller meals and/or snacks frequently throughout the day will keep the body fueled while moderat-

ing calorie intake. Eating three to five times per day or approximately every 3–4 hours will sustain metabolism and energy levels. This schedule of eating can prevent athletes from becoming too hungry and subsequently overeating when a meal is finally consumed. Eating based on physical needs for food (hunger) helps the athlete fuel up when energy levels are low and provides regular intake of calories without overconsumption.

Consuming carbohydrate calories from sports beverages may be indicated for athletes during high-intensity workouts or during training or competition sessions lasting more than an hour. Some athletes avoid sports drinks during long-duration training or competition events for fear that the calories in these products will prevent weight loss; however, this concern is not valid. Sports beverages have multiple benefits, including enhanced endurance and sport performance, as well as the prevention of dehydration and electrolyte imbalances. Emphasis should be placed on helping the athlete improve performance by using these products. Sports nutrition professionals can weave these calories into an athlete's training diet, thereby providing the performance benefit of sports beverages while keeping on track for weight loss.

After exercise, athletes trying to lose weight must consume a postexercise meal or snack. Many athletes find the elimination of the postexercise meal or snack an easy way to decrease calorie intake. However, by neglecting to replenish the body, the athlete will feel sluggish, fatigued, and sore during subsequent workouts. Therefore, athletes should consume moderate amounts of nutrient-dense grains, vegetables, fruits, low-fat dairy products, and lean protein sources after exercise while limiting calorie-dense high-fat and high-sugar foods.

A sample meal plan for weight loss is listed in **Training Table 11.2**. Notice that substitutions of lower-fat, higher-fiber foods created the 500-calorie decrease. This method of modification retains the athlete's basic dietary pattern while selecting foods that have lower levels of calories.

How do exercise and physical activity influence weight loss for athletes?

Most athletes engage in more exercise than is recommended for the overall population in regard to health, prevention of weight gain, and to aid in weight loss. The updated physical activity recommendations for adults from the American College of Sports Medicine (ACSM) and the American Heart Association

Training Table 11.2: Sample Meal Plan for Weight Loss

2500 Calories	2000 Calories
Breakfast	*Breakfast*
1 cup dry cereal	1 cup dry cereal
¼ cup raisins	¼ cup raisins
1 cup, 2% milk	2 tbsp slivered almonds
1 cup orange juice	1 cup skim milk
	1 small orange
Lunch	*Lunch*
1 small whole grain pita sandwich	1 small whole grain pita sandwich
3 oz deli meat	3 oz deli meat
Tomato slices, sprouts, lettuce	Tomato slices, sprouts, lettuce
1 tbsp mayonnaise	1 tbsp low-fat mayonnaise
1 bag potato chips	1 bag baked chips
12 oz soda	10 baby carrots
	12 oz water
Snack	*Snack*
Frozen yogurt with chocolate sprinkles	2 graham cracker sheets
Dinner	*Dinner*
1½ cups pasta	1 cup whole wheat pasta
1 cup tomato/vegetable spaghetti sauce	1 cup tomato/vegetable spaghetti sauce
3 small meatballs (5 oz)	2 small meatballs (3 oz)
1 cup cooked broccoli	1 cup cooked broccoli
1 cup 2% milk	1 cup skim milk
Snack	*Snack*
1 cup lowfat yogurt	1 cup lowfat yogurt
1 large banana	1 small banana

(AHA) state that to promote and maintain health, adults need the following amounts of activity:

- A minimum of 30 minutes of moderate intensity aerobic physical activity on 5 days each week *or* 20 minutes of vigorous intensity aerobic physical activity on 3 days each week.
- A combination of these two aerobic intensity levels of exercise is acceptable.
- In addition to the aerobic activity, adults should perform activities that maintain muscular strength and endurance a minimum of 2 days per week.[29]

This amount of exercise may be challenging for nonathletes to achieve in one week, but athletes could easily attain this amount of physical exercise in only 2 or 3 days of training. The updated guide-

lines are outlined for the adult population to maintain health, prevent chronic disease, and prevent weight gain.

To lose weight, additional exercise and physical activity are needed, along with dietary reductions in calories. The updated ACSM and AHA guidelines further delineate that to lose weight or to maintain a significant weight loss, as much as 60–90 minutes of physical activity 5 days per week may be necessary. Typically, athletes who are training for competition are going to get that amount of exercise in 1 week. So, for athletes to benefit from exercise to lose weight, they may need to alter their training routine and try to get more activity as part of their daily routine. Activities such as walking to class or work, using the stairs instead of elevators, yard work, active housework, and getting off the bus one stop early and walking could produce modest calorie burning that, when combined with sport training, could help produce weight loss. Making sure they are getting the right amount of aerobic and strength training in each week can also help athletes achieve weight loss. Aerobic exercise (e.g., cycling, running, swimming, aerobic dance) increases energy expenditure. Anaerobic exercise (e.g., resistance training, sprint training) increases and helps maintain lean body mass, which is the most metabolically active tissue in the body. This raises and helps sustain RMR dur-

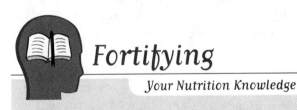

Fortifying
Your Nutrition Knowledge

Exercise Is Medicine

The American College of Sports Medicine and the American Medical Association launched Exercise Is Medicine in November 2007. It is a program designed to "encourage America's patients to incorporate physical activity and exercise into their daily routine." In addition, the program calls on doctors to prescribe exercise to their patients.

The program's Web site is www.exercise ismedicine.org and contains educational information for physicians to use in their practice and information for patients, the media, and policy makers as well as links to supporting organizations.

ing weight loss and weight management. Table 11.6 describes the amount of calories burned in many sport activities.

Similar to dietary modifications, athletes should attempt changes in exercise and physical activity during the off-season. Athletes are not necessarily focused on competitive performance in the off-season and therefore may be more willing to spend additional time on activities that may produce weight loss. To increase energy expenditure, an athlete can modify his or her workouts in several ways. Exercising at higher intensities or for longer durations can produce higher energy expenditure. Changing the type of aerobic workout performed can also help the body burn more calories per workout. Strength training is an important part of any athlete's exercise regimen for weight loss. Although strength training generally does not produce a large calorie expenditure, it helps maintain muscle mass, which is essential for maintaining a high RMR. Athletes should be encouraged to make gradual increases in workout intensity or duration to avoid overuse injuries.

How does goal setting help athletes lose weight?

It is difficult sometimes for athletes to make the necessary changes to help them achieve weight loss and maintain the weight loss over time. In Chapter 10, assessing readiness to change is outlined as one way to help nutrition professionals and athletes work together to make dietary changes. Once the athlete is ready to make changes in dietary behaviors, the athlete and nutrition professional should set goals and a method to measure the progress toward those goals for weight loss. Short- and long-term goal setting was discussed in Chapter 10. The following section provides a brief overview of goal setting as it relates to athletes attempting to lose weight.

What types of goals should athletes set for weight loss?

The NIH recommends initially losing 5–10% of current body weight over a period of 3–6 months. It then recommends maintaining that lost weight for 3–6 months before attempting further weight loss. If the athlete is able to maintain the initial weight loss and it is deemed appropriate to lose additional weight, then a goal of an additional 5–10% of current body weight is recommended. Using this recommendation, an athlete weighing 220 pounds would have a goal of losing 11–22 pounds in the first 3–6 months. If the weight loss is successfully maintained, then a reevaluation of weight and sport performance goals is appropriate. A total calorie deficit of 500–1000 kcal/day should produce this amount of weight loss gradually over the recommended time period. Weekly weight loss should not exceed 2 pounds per week. Rapid weight loss can contribute to muscle mass loss, fluid/electrolyte imbalances, and possibly cardiovascular complications. Therefore, if weight loss occurs too quickly, an increase in calorie intake or a decrease in physical activity may be indicated to slow the progression. Slow, gradual weight loss is safer for overall health, is more likely to target the loss of body fat versus muscle mass, is less likely to negatively affect sport performance, and has been shown to have a greater success rate long-term.

Setting a weight loss goal is essential to any weight loss plan, but goals for how to accomplish the weight loss are also needed. Goals should be developed that are short term or "process oriented" and long term or "outcome oriented." Short-term goals help the individual design a specific plan for dietary, exercise, or behavior changes needed to meet the long-term weight loss goal. These might include eating a high-fiber breakfast cereal every day for the next 7 days or spending an additional 15 minutes on strength training at practice twice per week. Long-term goals might include a weight loss goal or a body composition goal such as a reduction in body fat percentage. Once a short-term goal has been maintained for several weeks, a different goal can be established to further progress toward the long-term goal.

Other goals such as those that focus on changes in sport performance may motivate athletes to continue healthful eating behaviors. A goal of achieving a personal best in a sprint or long-distance event may motivate the competitive runner to continue with healthy eating behaviors. Realizing improvements in sport performance typically keeps athletes motivated, especially if weight loss is slow. Similarly, using both body composition and weight as measures of success is beneficial to the athlete. Because dietary and physical activ-

gaining the performance edge

Healthful weight loss programs for the general population and for athletes include a combination of diet and exercise changes to induce weight loss. A calorie deficit is essential to any weight loss plan. Athletes trying to produce a calorie deficit need to be careful to eat enough calories to continue optimal sport performance, while allowing for gradual weight loss. Weight loss should be attempted during the non-competitive season when possible.

ity recommendations for weight loss produce slow, gradual weight loss, it may be difficult for athletes to stay motivated when the scale does not show big losses. However, if body composition changes occur, the athlete can be confident that improvements are being made, despite slower weight loss. By setting both short- and long-term goals based on physical health or improving sport performance, the athlete establishes several ways to monitor success besides body weight.

How do athletes monitor progress toward goals?

Monitoring of goals and progress toward those goals is essential for continued weight loss success. Self-monitoring helps athletes identify the behavior they are attempting to change, track progress toward their goals, and regularly review the behavior and adjust as needed. Food diaries are helpful monitoring tools. Monitoring food intake by recording foods and portion sizes helps athletes become more conscious of food intake as well as the types of foods eaten. Athletes are often surprised at how often they eat without realizing it and how much is consumed at meals. Noting the level of hunger and satiation before and after eating can also add value to the food diary process. Athletes with already full exercise schedules might monitor intensity level of exercise or ability to train longer or harder once modest weight loss is achieved.

Monitoring weight or body composition is another useful tool for weight management success. Weighing once each week and plotting the progress over time can help individuals see gradual progress toward the long-term weight loss goal. Daily weighing is not recommended because it can become obsessive, and daily fluctuations in weight can occur regardless of food eaten or how much exercise is completed, leading to a false impression of weight loss or gain. Ideally, weight should be measured only once per week, on the same day of the week, and at the same time of day, to achieve consistency. Body composition measurements should be taken monthly or quarterly to evaluate progress. Evaluation of the effectiveness of an athlete's weight loss plan should include regular weight or body composition information as well as other measures of sport performance, energy levels, and satisfaction with the diet and exercise plan.

Evaluation of sport performance is another measure of success or failure of the weight loss plan. If sport performance declines, it could mean calorie intake is too low to sustain training levels and re-plenishment of glycogen stores. If sport performance is maintained or improves, the athlete is likely on the right track for weight loss success.

What are the summary recommendations for athletes regarding weight loss?

Successful weight loss practices for athletes include a combination of dietary, exercise, and behavior changes that can be maintained for a lifetime. Meal planning that encourages healthful eating at regular intervals while being mindful of portion sizes can provide the appropriate amount of calories and nutrients to maintain sport performance and allow for gradual weight loss. Exercise and physical activity levels are generally high in athletes, but slight modifications in the amount, type, or intensity of exercise can help produce a calorie deficit to achieve weight loss. **Table 11.7** provides a summary of recommendations for athletes trying to lose weight.

TABLE 11.7	**Weight Loss Recommendations for Athletes**

Determine Energy Needs
- Measure height, weight, waist circumference, and body composition
- Calculate athlete's estimated daily energy needs
- Determine calorie deficit appropriate for individual athlete to lose weight
- Calorie deficit of 250–1000 calories per day via diet and/or exercise

Dietary Modifications
- Emphasize healthful eating patterns and foods, not a "diet"
- Eat more often to fuel activities and avoid extreme hunger
- Enjoy small amounts of favorite foods occasionally
- Exercise portion control
- Choose nutrient-dense foods with more fiber for better nutrient intake and satiety
- Choose lower-fat foods

Set and Monitor Goals
- Attempt weight loss during the noncompetitive part of sport season
- Aim for a loss of 5–10% of current body weight
- Lose at a rate of no more than an average of 1–2 lb per week
- Monitor weight weekly
- Measure body composition monthly
- Assess training and sport performance level

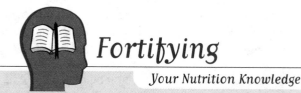

Should Athletes Go on a "Diet"?

There are many popular diet plans promoted for weight loss. These popular diets are often the first thing individuals try when aiming to lose weight. Unfortunately, most of these plans either are deficient in the nutrients required by athletes or do not promote long-term weight loss success, causing an athlete's performance to suffer and body weight to fluctuate over time. Athletes should be educated on how to decipher between a well-balanced, credible approach to weight loss and a quick-fix "fad" diet.

Diet books are a main source of popular diet information for consumers. Freedman et al.[27] reported in 2001 that a search of Amazon.com using the key words "weight loss" revealed 1214 matches. It seems that every year several "revolutionary" new diet books are published that claim to be the best new weight loss method. From low carbohydrate to high fat to cabbage soup to getting in the "zone," there seems to be no end to the number of weight loss diets available. One thing that all of these plans have in common is that they are low-calorie diets.

If fewer calories are consumed than expended, weight loss will occur over time. Therefore, in most cases, people who follow a popular diet plan lose weight. The problem is that weight loss is usually not sustained over time with these diets. Individuals may have success when "on" the diet but return to an equivalent or higher prediet body weight once they go "off" the plan. Athletes should be encouraged to avoid fad diets. Fad diets are too low in energy, do not provide enough nutrition for recovery needs, and will only decrease sport performance in the long run. Therefore, athletes should look for a diet and exercise regimen that they can continue long term and develop into a habit.

The main differences among popular diet programs are the macronutrient composition and the way foods are eaten or combined. Some plans suggest that a certain macronutrient composition is the key to weight loss success. Several current popular diets recommend lowered carbohydrate intake with subsequent higher fat and/or protein intake. Other plans suggest the opposite—low fat and high complex carbohydrates. Still others tout the benefits of a precise ratio of carbohydrates, protein, and fat eaten at every meal. In addition, some diets recommend a certain eating style, the combination of foods, or the avoidance of certain foods altogether. Athletes should look for weight loss plans that maintain a balance in macronutrients, allowing all foods to fit into a healthy diet, with a focus on portion control of all foods.

Being a good consumer of health and dieting information will improve an athlete's chances of success in weight management. There are many clues that athletes can use to determine whether a diet is a fad or has potential for long-term weight loss success. A credible diet should:

- Provide slow, progressive weight loss
- Emphasize health and emotional benefits, not aesthetics
- Include a sound, nutritionally balanced eating plan
- Include physical activity and exercise
- Include favorite foods in small amounts as part of the regular meal plan
- Include behavior modification changes and skill development for lifelong habits
- Include reasonable short- and long-term goals for weight loss, physical activity, nutrition, and health
- Be developed or monitored by credible medical personnel with experience in nutrition, exercise, and health

What are the weight loss issues for athletes in weight classification sports?

Weight classifications are typically found in sports such as wrestling, martial arts, crew (rowing), boxing, and horse racing (jockey). Athletes participating in these sports often try to perform in a weight class lower than their typical body weight to potentially gain a competitive edge over their competition. Athletes in these sports often struggle with their weight during the season and potentially use drastic weight loss measures to achieve their weight class goals.

Rapid weight loss prior to weighing in before an event, or **weight cutting**, is common for these athletes. Cutting weight is a practice of self-induced dehydration and starvation to reach a certain predetermined weight. It occurs often during a season, depending on how many events the athlete competes in and how well weight loss is maintained over the course of the season. Common weight cutting or rapid weight loss practices include excessive exercise, exercising in rubber or plastic suits, exercising in saunas or hot environments, fluid restriction, food restriction, spitting, fasting, self-induced vomiting, and laxative and diuretic abuse. Alderman reported that the most common rapid weight loss practices of wrestlers were excessive running, using saunas, and wearing vapor-impermeable suits.[30] These methods are usually undertaken immediately prior to the event so that rapid weight loss occurs in time for the weigh-in. Once the weigh-in is completed, rapid weight regain typically occurs through rehydration and food intake.

Some of these rapid weight loss methods can have significant health consequences. Dehydration and electrolyte imbalances caused by fluid restriction, exercising in saunas, and/or the use of diuretics and laxatives can negatively affect the cardiovascular system. Rapid weight loss, induced by a variety of methods, can quickly decrease plasma volume, thus acutely straining the cardiovascular system, thermoregulation system, and renal function. Food restriction can cause hypoglycemia, resulting in fatigue, an inability to mentally focus, and a decrease in physical stamina.[31] Clearly, all of these consequences are a detriment to sport performance, the safety of the athlete, and overall health.

Wrestling has been a very popular sport for years and is one of the sports most commonly known for weight loss practices. Significant research has been conducted on wrestlers' weight loss methods and the associated concerns. In 1997, three collegiate wrestlers died trying to cut weight for competition.[32] This unfortunate event prompted the National Collegiate Athletic Association (NCAA) to change collegiate wrestling rules in part to curb excessive weight-cutting practices. The new rules include adding 6 pounds to each of the 10 weight class categories, holding weigh-ins closer to the start of the competition, starting a wrestling weight certification program including a body fat assessment at the beginning of the season, and requiring the minimum competitive weight classification to be determined by December. Wrestlers can move up in a weight classification after December, but not down to a lower weight classification (see Figure 11.10). These new rules were implemented in full for the 1998–99 NCAA season. The wrestling weight certification program (WWCP) requires the weigh-in at the beginning of the season to be a hydrated weight.[33] The program uses the specific gravity of urine to determine hydration status. If specific gravity is at or below 1.02, then the athlete is well hydrated; if specific gravity is above 1.02, the athlete must come back the next day for a retest and weigh-in. Chapter 8 provides a more in-depth discussion of how hydration level affects urine specific gravity. High schools now have similar weight management guidelines to discourage rapid weight loss. Beginning with the 2006–7 season, the weight certification program includes a hydration level not to exceed 1.025 urine

weight cutting The practice of losing weight, usually in preparation for a competitive event in hopes of making a lower weight class and thus improving performance.

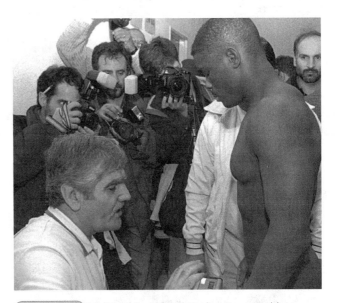

Figure 11.10 Weighing in. The NCAA discourages athletes from reducing their weight through intentional dehydration, a dangerous and potentially deadly practice.

specific gravity and minimum body fat percentage no lower than 7% for male wrestlers and 12% for female wrestlers.[34]

Opplinger et al.[35] studied 741 responses to questions from 43 collegiate wrestling teams about weight loss practices since the institution of the new rules. They reported that 40% of wrestlers in the study indicated that the new NCAA rules influenced their weight management practices; however, more than 25% of the wrestlers continued to use saunas and rubber/plastic suits and fasting as weight loss techniques. They also found that weight management behaviors were more extreme among wrestlers in lighter weight classes and became less extreme at the heavier weight classes. Little evidence existed for disordered eating in this sample. Davis reported that, based on their data, they believe the new NCAA WWCP and corresponding rule changes have begun to break the sport's historical cycle of weight cutting.[33]

Weight cutting can have both physical and emotional consequences. There is concern that athletes in sports that use weight-cutting practices may be at increased risk for eating disorders. Dale and Landers used the Eating Disorders Inventory (EDI) and Eating Disorders Examination (EDE) to assess wrestlers for eating behaviors.[36] The EDI is made up of eight different subscales. Only data collected from the first three subscales—drive for thinness, bulimia, and body dissatisfaction—were used. These three subscales examine attitudes and behaviors relating to body image, eating, and dieting. The EDE is a semistructured interview that was used on participants identified as being at high risk based on EDI scores. The researchers found that there was an increased drive for thinness in wrestlers but not an increase in actual eating disorders or eating disorder risk. Wrestlers in the study actually had a better body satisfaction rate than the matched nonwrestler controls. Wrestlers are more weight-conscious than nonwrestlers, but this does not mean they have eating disorders. Often the worrisome weight control practices occur only in-season. During the off-season, eating and weight control issues are not a concern. It is clear, however, that weight-cutting practices can be harmful to physical health, and focusing research and education on the physical consequences of weight-cutting practices may help alleviate these harms to athletes in the future.

Similar concerns for making weight are seen in other sports. Lightweight crew (rowing) is a team sport that requires the entire team to meet a weight standard to compete. If one athlete does not make the weight, then the entire team may be excluded from the event. Athletes in sports that require weigh-ins should focus their nutrition and exercise plans on maintaining a consistent weight throughout the season, rather than struggling to make weight prior to each event. Although dramatic weight loss methods are used less frequently by rowers than by wrestlers, they still may use unhealthy nutrition and weight loss practices during their training and competitive seasons. Coaches, trainers, and dietitians working with these athletes need to be aware of fast weight loss methods the athletes may be using and encourage healthful weight loss that can be maintained during the season.

When competing in events where weight must be measured, the best defense is a good offense. Athletes should attempt to maintain body weight year round within a few pounds of the weight class in which they compete. Some athletes may need to move up a weight class to comfortably maintain weight year round, which potentially means competing against tougher opponents. However, weight classes are designed to even out the competition from a weight standpoint. An athlete that moves up a weight class is likely to have more muscle mass and competitively should be on the same playing field as other athletes in the same weight class.

In summary, athletes in weight class sports face additional challenges in maintaining a competitive weight. Strategies for athletes to lose and maintain a healthy, competition weight are similar to the strategies used by other athletes. Establishing an appropriate, achievable weight early in the season or in the off-season, and then aiming to maintain that weight within a few pounds over the entire year, can help athletes avoid drastic weight loss measures to make weight. Coaches, strength trainers, dietitians, and athletic trainers can help the athlete decide the best competition weight to work toward. A sports diet and exercise plan that helps achieve that weight in a healthy manner can help the athlete achieve and maintain a stable competitive weight throughout the competitive season.

What happens when weight loss efforts develop into disordered eating patterns?

Problems with eating behaviors have become more prevalent in the last decade in the United States and in other parts of the industrialized world. Athletes not only face the same sociocultural influences on eating behaviors, size, and shape as the general population, but also have the pressure of fitting into the "ideal" for their sport. They see other athletes in their sport and assume they should look a certain way. Coaches, parents, and trainers may also suggest that a certain body type is advantageous and encourage changes in the athlete's body size or shape to help them excel in their sport. In many sports, athletes and coaches believe excess weight inhibits speed, agility, and endurance while increasing fatigue.[37] Although optimal body types may exist in general for certain sports, some athletes simply cannot achieve these stereotypes. Disordered eating develops when athletes continue to strive for that "ideal" at the expense of overall health and sport performance. As the obsession to achieve or maintain a certain ideal continues, athletes may develop eating disturbances that can lead to diagnosable eating disorders. Eating disorders have serious health consequences. Athletes with full-blown eating disorders often have decreased sport performance, are more likely to become injured, and suffer emotional and psychological consequences that affect life functioning.

Certain sports have an increased likelihood of encouraging negative body image and eating disorders. These sports place more emphasis on a certain body type as ideal or emphasize lean body shape or low body weight as optimal for the sport. Casual comments from coaches, officials, judges, and peers within competitive or practice environments can lead to negative self-perceptions associated with disordered eating.[38] **Social physique anxiety**

social physique anxiety A feeling of personal uneasiness or nervousness about how other people view or perceive the athlete's body shape or fatness level.

is a sense of anxiety resulting from situations in which one's physique or figure is being observed or evaluated by others.[39] Monsma and Malina, in a study of female figure skaters, found that after controlling for age and BMI, social physique anxiety was related to the Eating Disorders Inventory (EDI) score.[38] The authors suggest that disordered eating may be a response to social physique anxiety stemming from the subjective evaluative nature of figure skating. Clothing choices within sports can place athletes at greater risk for developing body image issues and disordered eating patterns, especially when not only the body but also the clothing can be subjected to judgment.

The American College of Sports Medicine developed the following list of sports likely to place women athletes at risk for developing eating disorders:

- Sports where the athlete is subjectively judged, such as diving, skating, gymnastics, and ballet
- Sports where minimal, tight, or revealing clothing is required, such as track, swimming, diving, gymnastics, and volleyball, which can make athletes uncomfortable
- Endurance sports such as long-distance running, cycling, and triathlons, where excess body weight may hinder performance, and therefore emphasis is placed on a lean body type
- Sports where weigh-ins are required, such as wrestling, horse racing, boxing, martial arts, and rowing[40]

These sports by their nature can place athletes, female or male, at greater risk for developing disordered eating. However, many women and men in these sports have normal dietary and exercise patterns, maintain their weight in a comfortable range, and never develop eating disorders. The sports listed are not the only sports in which athletes could potentially develop disordered eating patterns. Any athlete in any sport can succumb to the pressures of their sport or other issues in their lives and ultimately develop an eating disorder.

What are the different types of eating disorders?

The prevalence of eating disorders is difficult to determine because many individuals do not seek treatment. There are no national research projects or databases that gather statistics about eating disorders, and treatment can be sought from a variety of professionals—medical, nutrition, or mental health. Studies of the prevalence of eating disorders in athletes suggest an increased risk and incidence in athletes compared to the general population. Sundgot-Borgen and Torstveit reported a 13.5% incidence of eating disorders in athletes compared to a 4.6% incidence in nonathlete controls.[41] They studied a large group of elite Olympic athletes in Norway and a comparable control group. The researchers found the incidence of athletes who exhibited eating disorders was different based on the sport. In females, those in aesthetic sports had a 42% incidence, endurance sports 24%, technical sports 17%, and ball game sports 16%. Among male athletes, the prevalence of eating disorders was more common in anti-gravitation sports such as gymnastics or skating (22%) than in ball game sports (5%) and endurance sports (9%).[41]

The major classifications of eating disorders are defined by specific medical and emotional criteria. The American Psychiatric Association's *Diagnos-*

anorexia nervosa A clinical condition manifested by extreme fear of becoming obese, a distorted body image, and avoidance of food. Anorexia nervosa can be life-threatening and requires medical and psychiatric treatments.

amenorrhea The absence or abnormal cessation of menstruation; defined as less than four cycles per year.

bulimia nervosa A clinical condition characterized by repeated and uncontrolled food bingeing in which a large number of calories are consumed in a short period of time, followed by purging methods such as forced vomiting or use of laxatives or diuretics.

tic and Statistical Manual of Mental Disorders, 4th edition (DSM-IV), defines the classifications for diagnosis of three different eating disorder categories: Anorexia Nervosa, Bulimia Nervosa, and Eating Disorder—Not Otherwise Specified.[42]

Anorexia nervosa is a complex disorder with many causes and manifestations in behaviors. The main dietary concern with anorexia is severe calorie restriction leading to weight loss. Individuals with anorexia refuse to maintain body weight at or above a minimum level that would be normal for height versus weight, have an intense fear of weight gain, have a distorted body image, and have **amenorrhea** or the absence of menstrual cycles. Severe restriction of energy intake resulting in a significant calorie deficit and weight loss is commonly seen in individuals with anorexia. Some of these individuals also binge and purge the food they consume, while others maintain a constant low energy intake.

Complications of anorexia can be quite severe. Amenorrhea and energy deficit can lead to decreased bone density. Irregular and slow heart rates are commonly observed in anorexic patients. Dehydration, nutritional deficiencies, dizziness, fatigue, and social withdrawal are other common complications of anorexia. These complications can be dangerous to the overall health of the athlete and can significantly reduce sport performance levels.

Bulimia nervosa is characterized by an individual who binges on larger-than-normal amounts of foods and then uses inappropriate compensatory methods to rid him- or herself of the food consumed. The binge episodes are characterized as being out of control, with an inability to stop eating despite being overly full. The common misconception of bulimia is that purging is done exclusively through vomiting. The inappropriate compensatory behaviors after a binge can be any one of the following: vomiting, laxative abuse, excessive exercise, fasting, or any combination of these behaviors. Bulimia, similar to anorexia, is also characterized by a distorted body image and appearance having undo influence on self-esteem, eating, and exercise behaviors.

The prevalence of bulimia is higher in all population groups than anorexia is. Complications of bulimia nervosa can be quite severe. Erosion of tooth enamel, tears in the esophagus, chronic reflux, heart abnormalities, aspiration pneumonia, and even death can occur with vomiting as the main purging method. If laxatives are abused as a purging method, the intestinal tract becomes dependent on laxatives to move the bowels. This can lead to chronic constipation. Excessive exercise places the individual at greater risk for athletic-related injuries. Emotional and psychological concerns of lack of self-worth, self-loathing, anxiety, and depression can be concurrent conditions with bulimia nervosa.

In many cases, one or more of the criteria for bulimia nervosa or anorexia nervosa are not met. Thus, a diagnosis of bulimia or anorexia cannot be made. Another diagnosis listed in the DSM-IV called **Eating Disorder–Not Otherwise Specified (ED-NOS)** was created for disorders of eating that do not meet the criteria for anorexia or bulimia. For example, a female may have all of the criteria for anorexia nervosa, but the athlete is having regular menses. This category allows for the description of a variety of eating disturbances that can significantly affect the afflicted person's life but do not completely meet the criteria for anorexia or bulimia. With any type of eating disorder, the effects of low energy intake and/or the binge/purge cycle can eventually be detrimental to sport performance.

Eating Disorder–Not Otherwise Specified (ED-NOS) An eating disorder that does not meet all the criteria needed for it to be diagnosed as either bulimia nervosa or anorexia nervosa but that meets enough of the diagnostic criteria to be labeled as a true eating disorder.

anorexia athletica (AA) A subclinical condition in which individuals practice inappropriate eating behaviors and weight control methods to prevent weight gain and/or fat increases. Anorexia athletica does not meet the criteria for a clinically defined eating disorder, but the behaviors exhibited are on a continuum that could lead to the more severe clinically recognized eating disorders.

Anorexia athletica (AA) is not in the DSM-IV manual but is important in the discussion of athletes and eating disorders. There are many similarities to both bulimia and anorexia in the description of anorexia athletica; however, athletes are a unique population, and interpretation of symptoms that may meet criteria for ED-NOS may be somewhat different from those in the nonathlete population. Several factors distinguish anorexia athletica from the other eating disorders. Often athletes (both male and female) with anorexia athletica show a reduced energy intake and reduced body weight but maintain high levels of physical performance; athletes with other eating disorders typically have a diminished capacity or tolerance for training and competition. Another distinguishing factor of AA is that the reduction in body weight or loss of body fat is based on performance rather than appearance or concern with body shape or size.

The actual criteria for defining anorexia athletica are still not completely agreed upon by researchers in this area. However, several reviews of the characteristics of anorexia athletica have been published by different authors working with athletes in the eating disorder arena. With anorexia athletica, the athlete often has a rigid training schedule, tries to delay eating to save calories, and then often binges because of excessive hunger and lowered glucose levels. The common characteristics of anorexia athletica are listed in **Table 11.8** and are similar to anorexia nervosa, but with some additional characteristics related specifically to female athletes.[41,43]

Many athletes do not meet the criteria for anorexia, bulimia, or eating disorders not otherwise specified but still struggle with eating issues. These may be athletes who rarely binge and use compensatory behaviors, but might do so in a particularly stressful situation. They may also chronically diet; be overly concerned with their weight, body composition, and appearance; and make judgments about themselves based on the types of foods they have eaten or the number on the scale. Sport performance can suffer if the athlete does not eat enough calories to maintain energy levels during practice or competition. Some athletes may avoid carbohydrates as a way to diet, and glycogen stores will chronically be low, resulting in poor sport performance. Excessive exercise as a means to burn more calories could lead to injuries that keep the athlete out of competition. Although athletes with these types of eating behaviors do not meet the criteria for an eating disorder, the behaviors can negatively affect daily life and inhibit maximal sport performance.

What are the effects of eating disorders on athletic performance?

Athletes with eating disorders may appear normal and healthy and be able to maintain training levels for a period of time before any concerns develop. Typically, a change in weight is noticed that may not initially affect performance. Behavioral changes, such as withdrawal from teammates and coaches or atypical behaviors relating to other members, can also occur. Mental toughness and typical competitiveness may decrease, especially as caloric intake is decreased. Self-esteem and self-confidence may be reduced, and depression or anxiety can occur.

Physically, once the eating disorder has progressed, the athlete's performance during training and competition suffers. In some athletes this happens within a few months of restricting intake or bingeing and purging, whereas others can maintain a low caloric intake or binge and purge for many months before performance is altered. Eating-disordered athletes may develop nutritional deficiencies over time as a result of reduced caloric intake, chronic vomiting, or laxative abuse. If calories are significantly decreased, carbohydrate levels are often low. This causes an increased reliance on fat and protein as energy sources. When more protein is used for energy, less is available to maintain muscle mass. A decreased muscle mass almost certainly will decrease sport performance. Calcium, iron, and other vitamins and minerals may be lacking in the diet. This may eventually lead to iron deficiency, bone loss, and other consequences of vitamin and mineral deficiencies. Possibly most significant is the effect that reduced energy availability has on physical performance and health. When too few calories are consumed, energy expenditure from exercise is extreme, or a combination of both occur, the body lacks the energy necessary to sustain high levels of

TABLE 11.8	Characteristics of Anorexia Athletica

- Decreased energy intake
- Decreased weight in the absence of medical illness or affective disorder explaining the weight reduction
- Maintenance of high physical performance
- Desire to lose weight not based on appearance
- Desire for weight loss based on performance or perceived performance improvements
- Intense fear of weight gain
- Weight cycling based on training levels
- Dietary restraint
- Bingeing and purging
- Gastrointestinal complaints
- Menstrual dysfunction
- Compulsive exercise despite illness or injury
- View self-worth by athletic ability or performance
- Individual does not meet DSM-IV criteria for eating disorders, but possesses many eating-disorder characteristics

exercise intensity. In addition, this "energy drain" affects hormone responses that lead to menstrual irregularities and potential issues with bone health described later in the section titled "What is the female athlete triad?"

Some of the health concerns and psychological effects that may be noticed in athletes with eating disorders include the following:

- Decreased fat-free mass
- Dehydration
- Glycogen depletion
- Hormonal disturbances
- Decreased BMR
- Increased risk of poor nutritional status
- Poor exercise performance
- Anxiety, rapid heart rate, inability to sleep, and dehydration caused by the stimulant effect of diet pills and diuretics
- Dehydration, electrolyte loss, and gastrointestinal complications resulting from laxative use
- Increased risk of overuse injuries and fatigue caused by excessive exercise
- Decreased concentration
- Increased likelihood of food and weight obsession

What are the main concerns regarding female athletes and eating disturbances/disorders?

Female athletes are at greater risk for developing eating disorders than age-matched nonathletes.[43–45] Identifying eating concerns in female athletes early on can keep the athlete from developing a diagnosable eating disorder in the future. Certain physical characteristics, strict training regimens, dietary restraint, and attitudes and behaviors toward food and body weight are accepted as normal for many female athletes, making it difficult to use the usual criteria for defining disordered eating in this population. Many different questionnaires are used to assess eating behaviors in this population (such as the EDI, EDI-2, and EDE discussed earlier), but few assessment tools have been designed specifically to determine early signs of eating problems in female athletes.

The Female Athlete Screening Tool (FAST), designed by Affenito et al.[46] and researched by McNulty et al.,[47] can be used as a screening tool for eating disorders in female athletes. The FAST is able to measure the purpose of aberrant exercise and eating behaviors in those athletes with eating disorders, whereas the EDI-2 and EDE do not consistently differentiate between athletes and nonathletes

with eating disorders. Athletic programs in which female athletes participate at a highly competitive level should screen these athletes for eating disorders as part of the annual physical process.

What is the female athlete triad?

The **female athlete triad** (see Figure 11.11), typically observed in young female athletes, consists of three definable symptoms: disordered eating, menstrual irregularities, and osteopenia/osteoporosis. Cobb et al. reported that the actual existence of all three parts of the triad at the same time has not been well documented in the research.[48] These authors report that the relationship between disordered eating and menstrual irregularities, as well as separate studies that establish the relationship between menstrual irregularities and low bone mineral density, are well documented. Regardless of the ability to document all or some of the three

female athlete triad A group of three interrelated conditions, typically diagnosed in young female athletes—disordered eating, menstrual irregularities, and osteopenia/osteoporosis.

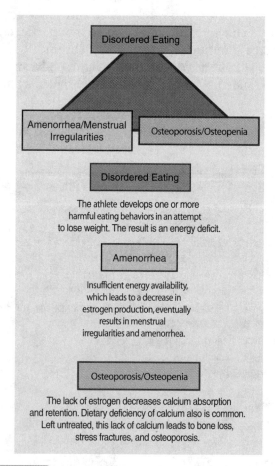

Figure 11.11 Female athlete triad. Disordered eating in female athletes that results in significant weight loss, energy drain, amenorrhea, or menstrual irregularities can also cause a loss of bone mineral density or osteoporosis.

components of the female athlete triad existing simultaneously, female athletes with one or more of the triad symptoms need early diagnosis and treatment for these concerns.

Disordered eating includes restrictive eating behaviors associated with eating disorders but may not meet the actual diagnostic criteria for eating disorders. Female athletes that exhibit disordered eating behaviors often restrict caloric intake and fat intake. They maintain a high training intensity and duration, thus producing a high energy expenditure and calorie deficit. Loucks and others have researched issues of energy availability and its effects on female athlete menstrual function. This research consistently reports that amenorrhea occurs because of insufficient energy availability or ingestion of too few calories to fuel both physical activity and normal body functions.[49–51] The disordered eating patterns seen in the triad are similar to those described earlier in this chapter for anorexia and anorexia athletica.

Irregular menstruation can be defined based on the number of menstrual cycles in 1 year. **Eumenorrhea** is defined as at least 10 or more menses per year and is considered normal. **Oligomenorrhea** is defined as 4–6 cycles per year, and amenorrhea is

eumenorrhea A term used to describe normal menstruation consisting of a least 10 menstrual cycles per year.

oligomenorrhea A condition in which the female menstrual period is irregular, with cycles occurring only four to six times per year.

defined as less than 4 cycles per year. Amenorrhea is part of the diagnostic criteria for anorexia. Oligomenorrhea and amenorrhea both are seen with the female athlete triad. These menstrual irregularities often cause changes in sex hormone secretion. Changes in hormone regulation are one of the causes of the decrease in bone mineral density found with dysmenorrheic female athletes.

The third part of the female athlete triad, osteopenia/osteoporosis, can occur when female athletes decrease nutrient intake and lose significant body fat. A significant reduction in body fat to unhealthy levels can alter hormone levels that affect bone mineral density. A reduction in nutrients that are necessary for bone health, such as calcium, vitamin D, and magnesium, can also contribute to bone loss. Bone mineral density (BMD), as previously discussed in the body composition section, is often measured by a DEXA scan. BMD can be decreased in females exhibiting disordered eating and dysmenorrheic tendencies. Cobb et al. found that BMD was lower in the lumbar spine, hip, and whole body in

oligomenorrheic and amenorrheic female athletes in their study.[48]

The relationship among all components of the triad is complex. Cobb et al.[48] completed an extensive study of all three components separately as well as the interrelationship of each component. Ninety-one female competitive runners 18–26 years old were surveyed by questionnaire and EDI to assess disordered eating, and BMD testing was performed using DEXA. The authors confirmed that the triad exists and that in female runners: (1) disordered eating is correlated with oligomenorrhea, (2) the association between oligomenorrhea and amenorrhea and low BMD is independent of body weight and composition, and (3) new evidence reveals that disordered eating is associated with low BMD in eumenorrheic women. The female athletes with elevated EDI scores reported 19% lower daily caloric intakes compared with the female athletes with normal EDI scores. Both groups had adequate calcium intakes. Of the 23 women with increased EDI scores, 65% had oligomenorrhea versus 25% of the 67 with normal EDI. Total energy intake was not associated with menstrual disturbance; however, a positive correlation was found with low percent fat intake. BMD was lower in the oligomenorrheic/amenorrheic women when compared to eumenorrheic women. When adjusted for body weight and composition, women with increased EDI scores had significantly lower BMD compared to women with normal EDI.

In summary, female athletes are at higher risk for developing eating disorders than female nonathletes. Disordered eating is one part of the triad, and the decrease in nutrient intake seen in disordered eating can lead to the other two parts of the triad. A reduction in body fat percentage and the hormone abnormalities occurring with this reduction can lead to the development of menstrual irregularities and decreased bone mineral density. Early detection and treatment of one or all of the triad components can help the athlete avoid chronic health issues and poor sport performance.

What are the main concerns regarding male athletes and eating disturbances/disorders?

Most research, public concern, and prevention and treatment strategies for eating disorders are aimed at females. However, as many as 1 million men and boys have eating disorders. As with female athletes, male athletes may be at higher risk for developing eating disorders than their sedentary counterparts.

However, it is difficult to determine the actual prevalence of eating disturbances and disorders in male athletes because there is a lack of research in this area. As with females, there is also a lack of reporting, and men are even less likely than women to seek help for their eating or body image concerns.

Certain sports may place male athletes at higher risk for eating disturbances. Sports with established weight classifications and those where low body weight is emphasized, such as distance running, are considered higher-risk sports. Body builders and weight lifters also appear to be at high risk for developing disordered eating and body image distortion/disturbance. These athletes are more concerned with a "drive for bulk" rather than a "drive for thinness" as described in anorexia.

muscle dysmorphia A type of distorted body image in which individuals have an intense and excessive preoccupation and/or dissatisfaction with body size and muscularity. Muscle dysmorphia is most prevalent in male body builders and weight lifters.

Muscle dysmorphia is a newly defined syndrome characterized by highly muscular individuals (usually men) having a pathological belief that they are of very small musculature.[52] Pope et al.[53] first coined this phrase and defined it as an intense and excessive preoccupation or dissatisfaction with body size and muscularity.[54] This concept also is referred to as reverse anorexia or bigorexia[55] because it is characterized as seeing oneself as small or frail, when in fact the individual is large and muscular. Athletes with muscle dysmorphia exhibit a strong drive for muscularity.[56] They have a strong compulsion for spending hours resistance training, purchasing nutritional supplements, and following diets that supposedly help increase muscle mass. Similar to those with anorexia and bulimia, they have a preoccupation with body size and weight and demonstrate pathologic eating patterns and behaviors. Pope et al.[54] have determined a list of characteristic features suggesting muscle dysmorphia in males. **Table 11.9** describes this list of features.

What are the best treatment options for eating disorders?

Treatment of eating disorders is best accomplished with a team approach to assessment and management of the condition.[57] A multidisciplinary team made up minimally of the team physician, psychological and psychiatric staff, and dietitians who can assess and provide treatment for the athlete is necessary. Including athletic trainers, coaches, and parents, if indicated, will give the eating-disordered

TABLE 11.9	Signs of Muscle Dysmorphia

1. Preoccupation with body shape and size. Feels insufficiently lean and/or muscular. Common signs of preoccupation exhibited include appearance checking; frequent weighing; criticizing self about weight, size, and shape; camouflaging body with baggy clothing.

2. Preoccupation with muscularity causes significant distress or impairment of social, occupational, or other life functioning such as personal relationships. This is demonstrated by two or more of the following:
   - Avoids social, occupational, or recreational activities to maintain compulsive exercise or diet regimens
   - Avoids situations where body would be exposed (pool, beach) or is very anxious in these situations
   - Preoccupation about inadequacy of size/muscularity causes clinically significant distress or impairment in social, occupational, and personal functioning
   - Individual continues to exercise, diet, and use performance-enhancing drugs/supplements despite knowledge of or experience with adverse physical or psychological consequences

3. Individual engages in excessive exercise, demonstrates preoccupation with food, follows strict diet regimen, or abuses steroids or other supplements.

Source: Adapted from Pope HG, Gruber AJ, Choi P., et al. Muscle dysmorphia: an underrecognized form of body dysmorphic disorder. *Psychosom.* 1997;38:548–557.

athlete the best chance of regaining physiological and psychological health.

A thorough medical examination including medical history, weight assessments, laboratory tests, bone scans if needed, electrocardiogram, and patient history should be conducted. This information can be used to determine whether it is safe for the athlete to continue sport activities or whether restrictions in activity are necessary. Most athletes with diagnosable eating disorders will not be allowed to continue to compete if medical information obtained suggests that training and competition could compromise their health status. Medical staff should provide ongoing monitoring of physical health, especially if the athlete continues to train.

Eating disorders are not about food; they are based on emotional and psychological issues in the athlete's life that manifest themselves in disordered eating and exercise behaviors. An evaluation with a psychologist, clinical social worker, or psychiatrist is encouraged to assess emotional issues that underlie the eating problems. Athletes with eating disorders require regular counseling for long-term recovery. Without help from a therapist to discover the root of the problem, athletes are unlikely to be able to make the necessary dietary and behavior changes to recover from the eating disorder. It may also be necessary to consult with a psychiatrist to evaluate the need for psychotropic medications to improve the eating disorder recovery process.

The dietitian should assess current dietary intake and compare that to estimated calorie needs, assess weight status, and determine any nutritional deficiencies. Dietitians play an integral role in the treatment team to help athletes understand the need for food as fuel as well as to help them make dietary behavior changes. Many athletes with eating disorders are very knowledgeable about nutrients, vitamins, minerals, and calories; however, their knowledge is not enough to translate needed changes into action plans to improve nutrition intake. Dietitians need to establish rapport with the athlete and work with him or her to develop a plan that aids in treatment of the disorder and also provides the nutrients required for exercise and competition.

How can eating disorders be prevented?

Prevention of eating disorders is the best defense against the development of an unhealthy relationship with food, medical problems, and the associated negative effects on sport performance. Prevention of eating disorders, including the diagnosable eating disorders, anorexia athletica, and muscle dysmorphia, occurs on three levels—primary, secondary, and tertiary. Each of these levels can help the athlete prevent the development of disordered eating patterns, recognize that problems are occurring, or seek out medical and psychological treatment to prevent the problem from becoming chronic and debilitating.

Primary prevention includes practices that help identify, eliminate, and reduce personal, social, and cultural factors that contribute to eating disorders. Nutrition strategies for primary prevention include nutrition education focused on healthful eating to fuel sport activities, including eating nutrient-dense foods for adequate dietary intake. Nutrition education that emphasizes health and improved performance, not weight loss, encourages a healthy relationship with food and a well-balanced diet. Coaches, parents, and athletic trainers can influence athletes using various primary prevention strategies, including the following:

- Taking the emphasis off weight and body composition by eliminating weekly weigh-ins or body fat testing (unless it is required by the sport)
- Emphasizing skills and performance, and recognizing that athletes come in different shapes and sizes; this will encourage a positive sport-based atmosphere that helps prevent body image distortions and eating problems
- Discouraging the use of fad diets or quick weight loss methods
- Modeling of healthy eating and exercise behaviors by coaches, parents, athletic trainers, and other staff
- Preventing muscle dysmorphia through early identification of body image distortion that often occurs in strength athletes, as well as establishing standard prevention strategies for preventing eating disorders
- Developing a healthy gym environment where education about myths associated with physique, dietary supplements, and the ability to obtain the "perfect" body are not perpetuated
- Setting achievable goals, avoiding comments about specific parts of the body, and dispelling myths about certain supplements and dietary practices that are unhealthy; this can be done by personal trainers, athletic trainers, and strength coaches

Secondary prevention includes identifying and recognizing warning signs that suggest early development of eating disorders. Once warning signs are recognized, immediate referral to medical, psychological, and/or nutrition professionals is essential for the athlete. Coaches, athletes, dietitians, teammates, trainers, and parents of athletes should educate themselves about the warning signs of eating disorders. Knowing the resources available in the community and establishing relationships with these resource personnel will help the referral process proceed smoothly for the athlete. Early detection and treatment mean better outcomes. Education of high-risk teams and their coaches early in the season or during recruitment will help athletes and those who work with them recognize early warning signs in themselves and

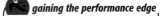

gaining the performance edge

Athletes are at higher risk for developing eating disturbances and disorders than the general population. Preventing eating disorders is essential for athletes to avoid negative consequences to health and sport performance. Regular screening of athletes at high risk for developing eating disorders helps identify problems early and prevents more serious complications later.

TABLE 11.10	Warning Signs of Eating Disorders in Athletes	
Behavioral Signs	**Physical Signs**	
Preoccupation with food, weight, or body composition	Normal, underweight, or overweight	
Criticism of weight, shape, body composition; comparisons of these to other teammates	Fatigue	
	Lethargy	
	Weakness	
Limited type and amount of food eaten	Impaired concentration	
Fear of becoming "fat"	Dizziness	
Excessive rigid exercise; exercise more than at scheduled practices	Abdominal pain	
	Faintness	
Recent switch to restrictive diet	Salivary gland enlargement	
Secretive eating (food disappears)	Sore muscles	
Consumption of large amounts of food inconsistent with athlete's weight	Chills or cold sweats	
	Frequent sore throat	
	Diarrhea	
Evidence of self-induced vomiting—bathroom smells, trips to bathroom immediately after meals	Constipation	
	Tooth enamel erosion	
	Esophagitis	
Laxative, diuretic, or diet pill abuse	Callus on fingers, back of hand	
Recurring injuries, especially overuse injuries	Oligomenorrhea	
	Amenorrhea	
Isolation from social situations, family, friends, teammates		
Withdrawal from team activities or change in interaction with teammates		
Mood changes, depressive signs, anxiety		

others. **Table 11.10** lists common warning signs that indicate an athlete may be moving toward disordered eating behaviors.

Tertiary prevention includes efforts to keep the disorder from becoming chronic. An athlete who is diagnosed with an eating disorder should get immediate evaluation and treatment from a physician and a mental health professional. These professionals should refer the athlete to a registered dietitian who can help the athlete with an appropriate nutritional plan. Obtaining professional assistance through either an inpatient or outpatient treatment facility is critical. Athletes with eating disorders may resist treatment because it means time away from their sport and requires them to realize they have

a problem. Pushing the athlete to accept and work at treatment with trained professionals to guide the process may save the athlete a lifetime of struggles with eating problems.

There are several nationwide resources available to help athletes prevent eating problems and to help sports professionals treat athletes with eating problems (see **Table 11.11**). Resources may also be available in the athlete's local community. Pro-

TABLE 11.11	Eating-Disorder Prevention and Treatment Resources
Organization	**Resources Offered**
National Collegiate Athletic Association www.ncaa.org/wps/portal/ncaahome	On the Web site under "Personal Welfare" is a section on Nutrition & Performance. This section contains sports nutrition information and under "Athletic Trainer" is a plan of action for a disordered-eating intervention protocol.
National Eating Disorders Association www.nationaleatingdisorders.org	Web site offers information on eating-disorder education, treatment, and links to referral sources for individuals struggling with eating concerns.
Harris Center, Massachusetts General Hospital www.harriscentermgh.org	Focuses on expanding knowledge of eating disorders, research, and education on identifying, treating, and preventing eating disorders.
American College of Sports Medicine www.acsm.org	Web site contains position papers on the female athlete triad, weight management, and sports nutrition. Other educational materials and resources are available at this site.
The Renfrew Centers and Foundation www.renfrew.org 1-800-renfrew	Residential treatment center for people with eating disorders. Several centers exist in various locations throughout the United States.
Sports, Cardiovascular and Wellness Nutritionists (SCAN) Dietetic Practice Group of the American Dietetic Association www.scandpg.org	Information on sports nutrition, eating disorders, rapid weight loss in wrestlers, and how to find a registered dietitian with sports nutrition experience.

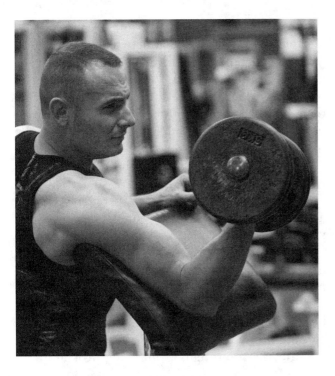

fessionals working with athletes should know the resources in their communities so that referrals can be made quickly to match the athlete's needs with the resources available.

How can athletes gain weight healthfully?

Although it seems that most athletes and the general public are spending most of their time trying to maintain or lose weight, there are some athletes who are interested in increasing body weight. As has already been discussed, gaining fat weight for most athletes is not desirable; therefore, any weight gain strategies should focus on increasing muscle mass. By increasing muscle mass, the athlete not only accomplishes his or her goal of gaining weight, but also becomes stronger, thereby increasing his or her strength-to-weight ratio, which is a desirable training adaptation for most athletes. Gaining weight via increases in fat mass decreases the strength-to-weight ratio, which is why weight gain should be aimed at increasing muscle mass with minimal contribution from added fat mass. There are three main requirements for increasing body weight, particularly in regard to muscle mass:

- Participation in an appropriately planned resistance-training program
- Achieving a positive energy balance
- Achieving a positive nitrogen balance

Each of these requirements is discussed in more detail in the following sections.

What kind of resistance training program is best for gaining weight?

Most athletes know that regular resistance training (also referred to as strength training) is effective for improving muscle mass, strength, and power. They also know that it can strengthen connective tissues such as tendons, ligaments, and bone, thus decreasing risk for injuries. However, many athletes do not know that not all resistance training programs produce the same results. The type of exercises performed, the amount of weight lifted, the number of repetitions performed in each set, the total number of sets completed for each exercise, and the amount of rest taken between sets can all affect the outcomes of a resistance training program.

The first criterion for any resistance training program designed to increase muscle mass is that it must challenge the muscles to work against resistances to which they are not accustomed. One of the basic principles of training, known as the "overload principle," states that resistance training must place a greater-than-normal stress on the muscle cells to stimulate adaptation. The amount of stress imposed on the muscle can be altered based on how much weight is being lifted and the number of repetitions and sets performed. When the muscle is challenged to contract against an appropriate resistance, the muscle cells respond and are stimulated to grow. The end result is muscle hypertrophy (i.e., the muscle gets bigger) and thus increased muscle mass.

The resistance training program chosen by an athlete wishing to gain weight should focus on stimulating muscle hypertrophy. As noted earlier, a common misconception is that all resistance training programs are created equal. Training for muscle hypertrophy is different from training for maximal strength or power. Resistance training programs designed to increase muscle mass should work all the major muscle groups with a training frequency of at least twice per week and incorporate weight loads that allow at a minimum 8, and a maximum 12, repetitions per set. Three to five sets should be performed for each exercise. Athletes should allow 48 hours between workouts for the same muscle groups so that the muscles can recover and adapt to the training. As the muscles adapt and become stronger, the amount of weight lifted should be increased to keep the repetitions performed per set in the 8 to 12 range. By progressively increasing the loads to accommodate the strength increases, the muscles will continue to be challenged and thus continue to hypertrophy. This format of resistance training is often referred to as "progressive" resistance training.

How can an athlete achieve a positive energy balance?

The second requirement of a weight gain program is that the athlete must attain a positive energy balance. In other words, calorie intake must exceed calorie expenditure for muscle gains to occur. A positive energy balance can be achieved by consuming more calories, decreasing energy expenditure, or both. In many instances, decreasing energy expenditure (i.e., training less) is not an option because of the necessity of training for the sport. Thus, increasing food intake is the most productive way for most athletes to gain weight; however, it should not be done indiscriminately. Doing so can result in higher levels of fat weight gain.

Approximately 2300 to 3600 calories above current requirements are needed to increase muscle mass by 1 pound. However, the body does not necessarily make more muscle solely because extra calories are consumed in the diet. The extra calories must be combined with the stimulus for muscle growth that results from resistance training. Even then, the body will use only what it needs to recover and adapt. A study involving individuals who were resistance training and consuming an extra 500 to 2000 calories per day indicated only 30% to 40% of the weight gained was lean body tissue.[58] The remaining calories are stored as energy, usually in the form of fat. In short, consuming large quantities of food will not result in increased muscle mass beyond what resistance training induces. The goal is to provide enough calories to cover the body's need to synthesize new muscle tissue without exceeding calorie requirements. The number of extra calories needed to support muscle growth is highly individual, and thus frequent body composition assessments should be performed so that caloric intake can be adjusted accordingly. Weight gain in the form of muscle is a gradual process, so increases in dietary intake should be modest to maximize muscle gain versus fat gain.

A weight gain goal of $\frac{1}{2}$ to 1 pound per week is generally considered appropriate. The amount of additional calories needed to accomplish weight gain depends on the individual's goals for rate of weight gain, the intensity and volume of their current training, the ability of the athlete to consume additional calories, and genetics. Consuming an additional 300 to 500 calories per day could provide for a weight gain rate of $\frac{1}{2}$ to 1 pound per week.

This modest increase in caloric intake can generally be consumed without the athlete feeling overly full or uncomfortable after meals. During the weight gain period, if increases in training volume occur, in particular any increases in aerobic-type exercise, then more than 300 to 500 additional calories may be needed to meet the additional energy demands of the training.

Finally, the composition of the additional calories is important. Many athletes assume that protein should make up the largest percentage of the additional calories because protein is essential for muscle synthesis. Protein intake is important, but it is more important to ensure that the total energy needs of the body are met regardless of the contributing macronutrients. As discussed in Chapters 2 and 3, carbohydrates are a critical energy source and must be present in the diet or the body will break down and use protein for energy. In other words, carbohydrates spare proteins from being broken down for energy, thus enabling them to be used for muscle tissue building. As a result, the largest proportion of the additional calories (55–60%) should be obtained from carbohydrate-rich foods. In summary, consuming 300 to 500 extra calories per day, primarily in the form of carbohydrates, will place the athlete in a positive energy balance and support a rate of weight gain that increases muscle mass and minimizes fat gain.

How can an athlete achieve a positive nitrogen balance?

With adequate additional caloric intake, athletes can successfully gain weight. Even though carbohydrates should contribute a majority of the extra calories needed for muscle mass gain, adequate protein intake is also necessary. As described in Chapter 5, protein needs for athletes are greater compared to sedentary individuals. During a targeted weight gain period, protein needs are also increased. Some of this additional protein is needed to support the energy costs of additional training. Most of the additional protein will be used to produce muscle hypertrophy. The RDA for protein is 0.8 gm/kg body weight for the average healthy individual. The recommendation for athletes during strength training activities ranges from 1.4 to 2.0 gm/kg body weight. This range provides a level of protein intake that is approximately twice the RDA and should be adequate to place the athlete in a state of positive nitrogen balance.

Attaining a daily protein intake of 1.4–2.0 gm/kg of body weight is not difficult for most athletes. In general, if an athlete is consuming enough food to meet his or her daily caloric needs and including protein-rich foods and beverages at each meal and snack throughout the day, obtaining adequate amounts of protein to support muscle mass gains is typically not of concern. For example, an 85 kg athlete who requires an estimated 3200 calories to meet daily energy demands and maintain weight will require approximately 3700 calories after adding 500 calories per day to support muscle mass gains (see **Training Table 11.3**). If the athlete wanted to boost protein intake to 1.8 gm/kg, then a total of 153 grams of protein would be required daily. When comparing total energy needs to protein requirements, only 16.5% of total calories would need to come from protein ([153 grams × 4 kcal per gram of protein] ÷ 3700 kcal = 16.5% of total calories from protein). The normal diet of most individuals consists of 10–20% of calories from protein. Clearly, an athlete who eats a diet on the high end of normal will more than likely meet the daily protein requirements to support muscle growth.

Do athletes need dietary supplements to gain weight?

Use of protein supplements is common in athletes desiring to gain weight, primarily because the popular press touts the importance of supplementation for muscle growth (see Figure 11.12). The marketing efforts of supplement companies that promote high protein intake for muscle growth sway athletes into believing they need supplements to meet protein demands. However, as demonstrated in the previous example, supplementation is not a necessity if the caloric needs of the athlete are being met and protein intake is on the upper end of the recommended range for athletes. Athletes need to keep in mind that any excess protein (i.e., protein not used for muscle growth) will be stored as fat. Conversely, if the athlete has food intolerances or preferences that challenge the adequate intake of protein from food sources, then supplementation may be recommended. If protein supplements are incorporated into the athlete's eating plan, they should be used in moderation with a continued focus on food sources of protein.

Training Table 11.3: Sample Meal Plan for Weight Gain

3200 Calories (166 g protein)	3700 Calories (183 g protein)
Breakfast	*Breakfast*
2 scrambled eggs, with salsa and shredded cheese	2 scrambled eggs, with salsa and shredded cheese
2 slices whole wheat toast with jelly	2 slices whole wheat toast with jelly
12 oz orange juice	12 oz orange juice
Mid-morning Snack	*Mid-morning Snack*
Granola bar	Granola bar
	Pear
Lunch	*Lunch*
3 oz turkey sandwich with Swiss cheese	3 oz turkey sandwich with Swiss cheese
Apple	Apple
Baked potato chips	Baked potato chips
12 oz 1% milk	4 small oatmeal cookies
	16 oz 1% milk
Mid-afternoon Snack	*Mid-afternoon Snack*
3 oz tuna with saltine crackers	3 oz tuna with saltine crackers
Dinner	*Dinner*
4 oz chicken breast	4 oz chicken breast
2 cups white rice	2 cups white rice
2 cups broccoli	2 cups broccoli
12 oz chocolate milk	16 oz chocolate milk
Evening Snack	*Evening Snack*
12 oz apple juice	2 oz ham sandwich
	12 oz apple juice

Weight gain or calorie supplements may also be helpful for athletes who have extremely high energy needs and just can't seem to eat enough food necessary to gain weight (see Figure 11.13). These calorie supplements typically provide between 300 and 500 calories and are usually sold as an 8-ounce drink or in powdered form. As with any dietary supplement, athletes should pay careful attention to the Supplement Facts label. Some weight gain or protein supplements may contain stimulants or other herbal or synthetic ingredients that may be banned by the NCAA, International Olympic Committee (IOC), and other professional sports organizations. Ignorance is not an excuse to these agencies, so reading the labels and asking about the ingredients of any supplement are very important.

How can athletes gain weight healthfully? **353**

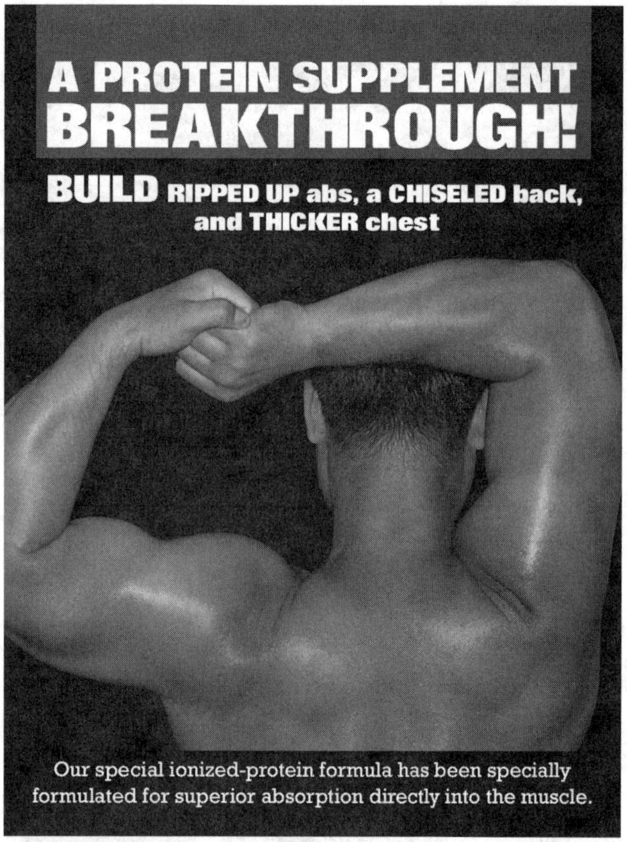

A PROTEIN SUPPLEMENT BREAKTHROUGH!

BUILD RIPPED UP abs, a CHISELED back, and THICKER chest

Our special ionized-protein formula has been specially formulated for superior absorption directly into the muscle.

Figure 11.12 Protein supplements are vigorously marketed to athletes. Adequate protein intake is necessary for muscle growth. If the athlete cannot meet daily protein needs through food sources, protein supplements might be appropriate. However, protein consumed in excess, whether from supplements or foods, can be stored as fat.

What other dietary practices might help an athlete gain weight?

For many athletes on a tight schedule, taking in extra calories during the day is not an easy thing to do. Likewise, there are other individuals who have to work very hard at consuming enough calories to gain weight. For these individuals and others wanting to add weight, **Training Table 11.4** lists some helpful dietary tips. Eating numerous small meals throughout the day and/or drinking juices or milk rather than water can help pack in the extra calories. This is especially helpful to athletes who already feel full after their meal and therefore need to add calories throughout the day versus solely at meals. Also, cutting back on drinking fluids during the meal, especially carbonated fluids, can leave more room for a few extra calories. For those athletes who are always on the go and find frequent snacking a bother, commercially prepared liquid meals can be an appropriate and easy-to-consume snack option. Alternatively, mixing up smoothies or calorie supplement drinks

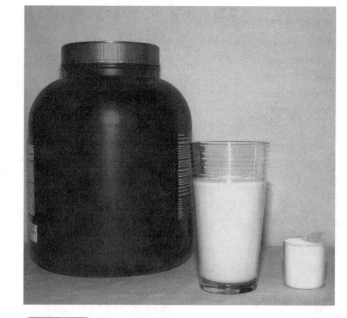

Figure 11.13 Weight gain powders and drinks. Athletes who have difficulty meeting high-energy demands and want to gain weight may benefit from easy-to-use powdered or liquid high-calorie supplements. Caution should be taken when using these supplements because they could contain banned or other substances the athlete does not want or should not consume.

before leaving home will make taking in extra calories throughout the day more convenient. Finally, late-night snacking is an excellent way to add the extra calories needed for weight gain. Regardless of the weight gain strategies chosen, it is important that the methods are not too disruptive to the normal routine of the athlete. Dietary strategies that look good on paper but do not fit the athlete's behaviors/habits will not result in the regular boost of calories required for attaining specific weight gain goals.

Training Table 11.4: Nutrition Tips for Weight Gain

- Consume fluids after meals to avoid becoming full on liquids.
- Avoid carbonated beverages that produce gas and bloating and the feeling of fullness.
- Use predetermined cues to eat (e.g., plan meals with friends, always have a 10:00 A.M. snack).
- Have small, frequent meals and snacks throughout the day.
- Consume a variety of nutrient-dense and energy-dense foods.
- Consume high-calorie beverages with meals.
- Use sports drinks instead of water during training.
- Include a bedtime snack approximately 1 hour prior to sleep.

The Box Score

Key Points of Chapter

- Athletes are concerned about weight loss for a variety of reasons. They may feel it will help improve their sport performance or make their appearance more attractive to judges. Many sports have a particular "look," such as the very thin appearance of long-distance runners. Athletes may aspire to change their weight to achieve a particular perceived ideal appearance for their sport.

- Body mass index (BMI) is equal to body weight (in kilograms) divided by height (in meters) squared. BMI measures can be calculated using the nonmetric pounds and inches conversions or the published nomogram charts as well. Although BMI is not a true measure of body composition, it is commonly used to provide an indication of body composition in the general population. Athletes should not solely use BMI as a measure of weight status because it is a crude indicator of body composition.

- Overweight and obesity are significant medical concerns for adults in the United States. Approximately two-thirds of the adult population has a BMI greater than 25, placing them in the overweight or obese category. Higher-than-normal BMI can result in increased risk for chronic illnesses such as diabetes, heart disease, and hypertension.

- A variety of methods to measure body composition is available. All have varying levels of cost, ease of assessment, and ability for use in the field with athletes. Skinfold measurements are a fairly accurate way to easily and inexpensively assess athletes' body composition in the training room. These measures can be done at intervals during the training season to track trends in body composition changes.

- Weight loss success is hard to achieve in many cases. Success depends on creating an energy deficit (i.e., negative energy balance) by reducing calorie intake, increasing energy expenditure, or a combination of both. The energy deficit created for weight loss in athletes should be small (approximately 500 calories per day). By creating a slight energy deficit, athletes losing weight will continue to have the energy needed to train and will minimize loss of muscle mass.

- Athletes in weight classification sports are at higher risk for using weight loss measures that are unhealthy. Athletes in these sports should attempt to maintain their training weight at competition weight to avoid having to "make weight" and use rapid weight loss measures that are detrimental to health.

- Eating disorders are more common in athletes than in nonathletes. Sports where appearance is judged or where subjective scoring occurs may impose a higher risk to athletes in developing eating disorders. Early detection of dieting or eating-disturbed behaviors will help prevent the associated consequences to health and sport performance.

- Weight gain for athletes can be as difficult to achieve as weight loss in some cases. Athletes need to consistently consume additional calories and adequate protein, and maintain or increase resistance training to gain weight. Because athletes already have high calorie needs, increasing food consumption may be difficult for some athletes. Consuming more calorie-dense foods and beverages and including high-calorie snacks can help athletes achieve increased mass in a healthy way.

Study Questions

1. What are some of the various ways to determine an athlete's body composition? Briefly discuss the pros and cons of each.

2. How is body mass index calculated? Is it truly a measure of body composition? Defend your answer.

3. Why do athletes tend to focus so much on body weight? Is this beneficial or detrimental? Defend your answer.

4. What is the significance of waist and hip measurements in regard to disease risk? What are the waist-to-hip ratios expected in individuals with gynoid and android fat distribution?

5. What is the difference between nonessential body fat and essential body fat? Do females have the same amounts of essential and nonessential fat as males?

6. What are the three major components of energy expenditure? Briefly explain each. Which component accounts for the largest portion of daily caloric expenditure?

7. How does the concept of energy balance pertain to weight gain or weight loss?

8. Discuss the various factors that can affect energy intake.

9. What is the recommended range of daily calorie deficit if weight loss is the goal?

10. What are some of the differences between credible diets and fad diets?

11. What are some dietary practices that will increase the chances of long-term weight loss success?

12. What are the commonly encountered eating disorders? Which athletes are at highest risk for eating disorders? Why?

13. What is muscle dysmorphia and what are some of its warning signs? Which athletes are at greatest risk for muscle dysmorphia?

14. What conditions make up the female athlete triad?

15. Discuss some of the ways that eating disorders can be prevented.

16. What are the three main requirements necessary for an athlete wanting to gain weight? What is an appropriate rate of weight gain for an athlete?

References

1. Ogden CL, Carroll MD. Prevalence of overweight, obesity and extreme obesity among adults: United States, trends 1976–1980 through 2007–2008. Available at: www.cdc.gov/nchs/data/hestat/obesity_adult_07_08/obesity_adult_07_08.htm. Accessed August 18, 2010.

2. Ogden C, Carroll M. Prevalence of obesity among children and adolescents: United States, trends 1963–1965 through 2007–2008. Available at: www.cdc.gov/nchs/data/hestat/obesity_child_07_08/obesity_child_07_08.htm. Accessed August 18, 2010.

3. Noel MB, Van Heest JL, Zaneteas P, Rodgers CD. Body composition in Division I football players. *J Strength Condition Res*. 2003;17(2):228–237.

4. Flegal KM, Graubard BI, Williamson DF, Gail MH. Excess deaths associated with underweight, overweight and obesity. *JAMA*. 2005;293:1861–1867.

5. Prentice A, Jebb SA. Beyond body mass index. *Obes Rev*. 2001;2(3):141–147.

6. National Heart Lung and Blood Institute, National Institutes of Health. The Practical Guide, Identification, Evaluation, and Treatment of Overweight and Obesity in Adults. Washington, DC: U.S. Department of Health and Human Services; 2002.

7. Centers for Disease Control and Prevention, National Center for Health Statistics. Prevalence of Overweight and Obesity Among Adults: United States, 1999–2000. Washington, DC: Centers for Disease Control. Available at: www.cdc.gov/nchs/products/pubs/pubd/hestats/obese/obse99.htm. Accessed September 14, 2005.

8. Keys A, Fidanza F, Karvonen MJ, Kimora N, Taylor, HL. Indices of relative weight and obesity. *J Chronic Dis*. 1972;25:329–343.

9. Deurenberg P, Weststrate JA, Seidell JC. Body mass index as a measure of body fatness: age- and sex-specific prediction formulas. *J Nutr*. 1991;65:105–114.

10. Gallagher D, Visser M, Sepulveda D, Pierson RN, Harris T, Heymsfield SB. How useful is body mass index for comparison of body fatness across age, sex and ethnic groups? *Am J Epidem*. 1996;143:228–239.

11. Chan J, Rimm EB, Colditz GA, Stampfer MJ, Willett WC. Obesity, fat distribution, and weight gain as risk factors for clinical diabetes in men. *Diabetes Care*. 1994;17:961–969.

12. Kuczmarski RJ, Carrol MD, Flegal KM, Troiano RP. Varying body mass index cutoff points to describe overweight prevalence among U.S. adults: NHANES III (1988–1994). *Obes Res*. 1997;5:542–548.

13. Nash NL. Body fat measurement: weighing the pros and cons of electrical impedance. *Physician Sports Med*. 1985;13(11):124–128.

14. Lohman TG. Basic concepts in body composition assessment. In: *Advances in Body Composition Assessment*. Champaign, IL: Human Kinetics; 1992:1–5.

15. Kohrt WM. Preliminary evidence that DEXA provides an accurate assessment of body composition. *J Appl Physiol*. 1998;84:372–377.

16. Van Loan MD. Is dual-energy X-ray absorptiometry ready for prime time in the clinical evaluation of body composition? *Am J Clin Nutr*. 1998;68:1155–1156.

17. Saunders MJ, Blevins JE, Broeder CE. Effects of hydration changes on bioelectrical impedance in endurance trained individuals. *Med Sci Sports Exerc*. 1998;30(6):885–892.

18. National Institutes of Health. Bioelectrical impedance analysis of body composition measurement. *NIH Technolog Assess State*. 1996;December 12–14:1–35.

19. Withers RT, Craig NP, Bourdon PC. Relative body fat and anthropometric prediction of body density of male athletes. *Eur J Appl Physiol Occup Physiol*. 1987;56(2):191–200.

20. McArdle WD, Katch FI, Katch VL. *Exercise Physiology: Energy, Nutrition, and Human Performance*. 5th ed. Philadelphia, PA: Lippincott Williams and Wilkins; 2001.

21. Manore M, Thompson J. *Sports Nutrition for Health and Performance*. Champaign, IL: Human Kinetics; 2000.

22. Borchers JR, Clem KL, Habash DL, Nagaraja HN, Stokley LM, Best TM. Metabolic syndrome and insulin resistance in Division 1 collegiate football players. *Med. Sci. Sports Exer*. 2009;41(12):2105–2110.

23. American Dietetic Association. Position of the American Dietetic Association, Dietitians of Canada, and the American College of Sports Medicine: nutrition and athletic performance. *J Am Dietet Assoc*. 2000;100:1543–1556.

24. Wildman REC, Miller BS. *Sports and Fitness Nutrition*. Belmont, CA: Thomson and Wadsworth; 2004.

25. Frankenfield D, Roth-Yousey L, Compher C. Comparison of predictive equations for resting metabolic rate in healthy nonobese and obese adults: a systematic review. *J Am Dietet Assoc*. 2005;105(5):775–789.

26. Lee RD, Nieman DC. *Nutritional Assessment*. 3rd ed. New York, NY: McGraw-Hill; 2003.

27. Zeman FJ. *Clinical Nutrition and Dietetics*. New York, NY: Macmillan; 1991.

28. Wilmore J, Costill DL. *Physiology of Sport and Exercise*. 3rd ed. Champaign, IL: Human Kinetics; 2004.

29. Haskell WL, Lee I-M, Pate RP, Powell KE, Blair SN, Franklin BA, Macera CA, Heath GW, Thompson PD, Bauman A. Physical activity and public health: updated recommendation for adults from the American College

of Sports Medicine and the American Heart Association. *Circulation*. 2007;116(9):1081–1093.

30. Alderman B, Landers DM, Carlson J, Scott JR. Factors related to rapid weight loss practices among international-style wrestlers. *Med Sci Sports Exerc*. 2004;36(2):249–252.

31. Choma C, Sforzo GA, Keller BA. Impact of rapid weight loss on cognitive function in collegiate wrestlers. *Med Sci Sports Exerc*. 1998;30(4):746–749.

32. Centers for Disease Control and Prevention. Hyperthermia and dehydration-related deaths associated with intentional rapid weight loss in three collegiate wrestlers—North Carolina, Wisconsin and Michigan, November–December 1997. *JAMA*. 1998;279(11):824–825.

33. Davis S, Dwyer GB, Reed K, Bopp C, Stosic J, Shepanski M. Preliminary investigation: the impact of the NCAA wrestling weight certification program on weight cutting. *J Strength Conditioning Res*. 2002;16(2):305–307.

34. National Federation of State High School Associations. Weight management program wrestling rules revisions. Available at: www.hfhs.org/2005/04/weightmanagement_program_headlines_wrestlingrules. Accessed July 20, 2007.

35. Oppliger RA, Steen SA, Scott JR. Weight loss practices of college wrestlers. *Int J Sport Nutr Exerc Metabol*. 2003;13(1):29–46.

36. Dale K, Landers DM. Weight control in wrestling: eating disorders or disordered eating? *Med Sci Sports Exerc*. 1999;31(10):1382–1389.

37. Krane V, Waldron J, Michalenok J, Stiles-Shipley J. Body image concerns in female exercisers and athletes: a feminist culture. *Women Sport Phys Activ J*. 2001; 10(1):17–54.

38. Monsma EV, Malina RM. Correlates of eating disorders risk among female figure skaters: a profile of adolescent competitors. *Psych Sport Exerc*. 2003;5(4):447–460.

39. Bartlewski PB, Van Raatle JL, Brewer BW. Effects of exercise on social physique anxiety and body esteem of female college students. *Women Sport Phys Activ J*. 1996;5(2):49–62.

40. Otis CL, Drinkwater B, Johnson M, Loucks A, Wilmore J. American College of Sports Medicine position stand: the female athlete triad. *Med Sci Sports Exerc*. 1997;29(5):1–10.

41. Sundgot-Borgen J, Torstveit MK. Prevalence of eating disorders in elite athletes is higher than in the general population. *Clin J Sport Med*. 2003;14(1):25–32.

42. American Psychiatric Association. *Diagnostic and Statistical Manual of Mental Disorders*. 4th ed. Washington, DC: American Psychiatric Association; 1994.

43. Sundgot-Borgen J. Risk and trigger factors for the development of eating disorders in female elite athletes. *Med Sci Sports Exerc*. 1994;26:414–419.

44. Beals KA, Manore MM. The prevalence and consequences of subclinical eating disorders in female athletes. *Int J Sport Nutr*. 1994;4:175–179.

45. Wiggins DL, Wiggins ME. The female athlete. *Clin J Sport Med*. 1997;16:593–612.

46. Affenito SG, Yeager KA, Rosman JR, Ludemann MA, Adams CH, Welch GW. Development and validation of a screening tool to identify eating disorders in female athletes. *J Am Dietet Assoc*. 1998;98(9 suppl 1):A78.

47. McNulty KY, Adams CH, Anderson JM, Affenito SG. Development and validation of a screening tool to identify eating disorders in female athletes. *J Am Dietet Assoc*. 2001;101:886–892.

48. Cobb K, Bachrach LK, Greendale G, et al. Disordered eating, menstrual irregularity, and bone mineral density in female runners. *Med Sci Sports Exerc*. 2003;35(5):711–719.

49. Loucks AB. Energy availability, not body fatness, regulates reproductive function in women. *Exerc Sport Sci Rev*. 2003;31:144.

50. Loucks AB, Verdun M, Heath EM. Low energy availability, not stress of exercise, alters LH pulsatility in exercising women. *J Appl Physiol*. 1998;84:37.

51. Sherman RT, Thompson RT. Practical use of the International Olympic Committee Medical Commission position stand on the female athlete triad: a case example. *Int J Eat Dis*. 39;3:193–201.

52. Choi PYL, Pope HG, Olivardia R. Muscle dysmorphia: a new syndrome in weightlifters. *Br J Sports Med*. 2002;36:375–376.

53. Pope HG, Gruber AJ, Choi P. Muscle dysmorphia: an unrecognized form of body dysmorphic disorder. *Psychosom*. 1997;38:548–557.

54. Pope HG, Katz DL, Hudson JI. Anorexia nervosa and "reverse anorexia" among 108 male body builders. *Comp Psychiatry*. 1993;34:406–409.

55. Mosley PE. Bigorexia: Bodybuilding and muscle dysmorphia. *Eur. Eat. Disorders Rev*. 2009;17:191–198.

56. Robert CA, Munroe-Chandler KJ, Gammage KL. The relationship between the drive for muscularity and muscle dysmorphia in male and female weight trainers. *J. Strength Cond. Res*. 2009;23(6):1656–1662.

57. Bonci CM, Bonci LJ, Granger LR, Johnson CL, Malina RM, Milne LW, Ryan RR, Vanderbunt EM. National Athletic Trainers' Association Position Statement: Preventing, detecting, and managing disordered eating in athletes. *J Athletic Training*. 2008;43(1):80–108.

58. Kreider RB. Dietary supplements and the promotion of muscle growth with resistance exercise. *Sports Med*. 1999;27:97–110.

Additional Resources

Miller WC, Niederprume MG, Wallace JP, Lindeman AK. Dietary fat, sugar and fiber predict body fat content. *J Am Dietet Assoc*. 1994;94(6):612–617.

Siri WE. The gross composition of the body. In: Lawrence JH, Tobias CA, eds. *Advances in Biological and Medical Physics*. 4th ed. New York: Academic Press; 1956:239–280.

Endurance and Ultra-Endurance Athletes

Key Questions Addressed

- What is different about endurance athletes?
- What energy systems are utilized during endurance exercise?
- Are total energy needs for endurance athletes different from energy needs of other types of athletes?
- Are macronutrient needs different for endurance athletes?
- How important are carbohydrates to endurance athletes?
- Are protein needs different for endurance athletes?
- Should endurance athletes eat more fats to meet their energy needs?
- Are vitamin/mineral needs different for endurance athletes?
- Why are fluids critical to endurance performance?
- What meal planning/event logistics need to be considered during endurance events?

You Are the Nutrition Coach

Adam is a 14-year-old distance swimmer. He swims with a club team and competes regularly. The team's weekly yardage ranges from 30,000–35,000 yards, with 2–3 days of dry land exercises. Several months ago, Adam decided to cut out all junk food from his diet in hopes of improving his swimming performance. After making the dietary change, his times for the 200 butterfly, 500 freestyle, and 1-mile freestyle began to improve, and he was feeling good. Another result of his dietary changes and hard efforts in the pool was a 28-pound weight loss in 6 months, dropping to a mere 140 pounds for his 5'11" frame. His mother and coach became concerned with his weight loss, afraid that he had lost too much and was also losing muscle mass, which would eventually hurt his performance. In addition to these concerns, Adam was approaching the time for a switch to the high school team, which meant more yardage in the pool and more dry land exercises. Adam was open to eating more food to keep his weight and strength stable, but was unsure of how to do it in a healthy way.

Questions

- What are Adam's daily calorie needs?
- Should Adam begin eating ice cream, candy bars, and other high-calorie "junk" foods again to increase his daily calorie intake?
- What advice would you give Adam?

What is different about endurance athletes?

In general, endurance is one of the basic components of physical fitness. As a result, most athletes have to possess some degree of muscular and cardiorespiratory endurance to perform in their respective sports. **Muscular endurance** is the ability of a muscle or group of muscles to repeatedly develop or maintain force without fatiguing. **Cardiorespiratory endurance** is the ability of the cardiovascular and respiratory systems to deliver blood and oxygen to working muscles, which in turn enables the working muscles to perform continuous exercise. In other words, a person who possesses good cardiorespiratory fitness will be able to perform higher intensity activity for a longer period of time than a person with poor cardiorespiratory fitness.

Obviously, endurance is important to almost all athletes, even those involved in sports requiring short, intermittent bursts of intense anaerobic activity that are repeated over the course of an hour or more. Because so many sports require endurance, clarification is needed regarding which athletes fall into the category of "endurance and ultra-endurance athletes." For the purposes of this chapter, **endurance athletes** are those who are engaged in continuous activity lasting between 30 minutes and 4 hours. **Ultra-endurance athletes** are a subgroup of endurance athletes who engage in extremely long bouts of continuous activity lasting more than 4 hours.

Because of the duration and continuous nature of their sports, endurance athletes expend a tremendous number of calories not only during competition, but also in their preparatory training. For example, energy expenditures of 6000 to 8000 kcals/day are not out of the ordinary for ultra-endurance athletes. This puts a tremendous drain on energy reserves that must be replenished after daily training bouts,

muscular endurance The ability of a muscle or group of muscles to repeatedly develop or maintain force without fatiguing.

cardiorespiratory endurance The ability of the cardiovascular and respiratory systems to deliver blood and oxygen to working muscles, which in turn enable the working muscles to perform continuous exercise. It is an indicator of a person's aerobic or cardiovascular fitness.

endurance athlete An athlete who participates in sports involving continuous activity (30 minutes to 4 hours, as defined in the chapter) involving large muscle groups.

ultra-endurance athlete A subgroup of endurance athletes who engage in extremely long bouts of continuous activity lasting more than 4 hours. Ironman triathletes and ultra-marathoners are examples of this group of endurance athletes.

making diet a key factor not only for athletic success, but also for overall health. Failure to maintain adequate dietary intake of nutrients can quickly result in chronic fatigue, dehydration, increased risk for illness (e.g., upper respiratory infection) and injuries, as well as muscle wasting.

Although endurance sports require high calorie intakes, they do not give athletes a license to eat indiscriminately. Although eating enough calories to offset the energy demands of their sport may sometimes be difficult, athletes must pay careful attention to dietary composition and the timing of consumption to help ensure their success. For the ultra-endurance athletes, not only is their training diet crucial, but so is their nutrient consumption during lengthy competitions. This chapter focuses on the dietary requirements of these "high caloric need" endurance and ultra-endurance athletes.

What energy systems are utilized during endurance exercise?

As with most sports, all three energy systems (i.e., phosphagen, anaerobic, aerobic) are working to contribute energy during endurance exercise. However, the primary energy system relied upon during endurance exercise is the aerobic system (shown on the right side of [Figure 12.1]). As discussed in Chapter 2, the chemical energy our bodies rely upon is adenosine triphosphate (ATP). The aerobic energy system has an almost unlimited capacity for producing ATP. The downside is that the aerobic system cannot produce ATP very quickly; as a result, the speeds at which endurance and ultra-endurance activities are carried out are slower relative to that of anaerobic athletes. However, with appropriately designed training programs, the aerobic energy system of muscles can be improved, thus enabling higher rates of ATP production. The rate of aerobic ATP production is known as **aerobic power**. The faster the rate of ATP production, the higher the aerobic power demonstrated by that athlete. Elite endurance athletes exhibit remarkable aerobic

aerobic power The rate of aerobic ATP production. It is usually represented by the fastest pace or rate of physical activity an athlete can sustain and is an indicator of cardiorespiratory fitness.

power. They can sustain relatively high-velocity movements for hours that an untrained individual may only be able to maintain for several minutes before fatiguing.

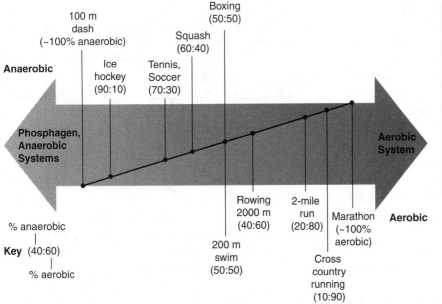

100 m dash (~100% anaerobic)

Boxing (50:50)

Squash (60:40)

Tennis, Soccer (70:30)

Ice hockey (90:10)

Anaerobic

Phosphagen, Anaerobic Systems

Aerobic System

Aerobic

% anaerobic

Key (40:60)

% aerobic

200 m swim (50:50)

Rowing 2000 m (40:60)

2-mile run (20:80)

Marathon (~100% aerobic)

Cross country running (10:90)

Figure 12.1 The anaerobic-aerobic continuum. The primary energy system relied upon during endurance exercise is the aerobic system.

Are total energy needs for endurance athletes different from energy needs of other types of athletes?

One of the main concerns for endurance athletes is matching energy consumption with energy expenditure. Long-distance, strenuous exercise requires a large number of calories. Elite athletes can potentially burn more than two to three times the number of calories as their untrained, weight-matched counterparts. If these calories are not replaced daily, energy for training and the ability to perform during competitions will decline.

How are daily energy needs calculated for endurance athletes?

To estimate the total energy needs for an endurance athlete, use the resting energy expenditure (REE) equations presented in Chapter 10 and reviewed in **Table 12.1**.

For example, Bill is a 35-year-old marathoner, running 60–80 miles a week. His weight has been stable at 140 pounds for the last 12 months. Using the calculation presented in Table 12.1, Bill's daily calorie needs are:

1. Calculation for 35-year-old men: REE = (11.6 × BW) + 879

2. Convert pounds of body weight to kilograms = 140 ÷ 2.2 = 63.6 kilograms
3. Bill's REE = (11.6 × 63.6 kg) + 879 = 737.8 + 879 = 1616.8 calories
4. Multiply the REE by the activity factor of 1.6–2.4 = 1616.8 × (1.6–2.4) = 2587–3880 calories per day

The daily calorie range calculated for Bill is quite large—a difference of 1293 calories. Bill can use this range to adjust his intake based on his daily volume of running. Rest and recovery days will require approximately 2500–2800 calories, whereas high mileage or hard workout days will require an intake of 3600–3900 calories. With a weekly mileage of 60–80 miles, Bill is running about 10–12 miles a day. Therefore, on most days he will need to consume a diet providing calories at the high end of his estimated range to perform well and recover completely from workouts.

Even though the activity factors of 1.6–2.4 will cover most recreational and competitive athletes, the

TABLE 12.1	Resting Energy Expenditure (REE) Calculations and Activity Factors	
Gender and Age	Equation (BW in kilograms)	Activity Factor
Males, 10–18 years	REE = (17.5 × BW) + 651	1.6–2.4
Males, 18–30 years	REE = (15.3 × BW) + 679	1.6–2.4
Males, 30–60 years	REE = (11.6 × BW) + 879	1.6–2.4
Females, 10–18 years	REE = (12.2 × BW) + 749	1.6–2.4
Females, 18–30 years	REE = (14.7 × BW) + 496	1.6–2.4
Females, 30–60 years	REE = (8.7 × BW) + 829	1.6–2.4

Source: World Health Organization. Energy and Protein Requirements. Report of a Joint FAO/WHO/UNU Expert Consultation. Technical Report Series 724. Geneva, Switzerland: World Health Organization; 1985:206.

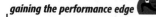

Knowing how to estimate the daily energy needs for an endurance athlete is a crucial first step to developing a dietary plan that provides enough calories to meet training and competition energy needs.

range may not estimate calories appropriately for all athletes. For example, cyclists participating in staged races that last from 1 to 3 weeks may burn calories in the 7000–8000 calorie per day range. If Bill, from the previous example, was a stage racing cyclist, to reach this calorie range, an activity factor of 4.3–4.9 would be appropriate. On the other end of the spectrum, endurance athletes who want to lose weight may find that an activity factor of 1.4–1.6 estimates an appropriate calorie level. Therefore, use the calculation guidelines while also making individualized adjustments for specific athletes.

It can sometimes be challenging for athletes to increase their daily intake to match their actual caloric needs. Training, work/school, sleep, and other nonsport activities take time away from preparing and eating meals and snacks. Some athletes also complain about feeling too full and not being able to comfortably add more calories to meet their needs. Also, strenuous effort during training or competition tends to decrease appetite, causing athletes to eat small meals and snacks. Athletes in these situations are looking for quick, easy, and nutrient-dense ways to increase their calories while enjoying their food and not spending all day in the kitchen. Meal plans should be created that fit the daily schedule of the athlete and incorporate nutrient- and calorie-dense meals/snacks that are within the cooking/preparation skills of the athlete.

When planning meals for individuals needing to increase calories, a balance of macronutrients is essential. If an athlete increases mainly carbohydrate- and fiber-rich foods, the result is a feeling of fullness and bloating. If protein-rich foods are the focus, the endurance athlete may neglect to fully replenish glycogen stores, ultimately hindering training and racing. Too many fat-rich foods can delay gastric emptying, potentially disrupting training sessions because of a sense of fullness, stomach cramps, or diarrhea. By balancing the macronutrients and increasing carbohydrates, protein, and fat in proportional amounts, athletes can reap the benefits of increasing total calorie intake while feeling good and performing well.

Training Table 12.1 presents sample meal plans for three different calorie levels—3000, 4000, and 5000 calories. Note that as the number of calories increases,

Training Table 12.1: Sample Meal Plans Providing 3000, 4000, or 5000 Calories per Day

3000 Calories

Meal/Snack	Food/Beverage	Carbohydrate Content (g)
Breakfast	2 cups raisin bran	94
	1 cup skim milk	12
	1 banana	28
Lunch	4 oz turkey and cheese sandwich	27
	6 oz low-fat yogurt	34
	¼ cup trail mix	23
	1 plum	9
	1 apple	21
During workout	20 oz sports beverage	48
Postworkout snack	½ peanut butter sandwich	15
	12 oz chocolate milk	39
Dinner	2 cups pasta	78
	¾ cup marinara sauce	15
	6 oz chicken breast	0
	2 cups steamed broccoli	9
	12 oz skim milk	18
	Total Calories = 2973	**Total Carbohydrates = 470 g**
		61% of total calories

4000 Calories

Meal/Snack	Food/Beverage	Carbohydrate Content (g)
Breakfast	Smoothie:	
	2 frozen bananas	55
	2 cups skim milk	24
	2 scoops protein powder	27
Snack	Orange	15
	Granola bar	29
Lunch	2 cups chili	54
	4 oz roast beef sandwich	25
	2 cups fruit salad	61
During workout	32 oz sports beverage	76
Postworkout snack	6 oz yogurt	34
	½ cup dry cereal	13
Dinner	6 oz salmon	0
	2 cups wild rice	70
	3 cups salad with dressing	17
	16 oz skim milk	24
Snack	1½ cups frozen yogurt	73
	½ cup frozen blueberries	9
	Total Calories = 4016	**Total Carbohydrates = 606 g**
		59% of total calories

5000 Calories

Meal/Snack	Food/Beverage	Carbohydrate Content (g)
Breakfast	2-egg omelet with cheese	5
	2 pieces of toast with 1 tbsp butter	47
	12 oz orange juice	39
Snack	1 cup mixed nuts and raisins	67
Lunch	2 hamburgers with buns	69
	16 oz skim milk	24
	2 pieces fresh fruit	52
Snack	Smoothie:	
	2 cups frozen mixed fruit	42
	1 cup pineapple juice	35
	8 oz yogurt	46
	2 scoops protein powder	27
During workout	48 oz sports beverage	114
Dinner	2 pieces lasagna	75
	2 pieces garlic bread	26
	2 cups green beans and carrots	22
	16 oz skim milk	24
Snack	8 oz skim milk	12
	3 oatmeal raisin cookies	23
	Total Calories = 4992	**Total Carbohydrates = 749 g**
		59% of total calories

the frequency of meals and snacks increases, as does the number of calorie-dense foods. Three meals plus several snacks distribute caloric intake throughout the day, preventing athletes from feeling "stuffed" or uncomfortable after eating. Calorie-dense foods increase energy intake considerably, without large increases in the volume of food consumed.

How many calories should be consumed during endurance training or competition?

The number of calories expended while participating in endurance sports varies. The energy requirements for an individual can be estimated based on the sport, the intensity and duration of activity, and the body weight of the athlete. However, often it is not physically or logistically possible for an athlete to fully match his or her energy expenditure with intake while exercising. Movement (e.g., running, biking), mental focus (e.g., mountain biking, race car driving), and lack of feasibility (e.g., swimming, rowing) can create circumstances where athletes are unable to meet their calorie needs. It can be not only extremely challenging for an athlete to physically consume enough food to match energy expenditure during activity, but also difficult for the body to digest high volumes of food without developing nausea or cramping. Therefore, it is more practical and realistic to develop a plan based on the nutrition basics needed for endurance performance: carbohydrates, fluids, and sodium.

For example, a 125-pound half-marathoner running a 6:30 minute/mile pace will burn approximately 775 calories in 1 hour of continuous running.[1] If this athlete were trying to match his energy needs by consuming a sports beverage (containing 50 calories per 8 ounces), he would need to drink 124 fluid ounces in 1 hour! An average range of fluid intake that can be consumed comfortably and safely for most athletes is approximately 24–48 ounces per hour—three to five times this amount is needed to obtain 775 calories. However, if the nutrition plan was based on fluid and carbohydrate needs, the requirements could be easily met. As mentioned in Chapter 3, it is recommended that athletes consume approximately 1.0–1.1 grams of carbohydrates per minute

during exercise. Therefore, this athlete would need approximately 60–70 grams of carbohydrates per hour. Assuming the sports beverage used contains 14–15 grams of carbohydrates per 8 fluid ounces, the runner would need to drink only about 34 fluid ounces per hour to meet his carbohydrate needs. Thirty-four fluid ounces per hour is much more manageable than 124 fluid ounces.

How many calories are required after a training session or competitive event?

A general guideline for endurance athletes is to consume 200–300 calories immediately following a training session or competitive event. This small snack should be followed by a substantial meal within the next 1 to 2 hours, supplying more calories, macronutrients, micronutrients, and fluids. Two hundred to 300 calories is not a large amount of food and can be easily obtained by eating half of a sandwich, a large glass of milk, or a glass of 100% juice. Often, athletes complain of not wanting to eat immediately following exercise—especially intense exercise. However, the suggestion of consuming a small snack versus a full meal is often perceived as more manageable, is generally well tolerated, and puts the recovery wheels in motion.

Are macronutrient needs different for endurance athletes?

The main difference between the diets of endurance athletes and those of athletes in other sports is in the quantity of food consumed, not necessarily the macronutrient composition of the diet. The extreme caloric demand of long-duration training, day in and day out, stresses the body's energy reserves, particularly the glycogen stores. Therefore, carbohydrates play a key role in the endurance athlete's diet. Similar to other athletes with high calorie needs, dietary fats are valuable for providing extra calories in a small volume of food. Another consequence of high calorie demands that is unique to endurance athletes is the use of protein for energy production. Proteins are not typically used by the body for energy production; however, they can play an energetic role, contributing up to 15% of the calories required during endurance and ultra-endurance sports. The bottom line is that endurance athletes need the same macronutrients as other athletes except in larger quantities so that the energy requirements of their sport can be met. The upcoming sections outline more specific recommendations and guidelines for carbohydrate, protein, and fat intakes for endurance and ultra-endurance athletes.

How important are carbohydrates to endurance athletes?

Carbohydrates are crucial to endurance athletes not only because they are an important energy source, but also because carbohydrates play a role in the rapid metabolizing of fats for energy. If the liver and muscles are depleted of glycogen, the endurance athlete experiences extreme fatigue (see Figure 12.2). This is called "hitting the wall," also known as **bonking**. When bonking occurs, the athlete can no longer generate the energy needed to maintain his or her race pace, and his or her perception of effort is greatly increased. The end result is a catastrophic decrease in performance.

Carbohydrate stores in the body are limited, and because of the long-duration and repetitive muscle activity involved with endurance training and sport performance, the need for carbohydrates is increased. In fact, the time to exhaustion during endurance exercise is directly related to the initial levels of stored glycogen in the muscles (see Figure 3.9 in Chapter 3). In addition, carbohydrates are also necessary for normal functioning of the central nervous system. Maintenance of blood glucose levels is important in

bonking A condition in which the endurance athlete experiences extreme fatigue and an inability to maintain the current level of activity. It is also known as "hitting the wall" and results when the body has depleted muscle and liver glycogen levels.

preventing mental fatigue because nerve cells rely on blood glucose for energy. For these reasons, it is difficult to overstate the importance of adequate carbohydrate intake for daily training as well as performance in competition. For the endurance athlete, carbohydrates are truly the "master fuel."

How are daily carbohydrate needs calculated for endurance athletes?

Current daily carbohydrate recommendations for endurance athletes range from 5–10 grams of carbohydrates per kilogram of body weight.[2–4] Applying this recommendation for Tony, a moderately active, 22-year-old male who weighs 150 pounds:

> 150 pounds ÷ 2.2 = 68.1 kilograms (kg) of body weight
>
> 68.1 kg × 5–10 g of carbohydrate per kg = 340–680 g of carbohydrates per day

The recommended 340–680 grams is a large range! To narrow the recommendation for practical purposes, the calculated carbohydrate requirements need to be compared to the total calorie requirements of the athlete. Using the equation from Table 12.1, Tony's calorie needs are estimated to be 2753–3442 calories per day:

> **1.** REE = (15.3 × BW) + 679
> **2.** REE = (15.3 × 68.1) + 679 = 1721
> **3.** Tony's total energy needs = REE × activity factor (for Tony's moderate activity level) = 1721 × (1.6–2.0) = 2753–3442 calories per day

To establish a narrower range for a carbohydrate recommendation, determine the percentage of total calories coming from carbohydrates at each end of the spectrum. For example, each gram of carbohydrates has 4 calories, and 340 grams of carbohydrates equals 1360 calories, which is about 50% of 2753 calories. Endurance athletes should generally aim for 50–65% of their total calories from carbohydrates. Therefore, the recommendation of 340 grams of carbohydrates providing 50% of the estimated total daily calories is appropriate. However, the high end of the carbohydrate recommendation would not be appropriate for a 2753-calorie diet, supplying nearly 99% of total calories ([680 grams × 4] ÷ 2753) × 100 = 99%! Even at the high end of the estimated calorie range (3442 calories), 680 grams of carbohydrate would be supplying 79% of

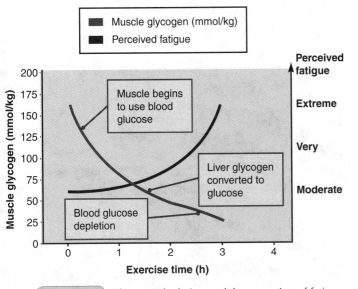

Figure 12.2 Glycogen depletion and the sensation of fatigue. If the liver and muscles are depleted of glycogen, the endurance athlete experiences extreme fatigue.

the total calories, which is generally too high for a balanced daily diet. Athletes should aim to meet both total calorie and carbohydrate requirements while maintaining a balance of all macronutrients. Recommendations for carbohydrates, as well as protein and fat, should always be compared to total calorie estimations.

How should endurance athletes carbohydrate-load before competition?

Carbohydrate loading is often cited as an effective way of maximizing muscle glycogen stores prior to an endurance event. As noted earlier, increasing muscle glycogen levels can increase the time to exhaustion and thus prevent or delay bonking (see Figure 3.9 in Chapter 3). In the 6 to 7 days leading up to a competition, endurance athletes should be **tapering** and resting their muscles. When tapering, endurance athletes decrease the volume and intensity of their training. During the taper, the percentage

> **tapering** A scheduled decrease in the volume and intensity of training 6 or more days prior to competition. The purpose is to allow for recovery from training and replenishment of glycogen stores in the liver and muscle.

of carbohydrates consumed each day should slowly increase from about 50–55% of total calories to 65–70%. This progression allows for carbohydrate storage within the muscles to be maximized while training time is minimized. The combination of rest and a full fuel tank produces an athlete who is mentally and physically fresh and nutritionally energized for race day.

A carbohydrate intake of approximately 8–10 grams of carbohydrates per kilogram of body weight, or about 500–600 grams of carbohydrates per day, is required to maximize glycogen stores. However, a further increase in carbohydrate intake may not necessarily further increase glycogen stores. Costill et al.[2] found that glycogen stores were similar when athletes consumed either 525 grams or 650 grams of carbohydrates per day. This study suggests that carbohydrate intake greater than 600 grams per day may not provide additional ergogenic benefits. For a 150-pound athlete, a range of 8–10 grams of carbohydrates per kilogram of body weight can be calculated as follows:

1. Convert pounds to kilograms: 150 ÷ 2.2 = 68.2 kg
2. Calculate carbohydrate needs: 68.2 kg × 8–10 grams carbohydrates/kg = 546–682 grams of carbohydrates per day

Because research has shown that consumption of greater than 600 grams of carbohydrates per day may

not be beneficial, it should be recommended that this 150-pound athlete consume 546–600 grams of carbohydrates in the days leading up to a competition. If the athlete feels that energy is running low during workouts, or recovery is slow, then the grams of carbohydrates can be increased gradually until an ideal quantity within the range is realized. Training Table 12.1 uses the 3000-, 4000-, and 5000-calorie per day sample meal plans to demonstrate the quantity of food needed to reach approximately 500–600 grams of carbohydrates per day.

During a tapering period, the decrease in calorie expenditure in the days leading up to an event needs to be realized and factored into a carbohydrate-loading plan. As previously mentioned, carbohydrate requirements increase during carbohydrate loading. However, due to a decrease in calorie needs, total calories need to be cut to prevent weight gain and a feeling of sluggishness. The best way to decrease calories without sacrificing overall nutrition or carbohydrate intake is to cut back on fat consumption temporarily (until the event). Protein is needed to repair muscle tissue and therefore should not be decreased dramatically to cut calories. Because fiber intake should be moderated in the days leading up

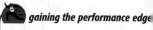

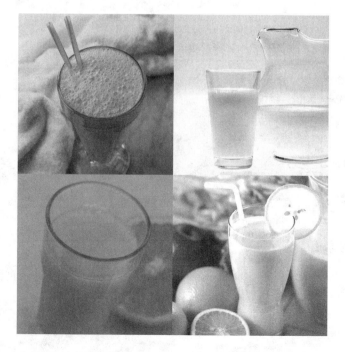

Training Table 12.2: Training Meal Plan vs. Carbohydrate-Loading Plan

Training Meal Plan
Breakfast
2 cups raisin bran
1 cup skim milk
1 banana

Lunch
Roast beef sandwich with cheese and mayonnaise
2 cups lentil soup
1 apple
16 oz water

Afternoon Snack
½ cup trail mix

Dinner
Stir-fry with 5 oz chicken, 1 cup broccoli, and 1.5 cup brown rice
3 cups tossed salad with 2 tbsp ranch dressing
1 cup skim milk
2 oatmeal cookies

Total Calories = 3000
Total Carbohydrate = 407 grams
Total Fat = 100 grams
Total Fiber = 50 grams

Carbohydrate-Loading Plan
Breakfast
2 cups Cheerios
1 cup skim milk
12 oz orange juice

Lunch
Roast beef sandwich, no cheese or mayonnaise
1 cup tomato soup
10 crackers
1 cup applesauce
16 oz water

Afternoon Snack
6 oz fruit-flavored yogurt
1 banana

Dinner
2 cups spaghetti with ¾ cup marinara sauce
3 oz ground turkey
2 slices French bread with 1 tbsp butter
½ cup green beans
1 cup skim milk
1 cup chocolate pudding

Total Calories = 2700
Total Carbohydrate = 462 grams
Total Fat = 54 grams
Total Fiber = 27 grams

to an event, juices, milk, smoothies, and other liquid forms of carbohydrates are ideal for use during a taper. Refer to **Training Table 12.2** for an example of how to increase carbohydrates while decreasing total calories, fat, and fiber in preparation for an endurance event.

Athletes who are competing several times a week do not have time to taper for 7 days while increasing carbohydrate intake. These athletes should ensure an adequate consumption of carbohydrates on a daily basis, which can also effectively keep glycogen stores near their maximum.

Should carbohydrates be consumed in the hours or minutes prior to endurance activities?

Research has demonstrated that consuming carbohydrates in the hours leading up to an endurance training session or competition is critical for optimal performance, especially during activities last-ing longer than 2 hours.[5,6] Carbohydrates consumed prior to exercise increase blood glucose, which leads to a sparing of muscle and liver glycogen, thus enhancing endurance performance. The question for endurance athletes is not whether they should consume carbohydrates prior to exercise, but rather when and how many carbohydrates should be consumed.

Even though it appears obvious in the research that preexercise carbohydrate consumption can prevent fatigue, the reality is that many athletes choose to forgo consuming any food, including carbohydrates, prior to training or competitions. Athletes need to be educated on the detrimental effects of this behavior. After an overnight fast, liver glycogen

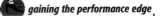

gaining the performance edge

Juices, milk, smoothies, and other liquid forms of carbohydrates are ideal for endurance athletes during a taper and carbohydrate loading.

stores are depleted, which can lead to premature fatigue during exercise.[7] Some athletes justify not consuming carbohydrates before training because they plan to consume carbohydrate-rich sports beverages, gels, or bars during exercise. Although consuming these products during exercise is clearly advantageous, it does not completely negate the need for a preexercise meal.[8]

A recent study by Chryssanthopoulos et al.[9] examined the effects of a preexercise meal and carbohydrate consumption during endurance running as compared with running on an empty stomach (no preexercise meal) and no carbohydrate supplementation during exercise. The authors reported a 9% increase in running capacity when a meal (containing 2.5 grams of carbohydrates per kilogram of body mass) was eaten 3 hours prior to exercise versus when no meal was consumed. An additional endurance benefit (22% increase) was observed when the subjects ate a carbohydrate-rich meal 3 hours prior to exercise and consumed a 6.9% carbohydrate beverage during running, as compared to those who did not eat a preexercise meal and did not drink the sports beverage during running. Endurance athletes are encouraged to consume a well-rounded, carbohydrate-rich preexercise meal, and then continue consuming carbohydrates during exercise to optimize performance.

When is the ideal time to consume carbohydrates prior to endurance training or competition?

The ideal time for consuming carbohydrates prior to exercise has been debated. Popular thought has led to the recommendation of consuming carbohydrate-rich foods in the 2–4 hours leading up to exercise and avoiding carbohydrates, specifically high glycemic foods/beverages such as glucose, in the hour immediately prior to activity. The reasoning for this advice has been that the combined effects of insulin (secreted in response to the high glycemic index products) and muscle contraction mediated glucose uptake (physical activity) would result in hypoglycemia immediately prior to or at the onset of exercise and thus negatively affect performance. However, a review of the current literature has revealed that only one study has reported a decrease in performance, whereas a majority of the studies have

shown either no impact or enhancement of up to 20% on subsequent endurance performance.[10]

A recent article studying the impact of precarbohydrate feedings on a series of 4000-meter swims performed by triathletes confirmed a positive impact on performance when carbohydrates are consumed within an hour of exercise. Smith et al.[11] examined the effect of consuming a 10% glucose solution 5 minutes prior to a 4000-meter swim, the same solution 35 minutes prior to the swim, or the equivalent volume of a placebo, on swim time to completion. Although no statistical significance was found between the trials, the findings were meaningful, revealing a difference ranging from 24 seconds to 5 minutes in 8 out of the 10 subjects studied when either glucose protocol was followed compared with placebo. The reported time difference would make an impact, for example, on the final placement of a triathlete performing a similar distance swim in an Ironman distance race (3.8 km swim distance).

The timing of a preexercise carbohydrate meal will vary greatly based on the quantity of carbohydrates consumed and an athlete's individual tolerance. Athletes typically consume their preexercise meal as close as 30 minutes before the initiation of endurance exercise to as long as 4 hours prior. In general, the greater the quantity of carbohydrates consumed, the longer an athlete should leave between eating and the beginning of an exercise session. It has been suggested that athletes consume greater than 2 grams of carbohydrates per kilogram of body weight prior to endurance exercise to have a positive impact on performance.[12,13] For a female endurance athlete weighing 125 pounds, the minimum quantity of carbohydrates required prior to a long-duration training session or competition would be 114 grams, calculated as follows:

1. Convert pounds to kilograms = $125 \div 2.2 = 56.8$ kg of body weight
2. The minimum amount of carbohydrates needed prior to exercise = 2×56.8 kg = 114 g

As noted in the 3000-calorie meal plan presented in Training Table 12.1, 114 grams can easily be obtained by eating 2 cups of raisin bran, 1 cup of skim milk, and a banana, which provides a total of 133 grams of carbohydrates.

Once an athlete knows the optimal quantity of carbohydrates to eat before endurance training, the athlete can then experiment with varying time periods between eating and exercise. The athlete should aim to eat far enough in advance to ensure that the food digests well before exercising, thus minimizing

gaining the performance edge

Endurance athletes should experiment and aim to eat far enough in advance that food digests well before competition, thus minimizing stomach and intestinal discomfort, but not so far in advance that hunger ensues.

stomach and intestinal discomfort, but not so long that hunger ensues. Therefore, the optimal timing of a preexercise carbohydrate-rich meal or snack will ultimately be determined by each athlete.

Should the endurance athlete consume carbohydrates during endurance activities?

As glycogen stores in the body are depleted, muscles rely more heavily on blood glucose for fuel, especially after 2–4 hours of continuous physical activity.[14] To maintain blood glucose for oxidation and continued energy production, athletes need to ingest carbohydrates while exercising. Although consuming enough carbohydrates during exercise can enhance endurance performance, ingesting too many carbohydrates can lead to stomach cramping, intestinal discomfort, and diarrhea, all of which can hinder performance. It is critical that athletes know their carbohydrate needs during activity and practice the ingestion of carbohydrate-rich foods and fluids during training to establish a nutrition plan based on personal preferences and tolerances.

As stated earlier in this chapter, carbohydrate needs during exercise are estimated at 1.0–1.1 grams of carbohydrates per minute of activity, or approximately 60–70 grams of carbohydrates per hour. Some athletes can easily consume and digest upward of 75–85 grams of carbohydrates per hour, whereas others can barely tolerate 45–55 grams. Athletes need to experiment with varying quantities of carbohydrates surrounding the 60–70 gram range to determine the best estimate for them individually. Carbohydrates can be consumed through a variety of foods and fluids such as sports drinks, energy bars, energy gels, fruits, granola bars, fig cookies, and even sandwiches. In addition to individual preferences, a nutrition plan needs to be developed with the limitations of the sport in mind. Refer to the section "What meal planning/event logistics need to be considered during endurance events?" at the end of this chapter for several examples of nutrition plans developed to meet the nutritional needs of endurance athletes while factoring in the inherent limitations of the sport.

Is carbohydrate intake important during the recovery period after endurance training or competition?

Carbohydrates are critical for recovery from endurance exercise. Repeated exercise sessions of long duration can deplete muscle glycogen stores. If glycogen stores are not replenished, performance in subsequent training or competitive sessions will suffer. Carbohydrates should be consumed as soon as possible after exercise in adequate amounts for glycogen replenishment, based on individual needs.

To optimize the replenishment of glycogen after endurance exercise, carbohydrates should be consumed as soon as possible after exercise—ideally within 15–30 minutes after exercise. The short time between cessation of exercise and carbohydrate consumption allows for digestion, absorption, and delivery of carbohydrates to the muscles for replenishment when muscles are most receptive to glycogen storage. Endurance athletes who train daily at high intensity levels or for a long duration need to consume adequate amounts of carbohydrates within this time frame to be prepared for the next exercise session.

Endurance athletes should consume approximately 1.2 grams of carbohydrates per kilogram of body weight per hour for 3–4 hours postexercise. The first dose of carbohydrate should be consumed within 15–30 minutes of the end of the training session. For example, a 130-pound athlete in training for a marathon should consume approximately 71 grams of carbohydrates per hour after exercise, and a 160-pound marathoner would need 87 grams of carbohydrates per hour. Whenever possible, athletes should focus on consuming whole food carbohydrates, juices, and low-fat dairy products to meet postexercise carbohydrate needs. Some athletes are not hungry after a long exercise session and may feel uncomfortable eating within 30 minutes after exercise cessation. In this case, athletes can consume high-carbohydrate beverages that are usually more tolerable than whole foods. This encourages rehydration as well as carbohydrate replenishment. **Table 12.2** provides some examples of both fluid and whole food combinations of carbohydrate sources to help endurance athletes meet their needs immediately postexercise. By following the guidelines for both the amount and timing of carbohydrate consumption after endurance exercise, athletes will recover quickly and perform well in their next training session.

Many supplements are marketed to endurance athletes for recovery from training sessions and competitive events. Before purchasing and using one of these supplements, consider the following:

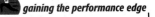

gaining the performance edge

Carbohydrates are truly the master fuel for endurance athletes. Individual needs should be calculated for daily consumption, as well as for before, during, and after training. Through trial and error, athletes will discover their individual tolerances, which should be built into the overall nutrition plan.

TABLE 12.2 Sample Postexercise Carbohydrate Options

Food	Carbohydrates (in grams)
1 orange	15
1 cup soy milk	15
2 sheets graham crackers	20
2 small fig cookies	22
1 cup animal crackers	24
½ cup applesauce	25
1 cereal bar	25
1 cup chocolate milk	26
½ whole grain bagel	26
1 cup apple juice	27
1 whole banana	28
1 cup cranberry juice	36
1 cup fruit yogurt	40
12 oz carbohydrate energy drink	78

Note: Combine a high-carbohydrate fluid with a high-carbohydrate solid food to obtain approximately 1.2 g carbohydrates per kilogram of body weight within 15–30 minutes after exercise.

- *How much carbohydrate is supplied in the supplement?* Some of the recovery supplements do not provide an adequate amount of carbohydrates. Athletes should calculate the number of grams they require and then determine whether the supplement is adequate.

- *What are the levels of other nutrients in the supplement?* Look on the Supplement Facts label for the %DV (% Daily Value) of the various nutrients supplied in one serving of the product. If specific vitamins or minerals are present in quantities greater than 100–200% DV, the quantities are excessive and in general should be avoided.

- *How much does the supplement cost?* Supplements of any kind can cost two to three times as much as whole foods, milks, and juices. If an athlete is on a limited budget, whole foods are generally more affordable and often supply a variety of nutrients.

- *Are foods and beverages available?* Supplements, especially those that do not require refrigeration, are very useful when athletes are traveling or away from home. Powders, bars, and liquids can be transported easily, carried in a gear bag, and consumed quickly after exercise when other options are not available. However, if whole food, juice, or dairy/alternative options are available, athletes should choose these items over supplements.

Are protein needs different for endurance athletes?

The dietary protein requirement for athletes has been a subject of debate for years, particularly for strength and power athletes. However, protein is important to the endurance athlete as well. Contrary to popular belief, recent research suggests that endurance athletes may actually require more protein than their resistance training counterparts. Tarnopolsky et al.[15] found that endurance athletes required approximately 1.4 grams of protein per kilogram of body weight to maintain nitrogen balance—a level higher than that needed by the resistance-trained subjects in the study. Although endurance athletes do not possess or strive to build the muscle mass of strength and power athletes, research has clearly demonstrated that endurance training results in increased protein turnover in the body. The trauma of repeated contractions and high-impact activities can increase protein breakdown during exercise. In addition, because of the huge energetic demands of endurance training it is now realized that some proteins are mobilized for energy. Protein is not typically used as a source of energy for the body; however, when caloric expenditure is high, the body will turn to proteins to supplement its energy needs. This reliance on proteins for energy is exacerbated when an athlete's diet is not adequate to maintain energy balance and/or carbohydrate intake is low. After endurance exercise, protein synthesis has been shown to increase 10–80% within 4–24 hours.[16] Because of the rise in protein catabolism during activity and protein synthesis after exercise, appropriate daily protein intake is important. Endurance athletes should focus on consuming adequate quantities of protein daily to achieve a positive protein balance, which is important for muscle maintenance and recovery after daily training and competition.

How are daily protein needs calculated for endurance athletes?

Several factors need to be considered when determining daily protein needs for endurance athletes. A general recommendation proposed by Lemon[17,18] based on a review of the literature, as well as Tarnopolsky et al.'s finding stated previously, suggests endurance athletes should aim to consume approximately 1.2 to 1.4 grams of protein per kilogram of body weight daily. Others have recommended a higher daily intake ranging up to 1.8–2.0 grams per kilogram of body weight for a greater safety margin.[19,20] Anywhere from 1.2 to 2.0 grams per kilogram can be appropriate for endurance athletes. The final recommendation for an individual should be based on the following:

- *How many hours a week and how intensely is the athlete training?* The greater the number of hours and the higher the intensity, the more protein an athlete will need. Recreational athletes should be encouraged to consume approximately 1.2–1.4 grams of protein per kilogram of body weight, whereas elite athletes should aim for daily intakes closer to 1.8–2.0 grams per kilogram.

- *Is the athlete aiming to lose, maintain, or gain weight?* Often endurance athletes are trying to lose weight in an attempt to increase their speed in sports such as long-distance running, duathlons, or cycling. When combining intense training and weight loss, protein needs will increase to the higher end of the spectrum (1.6–2.0 grams per kilogram). Athletes attempting to gain weight will also need more protein daily to build new tissue (1.6–2.0 grams per kilogram). Those with the goal of maintaining their weight will require a more moderate level of protein (1.2–1.5 grams per kilogram).

- *Is the athlete in a state of overtraining?* Because of the nature of endurance sports and the higher volume of training, endurance athletes are more likely than other athletes to experience the effects of overtraining. Individuals who are overtrained feel fatigued, sore, and stale because of the inability of muscles to completely recover from long, intense training sessions. These individuals can benefit from higher daily intakes of protein, aiding in the repair and recovery of muscles and tissues.

- *Is the athlete consuming adequate carbohydrates?* For all endurance athletes, emphasis should be placed on consuming enough carbohydrates, as well as adequate total calories, to spare protein. Without adequate carbohydrates and total energy, proteins are used at a higher rate for energy production, thus increasing total daily requirements for dietary protein. However, if glycogen stores are high, carbohydrates are consumed during activity, and total calorie needs are met, protein can be spared and daily intake

will remain moderate. The importance of carbohydrates for protein sparing was demonstrated in a study conducted by Lemon and Mullin.[21] The researchers revealed that protein accounted for 4.4% of the energy needed to complete 1 hour of cycling at 60% VO$_2$max in a glycogen-loaded state versus 10.4% of the energy required in a glycogen-depleted state. The bottom line: Athletes should ensure that carbohydrate intake is adequate while incorporating moderate amounts of protein on a daily basis. Refer to **Table 12.3** for daily protein recommendations for endurance athletes.

How can a daily meal plan be developed to meet the protein needs of an endurance athlete?

Dave is a competitive cross-country skier who trains 3 hours a day, 6–7 days a week. Dave is 22 years old and weighs 170 pounds. To develop a sample meal plan for Dave, the first step is to determine Dave's daily energy needs and protein requirements. The second step is to show Dave how he can put the recommendations into practice by developing a sample meal plan that provides adequate calories and protein. Following the energy requirement equations listed in Table 12.1 and the protein requirement calculations presented in Table 12.3, Dave's needs can be calculated as follows:

1. *Determine Dave's calorie and protein needs:*
   a. For a 22-year-old male, the energy estimation equation is:

   $$REE = (15.3 \times BW) + 679$$

   Dave's body weight is 170 pounds, or 77.2 kilograms

TABLE 12.3 Daily Protein Recommendations for Endurance Athletes

Activity Level	Daily Protein Recommendation (g protein/kg body weight)
Recreational athlete, *exercising 10–12 hours per week*	1.2–1.4
Competitive amateur athlete, *training 12–20 hours per week*	1.4–1.7
Elite athlete, *training and competing 20+ hours a week*	1.7–2.0

REE = (15.3 × 77.2) + 679 = 1860 calories × (activity factor of 1.6–2.4)

Total energy needs = 1860 × (1.6–2.4) = ~3000–4500 calories per day

Dave's average energy needs = (3000 + 4500) ÷ 2 = 3750 calories per day

b. For an athlete exercising about 20 hours per week, the protein needs are:

Protein needs = 1.7–2.0 grams of protein per kilogram of body weight

Protein needs = (1.7–2.0) × 77.2 kilograms = 131–154 grams of protein per day

Dave's average protein needs = (131 + 154) ÷ 2 = 143 grams of protein per day

(15% of total calories)

2. *Develop a meal plan to supply adequate calories and protein per day:* Modifying the 4000-calorie example meal plan presented earlier in this chapter, a meal plan can be developed that meets Dave's needs for 3000–4500 calories per day as well as his requirement for 131–154 grams of protein each day. See Training Table 12.3 for a sample meal plan that meets Dave's total calories and protein requirements.

What is the effect of consuming protein prior to endurance activities?

As established earlier in this chapter, carbohydrates consumed prior to endurance activities are critical to optimal endurance performance. Is protein intake just as important? The answer depends on when the protein is consumed.

Protein-rich foods consumed in the preactivity meal 2–4 hours prior to the initiation of endurance exercise contribute to a feeling of satiation and a slowing of digestion, thus maintaining energy levels for a longer period of time. In addition, some studies have suggested that protein consumption prior to exercise is beneficial in regard to the provision of **branched-chain amino acids (BCAAs)**.

> **branched-chain amino acids (BCAA)** A group of amino acids whose carbon side chain, unlike other amino acids, is branched. The branched-chain amino acids include leucine, isoleucine, and valine.

Training Table 12.3: Dave's Meal Plan

Meal/Snack	Food/Beverage	Protein Content (grams)
Breakfast	Smoothie:	
	2 frozen bananas	2
	2 cups skim milk	16
	1 scoop protein powder	8.5
Snack	2 oranges	2
	Granola bar	4
Lunch	1 cup chili	22
	3 oz roast beef sandwich	22.5
	2 cups fruit salad	4.5
During workout	48 oz sports beverage	0
Postworkout snack	6 oz yogurt	8
	1 cup dry cereal	2
Dinner	4 oz salmon	21
	2 cups wild rice	13
	3 cups salad with dressing	5
	16 oz skim milk	16
Snack	1½ cups frozen yogurt	10
	1 cup frozen blueberries	0
	Total Calories = 3750	**Total Protein = 156 grams**
		16% of total calories

It has been suggested that consuming BCAAs before exercising might delay fatigue during exercise via a mechanism involving the attenuation of central fatigue; however, the effect of consuming BCAAs immediately prior to exercise has so far been shown to be small at best.[22,23] Carbohydrate-rich foods should still take center stage in the preactivity meal to supply the muscles with glucose for energy, while protein assumes a supporting role. Consuming too much protein before exercise can lead to a sluggish feeling resulting from a lack of carbohydrates as well as dehydration because of increased urine production to flush out the by-product of protein breakdown, urea.

If protein-rich foods are consumed within an hour of endurance exercise, some researchers have shown a negative impact on performance. Wiles et al.[24] reported a higher oxygen consumption rate during various exercise intensities as well as an increased rating of perceived exertion when subjects consumed a moderate to high protein meal within 1 hour of exercise. No negative effects were shown when the same quantity of protein was consumed 3 hours prior to exercise. Therefore, it appears that moderate protein intake before exercise is beneficial if consumed with adequate quantities of carbohydrates several hours prior to exercise. By consuming carbohydrates, protein, and very small amounts of fat before exercise, athletes can maintain a balance and variety of foods within one meal, which is the goal for all meals throughout training.

Should proteins be ingested during endurance activities?

A significant amount of research has demonstrated that amino acids are secreted from the muscle, oxidized, and metabolized during exercise, thus implying their usage and importance during endurance activities.[25,26] A majority of this research has focused on the BCAAs—leucine, valine, and isoleucine.

The magnitude of BCAA usage is an important consideration for endurance athletes. It has been reported that a mere 2 hours of exercise at 55% VO_2max oxidizes close to 90% of the daily total requirement for at least one of the BCAAs.[27] It appears that as endurance training intensity increases, the use of BCAAs also increases proportionately.[28] These studies reveal that amino acids are used during endurance exercise and thus suggest a need for increased overall daily protein intake for athletes. However, is it essential and beneficial to be consum-ing protein *during* an activity versus before and after training and competitions?

Some research has suggested that the consumption of protein during exercise may enhance endurance performance. Several theories have arisen:

- *Usage of protein for energy production*: Utilization of BCAAs and provision of Krebs cycle intermediates have been suggested as the pathways for energy production and metabolism with protein ingestion.[29]

- *Increased stimulation of insulin secretion*: A combination carbohydrate–protein supplement has been found to stimulate insulin secretion after prolonged exercise.[30,31] This rise in plasma insulin has been hypothesized to lead to an increased glycogen synthesis, thus aiding in recovery from exercise. Recent researchers have suggested that it is possible that a similar action may occur during exercise—that protein (with carbohydrate) ingestion during exercise might increase insulin secretion and in turn spare muscle and liver glycogen usage during exercise. Some studies have found an ergogenic effect of adding protein to a carbohydrate supplement during exercise; however, they have failed to directly correlate insulin levels or any other plasma or metabolic reason for the enhanced performance.[32]

- *Suppression of central fatigue* (see Figure 12.3): During endurance exercise there is a decrease in plasma BCAAs. At the same time, tryptophan is unloaded from albumin at a higher rate into the plasma. BCAA and tryptophan compete for the same transporters across the blood–brain barrier; therefore, when BCAA levels decrease, a higher percentage of tryptophan can attach to the transporters, increasing the brain's uptake of tryptophan. Tryptophan converts into serotonin, which has a relaxation effect, ultimately causing an athlete to feel fatigued and eventually cease exercising.[33] Some researchers have suggested that the ingestion of BCAAs during exercise will maintain the plasma concentration and thus delay fatigue and enhance endurance performance. This theory has been supported in some studies and refuted in others.[34–37] More research is needed to draw definitive conclusions.

These theories and relevant research are still in their infancy and require more studies to clarify the actions of ingested proteins and amino acids during exercise and their associated mechanisms and effects on performance.

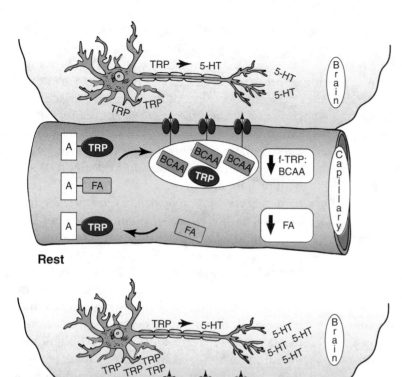

Rest

Exercise

Figure 12.3   Suppression of central fatigue. A decrease in branched-chain amino acid (BCAA) levels can cause an increase in the brain's uptake of tryptophan (TRP). Tryptophan converts into serotonin (5-HT), which has a relaxation effect, resulting in fatigue and ultimately the cessation of exercise. A = albumin, FA = Fatty acid, f-TRP = Free tryptophan.
Source: Davis JM, Alderson NL, Welsh RS. Serotonin and central nervous system fatigue: nutritional considerations. *Am J Clin Nutr.* 2000;72:573S–578S. Used with permission from American Society for Nutrition.

Regardless of actual performance benefits from ingesting amino acids, foods and drinks containing protein can be beneficial to consume during endurance activities, especially ultra-endurance events, from a practical standpoint. Items containing some protein in general will be less sweet but more salty than the typical endurance sport fare. When a training session or competition continues for 4–24 hours, flavor fatigue is of great concern because when an athlete stops ingesting calories, energy levels will soon plummet. Many sports nutrition products have a sweet flavor, and therefore salty foods are generally a welcomed change of taste. Conversely, if too

much protein is consumed, gastric emptying can be delayed, which can cause stomach cramping and delayed absorption of nutrients. Some practical ideas for items that have moderate amounts of protein, are easily digestible, and are compact for carrying during activities such as hiking, day-long bike trips, or adventure races include energy bars, sesame sticks, peanut butter sandwiches, peanut butter crackers, meat jerky, trail mix, and mixed nuts.

Is protein needed for recovery from endurance exercise?

Although not as critical as carbohydrate consumption, protein consumption after endurance exercise aids in the recovery process. Several proposed roles of protein after endurance exercise include enhancing the insulin response to accelerate glycogen synthesis and rebuilding damaged muscle tissue.

Research began with the investigation and discovery that protein added to a carbohydrate supplement can enhance the insulin response, suggesting a hastened delivery of nutrients into the cells versus carbohydrates alone.[38,39] Further studies then explored whether the increase in insulin levels correlated with greater amounts of glycogen several hours postexercise. A study completed by Zawadzki et al.,[31] mentioned in Chapter 5, often is cited when justifying the need for protein after exercise to maximize glycogen levels. The researchers reported that after several hours of cycling, the athletes who consumed a combination carbohydrate and protein supplement had higher levels of glycogen than the cyclists who consumed only carbohydrates. However, it should be noted that the combination supplement had more total calories than the carbohydrate-only supplement, which may have contributed to the enhancement, not necessarily the pairing of protein and carbohydrates. Regardless, protein-rich foods consumed after exercise will provide a unique profile of nutrients as well as supply amino acids needed for muscle repair.

Researchers at Indiana University (Karp et al.[40]) studied chocolate milk compared to traditional carbohydrate replacement beverages as a recovery aid following exhaustive exercise in nine endurance-trained cyclists. Subjects performed an interval

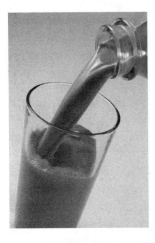

workout to deplete muscle glycogen, followed by 4 hours of recovery, and then an endurance performance trial to exhaustion. Subjects consumed an equivalent amount of carbohydrates (1 g/kg body weight) from a traditional ready-to-drink carbohydrate replacement drink or chocolate milk immediately after the depletion exercise and again 2 hours later. Results showed that consumption of chocolate milk after exercise was equal to or better than traditional carbohydrate drinks in time to exhaustion and total work for the endurance trial to exhaustion. More research is needed to determine whether the combined protein and carbohydrates in chocolate milk, instead of carbohydrates alone, helped improve these athletes' performance during the endurance trial phase of the study. Chocolate milk is highly palatable and inexpensive compared to many ready-to-drink sport supplements. This research could prove valuable for athletes to practically and inexpensively apply recovery nutrition to their daily diet.

The repetitive nature of endurance sports has led to the recommendation to consume protein after exercise to repair muscle tissue. Especially after repetitive eccentric movements, such as running, muscles may experience microtrauma, requiring amino acids as building blocks to repair the damage. Some research suggests that the microtrauma to the muscle cells contributes to muscle soreness after exercise. Therefore, if protein-rich foods consumed immediately after endurance exercise supply amino acids for hungry muscles, muscle soreness may be decreased.

Similar to carbohydrate foods, protein-rich foods should be consumed within 15–30 minutes postexercise to maximize the delivery of nutrients to the muscles. Approximately 6–20 grams of essential amino acids from an appropriate protein source immediately following endurance exercise appear to be sufficient to initiate the recovery process. Continuing to consume protein in subsequent meals throughout the day will supply the total daily requirements of protein for an athlete and thus aid in the continuous rebuilding and repair of tissues before the next endurance exercise bout.

Should endurance athletes eat more fats to meet their energy needs?

Because the body relies on fats for energy and the energy requirements for endurance athletes are high, one might be foolishly misled into thinking that fat intake should be of prime importance in the diet of endurance athletes. Numerous studies have demonstrated that endurance training does indeed cause metabolic adaptations that enable the body to rely more heavily on fat metabolism for energy during exercise (see Figure 3.8 in Chapter 3). This is an important adaptation because it decreases the drain on the body's somewhat limited carbohydrate reserves (Figure 12.4). However, the onset of fatigue during endurance training and competition is not caused by exhausting the body's fat reserves; in most cases it is caused by depletion of carbohydrate stores. Therefore, increasing the percentage of calories from fats in the diet does little to enhance performance because it is the availability of carbohydrates that ultimately limits the metabolizing of fats in relation to delaying the onset of fatigue.

However, some researchers have suggested that a high-fat diet, consumed either for a single meal or for several weeks, may actually be advantageous to endurance athletes. The theory is that because fat usage during exercise is caused in part by the concentration of free fatty acids in the plasma, if blood levels can be increased, more fats will be used for en-

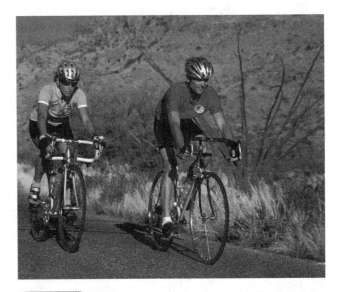

Figure 12.4 Endurance training causes metabolic adaptations that enable the body to rely more heavily on fat metabolism for energy during exercise. This is an important adaptation because it decreases the drain on the body's somewhat limited carbohydrate reserves.

ergy, sparing carbohydrates and possibly enhancing endurance performance. Studies have investigated the ergogenic benefit of short-term and long-term, high-fat diets to determine whether increasing the fat content of one meal or the daily diet can cause the body to adjust and adapt to become a higher fat-burning machine.

Several methodical strategies have been used in short-term, high-fat studies. Most of the research showing a positive result from a single high-fat meal has included the infusion of heparin. Heparin stimulates lipoprotein lipase activity, which in turn increases the plasma levels of free fatty acids in the blood. Because the infusion of heparin before endurance activities is not considered a sound medical practice, these studies provide little relevant information to the practical world of endurance sports. In the studies that involve strictly high-fat meals and subsequent tests of endurance (without heparin injections), most show no benefit over a high-carbohydrate meal.[41,42]

fat loading The dietary practice of eating a diet high in fats (i.e., >60% of total daily calories) 3 to 5 days prior to competition.

The effect of **fat loading** (i.e., consuming high levels of fat in the diet) on endurance performance has been evaluated in studies of high-fat diets consumed for 3–5 days prior to exercise. Studies have compared the effect of a high-fat diet (more than 74% of total calories) versus a high-carbohydrate diet (more than 77% of total calories) on performance tests to exhaustion. Results have consistently shown that high-fat diets have a negative impact on endurance performance.[12,43,44] At this time, fat loading cannot be recommended as a method of improving performance in endurance activities.

Another set of studies has focused on the effect on endurance performance of a high-fat diet consumed for 1–4 weeks. It appears that individuals consuming a high-fat diet for this moderate length of time can adapt to using more fat for fuel, and thus increase time to exhaustion in endurance tests. Lambert et al.[26] studied five endurance cyclists who consumed either a high-fat diet (76% of total calories) or a high-carbohydrate diet (74% of total calories). After 2 weeks on the diet, the subjects consumed a normal diet for 2 weeks and then consumed the opposite diet plan for 2 weeks. After each 2-week experimental set, the cyclists performed a Wingate power test, a high-intensity exhaustion test (90% of VO$_2$max), and a moderate-intensity exhaustion test, cycling at 60% of VO$_2$max. No difference was noted on the power test or the high-intensity test.

However, the cyclists performed better in the moderate-intensity cycle test (increased endurance) when consuming the high-fat diet. The authors attributed the benefit to a lower respiratory exchange ratio, meaning the individuals were relying more on fats for energy than carbohydrates. However, it should be noted that the endurance test was performed after two other intense physical tests, with little rest between tests, which can affect endurance performance and thus make the interpretation of these results difficult. Other studies have suggested a benefit from a moderate- or high-fat diet, but with varying levels of fat intake, the use of trained and untrained subjects, and different testing/diet protocols, comparisons are difficult and drawing conclusions has been challenging.[45,46]

Finally, long-term studies (>7 weeks) on the effects of a high-fat diet on endurance performance have failed to show an ergogenic benefit.[47] In addition to inconsistent results from short-term to long-term, high-fat consumption, high-fat diets should be evaluated based on the following:

- Fat takes longer to digest, and therefore high-fat meals put the athlete at higher risk for gastrointestinal issues during exercise.
- High-fat diets can lead to flavor fatigue relatively quickly, causing an athlete to stray from the prescribed diet, thus making a long-term plan impractical.
- High-fat diets have been shown to negatively affect cardiovascular health long term, and therefore are not generally recommended.

Currently, the available research does not support a widespread recommendation for athletes to consume a high-fat meal prior to endurance exercise or to follow a high-fat diet plan. More research is needed to fully understand the effects of high-fat meals on endurance athletes and the mechanisms involved. Dietary fat provides additional calories necessary for athletes with high daily energy expenditures. Foods that contain fat also provide vitamins and minerals that are essential to optimal sport performance in endurance events. Endurance athletes can consume moderate amounts of fat, if desired, so long as dietary fat does not replace the carbohydrates and protein necessary for success in endurance exercise.

How are daily fat needs calculated for endurance athletes?

For endurance athletes, fat requirements are generally calculated after determining carbohydrate and protein needs. Carbohydrates are the main fuel in the body for endurance sports, and protein is critical for repairing muscle tissue after long-duration activities, especially weight-bearing sports. Therefore, both macronutrients take precedence over fat. However, the importance of dietary fat should not be downplayed—fatty acids are critical for meeting total energy needs, obtaining essential fatty acids, and absorbing fat-soluble vitamins from foods and beverages.

One of the main functions of fat in the endurance athlete's diet is to provide a concentrated source of energy. For athletes training 3–6 hours or more a day, energy needs can climb into the 4000–6000 calorie range. Consuming enough food to meet these energy needs can be challenging, especially if an athlete is aiming to meet these needs with predominantly carbohydrates and protein. Meeting high energy needs with mainly carbohydrate- and protein-rich foods will require an athlete to eat very large volumes of food that can cause gastrointestinal discomfort. The large volume of food may also be challenging from a schedule standpoint, requiring an athlete to eat 6+ meals and snacks a day; eating that frequently becomes difficult when 3–6+ hours a day are spent exercising. Conversely, fat-rich foods are calorie-dense, allowing an athlete to consume more calories with less food and without feeling too full or bloated.

As with any athlete, moderate amounts of fat must be consumed on a daily basis to obtain the essential fatty acids provided in food. Endurance athletes—especially those trying to lose weight or body fat—often become too focused on carbohydrates and lean protein sources, while attempting to minimize or eliminate fat intake. Athletes need to remember that fat is a healthy part of a daily diet. Essential fatty acids provide energy, help to produce hormones in the body, surround all nerves contributing to proper nerve function, and aid in the absorption of fat-soluble vitamins and antioxidants.

Fat-soluble vitamins—vitamins A, D, E, and K—are all critical nutrients for an endurance athlete. Vitamins A and E are classified as antioxidant vitamins, helping to neutralize oxidative damage that occurs during exercise. Vitamin D works closely with calcium to provide structure and strength to bones—essential for weight-bearing activities and the prevention of stress fractures. Vitamin K has the role of helping blood to clot. Cuts and gashes can occur during some endurance sports, such as mountain biking or adventure racing, and an athlete will be thankful that their blood can clot properly, ceasing the flow of blood and allowing the injury to heal. All of these vitamins cannot be absorbed to their full capacity if not consumed with a small amount of dietary fat.

In summary, fat is important in an endurance athlete's diet, but only moderate amounts are needed. If carbohydrate needs are calculated at 50–65% of total calories, and protein needs fall between 12% and 18%, then the remaining calories should be contributed by fat—approximately 20–35% of total calories. Most often, fat needs for endurance athletes will be calculated at the lower end of this range. However, if calorie needs are very high, fat intake at 30–35% of total calories will ensure adequate total calories, a feeling of satiety, and a decrease in the total volume of food that needs to be consumed in one day.

To estimate fat requirements for endurance athletes, calculate total energy needs first. Then, determine carbohydrate and protein requirements in total grams as well as a percentage of total calories. The remaining percentage of calories should come from fat. Double-check the calculations to ensure that fat intake does not fall below 20% of total calories, to prevent fatty acid deficiencies, and does not exceed 30–35%, for heart health and overall dietary balance. The ranges for carbohydrates, protein, and fat provide a wide spectrum of appropriate options to develop a nutrition plan that incorporates balance, variety, and moderation while simultaneously providing enough fuel for an athlete to remain energetic, fresh, and recovering well from hard workouts and competitions.

For example, Brooke is a cyclist, riding 150–200 miles a week. She is 30 years old, is 5'8", weighs 132 pounds, and wants to maintain her weight. To calculate her fat needs:

1. *Determine her total energy needs:*

$$REE = (14.7 \times 60 \text{ kg}) + 496$$
$$= 1378 \times (1.6 - 2.4) = {\sim}2200 - 3300$$

Brooke's average calorie needs
= 2750 calories per day

2. *Determine her carbohydrate (CHO) needs:*

5–10 grams carbohydrates × kilograms of body weight = 5–10 g × 60 kg = 300–600 grams

Brooke's average carbohydrate needs = 450 grams of carbohydrates per day (65% of total calories)

3. *Determine her protein needs:*

Training 12–20 hours per week = 1.4–1.7 grams of protein per kilogram of body weight

(1.4–1.7) × 60 kg = 84–102 grams of protein

Brooke's average protein needs = 93 grams of protein per day (14% of total calories)

4. *Determine her fat needs:*

Remaining calories based on percentage = 100 – 65 (CHO) – 14 (protein) = 21% of total calories from fat

21% of 2750 = 577.5 calories ÷ 9 kcal/gram of fat = ~64 grams of fat per day

Should fats be eaten while performing endurance activities?

During low-to-moderate-intensity activities, a majority of energy is derived from fatty acids in the blood. Because fats are such an important fuel source, it would seem logical that consuming fats (long-chain triglycerides) while competing in endurance sports would be a good practice. However, other factors must be taken into consideration regarding fat intake during competition. First, depleting the body's fat stores, even on the leanest of individuals, is not a likely scenario and thus not an energetic cause of fatigue. In addition, fatty foods are slow to digest, delay gastric emptying, and may cause gastrointestinal cramping and diarrhea—none of which will enhance performance. Despite the negative effects of consuming dietary fats during endurance exercise, some researchers have suggested that ingestion of **medium-chain triglycerides (MCTs)** may be beneficial by sparing endogenous carbohydrate stores and enhancing endurance performance. MCT supplements marketed to endurance athletes have suggested benefits such as increased energy levels, enhanced endurance, increased fat metabolism, and lower body fat levels. Although these claims sound appealing, research has not been able to consistently support these statements.

An early focus of research was centered on the fact that MCTs can be oxidized as rapidly as exogenous glucose. The theory derived from this fact was that MCTs could potentially spare the usage of muscle glycogen as well as exogenous glucose during endurance exercise, thus delaying fatigue. Two different studies[48,49] from the early 1980s with similar

medium-chain triglycerides (MCT) A glycerol molecule with three medium-chain fatty acids attached.

methodology revealed similar results. Both studies compared the effects of consuming 25–30 grams of MCTs or 50+ grams of carbohydrates before 1 hour of exercise at 60–70% VO_2max on substrate utilization and glycogen sparing. The amount of carbohydrates and fat used during the hour of exercise was virtually identical across experimental groups, and glycogen stores were not spared.

The next step was for researchers to investigate the effects of larger quantities of MCTs to determine whether earlier studies did not find a benefit because of low dosages. It should be noted that earlier studies documented preliminary findings of gastrointestinal intolerances of MCTs at doses higher than 50–60 grams.[49] Despite this information, future studies were completed with doses upward of 85 grams of MCTs. The first study performed by Van Zyl and associates[50] studied the effects of glucose, MCT, or glucose plus MCT ingestion during cycling. Six endurance-trained cyclists performed a 2-hour bout of cycling at 60% VO_2max, followed by a 40-kilometer time trial. While cycling on separate occasions, the subjects consumed one of three beverages in random order: 10% glucose, 4.3% MCT, or 10% glucose + 4.3% MCT solution. The MCT-only beverage negatively affected the time trial performance by 5.3 minutes, while the combination beverage improved performance by 1.7 minutes compared to glucose alone. Unfortunately, muscle glycogen levels were not directly measured in this study, and therefore the glycogen sparing theory of MCTs could not be confirmed.

A follow-up study was performed by Jeukendrup and associates,[51] once again testing cyclists consuming glucose only, MCT only, or a combination beverage. Several differences in experimental design were implemented as compared to the Van Zyl study:[50]

1. A 5% MCT solution was used instead of a 4.3% solution (the 10% glucose solution remained the same).
2. A placebo group was included.
3. The time trial after the 2 hours of cycling at 60% VO_2max involved the maximum amount of work produced in 15 minutes versus the time to complete a 40-kilometer distance.
4. Carbohydrate and protein utilization during exercise was measured.

The authors found no difference in performance among the placebo, glucose, and glucose + MCT trials. However, they did find a 17–18% decrease in performance when cyclists consumed the MCT-only beverage. The MCT beverage also did not alter carbohydrate or protein utilization during exercise, thus not sparing glycogen stores. It was documented that several subjects vomited during the MCT trials, and others suffered from diarrhea.

In conclusion, long-chain triglycerides are not recommended for consumption during endurance sports. Small amounts may be consumed during ultra-endurance events lasting more than 4–6 hours without consequence; however, the amount should remain minute, with the focus placed primarily on carbohydrates and secondarily on protein. Some examples of fat-containing foods that may be tolerated during long-duration activities include peanut butter sandwiches, trail mixes, and sesame sticks. Intake of these foods should be tested during training and incorporated based on individual tolerance. Although a few researchers suggest a benefit of consuming small amounts of MCTs during endurance activities, the results have not consistently shown improvements in endurance performance. Although greater amounts may have a more significant impact on substrate utilization, large quantities of MCTs have also been shown to increase gastrointestinal distress. At this time, a recommendation cannot be made for endurance athletes to consume MCTs prior to and during training or competition.

Is fat needed for recovery from endurance exercise?

Unlike carbohydrates and protein, it is not essential to replace fat used during endurance exercise by consuming certain quantities or types of fat immediately following training or competition. The body's stores of fat are so great that they will not be depleted in an exercise session, even after prolonged endurance events. Because ingesting carbohydrates and protein is the main priority after endurance training, allowing the replacement, restoration, and replenishment of muscles, fat should be kept to a minimum. Fat causes the stomach to empty more slowly than do carbohydrates and protein, which could potentially delay the delivery of nutrients to the muscles in a timely fashion. However, fats add flavor to foods and create a sense of satiety, and therefore can be included in small amounts in the postexercise meal or snack.

Are vitamin/mineral needs different for endurance athletes?

Endurance athletes need higher levels of various nutrients, including some vitamins and minerals, as compared to their sedentary counterparts. But are specific vitamins and minerals of greater importance to endurance athletes versus team sport or strength/power athletes? Although all vitamins and minerals are needed in adequate amounts for proper health and bodily functioning, a handful of vitamins and minerals are in the spotlight for endurance athletes: B vitamins, iron, calcium, vitamin C, vitamin E, sodium, and potassium.

Why are the B vitamins important for endurance athletes?

B vitamins, specifically thiamin, riboflavin, and niacin, are involved in energy production pathways and thus are required in higher amounts for endurance athletes.[52] Thiamin plays a role in the conversion and utilization of glycogen for energy and the catabolism of branched-chain amino acids. Riboflavin is highly involved in the production of energy from carbohydrates, proteins, and fats for both health and performance. Niacin is a component of two coenzymes: nicotinamide adenine dinucleotide (NAD) and nicotinamide adenine dinucleotide phosphate (NADP). These coenzymes are involved in oxidation-reduction reactions required for the progression of metabolic pathways toward the synthesis of fatty acids and glycogen.

Increased intake of these B vitamins is important on a daily basis but is not necessarily required during exercise. The key is for endurance athletes to consume thiamin-, riboflavin-, and niacin-rich foods throughout the day, at meals and snacks. See **Table 12.4** for examples of thiamin-, riboflavin-, and niacin-rich foods.

Why is iron important for endurance athletes?

Iron is best known for aiding in the formation of compounds essential for transporting and utilizing oxygen (myoglobin and hemoglobin) and is therefore critical for aerobic activities and endurance training. Iron deficiency is one of the most common nutrient deficiencies in the United States and therefore deserves special mention. Because of the nature of endurance sports, athletes experience an increased loss of iron. **Hematuria,** or the presence of hemoglobin or myoglobin in the urine, is caused by a breakdown of red blood cells. The breakdown of red blood cells, also known as **hemolysis,** results in the release of hemoglobin and ultimately its elimination from the body via urine.

hematuria The presence of hemoglobin or myoglobin in the urine. Hematuria is an indicator of hemolysis.

hemolysis The breakdown of red blood cells in the body. This, in turn, results in the release of hemoglobin into body fluids.

TABLE 12.4	Key Vitamins and Minerals for Endurance Athletes		
	Importance Related to Endurance Sports	Food Sources	Critical Consumption Time Frame
Vitamins			
Thiamin	Energy production	Fortified and whole grains, legumes, wheat germ, nuts, pork	Daily meals and snacks
Riboflavin	Energy production	Milk, yogurt, bread and cereal products, mushrooms, cottage cheese, and eggs	Daily meals and snacks
Niacin	Energy production	Beef, poultry, fish, legumes, liver, seafood, fortified and whole grain products, mushrooms	Daily meals and snacks
Vitamin C	Antioxidant	Citrus fruits, berries, melon, tomatoes, green leafy vegetables, bananas, sweet potatoes	Daily meals and snacks as well as after intense, long training sessions
Vitamin E	Antioxidant	Nuts, seeds, wheat germ, fortified cereals, strawberries	Daily meals and snacks as well as after intense, long training sessions
Minerals			
Iron	Oxygen-carrying compounds and energy-producing enzymes	Beef, poultry, fish, soy products, dried fruits, legumes, whole grains, fortified cereals, green leafy vegetables	Daily meals and snacks
Calcium	Bone strength	Milk, yogurt, cottage cheese, hard cheese (and nondairy alternatives), fortified foods, and juices	Daily meals and snacks
Sodium	Electrolytes lost in sweat	Table salt, condiments, canned foods, processed foods, fast foods, smoked meats, salted snack foods, soups	Daily meals and snacks, during workouts lasting longer than 4 hours, after exercise to replenish sodium losses
Potassium	Electrolytes lost in sweat	Fruits, vegetables, coffee, tea, milk, and meat	Daily meals and snacks, small amounts during exercise, after exercise to replenish potassium losses

Hemolysis, which is believed to be at least partially caused by repeated impact, is common in distance runners.[53] Nonimpact endurance sport athletes, such as rowers or cyclists, can also experience hemolysis resulting from a loss of iron from the intestinal wall, in urine or feces, because of an irritation caused by equipment and body friction, oxidative stress caused by the formation of free radicals, and/or the consumption of nonsteroidal anti-inflammatory drugs.[53,54] Iron can also be lost through sweat. Endurance athletes lose a lot of sweat on a daily basis, further justifying an increased emphasis on adequate daily intake of iron.

Endurance athletes should focus on consuming iron-rich foods on a daily basis during meals and snacks. Similar to B vitamins, it is not necessary to consume iron-rich foods during activities. See Table 12.4 for examples of iron-rich foods.

Why is calcium important for endurance athletes?

Calcium is widely recognized as a bone-strengthening mineral. However, calcium's role in endurance performance extends beyond the skeleton. Calcium helps to produce fibrin, the protein responsible for the structure of blood clots. It is required for proper nerve function, releasing neurotransmitters that facilitate the perpetuation and activation of nerve signals. Calcium is pumped into and out of muscle cells to initiate both muscle contraction and relaxation in smooth muscle, skeletal muscle, and the heart. These functions are all essential for endurance athletes to maintain the intensity and duration of training and competition. During exercise, heart rate, muscle contraction and relaxation, and nerve impulse activity are all increased at incredible rates for sustained periods of time. Calcium also activates several enzymes that affect the synthesis and breakdown of muscle and liver glycogen, which is the main energy source during endurance exercise. Although critical in many ways for peak performance, many athletes are consuming suboptimal amounts of calcium on a daily basis. By striving for three to four servings of dairy/ alternatives, or other calcium-rich sources every day, athletes can meet their calcium needs. Calcium intake is not required during training sessions or competitions. Calcium stored within the body and the small amounts consumed in preexercise meals will provide the calcium needed during activity for proper nerve function and muscle contraction. See Table 12.4 for examples of calcium-rich foods.

Why are vitamins C and E important for endurance athletes?

Vitamins C and E have recently been acknowledged as potent antioxidants, helping to combat the oxidative damage that can occur during intense endurance exercise. Some research has shown that vitamins C and E actually work in concert with one another, enhancing each other's antioxidant properties.

Megadose supplements of vitamins C and E are often marketed to endurance athletes, touting enhanced recovery from intense workouts. Although these vitamins can make an impact on the recovery process, there is a safe and acceptable limit to daily intake. Vitamin C intake of 250–500 mg per day is above the RDA of 90 mg for males and 75 mg for females, yet far below the tolerable upper intake level (UL) of 2000 mg daily for adults.[55] Intake of 250–500 mg will ensure that endurance athletes are meeting minimum needs and also possible additional antioxidant needs from the added stress of physical activity. This level is easily obtained through a balanced, calorie-sufficient diet including plenty of fruits and vegetables.

Supplementation of vitamin E has become quite popular with endurance athletes because of recent studies touting its antioxidant abilities.[56] This research is conflicting (see Chapter 6); a prudent approach to vitamin E intake is to remain below the UL of 1000 mg (1500 IU) daily. Endurance athletes who may not meet daily energy needs or are restricting dietary intake for weight control may require vitamin E supplementation. Because large amounts of vitamin E are rarely toxic, supplementation at far higher than the 15 mg (23 IU) RDA is not a concern for most endurance athletes. However, it is also not clear whether and at what level of supplementation vitamin E might enhance endurance athletes'

performance. Combined dietary and supplemental vitamin E intakes of 100–270 mg daily (or approximately 150–400 IU) are appropriate and will ensure adequate intake without concern for negative side effects. See Table 12.4 for examples of vitamin C– and vitamin E–rich foods.

Why are sodium and potassium important for endurance athletes?

Sodium and potassium are crowned as heroes for their critical roles during endurance exercise. Sodium, one of the extracellular electrolytes, acts in conjunction with potassium, one of the intracellular electrolytes, to maintain proper fluid balance throughout the body during long-duration exercise. The interchange and flow of these electrolytes into and out of cells are responsible for the transmission of nerve impulses and muscle contractions. Sodium and potassium are both lost in sweat; however, sodium losses are of greater magnitude and significance. If sodium loss during exercise is excessive, without replacement, a life-threatening condition called hyponatremia can result. Sodium also aids in the absorption of glucose, which makes it a key component to any sports beverage.

Most Americans, including athletes, consume plenty of sodium on a daily basis. For athletes participating in ultra-endurance events, adding a little more sodium to meals and snacks in the days leading up to an event can help to "stockpile" a little extra sodium for race day. Sodium consumption during endurance training and competitive events is important for health and performance. Refer to the following section titled "Why are fluids critical to endurance performance?" for more information on calculating sodium needs for athletes during endurance events as well as guidelines for developing a nutrition plan that includes sports beverages, foods, and sodium supplements. The replacement of sodium after endurance exercise is easily accomplished by consuming salty foods and beverages.

On the other hand, most Americans, including athletes, are not doing a good job of consuming enough potassium on a daily basis. This suboptimal intake has been attributed to a low consumption of fruits, vegetables, and low-fat dairy products. Endurance athletes should be encouraged to eat more of these foods every day. During exercise, potassium can be obtained from sports beverages, as well as commonly consumed endurance fare such as bananas and oranges. See Table 12.4 and Figure 12.5 for examples of sodium- and potassium-rich foods.

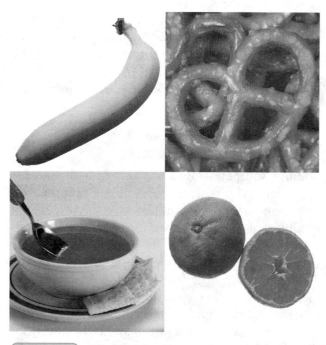

Choose foods with potassium and sodium after long exercise bouts to replenish these lost electrolytes.

Why are fluids critical to endurance performance?

As discussed in Chapter 8, 60% of our body weight is water. Fluid intake and maintenance of body water levels are critical to the endurance athlete for several reasons, in particular for the regulation of body temperature and maintenance of blood plasma volume. During exercise, the body's primary means of cooling itself is through the evaporation of sweat. Failure to adequately rehydrate during and after training leads to dehydration, which in turn results in elevated body temperatures during exercise. Elevated body temperatures cause an increased strain on the cardiovascular system, which is already a weak link in the aerobic power of most athletes, and leads to overheating of the body, which has negative and sometimes deadly consequences.

Blood plasma volume is one of the most important determinants of aerobic capacity because the cardiovascular system's ability to deliver oxygen is rate-limiting in regard to exercise intensity. The more blood that can be delivered to working muscles, the faster oxygen can be used for the aerobic production of ATP. The direct consequence of this is that the athlete can perform or maintain a faster race pace without the buildup of lactic acid, which ultimately can cause fatigue. If an athlete becomes dehydrated, the blood plasma volume decreases to support sweat

formation for evaporative cooling purposes. The resulting decrease in blood plasma volume leads to a decrease in the cardiac output of the heart, which in turn decreases delivery of oxygen to the working muscles and slows aerobic performance. Obviously, maintenance of hydration is of utmost importance to the endurance athlete because of the direct negative consequences inadequate fluid intake can have on performance.

How are daily fluid needs calculated for endurance athletes?

An endurance athlete cannot rely on becoming well hydrated during activity by drinking copious amounts of fluids if he or she is not well hydrated at the onset of exercise. To be well hydrated at the onset of exercise, endurance athletes should follow the daily hydration guidelines stated in Chapter 8 of this book. As a reminder, the AI of water for men and women over age 19 is 3.7 liters and 2.7 liters of water per day, respectively. Basic fluid needs can also be estimated based on an athlete's total daily calorie needs (see Chapter 8 for the estimation calculation). Remember, fluid losses during exercise are in addition to daily fluid recommendations. Because of the frequency and duration of endurance athletes' training and competition sessions, maintaining euhydration is of utmost importance and should be a dietary focus every day.

How are fluid and electrolyte needs during endurance activities determined?

Maintaining euhydration during endurance activities is dependent on making accurate estimations of individual sweat rates and electrolyte losses, practicing the consumption of the estimated amounts of fluid while exercising, and overcoming any logistical barriers to fluid availability.

How do endurance athletes determine their individual fluid needs?

If left to their own devices, endurance athletes will typically not drink enough fluid during exercise to maintain euhydration.[57,58] In a study conducted by Iuliano et al.,[59] female and male junior elite triathletes performed a simulated duathlon event consisting of either a 2-km run, 12-km bike ride, and 4-km

gaining the performance edge

Endurance athletes should make it a habit to carry a water bottle throughout the day. The physical reminder of holding a water bottle and the immediate availability of water will help athletes meet their daily fluid needs.

run, or a 1-km run, 8-km bike ride, and 2-km run based on age. All subjects were allowed to drink ad lib of their chosen beverage during all three segments of the simulated duathlon. All groups drank suboptimally, as revealed by a loss of body mass, in both absolute and relative terms. Many endurance athletes are not aware of how much fluid they are losing during exercise; therefore, the first step in promoting an athlete's awareness is to perform a sweat trial and then to practice his or her "ideal" fluid consumption frequently in training sessions. To review the sweat trial calculations presented in Chapter 8:

1. *Determine body weight (BW) lost during exercise:*

   BW before exercise – BW after exercise = pounds of water weight loss

2. *Determine the fluid equivalent, in ounces, of the total weight lost during exercise:*

   Pounds of water weight lost during exercise × 16–24 ounces = number of ounces of additional fluid that should have been consumed to maintain fluid balance during the exercise session

3. *Determine the actual fluid needs of the athlete during an identical workout:*

   Ounces of fluid consumed + ounces of additional fluid needed to establish fluid balance = total fluid needs

4. *Determine the number of fluid ounces needed per hour of exercise:*

   For practical purposes, total fluid needs ÷ duration of the sweat trial, in hours = number of fluid ounces needed per hour of exercise

For example, Jack is preparing for an ultra-endurance bike ride called the RAIN ride (Ride Across INdiana), which consists of riding 162 miles across the state of Indiana in one day. As part of his training, he participates in a 110-mile group bike ride. The ride takes 7.5 hours. During this time he drinks 224 fluid ounces of a sports drink. By the end of his workout, he had lost 8 pounds of body weight. What is the ideal amount of fluid he should be consuming per hour?

Using the steps stated previously:

1. His body weight loss during the workout was 8 pounds.
2. The fluid equivalent of his loss was 128–192 ounces (8 × 16–24 oz).

3. His total fluid needs for the 7.5 hours of cycling are 352–416 ounces (224 oz + 128–192 oz).
4. Jack needs 47–55 ounces of fluid per hour to match his sweat losses (352–416 ÷ 7.5).

For practical purposes, 47–55 ounces of fluid per hour is equivalent to 2.3–2.75 bottles per hour (assuming 20 oz bottles). For Jack, it would be in his best interest to install at least four water bottle holders on his bike so that he could carry enough fluid for several hours of riding. Because Jack was only drinking about 30 ounces per hour during the 110-mile training ride (224 oz ÷ 7.5 hours = 29.8 oz/hour), he will need to practice drinking 60–80% more fluid per hour before participating in the RAIN ride. A change in drinking behavior of this magnitude should be incorporated over time and not made overnight, to allow the body to adjust.

It is ideal for an athlete to consume mainly—if not solely—sports beverages during endurance activities lasting longer than an hour. A sports beverage delivers not only fluids, but also carbohydrates, sodium, and other electrolytes to the body. Generally, liquids or semi-solid foods consumed while exercising settle better than solid food. Therefore, if calories, carbohydrates, and electrolytes can all be obtained while maintaining hydration, the athlete will minimize the gastrointestinal issues that often result from eating solid foods during exercise.

How do you determine fluid and electrolyte needs for "big sweaters"?

Athletes who lose excessively large quantities of fluid and/or sodium during endurance exercise are often classified as "big sweaters." Although sports beverages are critical for the health and performance of these athletes, plain water can also be added into the nutrition/hydration plan for during activity. Some individuals require 64 fluid ounces or more per hour—that is a lot! If an athlete was to consume solely sports drinks in quantities to match fluid needs, the total amount of carbohydrates consumed could potentially reach a level that exceeds the recommended range of 1.0–1.1 grams of carbohydrates per minute. For example, if an athlete requires 54 ounces of fluid (based on sweat trials), this quantity of most sports

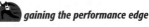
gaining the performance edge

Suggest endurance athletes start performing sweat trials months in advance of an important athletic event or competition. Changing fluid (as well as food) intake while exercising should be incorporated over time. Gradual increases in fluid are perceived as less challenging and overwhelming.

beverages would supply approximately 94–101 grams of carbohydrates in 1 hour—far exceeding the recommended range of approximately 60–70 grams of carbohydrates per hour. In this example, the athlete should consume 36–40 fluid ounces of a sports beverage and then drink an additional 14–18 ounces of water to meet his or her total fluid needs without exceeding carbohydrate recommendations.

"Big sweaters" will often complain of muscle cramps during training sessions and competitions. Muscle cramping is mainly caused by inadequate fluid consumption and dehydration. By performing a sweat trial and developing a hydration plan based on individual needs, cramping issues are often resolved. After an inquiry on the fluid choices of big sweaters, it is often revealed that they are drinking mainly water (versus a sports beverage) during training sessions. By switching from water to sports drinks, thereby supplying sodium, potassium, and other electrolytes lost in sweat, a second line of defense against muscle cramps is established. If these two approaches do not work, the athlete should seek professional help from a dietitian, physician, and athletic trainer. In some cases, athletes are not only "big sweaters" but also "big salt sweaters," meaning they are losing excessive amounts of sodium and other electrolytes because of higher concentrations in their sweat, which in turn cause muscle cramps. For big salt sweaters, an electrolyte supplement in addition to a sports beverage may be indicated. The provision of specific electrolyte supplements on a regular basis should be monitored by a physician to avoid any complications and to ensure that supplements are taken safely. The excessive consumption of electrolyte supplements can disrupt the electrolyte balance in the body and ultimately alter heart function.

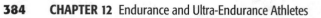

gaining the performance edge

Remember that each athlete is different. Some athletes can digest and tolerate more carbohydrates and fluid than the recommended ranges. Trial runs and practice will fine-tune a nutrition plan in preparation for hard training days and competitions.

How do you determine electrolyte needs for ultra-endurance athletes?

Ultra-endurance athletes, even those who are not considered big salt sweaters, may require additional sodium during long-duration training sessions and competitive events. Sodium losses are estimated at 50 mmol per liter of sweat, or 1 gram per liter, during exercise, with a range of 20–80 mmol per liter.[60]

Therefore, sodium requirements for athletes participating in training sessions and competitions lasting longer than 4–6 hours require approximately 500–1000 milligrams of sodium per hour of exercise, based on sweat rate.[60] If the sodium lost in sweat is not replaced in adequate amounts, blood levels of sodium begin to drop, and hyponatremia can ensue.

As mentioned in Chapter 8, hyponatremia is defined as blood sodium levels below 130–135 mmol/L. As the duration of an endurance event increases, the risk for hyponatremia also increases. However, with proper nutrition and hydration planning, it can be avoided. Salt tablets are commonly used to boost sodium intake above what is supplied in a sports beverage for events lasting longer than 4 hours. The quantity of sodium in a salt tablet can range from as little as 40 milligrams up to 1000 milligrams per tablet. Salt tablets are sold online and in local pharmacies. Salt tablets should be used in moderation and used only to supplement the sodium obtained from sports beverages during training sessions and competitive events lasting longer than 4 hours. Consuming sports drinks alone, in adequate amounts, is sufficient for endurance activity lasting less than 4 hours.

To reiterate the importance of monitoring intake, caution should be taken to ensure that excessive sodium is not ingested. Salt tablets are not required on a daily basis. The average American diet provides adequate sodium to replace losses through sweat. If necessary, additional salt can be consumed by using the salt shaker at the table in small amounts. Refer to the example in the **Fortifying Your Nutrition Knowledge** section regarding Mark, a half-Ironman triathlete, which demonstrates the development of a race-day nutrition plan including the appropriate use of salt tablets.

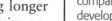

gaining the performance edge

Some sports beverage companies have recently developed formulas containing almost twice as much sodium as regular sports beverages. Endurance athletes regularly engaging in training and competitive sessions lasting longer than 4 hours should use the higher-sodium versions. Look for beverages containing approximately 175–200 mg of sodium per 8 fluid ounces of the beverage.

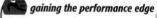

gaining the performance edge

Remember to use moderation with sodium intake. Replacing sodium losses is important for the prevention of hyponatremia; however, excessive amounts of sodium intake on a regular basis can contribute to high blood pressure. Use salt tablets discriminately and consume salty foods and table salt in moderation.

Mark contacted a dietitian to help him determine how to prevent the cramping he was experiencing during long bike rides and runs while training for a half-Ironman triathlon (1.2-mile swim, 56-mile bike ride, 13.1-mile run). He was baffled regarding the source of the problem because he had been taking three salt tablets an hour (150 milligrams of sodium per tablet) during long workouts since a training partner had suggested that low sodium levels were most likely the culprit of his cramps. Mark also reported that he was drinking plenty of water—consuming a full 20-ounce water bottle per hour during training.

The dietitian asked Mark to perform a sweat trial to determine the amount of fluid loss he was experiencing during training. After performing the trial and reporting the results, the dietitian informed Mark that he was only meeting a portion of his fluid needs. Mark was losing 32–36 ounces of fluid per hour and only replacing 20 ounces. In addition to not meeting his fluid needs, he was also falling short on his sodium intake. Even though he was taking salt tablets, he was consuming only 450 milligrams of sodium per hour because he was drinking solely water, which provides no sodium. The dietitian calculated his total fluid, carbohydrate, and sodium requirements and helped Mark develop a nutrition and hydration plan for the race using the following steps:

1. The first step was to determine his fluid needs. As stated earlier, the sweat trial results revealed a fluid loss of 32–36 ounces of fluid per hour.
2. The next step was to determine how much carbohydrate and sodium would be supplied if all of his fluid needs were met by a sports beverage. Thirty-two to 36 ounces of a sports beverage per hour supplies approximately 56–63 grams of carbohydrates and 440–495 milligrams of sodium per hour, depending on the brand used. A sports beverage is preferred over water because fluid, carbohydrates, and sodium can all be provided, versus only fluid supplied in water.
3. The quantity of carbohydrates supplied through the sports beverage was sufficient to meet his needs during exercise, although on the low end of the range. Mark can consume carbohydrate gels, energy bars, bananas, or other foods to supplement the carbohydrates supplied through the sports beverage.
4. Mark had been consuming approximately 450 milligrams of sodium through salt tablets. This quantity of sodium was just slightly below the minimal level of sodium recommended per hour, which may have been contributing to his muscle cramps in addition to dehydration. Preferably, sodium would be obtained by drinking a sports beverage that simultaneously supplies fluid, sodium, and carbohydrates for optimal performance and hydration. In Mark's case, basing his intake of a sports beverage solely on fluid needs, the quantity of sodium supplied by the sports beverage is slightly below the 500-milligram minimum level recommended per hour. If he consumes 440–495 milligrams of sodium in the sports beverage, an additional 150–500 milligrams need to be obtained from other sources. If he chooses to use an energy gel, bar, or peanut butter/cheese crackers for food during the bike portion of the triathlon, then additional sodium will be supplied in small quantities from these foods. By also planning on taking 1–2 salt tablets per hour, 150 milligrams of sodium per tablet, Mark can easily reach the goal of 500–1000 milligrams of sodium per hour.

See **Training Table 12.4** for an excerpt of Mark's half-Ironman plan focused on his needs during the race. The plan is designed to prevent muscle cramps by supplying adequate fluids and sodium while also providing the carbohydrates needed to keep him performing at his best.

Training Table 12.4: Mark's Half-Ironman Nutrition/Hydration Plan

Swim 1.2 miles
Total Time = 45 minutes
no food or drink

Bike 56 miles
Total Time = 3:18 (~17 mph)

Hour Elapsed on the Bike	Food/Fluid	Fluid (oz)	Carbohydrates (g)	Sodium (mg)
1	32–36 oz sports beverage*	32–36	56–63	440–495
	1 salt tablet**			150
2	32–36 oz sports beverage	32–36	56–63	440–495
	½ energy gel***		14	25
	1 salt tablet			150
3	32–36 oz sports beverage	32–36	56–63	440–495
	1 salt tablet			150
18 minutes	10–12 oz sports beverage	10–12	18–21	138–165
Average intake on bike		*32–36 oz/hour*	*60–67 g/hour*	*580–638 mg/hour*

Run 13.1 miles
Total Time = 1:51 (~8:30 min/mile pace)

Aid Stations on Course at Mile Markers	Food/Fluid	Fluid (oz)	Carbohydrates (g)	Sodium (mg)
1	5 oz sports beverage	5	9	69
2	5 oz sports beverage	5	9	69
	1 salt tablet			150
3	5 oz sports beverage	5	9	69
4	5 oz sports beverage	5	9	69
5	5 oz sports beverage	5	9	69
	1 salt tablet			150
	½ energy gel		14	25
6	5 oz sports beverage	5	9	69
7	5 oz sports beverage	5	9	69
	1 salt tablet			150
8	5 oz sports beverage	5	9	69
9	5 oz sports beverage	5	9	69
10	5 oz sports beverage	5	9	69
	1 salt tablet			150
11	5 oz sports beverage	5	9	69
12	5 oz sports beverage	5	9	69
13.1—strong to the finish!				
Average intake on run		*32 oz/hour*	*66 g/hour*	*785 mg/hour*

* Using a sports beverage with 14 grams of carbohydrates and 110 milligrams of sodium per 8 oz serving

** Using a salt tablet with 150 milligrams of sodium per tablet

*** Using an energy gel with 28 grams of carbohydrates and 50 milligrams of sodium per gel

Are fluids needed for recovery from endurance exercise?

Absolutely! Endurance athletes can potentially lose huge quantities of fluid while exercising, which need to be replaced as quickly as possible after exercise. As highlighted in Chapter 8, endurance athletes should:

- Drink fluids to replace any weight loss during endurance exercise. For every pound lost, an athlete should consume 16–24 ounces of fluid.
- Consume fluids slowly and gradually, instead of through a large bolus of fluid in one sitting. Athletes should begin drinking immediately after exercise and then continue to drink throughout the day.
- It is ideal to consume fluids containing carbohydrates, sodium, and potassium, which help to maximize not only fluid replenishment, but also glycogen stores and lost electrolytes. Sports drinks, vegetable and fruit juices, milk, and smoothies are examples of fluids containing more than just water.

Fluid replenishment ranks as high as carbohydrate replenishment on the recovery importance list for endurance athletes. Athletes should strive for consuming individually optimal amounts of fluids in a timely manner.

What meal planning/event logistics need to be considered during endurance events?

The nature of the sport will be a major factor in determining a specific nutrition plan for an endurance athlete. Endurance training prepares athletes for events that can last minutes, hours, or days. Training may occur in a controlled environment or can be held in a remote area with limited access to facilities. When developing a nutrition plan for endurance athletes, the feasibility of consuming foods or fluids, length of the event, availability of refrigeration/heating equipment, and space for carrying supplies must be considered.

How can a nutrition plan be developed for sports that are not conducive to consuming foods or fluids while exercising?

Long-distance swimming, mountain biking, and rowing events are examples of sports that do not lend themselves to easily consuming foods and fluids during an event. Swimming and rowing involve both upper and lower body movement, requiring an athlete to come to a complete stop to eat or drink.

In a competitive environment, coming to a halt will translate into the loss of precious seconds or minutes to competitors. In rowing, carrying any food or fluid will add weight to the boat, thus potentially slowing the athlete and negatively affecting performance. Mountain biking requires concentration and attention to the course, with legs needed for pedaling while arms and hands are steering the bike and keeping it upright and on course. In these situations, proper nutrition before and after the event will be critical in supplying nutrients and fluids to the athlete, because minimal consumption will occur during exercise.

Several factors should be considered in the days prior to and immediately before training or competition. Consuming higher levels of carbohydrates in the 3–4 days prior to an endurance competition can super-compensate muscle and liver glycogen stores. This allows additional energy stores to be available during long events where carbohydrate consumption is logistically impossible. The nutrients and fluid supplied in the hours leading up to the event will be the fuel used during exercise. If an athlete runs short on calories, carbohydrates, or fluids, performance will suffer because additional nutrients will not be consumed during the activity. Athletes should consider eating a larger preactivity meal, which might also mean planning additional time before a training session or event to allow for the digestion of the meal. Athletes should continue to sip on fluids between the preactivity meal and the beginning of a training session or competition to ensure proper hydration. Athletes also need to plan ahead and pack food and beverages to be consumed immediately following the activity to replenish lost nutrients and fluids.

There are some exceptions to the rule. For example, several ultra-endurance open-water swimming events

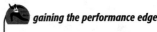

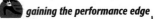

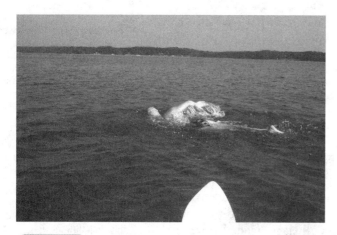

Figure 12.6 Swimmer Amy Krauss during the Key West Open Water Swim. Having support staff carry fluids and foods in long-distance endurance races makes adequate replenishment of needed nutrients more likely.

allow support boats to follow swimmers, giving the athletes a chance to stop, drink or eat, and then continue swimming. The following is an example of a swimmer, Amy Krauss (see Figure 12.6), who is a four-time competitor in the Key West Open Water Swim—a 12.5-mile event circling the island of Key West in 1 day.

Key West 12.5-Mile Open Water Swim

Most open-water swims consist of a 1-, 2-, or 6-mile course. The Key West Open Water Swim is an incredible 12.5-mile swim completed in one session. During the event, each swimmer must have a kayaker following alongside for safety reasons. The accompanying kayak also provides the opportunity for the competitors to have access to fluids and food during the event. On average, it will take a swimmer 4–6 hours to complete the race. By maintaining proper hydration and supplying a steady stream of energy to the body, the swimmer can perform at his or her best.

Over the years Amy has experimented with various hydration/fueling schedules, including different fluids, food, and nutrition products, to determine which options taste appealing and digest easily while swimming. Her hydration goal has been to drink 24 ounces of fluid per hour, which is achieved by stopping to drink every 15–20 minutes. Amy alternates between water, sports drinks, and more concentrated recovery-type nutrition drinks to supply fluids, carbohydrates, and electrolytes. In addition to fluids, Amy consumes sports gels and small pieces of energy bars to supply more calories and carbohydrates to her muscles.

Although the kayaker makes it easy to have fluids and food available at any time, it is not always easy to eat and drink. Depending on the roughness of the water, actual ingestion of fluid and food can be challenging. The constant bobbing of the body in the waves can lead to seasickness and vomiting, which is obviously detrimental to athletic performance. Amy experienced this scenario in the 2000 race when she had to stop to tread water for 90 minutes while vomiting. She now takes medication several days before the race to prevent the seasickness, allowing her to consume fluids and food comfortably, which has led to several great race performances.

How can a nutrition plan be developed for sports lasting 24 hours or longer?

Ultra-endurance events once reserved for really "crazy" people are now becoming more mainstream. Ultra-marathons and adventure races have exploded in popularity, drawing recreational and elite athletes into events lasting 8–24 or more hours. When events are spanning the majority of 1 day, energy expenditure increases dramatically while simultaneously making it challenging to consume enough fuel because regular meals are essentially skipped.

Fortunately, these ultra-endurance sports are conducive to eating and drinking while moving, though only in small quantities at a time. In some cases, aid stations with supplies may be available on the race course, whereas other events are self-sustaining.

In cases when an athlete is planning on relying on aid stations for food and fluids, planning and practicing before an event are paramount. Athletes should contact the race director or consult the race information packet or Web site to discover what type of food and fluids will be available on the course. Athletes should then consume the same type of food and fluid throughout their training. For example, Barbara, an ultra-marathoner, typically uses All-Sport, oranges, and PowerBars during her training. She registers for a race and discovers that Gatorade, bananas, and fig bars are going to be supplied on the course. Barbara should immediately switch to using these products and foods during her training. Even though All-Sport, oranges, and PowerBars are nutritionally similar to Gatorade, bananas, and fig bars, they are not identical and can potentially cause taste aversions and gastrointestinal problems if an athlete is not accustomed to the products. As the length of an endurance event increases, nutrition becomes even more critical to performance. As with any sport, there should be no surprises on race day! Athletes should find out what products are going to be supplied during their scheduled races and then practice, practice, practice during training.

Another issue to address during 8–24+ hour events is the variety of flavors and textures of food consumed. A common complaint of ultra-endurance athletes is flavor fatigue for sweet products. Sports drinks, bars, and gels are made of carbohydrates that taste sweet—some more intensely than others. When an athlete is consuming these foods over 1–4 hours, flavor fatigue is not typically a concern. However, when athletes are consuming large quantities of food to meet the energy needs of events lasting more than 8 hours, flavor fatigue is a reality that must be addressed during training. If an athlete gets "tired" of the sweet taste, and all he or she has practiced consuming during training is sports drinks, fruits, and bars, then a switch to different foods or fluids during a race can be disastrous. Athletes should practice consuming foods and fluids with salty or bland flavors to balance with sweet items. Examples of salty items that are commonly used in races are pretzels, peanut butter crackers, chicken broth, sesame sticks, and even lunchmeat sandwiches. Continuing the ingestion of calories will ensure that an athlete keeps moving forward on pace and feeling good.

In an adventure race, when many different sports are involved in one event and athletes are typically self-supporting, the timing of food and fluid intake as well as the reliance on nonperishable items makes the nutrition plan unique. Keep in mind that nutrition plans need to include an athlete's favorite training foods and fluids, while maintaining the feasibility of transporting the items while moving and ensuring food safety. For example, an adventure racer might really enjoy eating a turkey and cheese sandwich 10 hours into a race. However, if the race is self-sufficient and without access to refrigeration, keeping a lunchmeat and cheese sandwich outside refrigeration for more than 2 hours will increase the risk for a foodborne illness. A peanut butter and jelly sandwich or turkey jerky might be better options.

How can a nutrition plan be developed for a multiday event that will be fully supported?

Multiday endurance events, or stage events, may be fully supported with team vehicles and overnight accommodations supplying refrigeration and cooking capabilities. These types of events are logistically much easier to plan for because athletes can in some cases stay on a "normal" schedule of eating meals and snacks. The variables to consider in this type of scenario are the refrigeration, preparation, and storage space for supplies as well as the length and frequency of exercise during the multiday event.

An example of this type of event is the Race Across America (RAAM). RAAM, first held in 1982, is a nonstop cycling event across the United States. The 2900–3000 mile race begins on the West Coast and travels across the mountains and plains to the East Coast. Racers can enter the event as a solo rider or as a 2-, 4-, or 8-person team. Individuals and teams are allowed to have multiple support vehicles throughout the race and along the course. Most competitors will have a motor home to allow for meal preparation and vans to fetch additional supplies while the cyclists continue to progress en route. **Training Table 12.5** gives a sample day of meals, snacks, and fluids consumed by a rider on the 4-man Team 70+ in 1996.

How can a meal plan be developed for a sport such as a long-distance triathlon that includes a nonconducive eating environment, a length of time spanning several meals, and race course support?

The sport of triathlon has exploded in popularity in the past decade. Triathlons can be categorized into four distances: Sprint (500-meter swim, 10-mile bike ride, 5-kilometer run), Olympic (1.5-kilometer swim, 40-kilometer bike ride, 10-kilometer run), half-Ironman (1.2-mile swim, 56-mile bike ride, 13.1-mile run), and Ironman (2.4-mile swim, 112-mile bike ride, 26.2-mile run). Sprint and Olympic distance races can be completed within 1–3 hours for a majority of competitors, requiring a proper prerace meal, a strong focus on hydration, and minimal amounts of sports bars, gels, and other foods during the race. However, the half and full Ironman distance races can last 4–17 hours, making nutrition a critical component of race day success. Triathlon is unique because of the three sports included, each

Training Table 12.5: Jack's Meal Plan during RAAM

Jack Boyer was a 70-year-old member of Team 70+. He was 5'8" and weighed 158 pounds. His daily energy and carbohydrate needs, accounting for 4–8 hours of cycling per day, were estimated at 5422 calories and 990 grams of carbohydrates. To meet this goal, he was instructed to consume the following each day:

- 6 liters of Cytomax sports beverage, supplying 1278 calories and 360 grams of carbohydrates
- 1 "Meal A," supplying 1100 calories and 150 grams of carbohydrates
- 2 "Meal Bs," each supplying 800 calories and 120 grams of carbohydrates
- 12 snacks, each supplying 120 calories and 20 grams of carbohydrates

Meal options included, but were not limited to: oatmeal, dry cereal, spinach lasagna, turkey chili, stuffed potatoes, bagel sandwiches, and pasta dishes. Snacks were eaten during breaks from cycling. Snacks included, but were not limited to: PowerBars, granola bars, GatorPro, Gatorlode, pretzels, bagels with jelly, dry cereal, trail mix, peanut butter crackers, and Ritz snack crackers. The four-man team was split into two subteams. The subteams alternated 8-hour shifts—8 hours in the motor home resting, eating, and getting massages, alternating with 8 hours of cycling. The 8 hours of cycling by each subteam of two men was then split into alternating 1-hour time blocks of riding and then resting in the van following directly behind the cyclist on the road. All meals were eaten in the motor home while sports beverages and snacks were consumed during the 8-hour shift of cycling.

Because the motor home had a refrigerator and a microwave, foods could be prepared for the team on-site. However, most of the food was prepared before leaving on the adventure and frozen, minimizing the time and effort of meal preparation during the race. Therefore, the menu was planned around foods that could be reheated well, made from scratch in a microwave, or prepared with no cooking. A small cooler was taken during the 8-hour shift of cycling, allowing for drinks and other foods to stay cold.

Jack, as well as the other three riders, was monitored daily through a food record and by obtaining body weights before and after 8-hour riding shifts. The riders stayed on plan for the entire race, feeling good and riding strong. Tastes changed during the ride, requiring the menu to be flexible, allowing for foods from restaurants and "interesting" requested combinations such as baked potatoes with raisins, milk, and salt. The nutrition plan fueled Jack and the rest of the 70+ Team to a successful RAAM finish of 9 days, 2 hours, and 27 minutes.

providing a different environment and plan for hydration and fuel consumption. No food or drink is available during the swim portion of a triathlon, making prerace nutrition and hydration a top priority. The bike segment of the race is most conducive to drinking and eating. Bikes can carry fluids in bottles attached to the bike frame, behind the seat, and in specialized bottles that fit within the aerobars placed on the front of the bike. Athletes can pack their own food to be carried in the back pockets of a bike jersey or in a variety of bike bags, pouches, or "boxes" that attach to the bike frame or seat. This allows an athlete to drink and eat gradually throughout the bike segment of the race, playing a little "catch-up" from the swim and "stocking up" before the run. Because biking is nonimpact, athletes experience fewer gastrointestinal issues with eating and drinking while cycling as opposed to running, and therefore the second segment of a triathlon is an ideal time for fueling. The nutrition plan for the run is typically developed around what is available on the course at aid stations. Some athletes choose to rely mainly on their own fluid and food choices by wearing belts with bottle holders and pouches for food. However, for the Ironman distance races, the amount of fluid and fuel needed during the marathon will exceed the carrying capacity of the belt. Therefore, a combination plan of self-support and race course support may work best. One other opportunity for food and fluid consumption occurs during the two transitions during a triathlon—one after the swim and the second after the bike segment. During shorter triathlons, athletes aim to keep transition time to a minimum, often choosing not to take time to consume anything during transition. In longer-distance triathlons, during transition is an ideal time for changing clothes, taking a minute to rest before the next segment of the race, and consuming small amounts of food or fluids.

The Ironman distance is by far the most taxing and most reliant on proper nutrition and hydration. **Training Table 12.6** provides a sample of the Ironman plan followed by Heather Fink when she completed Ironman Coeur d'Alene in 2003. Her race and nutrition plan progressed flawlessly, allowing her to qualify for the Hawaii Ironman in the fall of 2003.

After 5 years of competing in sprint through half-Ironman distance triathlons, in 2003 Heather decided to participate in an Ironman distance race. Ironman Coeur d'Alene, held in late June and located in northern Idaho, involved a cold swim in Lake Coeur d'Alene; a challenging bike course with several tough, steep hills; and a relatively flat run course. Heather, being a dietitian, knew the importance of practicing her race day nutrition throughout her training, and therefore developed a proposed plan by January and spent the next 4–5 months refining the plan for race day. From past experience in triathlons, she knew sports beverages, gels, and bars worked well and settled well for her during races. However, she knew she would need to take in more energy and sodium during Ironman and therefore began experimenting with other foods, drinks, and products. The schedule below was the result of using tried-and-true products, newly discovered products, and beverages/foods known to be available on the race course:

Breakfast (4 hours prior to race start)

- 1½ cups dry cereal with one scoop of protein powder and 1 cup soy milk
- 1 banana and 8 ounces of orange juice
- Sips of Gatorade between breakfast and race start

2.4-Mile Swim (total time = 1:05:00)

- No food or drink

Transition #1 (after swim, before bike; total time = 3:36)
- ½–1 can of Ensure

112-Mile Bike Ride (total time = 6:02:00)

Nutrition Goals During the Bike Ride: 32 ounces of fluid per hour (specifically, Gatorade), 70–75 grams of carbohydrates per hour, and 500–750 mg sodium per hour. Plan was broken down into 10-mile increments because aid stations were located every 10 miles on the bike course. Three 24-ounce bottles of Gatorade were placed on the bike at the beginning of the race and replaced throughout the course. A Bento box was attached to the bike frame holding salt tablets, Baker's Breakfast Cookies, peanut butter crackers, and one gel. The specific nutrition plan for the bike ride progressed as follows:

- 10 miles—Bottle pick-up
- 20 miles—¾ of a Baker's Breakfast Cookie
- 30 miles—Bottle pick-up
- 40 miles—3 peanut butter crackers
- 50 miles—Bottle pick-up + one sodium tablet (1000 mg)
- 60 miles—1 gel
- 70 miles—Bottle pick-up
- 80 miles—¾ Baker's Breakfast Cookie
- 90 miles—Bottle pick-up
- 100 miles—3 peanut butter crackers + one sodium tablet
- 110 miles—Bottle pick-up

Transition #2 (after bike, before run; total time = 2:51)
- ½–1 can of Ensure

26.2-Mile Run (total time = 3:43:00)

Nutrition Goals During the Run: 28 ounces of fluid per hour, 60–65 grams of carbohydrates per hour, and 500–750 mg sodium per hour. The plan was broken down into 1-mile increments because aid stations were located every mile on the run course. A gel flask filled with four gels was carried during the run with a small plastic pouch attached to the flask to hold several sodium tablets.

- 4–6 ounces of fluid were consumed every mile on the course, mainly Gatorade, with a little water, cola (for a flavor change), and ice cubes.
- Half of a gel was originally planned to be consumed every 3 miles during the race for a total of four gels over the 26.2 miles. However, only one to two gels were actually consumed. The temperatures on race day climbed to 97 degrees, increasing the need for fluids during the race. Because of an increased ingestion of fluids, which contained calories, fewer gels were consumed to stay on track with the planned quantity of carbohydrates needed per hour.

Total Ironman race time = 10:58

Second female in 30–34 age group, qualifying Heather for the Hawaii Ironman in October 2003.

2.4-Mile Swim (Total time = 1:05:00)

112-Mile Bike Ride (Total time = 6:02:00)

26.2-Mile Run (Total time = 3:43:00)

The Box Score

Key Points of Chapter

- Endurance athletes expend a tremendous number of calories not only during competition, but also in preparatory training. Energy expenditures of 6000–8000 kcals/day are not out of the ordinary for ultra-endurance athletes. This puts a huge drain on energy reserves that must be replenished after daily training bouts and thus makes diet a key factor in athletic success.

- Of the three energy systems, endurance athletes rely most heavily on the aerobic energy system. Appropriately designed training programs challenge the aerobic system and increase the athlete's aerobic power so that he or she can maintain a faster race pace.

- It is critical for endurance athletes to consume sufficient calories on a daily basis to supply the energy for daily training and competition, ensure the delivery of nutrients needed for complete recovery from workouts, and stay healthy and injury-free. Daily energy needs can be estimated using the following formula: Resting energy expenditure × Activity factor.

- Often it is not physically or logistically possible for an endurance athlete to fully match his or her energy expenditure with intake during actual training or competition. As a consequence, the event nutrition plan should be based on meeting the performance requirements of carbohydrates, fluids, and sodium.

- The main difference between diets of endurance athletes and those of other sports is in the quantity of food consumed, not necessarily the macronutrient composition of the diet.

- Carbohydrate intakes of 5 to 10 grams per kilogram of body weight are recommended for endurance athletes. When expressed as a percentage of their total daily caloric intake, carbohydrates should be approximately 50–65% for daily training and approximately 65–70% during carbohydrate loading.

- Research has demonstrated that consuming carbohydrates in the hours leading up to an endurance training session or competition is critical for optimal performance, especially during activities lasting longer than 2 hours. Endurance athletes should be encouraged to consume a carbohydrate-rich preactivity meal 2–4 hours prior to a training session or event and then continue consuming carbohydrates throughout exercise to optimize performance.

- Carbohydrate needs during exercise are estimated at 1.0–1.1 grams of carbohydrates per minute of activity, or approximately 60–70 grams carbohydrates per hour for endurance athletes. Some athletes can easily consume and digest upward of 75–85 grams of carbohydrates per hour, whereas others can barely tolerate 45–55 grams. Athletes need to experiment with varying quantities of carbohydrates surrounding the 60–70 gram range to determine the best estimate for them individually.

- Carbohydrate intake is also important after competition to help replenish glycogen stores. Consuming 1.2 grams of carbohydrates per kilogram of body weight per hour for 3–4 hours after the cessation of exercise provides glucose to muscles at a time when they are most receptive to absorbing and storing glucose as glycogen.

- Although protein is not typically used by the body to provide energy, the extreme energy demands of endurance training and competition do result in the metabolizing of some protein for energy. As a result, the protein intake recommendation for endurance athletes is higher than the current RDA and falls in the range of 1.2–2.0 grams per kilogram of body weight.

- The effect of protein intake during competition and its impact on performance require more research; however, for ultra-endurance athletes, the consumption of protein seems prudent.

- Despite the fact that fats are a major energy source during endurance sports, high-fat diets have not been shown to improve endurance performance. The diet of endurance athletes should include enough fat to account for approximately 20–35% of total daily calories consumed. Immediately prior to training, during exercise, and immediately after training, fat intake should be kept to a minimum while focusing primarily on carbohydrates and secondarily on protein.

- Vitamin and mineral needs of endurance athletes are similar to those of other athletes. However, there are a few vitamins and minerals that should be given particular attention. These include the B vitamins, iron, calcium, vitamin C, vitamin E, sodium, and potassium.

- Adequate fluid intake is important for maintaining the hydration status of endurance athletes during their prolonged training bouts and during competition. Failure to do so can have deadly consequences.

- An excellent way to monitor hydration status is to weigh athletes before and after training or competition. For every pound of body weight lost, the athlete should drink 16–24 oz of fluid.

- The risk for hyponatremia increases as the duration of an endurance event lengthens. As a result, the sodium intake of ultra-endurance athletes should be considered when developing a nutrition plan. Sports beverages can provide both fluid and sodium; however, pre-event experimentation is critical for successful use.

- Each endurance athlete requires an individualized nutrition plan. Sport-specific logistics must be considered to plan food and fluid intake appropriately and to implement the plan successfully.

Study Questions

1. Can endurance athletes adopt an "eat-as-you-like attitude"? Defend your answer.

2. Of the three energy systems, which one do endurance athletes rely upon most for energy? Under what circumstances would the other two energy systems play a bigger role during endurance competition?

3. What pieces of information would you need as a dietitian to estimate an endurance athlete's daily caloric needs?

4. What is the reasoning behind the statement "An athlete who cuts back on carbohydrate intake is committing performance suicide"?

5. What should the percent composition of carbohydrates, proteins, and fats be for an endurance athlete's diet?

6. How does the combination of tapering and carbohydrate loading affect endurance performance?

7. What role do proteins play in regard to the needs of the endurance athlete? What is the current recommendation for protein intake in endurance athletes?

8. For ultra-endurance athletes, is there a training or performance benefit to eating a high-fat diet? Should you recommend eating higher-fat foods during and after training or competition? Discuss why or why not.

9. What are BCAAs and MCTs? What role, if any, do they play in meeting the needs of the endurance athlete?

10. What is hyponatremia? Which athletes are at greatest risk for developing it (be very specific)? What nutritional strategies would you use to prevent it?

11. Which vitamins and minerals are of special concern to endurance athletes?

12. What strategies could be employed to help ensure the hydration status of endurance athletes?

13. What is a "sweat trial," and why is it important to the endurance athlete?

14. What are some of the logistical and nutritional issues that must be dealt with when working with ultra-endurance athletes who are competing in 8+ hour events?

References

1. Wolinsky I. *Nutrition in Exercise and Sport*. New York: CRC; 1998.

2. Costill DL, Sherman WM, Fink WJ, Maresh C, Witten M, Miller JM. The role of dietary carbohydrate in muscle glycogen resynthesis after strenuous running. *Am J Clin Nutr*. 1981;34:1831–1836.

3. Sherman WM, Doyle JA, Lamb DR, Dernbach AR, Doyle JA, Strauss R. Dietary carbohydrate, muscle glycogen and exercise performance during 7 d of training. *Am J Clin Nutr*. 1991;57:27–31.

4. Sherman WM. Metabolism of sugars and physical performance. *Am J Clin Nutr*. 1995;62(suppl):228s–241s.

5. Costill DL, Hargreaves M. Carbohydrate nutrition and fatigue. *Sports Med*. 1992;13:86–92.

6. Foster C, Costill DL, Fink WJ. Effects of pre-exercise feedings on endurance performance. *Med Sci Sports Exerc*. 1979;11:1–5.

7. Nilsson LH, Hultman E. Liver glycogen in man—the effect of total starvation or a carbohydrate-poor diet followed by carbohydrate refeeding. *Scand J Clin Lab Invest*. 1973;32:325–330.

8. Chryssanthopoulos C, Williams C. Pre-exercise meal and endurance running capacity when carbohydrates are ingested during exercise. *Int J Sports Med*. 1997;18:543–548.

9. Chryssanthopoulos C, Williams C, Nowitz A, Kotsiopoulou C, Vleck V. The effect of a high carbohydrate meal on endurance running capacity. *Int J Sports Nutr Exerc Metab*. 2002;12(2):157–171.

10. Hawley JA, Burke LM. Effect of meal frequency and timing on physical performance. *Br J Nutr*. 1997;77(suppl 1):S91–S103.

11. Smith GJ, Rhodes EC, Langill RH. The effect of pre-exercise glucose ingestion on performance during prolonged swimming. *Int J Sport Nutr Exerc Metabol*. 2002;12(2):136–144.

12. Febbraio MA, Stewart KL. CHO feeding before prolonged exercise: effect of glycemic index on muscle glycogenolysis and exercise performance. *J Appl Physiol*. 1996; 81:1115–1120.

13. Febbraio MA, Keenan J, Angus DJ, Campbell SE, Garnham AP. Pre-exercise carbohydrate ingestion, glucose kinetics and muscle glycogen use: effect of the glycemic index. *J Appl Physiol*. 2000;89:1845–1851.

14. Coyle EF. Carbohydrate supplementation during exercise. *J Nutr*. 1992;122:788.

15. Tarnopolsky M, MacDougall J, Atkinson S. Influence of protein intake and training status on nitrogen balance and lean body mass. *J Appl Physiol*. 1988;66:187.

16. Carraro F, Stuart CA, Hartl WH, Rosenblatt J, Wolfe RR. Effect of exercise and recovery on muscle protein

synthesis in human subjects. *Am J Physiol*. 1990;259(4 Pt 1):E470–E476.

17. Lemon P. Is increased dietary protein necessary or beneficial for individuals with a physically active lifestyle? *Nutr Rev*. 1996;54:S169–S175.

18. Lemon P. Effects of exercise on dietary protein requirements. *Int J Sports Nutr*. 1998;8:426–447.

19. Kreider RB, Leutholz B. Nutritional considerations for preventing overtraining. In: Antonio J, Stout JR, eds. *Sport Supplements*. Philadelphia, PA: Lippincott Williams and Wilkins; 2001:199–208.

20. Tarnopolsky M. Protein metabolism in strength and endurance activities. In: Lamb DR, Murray R, eds. *The Metabolic Basis of Performance in Exercise and Sport: Vol. 12, Perspectives in Exercise Science and Sports Medicine*. Carmel, IN: Cooper; 1999:125–157.

21. Lemon P, Mullin JP. Effect of initial muscle glycogen levels on protein catabolism during exercise. *J Appl Physiol*. 1980;48:624–629.

22. Davis JM, Alderson NL, Welsh RS. Serotonin and central nervous system fatigue: nutritional considerations. *Am J Clin Nutr*. 2000;72:573S–578S.

23. Newsholme EA, Blomstrand E, Ekblom B. Physical and mental fatigue: metabloic mechanisms and importance of plasma amino acids. *Br Med Bull*. 1992;48:477–495.

24. Wiles J, Woodward R, Bird SR. Effect of pre-exercise protein ingestion upon VO$_2$, R, and perceived exertion during treadmill running. *Br J Sports Med*. 1991;25(1):26–30.

25. Graham TE, Turcotte LP, Kiens B, Richter EA. Training and muscle ammonia amino acid metabolism in humans during prolonged exercise. *J Appl Physiol*. 1995;78:725–735.

26. Lambert EV, Speechly DP, Dennis SC, Noakes TD. Enhanced endurance in trained cyclists during moderate intensity exercise following 2 weeks adaptation to a high fat diet. *Eur J Appl Physiol Occup Physiol*. 1994;69(4):287–293.

27. Evans WJ, Fisher EC, Hoerr RA, Young VR. Protein metabolism and endurance exercise. *Physician Sports Med*. 1983;11:63–72.

28. Tarnopolsky M, Atkinson S, MacDougall JD, Senor BB, Lemon P, Schwarcz H. Whole body leucine metabolism during and after resistance exercise in fed humans. *Med Sci Sports Exerc*. 1991;23:326–333.

29. Wagenmakers A, Coakley J, Edwards R. Metabolism of branch-chain amino acids and ammonia during exercise: clues from McArdle's disease. *Int J Sports Med*. 1990;11:S101–S113.

30. Van Loon L, Saris W, Kruijshoop M, Wagenmakers A. Maximizing post-exercise muscle glycogen synthesis: carbohydrate supplementation and the application of

amino acid and protein hydrolysate mixtures. *Am J Clin Nutr*. 2000;72:106–111.

31. Zawadzki K, Yaspelkis B, Ivy J. Carbohydrate-protein supplement increases the rate of muscle glycogen storage post exercise. *J Appl Physiol*. 1992;72:1854–1859.

32. Ivy JL, Res PT, Sprague RC, Widzer MO. Effect of a carbohydrate-protein supplement on endurance performance during exercise of varying intensity. *Int J Sport Nutr Exerc Metabol*. 2003;13(3):382–395.

33. Davis JM, Bailey SP. Possible mechanisms of central nervous system fatigue during exercise. *Med Sci Sports Exerc*. 1997;29:45–57.

34. Blomstrand E, Hassman P, Ekblom B, Newsholme E. Administration of branched-chain amino acids during sustained exercise—effects on performance and on plasma concentration of some amino acids. *Eur J Appl Physiol*. 1991;63:83–88.

35. Blomstrand E, Andersson S, Hassmen P, Ekblom B, Newsholme E. Effect of branched-chained amino acid and carbohydrate supplementation on the exercise-induced change in plasma and muscle concentration of amino acids in human subjects. *Acta Physiol Scand*. 1995;153:87–96.

36. Mittleman KD, Ricci MR, Bailey SP. Branched-chain amino acids prolong exercise during heat stress in men and women. *Med Sci Sports Exerc*. 1998;30:83–91.

37. Van Hall G, Raaymakers SH, Saris WHM, Wagenmakers AJM. Ingestion of branched-chain amino acids and tryptophan during sustained exercise in man: failure to affect performance. *J Physiol*. 1995;486:789–794.

38. Pallota JA, Kennedy PJ. Response of plasma insulin and growth hormone to carbohydrate and protein feedings. *Metabol*. 1968;17:901–908.

39. Spiller GA, Jenesen CD, Pattison TS, Chuck CS, Whittam JH, Scala J. Effect of protein dose on serum glucose and insulin response to sugars. *Am J Clin Nutr*. 1987;46:474–480.

40. Karp JR, Johnston JD, Tecklenburg S, Mickleborough T, Fly A, Stager JM. The efficacy of chocolate milk as a recovery aid. *Med Sci Sports Exerc*. 2004;36(5 suppl):S126, Abstract 0850.

41. Okano G, Sato Y, Murata Y. Effect of elevated blood FFA levels on endurance performance after a single high fat meal ingestion. *Med Sci Sports Exerc*. 1998;30(5):763–768.

42. Satabin P, Portero P, Defer G, Bricout J, Guezennec CY. Metabolic and hormonal responses to lipid and carbohydrate diets during exercise in man. *Med Sci Sports Exerc*. 1987;19:218–223.

43. Galbo H, Holst JJ, Christensen NJ. The effect of different diets and of insulin on the hormonal response to prolonged exercise. *Acta Physiol Scand*. 1979;107:19–32.

44. Karlsson J, Saltin B. Diet, muscle glycogen and endurance performance. *J Appl Physiol*. 1971;31:203–206.

45. Helge JW, Wulff B, Kiens B. Impact of a fat-rich diet on endurance in man: role of the dietary period. *Med Sci Sports Exerc*. 1998;30:456–461.

46. Venkatraman JT, Pendergast D. Effects of the level of dietary fat intake and endurance exercise on plasma cytokines in runners. *Med Sci Sports Exerc*. 1998;30:1198–1204.

47. Helge JW, Richter EA, Kiens B. Interaction of training and diet on metabolism and endurance during exercise in man. *J Physiol*. 1996;492:293–306.

48. Decombaz J, Arnaud MJ, Milon H, et al. Energy metabolism of medium-chain triglycerides versus carbohydrates during exercise. *Eur J Appl Physiol*. 1983; 52:9–14.

49. Ivy JL, Costill DL, Fink WJ, Maglischo E. Contribution of medium and long-chain triglyceride intake to energy metabolism during prolonged exercise. *Int J Sports Med*. 1980;1:15–20.

50. Van Zyl CG, Lambert EV, Hawley JA, Noakes TD, Dennis SC. Effects of medium-chain trigylceride ingestion on fuel metabolism and cycling performance. *J Appl Physiol*. 1996;80:2217–2225.

51. Jeukendrup AE, Thielen JJ, Wagenmakers AJ, Brouns F, Saris WH. Effect of medium-chain triacylglycerol and carbohydrate ingestion during exercise on substrate utilization and subsequent cycling performance. *Am J Clin Nutr*. 1998;67:397–404.

52. Williams MH. Vitamin supplementation and athletic performance. *Int J Vitam Nutr Res*. 1989;30(suppl):163–191.

53. Telford RD, Sly GJ, Hahn AG, Cunningham RB, Bryant C, Smith JA. Footstrike is the major cause of hemolysis during running. *J Appl Physiol*. 2003;94(1):38–42.

54. Shaskey DJ, Green GA. Sports haematology. *Sports Med*. 2000;29(1):27–38.

55. Institute of Medicine. *Dietary Reference Intakes for Vitamin C, Vitamin E, Selenium, and Carotenoids*. Food and Nutrition Board. Washington, DC: National Academies Press; 2000.

56. Takanami Y, Iwane H, Kawai Y, Shimonitsu T. Vitamin E supplementation and endurance exercise: are there benefits? *Sports Med*. 2000;29(2):73–83.

57. Gore CJ, Bourdon PC, Woolford SM, Pederson DG. Involuntary dehydration during cricket. *Int J Sports Med*. 1993;14(7):387–395.

58. Meyer F, Bar-Or O, Salberg A, Passe D. Hypohydration during exercise in children: effect on thirst, drink preference, and rehydration. *Int J Sports Nutr*. 1994;4(1):22–35.

59. Iuliano S, Naughton G, Collier G, Carlson J. Examination of the self-selected fluid intake practices by junior athletes during a simulated duathlon event. *Int J Sports Nutr*. 1998;8:10–23.

60. Maughan RJ, Shirreffs SM. Recovery from prolonged exercise: restoration of water and electrolyte balance. *J Sports Sci*. 1997;15:297–303.

Additional Resources

Bergstrom J, Hermansen L, Hultman E, Saltin B. Diet, muscle glycogen and physical performance. *Acta Physiol Scand*. 1967;71:140–150.

Christensen EH, Hansen O. Work capacity and diet. *Skandinavisches Archiv fur Physiologie*. 1939;81:160–171.

Davis JM, Alderson NL, Welsh RS. Serotonin and central nervous system fatigue: nutritional considerations. *Am J Clin Nutr*. 2000;72(2 suppl):573S–578S.

Key Questions Addressed

- What is different about strength/power athletes?
- What energy systems are utilized during strength/power exercise?
- Are the calorie needs of strength/power athletes different from those of other types of athletes?
- Are carbohydrate needs different for strength/power athletes?
- Are protein needs different for strength/power athletes?
- Are fat needs different for strength/power athletes?
- Are vitamin and mineral needs different for strength/power athletes?
- Are fluid needs different for strength/power athletes?
- What meal-planning/event-planning logistics need to be considered during strength/power events?

Robert is 45 years old and a competitive master's power lifter who competes in the 181-pound weight class. He has been having trouble keeping his body weight low enough to compete in the 181-pound class and is concerned that his body fat level is actually increasing despite his heavy weight-training regimen. He has a rather sedentary office job and tries to walk about a mile every weekday evening with his wife. He states that he eats well (approximately 3500 calories per day), and to help build muscle and enhance recovery he consumes about 250 grams of protein per day from natural food sources and supplementation. His carbohydrate intake is low because he has been experimenting with an Atkins-type diet to control his weight.

Questions

- Why is Robert having trouble controlling his body weight?
- What are the most glaring concerns about his diet?

What is different about strength/power athletes?

The terms **strength** and **power** are often used interchangeably when describing athletes. Although strength and power are important aspects of physical fitness, and strength is a component of power, they are not synonymous. Strength is the ability of a muscle or group of muscles to generate force. Strength is purely a measure of how much weight can be moved or lifted by an athlete. It is highly dependent on the amount of muscle tissue an athlete possesses. In other words, the bigger the muscle, the greater the strength. Power, on the other hand, is dependent not only on how much force is capable of being developed by the muscles (i.e., strength), but also on how fast the force can be generated. Because velocity of movement is an integral part of power, power is often referred to as **speed-strength**. Strength, and even more so power, is critical to performance in almost all sports; however, there are specific sports that are characterized as strength/power sports. For the purposes of this chapter, strength/power athletes are those involved in the explosive track and field events (i.e., javelin, shot put, discus, high jump, long jump, hammer, sprints), weight lifting, gymnastics, and wrestling, just to name a few. In short, strength/power athletes are athletes who participate in sports in which success is dependent primarily on demonstration of brute strength or relatively short bursts (i.e., ≤1.5 minutes) of near maximal muscle force production.

The pure strength/power athletes are different from many other athletes in that success in their sport relies on activities of short duration; for example, any of the throws in track and field take only a few seconds to perform. As a result, the energy needs and goals of training differ vastly from those of the endurance athlete (see Chapter 12). This chapter discusses the macro- and micronutrient needs along with issues regarding hydration and meal planning.

What energy systems are utilized during strength/power exercise?

As discussed in Chapter 2, the body's three energy systems (the phosphagen, anaerobic, and aerobic systems) are constantly working together to meet the immediate energy demands of the body. The short, high-intensity muscle contractions required to perform strength and power sports rely heavily on the phosphagen system, with increasing contribution from the anaerobic system as the length of the activity increases (see Figure 13.1). In the case of a strength athlete performing a one-repetition maximum bench press, the actual time the athlete spends performing the lift may be only 4 seconds. The time interval is even shorter for a javelin thrower or a person performing the shot put (i.e., corresponds to the left-most region of area 1 in Figure 13.1).

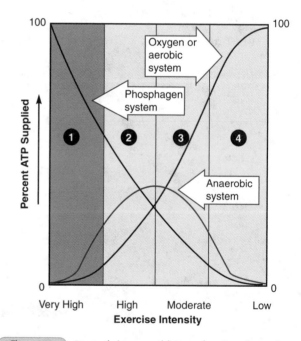

Figure 13.1 Strength/power athletes rely primarily on the phosphagen and anaerobic energy systems to provide ATP. The shaded area 1 in the graph represents all-out activities that progress in length from 1 second (i.e., left margin) to 30 seconds (right margin). Area 2 involves all-out efforts that progress from 30 seconds to about 1.5 minutes. Strength/power athletes tend to perform activities that fall in areas 1 and 2. Although the aerobic energy system is not a major provider of energy for these athletes, it is important for recovery afterward. *Source:* Bower RW, Fox EL. *Sport Physiology.* 3rd ed. Dubuque, IA: William C. Brown Publishers; 1992. Reprinted with permission of the McGraw-Hill Companies.

Muscle stores of adenosine triphosphate (ATP) and creatine phosphate (CP) enable the muscles of these athletes to meet the immediate demands for energy and thus complete a successful lift or throw. On the other end of the strength/power spectrum is an athlete such as an 800-meter sprinter. These athletes derive the majority of their energy from the combined efforts of the phosphagen and anaerobic energy systems (i.e., right-most region of area 2 in Figure 13.1).

Depending on the nature of the sport, it may be necessary to repeat the strength/power movement numerous times. Even though the phosphagen and the anaerobic systems supply the immediate energy need, the aerobic system should not be neglected or shrugged off as unimportant. In the case of a shot putter, aerobic metabolism is relatively unimportant because there is usually plenty of rest time between puts to recover; however, there are other strength/power sports that require the athlete to repeatedly perform strength/power movements over a period of time with relatively short intervals of rest in between. In these cases, the aerobic system is important for supplying the energy for recovery, which in turn indirectly affects performance by delaying the onset of fatigue. An example of a sport requiring repeated powerful bursts of muscle activity can be seen during gymnastics competitions. In competition and during training, skills requiring muscle strength and power are separated by short rest periods that occur during the event (e.g., between tumbling runs during floor exercise) or between apparatus as the athletes rotate from one to another. Muscle recovery and the associated recharging of the creatine and ATP stores are dependent on the aerobic system. Therefore, if strength/power athletes neglect the development of their aerobic system, their ability to recover will be impaired, and fatigue will ensue more quickly.

In summary, strength/power athletes rely primarily on the phosphagen energy system to provide ATP during strength/power events, with increasing contributions of ATP coming from the anaerobic energy system as the duration of the activity increases. Although the aerobic energy system contributes little ATP during the actual strength/power activity, it is important for recovery after the activity. During the recovery period, the aerobic energy system replenishes ATP and CP levels, thus recharging the phosphagen system and delaying the onset of fatigue.

Are the calorie needs of strength/ power athletes different from those of other types of athletes?

As with most athletes, the main dietary concern with individuals involved in strength/power sports is the consumption of adequate amounts of total daily calories. Energy needs are based on several factors, including age, gender, body mass, and sport-specific demands, which can vary tremendously between athletes. No single macronutrient is more important than the others; thus the dietary composition for strength/power athletes is not much different from the recommended healthy diet of nonathletes. This section will review calculating total calorie needs for strength/power athletes, and subsequent sections will focus on the roles of each of the macronutrients, micronutrients, and fluids.

How are daily calorie needs calculated for strength/power athletes?

For strength/power athletes, similar to other athletes, there are three main considerations when determining energy needs and developing an individualized meal plan: Does the athlete want to maintain, lose, or gain weight? In the category of strength/power athletes, weight goals span an enormous continuum. On one end of the spectrum are weight lifters who, in general, are trying to gain muscle tissue and build mass. At the other end are gymnasts who, in general, are attempting to minimize body mass while simultaneously aiming for increased strength and power. Therefore, nutrition plans need to meet the athlete's basic nutrient requirements while also reflecting the desires and goals of the athlete.

The energy needs for strength/power athletes can be calculated using the same equations presented in Chapter 10. Refer to **Table 13.1** for a reminder of the equations and activity factors. The following examples provide real-life scenarios of strength/power athletes who want to lose, maintain, or gain weight. Each scenario reviews how to calculate energy needs and provides recommendations based on the athlete's goals and objectives.

How can calorie needs be calculated for athletes aiming to lose/minimize body weight while increasing strength/power?

Female gymnasts are a category of strength/power athletes who are generally aiming to lose weight or maintain an already low weight. To obtain their

TABLE 13.1	Resting Energy Expenditure (REE) Calculations and Activity Factors	
Gender and Age	Equation (BW in kilograms)	Activity Factor
Males, 10–18 years	REE = (17.5 × BW) + 651	1.6–2.4
Males, 18–30 years	REE = (15.3 × BW) + 679	1.6–2.4
Males, 30–60 years	REE = (11.6 × BW) + 879	1.6–2.4
Females, 10–18 years	REE = (12.2 × BW) + 749	1.6–2.4
Females, 18–30 years	REE = (14.7 × BW) + 496	1.6–2.4
Females, 30–60 years	REE = (8.7 × BW) + 829	1.6–2.4

Source: World Health Organization. Energy and Protein Requirements: Report of a Joint FAO/WHO/UNU Expert Consultation. Technical Reprint Series 724. Geneva, Switzerland: World Health Organization; 1985:206.

goal, many gymnasts are eating suboptimal levels of not only total calories, but also a variety of nutrients. Several studies have examined the differential between recommended and actual calorie intake. The results are staggering—gymnasts are consuming only 47–84% of their daily calorie requirements![1–4] When working with female gymnasts or any other strength/power athlete whose goal is to lose weight, calculate energy needs and then compare the calculations to actual current intake before developing a meal plan and making recommendations.

Lyndsi's Case Study Kari, the mother of an 11-year-old gymnast named Lyndsi, calls to make an appointment with a sports nutritionist. Kari has grown increasingly concerned about her daughter's eating habits and weight loss over the past several months. Lyndsi has been part of a local club team for several years that practices 2–3 hours a day, 5–6 days a week. While on summer break, the club team hosted a 2-week gymnastic camp. Lyndsi was very excited about the opportunity to train and learn from the older girls on the team, commenting to her mother several times about how she envied their performance and abilities. At the end of camp, Kari noticed gradual changes in her daughter's eating habits—Lyndsi began to turn down her

favorite foods, and she had developed a strong aversion to any food containing fat. Lyndsi's eating habits subsequently became very routine, consisting of a plain bagel for breakfast, an iceberg lettuce and green pepper salad with nonfat dressing for lunch, and a chicken breast, baked potato, and broccoli every night for dinner (see **Training Table 13.1**). Lyndsi would usually have a small bowl of nonfat frozen yogurt or dry cereal for a snack in the evening. Kari has noticed a "drawn" look to Lyndsi's face and that her clothes seemed to just hang loosely on her body. The point at which she knew it was time to seek professional assistance was when Lyndsi went to the doctor for a routine check-up, and her 5'3" frame weighed only 95 pounds. She is certain Lyndsi is not eating enough but is unsure of how much she should be consuming and how she can get Lyndsi back on track to "normal" eating.

Making recommendations. In this situation, Lyndsi has made some drastic changes to her diet and, as a result, noticeable weight loss has occurred.

1. The first step is to estimate her total calorie needs:
   REE = (12.2 × BW in kg) + 749 = (12.2 × 43.2) + 749 = 1276
   Total calorie needs = REE × activity factor = 1276 × (1.6 − 2.4) = 2041–3062 calories/day
   Lyndsi needs at least 2041 calories per day on rest or easy days, and up to 3062 calories a day for heavy training days (3+ hours per day).

2. *The second step is to estimate her calorie intake.* Refer to Training Table 13.1 for Lyndsi's initial meal plan. After making changes to her diet, she was only consuming ~900 calories a day. It is obvious that she is not meeting her energy requirements—in fact, she is only consuming 45% of her bottom-level energy needs ([916 calories / 2041 calories] × 100 = 45%). One of the roles of a sports nutrition professional is to understand the client's perspective by determining why a client eats in a certain way. In this scenario, it is critical to determine why Lyndsi made changes to her diet in order to have a better feel for her potential risk of developing an eating disorder. Chapter 11 in this book reviews the steps to take when a client has developed disordered eating patterns. For this example, assume that Lyndsi is merely ignorant of how the changes she has implemented can potentially negatively affect her health and performance.

3. Because her calorie intake is low, she should increase her daily calories, but gradually. The sports nutrition professional should ensure that Lyndsi's questions, concerns, and fears are addressed prior to suggesting the revised meal plan. The revised meal plan (refer to Training Table 13.1) pro-

Training Table 13.1: Lyndsi's Initial and Revised Meal Plans

Meal/Snack	Lyndsi's Initial Meal Plan		Lyndsi's Revised Meal Plan	
	Food/Beverage	Calorie Content (kcal)	Food/Beverage	Calorie Content (kcal)
Breakfast	Bagel	195	Bagel	195
			with 2 tbsp peanut butter	190
			8 oz orange juice	112
Lunch	2 cups iceberg lettuce	13	2 cups iceberg lettuce	13
	with ½ green pepper	10	with ½ green pepper	10
	3 tbsp fat-free French dressing	68	½ tomato	13
			½ cup mushrooms	13
			3 tbsp fat-free French dressing	68
			3 oz turkey sandwich	388
			8 oz skim milk	85
Dinner	4 oz chicken	187	4 oz chicken	187
	1 baked potato	220	1 baked potato	220
	1½ cups broccoli	66	1½ cups broccoli	66
			cooked in 1 tbsp olive oil	119
			12 oz skim milk	128
Snack	1 cup fat-free frozen yogurt	157	1 cup Total raisin bran	180
			8 oz skim milk	85
	Total calories = 916		Total calories = 2072	
	Total carbohydrates = 153 g		Total carbohydrates = 290 g	

vides adequate nutrients for growth, development, health, and performance. Even though the revised plan is at the lower end of the recommended range, it may take a couple of weeks to gradually progress her intake to the new level. The more gradual the process, the easier it will be for Lyndsi to adapt physically and mentally to the increased number of calories. Once she reaches the minimum requirement for calories, the revised meal plan can be re-evaluated and adjusted accordingly.

How can calorie needs be calculated for athletes aiming to maintain body weight while increasing strength/power?

Nutrition becomes a focus for some athletes who are trying to bring their performance "to the next level" by optimizing their intake of macro- and micronutrients. Often, these athletes are satisfied with their current weight but feel something is missing in their daily dietary regimen. For these athletes, energy needs should be calculated to confirm an appropriate calorie level is being consumed, and then the focus should shift to establishing balance, variety, and moderation within the diet.

Jake's Case Study Jake is a 25-year-old 50-meter butterfly swimmer. He swam competitively in high school and college, and now trains and competes periodically with the master's swim team at the YMCA. During high school and college, he ate "whatever he wanted" and never gained an ounce because he was so active. He has been at the same weight (165 pounds) since graduation and he wants to maintain that weight. He works full-time, lives alone, swims 5–6 days a week, and volunteers as an assistant coach for a high school team. Since he has become so busy, he has been relying more on fast food (see **Training Table 13.2**), which he recognizes has affected his swimming performance and energy levels (unlike the "glory days" of his high school and collegiate career). He wants to stay fit, eat healthy, increase his energy levels, and compete at several upcoming swim meets.

Making recommendations. In this scenario, Jake has realized he needs to make some changes to his diet to keep his energy levels up, to meet his nutritional needs, to avoid weight gain, and to swim at his best.

1. The first step is to calculate his energy needs:
   REE = (15.3 × BW in kg) + 679 = (15.3 × 75) + 679 = 1827

Training Table 13.2: Jake's Initial and Revised Meal Plans

	Jake's Initial Meal Plan		Jake's Revised Meal Plan	
Meal/Snack	Food/Beverage	Calorie Content (kcal)	Food/Beverage	Calorie Content (kcal)
Breakfast	2 pieces wheat toast with butter	245	2 pieces wheat toast	160
	8 oz cranberry juice cocktail	144	with 2 tbsp peanut butter	190
			12 oz 100% cranberry juice blend	199
			½ cup Egg Beaters, scrambled	60
			with 2 tbsp shredded cheddar cheese	57
Snack	Granola bar	180	Granola bar	180
Lunch	2 McDonald's cheeseburgers	640	1 McDonald's cheeseburger	320
	Small french fries	210	McDonald's garden salad	35
	12 oz Diet Coke	2	with 1 pkt of fat-free dressing	50
			16 oz skim milk	170
			Banana	108
Snack	Banana	108	Orange	62
Dinner	12" Tombstone pizza	1550	2 cups instant brown rice	433
	16 oz 2% milk	242	6 oz stir-fry chicken	281
			2–3 cups stir-fry vegetables	98
			cooked in 2 tbsp olive oil	239
			16 oz skim milk	171
Snack			1 cup low-fat yogurt	258
	Total calories = 3321		Total calories = 3071	
	37% of calories from fat		25% of calories from fat	
	Total carbohydrates = 381 g		Total carbohydrates = 411 g	

Total energy needs = REE × activity factor = 1827 × (1.6–2.0) = 2922–3654 calories/day
Because Jake is not as active as he was in high school and college, a moderate activity factor can be used (1.6–2.0 versus 1.6–2.4).

2. The next step is to evaluate the adequacy of his current intake by analyzing a food record. An excerpt from Jake's food record is listed in Training Table 13.2. As noted by the nutrition analysis, Jake is consuming an appropriate number of total calories; however, he is eating 37% of his calories from fat. Therefore, dietary recommendations for Jake should focus on substituting some of the high-fat foods with lower-fat, more nutrient-dense options.

3. Jake maintains a busy schedule, so meal planning needs to be simple and easy to follow. By making a few adjustments to his food choices, keeping meal preparation to a minimum, and taking time to plan ahead, Jake's revised meal plan will help him maintain his weight while also rebalancing his daily macronutrient intake. See Training Table 13.2 for Jake's revised meal plan.

How can calorie needs be calculated for athletes aiming to gain muscle mass to increase strength/power?

Strength/power athletes who are aiming to gain weight need to consume extra calories each day to support basic energy needs, the energy demands of daily training, and the nutrient support for tissue growth and development. The success of a plan for weight gain depends on both the quality and quantity of the diet as well as an appropriate strength training and conditioning program. It is essential that these two components go hand in hand; if increases in training are not accompanied by extra calories, muscle mass can potentially be used as an energy source, resulting in weight loss, and if extra calories are consumed without the physical challenge of training, extra calories will most likely contribute to larger fat stores.

Tissue growth of approximately 1 pound requires approximately 5 to 8 calories per gram.[5,6] Because 1 pound of muscle weighs 454 grams, a reasonable estimate of total calories needed to produce 1 pound of muscle is a range of 2300–3600 calories. In general, no more than 1–2 pounds of weight gain is recommended per week. Therefore, an athlete would need to consume approximately 300–500 additional calories per day for a 1-pound lean weight gain per week, or 600–1000 additional calories for a 2-pound lean weight gain per week, assuming all calories are used for muscle construction. However, this assumption cannot always be made. Although increasing daily calories is an effective way to gain weight, researchers have found that only 30–40% of the weight gain is in the form of lean mass when study participants are consuming an extra 500–2000 calories per day.[7] It seems reasonable to assume that the more dramatic the increase in daily calorie consumption, the greater the percentage of gained weight will be in the form of fat. The body can construct only a finite amount of muscle tissue daily; above that level, extra calories are stored as adipose tissue. Therefore, strength/power athletes should aim for a modest increase in daily calorie consumption (300–500 calories/day) and be patient with gradual weight gain.

The extra calories needed for a 1-pound weight gain can be easily obtained by consuming a snack such as:

- 2 tablespoons of peanut butter on one slice of thick bread with 1 cup of milk = 370 calories
- A 6-ounce yogurt with ¼ cup of dry oatmeal and ¼ cup of mixed nuts = 310 calories
- A can of tuna with 4–6 crackers and a banana = 395 calories

For individuals needing 600–1000 calories, portion sizes should be increased at each meal and at least one or two snacks included throughout the day, such as:

- Any of the preceding snacks
- A smoothie made with 12 ounces of milk, 1 cup of frozen fruit, and a scoop of protein powder = 470 calories
- 4–6 ounces of turkey in a whole wheat pita with lettuce and tomato = 410 calories
- A canned nutrition drink or a large energy bar (no more than one supplement item per day—focus heavily on whole foods) = 255–360 calories

---

Leo's Case Study Leo is a 45-year-old recreational cyclist and weight lifter. He commutes to work on his bike daily and goes to the gym 4–5 times per week for weight-lifting sessions. His goal is to gain 5–10 pounds of muscle mass (current weight 170 pounds), but he is having a hard time gaining any weight. He follows a well-balanced strength-training program and changes his routine every 6–8 weeks. He is currently eating three meals a day and sometimes a snack. He wants to gain weight in a healthy way and not rely on candy bars and chocolate shakes to add calories to his diet. However, when he increases his intake through fruits and vegetables, he experiences some gastrointestinal bloating and discomfort. He is frustrated about his inability to gain weight and is looking for advice from a professional.

Making recommendations. Leo's complaints are common among strength/power athletes—he has attempted to gain weight with little to no success. Fortunately, he is dedicated to a healthy diet by focusing not only on weight gain, but also on long-term health. However, in his attempts to add more food to his normal regimen, he has chosen the two food groups with the lowest calorie density—fruits and vegetables. Although whole fruits and vegetables are certainly an important part of his overall diet, they may be contributing to his sense of fullness and discomfort, ultimately discouraging him from eating enough food to increase his total calorie intake.

1. The first step is to determine how much he is currently consuming. **Training Table 13.3** shows a typical day for Leo. An analysis of his current intake reveals a total calorie consumption of 3527 calories. Therefore, it is obvious that he needs to eat more than 3527 calories a day to make any progress in gaining weight.

2. The next step is to calculate total energy needs based on his age and activity level. Using the formulas stated in Table 13.1, his total daily energy needs are:
   REE = $(11.6 \times BW \text{ in kg}) + 879 = (11.6 \times 77.3) + 879 = 1775$
   Total calorie needs = REE $\times$ activity factor = $1775 \times (1.6 - 2.4) = 2840 - 4260$ calories/day
   Because he is currently consuming ~3500 calories and he is not gaining weight, the lower end of the spectrum can be eliminated. For him to gain weight gradually, he will need to consume approximately 3800–4200 calories per day. This range

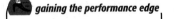
gaining the performance edge

Strength/power athletes must be provided with a sufficient amount of calories per day to meet energy needs or performance will suffer. Total energy requirements should be calculated on an individual basis and modified according to the athlete's goals and objectives. Take into consideration an athlete's current intake before making final recommendations to avoid drastic and unrealistic changes.

Training Table 13.3: Leo's Initial and Revised Meal Plans

Meal/Snack	Leo's Revised Meal Plan		Leo's Revised Meal Plan	
	Food/Beverage	Calorie Content (kcal)	Food/Beverage	Calorie Content (kcal)
Breakfast	Smoothie:		Smoothie:	
	16 oz skim milk	171	16 oz skim milk	171
	½ cup nonfat yogurt	78	½ cup nonfat yogurt	78
	Banana	108	Banana	108
	½ cup protein powder	180	1 packet instant breakfast mix	130
	2-egg cheese omelet	284	2 small blueberry muffins	316
Snack			8 pretzel twists	183
Lunch	Two 4–5 oz ham sandwiches	691	Two 4–5 oz ham sandwiches	691
	Apple	81	16 oz apple juice	233
	1½ cups melon balls	86	1½ cups melon balls	86
	16 oz skim milk	171	16 oz skim milk	171
Snack	2 cups carrots	104	2 cups carrots	104
	with 2 tbsp fat-free dressing	50	with 2 tbsp fat-free dressing	50
	Pear	98	5 oz tuna	181
	5 oz tuna	181		
Dinner	6 oz pork chops	408	6 oz pork chops	408
	1½ cups mashed potatoes	332	1½ cups mashed potatoes	332
	3–4 cups salad with veggies	93	3–4 cups salad with veggies	93
	3 tbsp oil/vinegar dressing	240	2 tbsp oil/vinegar dressing	121
	16 oz skim milk	171	2 dinner rolls	205
			16 oz skim milk	171
Snack			3 oatmeal cookies	240
			8 oz skim milk	85
	Total calories = 3527		**Total calories = 4157**	
	Total carbohydrates = 399 g		**Total carbohydrates = 612 g**	

would provide additional calories above his current intake, while staying within the calculated estimate.

3. Leo should be congratulated on adding fruits and vegetables to his diet. However, consuming more nutritious and calorie-dense foods should be the focus of his weight gain efforts. Foods that provide excellent nutrition and extra calories include items such as fruit juices, dried fruits, avocados, olives, thick breads, nuts, seeds, yogurt, instant breakfast mixes, granola bars, and fruit/milk smoothies. See **Table 13.2** for more ideas on how athletes can gain weight in a healthy way by eating nutrient- and calorie-dense foods. Leo should maintain balance in his diet by eating items from every food group of the MyPlate food guidance system. Discourage Leo from focusing on one type of macronutrient or food group as the sole source of added calories.

Balance, variety, and moderation are still his keys to success. Refer to Training Table 13.3 for Leo's revised meal plan, which provides 4157 calories per day.

How are calorie needs calculated during strength/power training and competition?

Energy needs for strength/power athletes can vary greatly between a training session and a competitive event. Training sessions can last several hours, whereas performance at a competition may last only seconds or minutes. Therefore, these two scenarios should be addressed differently.

Similar to endurance athletes, consuming appropriate amounts of energy, mainly in the form of

TABLE 13.2	Gaining Weight the Healthy Way Through Nutrient- and Calorie-Dense Foods
Foods	**Nutrient- and Calorie-Dense Options**
Grains	Oatmeal Cream of Wheat
	Thick, dense breads
	Bagels
	Wheat germ
	Muffins
	Cornbread
	Quick breads (e.g., banana bread)
Fruits	100% fruit juice
	Dried fruit
	Pineapple
	Bananas
Vegetables	Potatoes
	Corn
	Peas
	Squash
	Beets
	Avocados
	Olives
Dairy (milk alternatives)	Nonfat powdered milk
	Malt powder
	Instant breakfast mixes
	Fruited yogurts
	Canned shakes (e.g., Ensure)
Protein foods (meat alternatives)	Beans—pinto, black, kidney
	Lentils
	Split peas
	Nuts and nut butters
	Seeds
Desserts	Puddings
	Hot cocoa made with milk
	Oatmeal raisin cookies
	Fig bars
	Milk shakes made with low-fat dairy products

training session. This factor mandates the need for energy sources that are easily digestible to avoid gastrointestinal discomfort. Sports beverages are an ideal source of calories and are generally well tolerated even during high-intensity exercise. The consumption of solid food should be reserved for during breaks or at the end of a training session.

For some strength/power athletes, competition day consists of only one event that lasts less than a few minutes. In these situations, it is neither practical nor necessary to consume calories during the event. The body will not deplete its energy reserves in such a short burst of effort, and therefore immediate replenishment is not critical to performance. The exception to this rule is when an athlete is competing in multiple events at the same meet within one day. In this situation, the length of the meet can last several hours, with a small, but progressive, depletion of energy stores with each event. Therefore, to sustain a high level of performance throughout the day, an athlete should plan on consuming easy-to-digest snacks, beverages, and possibly small meals in between events to keep energy levels elevated. The quantity of food consumed will depend on several factors including time between events, length of each event, time elapsed since the last full meal, and personal preferences.

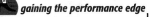 *gaining the performance edge*

A majority of required calories for strength/power activities should be consumed before or after exercise sessions to avoid gastrointestinal upset and the subsequent interference with training. Consuming sports beverages throughout a practice or eating a light snack during a break will provide the energy needed to fuel high-intensity performance.

gaining the performance edge

To meet calorie needs, strength/power athletes should focus on consuming calorie-containing beverages and easily digestible snacks during training sessions and half- or full-day competitive meets. However, during single-bout events it is neither practical nor necessary to consume any food or beverage.

Are carbohydrate needs different for strength/power athletes?

Consuming enough carbohydrates on a daily basis is critical for optimal strength/power performance. Because many strength/power sports rely on anaerobic metabolism, carbohydrates are the main fuel for these short, high-intensity bursts of energy. Anaerobic metabolism taps into glycogen stores for energy

carbohydrates, during training sessions will help to delay fatigue. Carbohydrate intake of 1.0–1.1 grams of carbohydrates per minute is appropriate, providing approximately 240–270 calories per hour. Strength/power athletes add the element of repeated high-intensity bursts of effort throughout a typical

during an activity; therefore, if glycogen stores are depleted, performance will suffer.

Similar to endurance exercise, strength/power exercise can deplete muscle glycogen, although not to the same degree. Several studies have examined the glycogen-depleting effects of strength training. Tesch and colleagues[8] found a 25% decline in muscle glycogen stores after subjects performed 5 sets of 4 different leg exercises for 6–12 repetitions each. Other protocols involving 5–6 sets of 6–12 repetitions at 35–70% of maximal strength produced a similar reduction in glycogen stores.[9,10] Therefore, it has been suggested that the ingestion of higher carbohydrate diets will improve performance through higher initial glycogen levels. Several studies have supported this recommendation after examining the effects of a high- versus low-carbohydrate diet prior to performing a single bout, as well as intermittent, high-intensity activities.[11–14] Strength/power athletes should strive for a moderate to high intake of carbohydrates daily to have fully loaded glycogen stores before training sessions and competitive events.

A possible exception to the rule of glycogen stores making an impact on strength/power performance is during a single sprint effort. During one sprint of about 400 meters or less, the quantity of muscle glycogen stored in the muscle is not necessarily the limiting factor in performance.[15] Carbohydrates are still the main source of fuel; however, because of the short duration of the effort, glycogen stores will not be depleted by one burst of sprinting. Therefore, carbohydrate loading for one sprint is not as critical as it would be before a training session or other repeated high-intensity exercise bout. Sprinters may train intensely several times per week, including repeated sprints per workout, so moderate carbohydrate consumption on a daily basis is a sound dietary practice.

In addition to fueling activity, carbohydrate intake can play an indirect role in building muscle mass. Carbohydrate ingestion stimulates the secretion of insulin. Insulin is considered an **anabolic** hormone, driving nutrients into the cells for the growth and development of tissues as well as preventing normal postexercise muscle protein breakdown.[16,17] Consuming adequate amounts of carbohydrates, as well as ensuring that total energy and protein needs are met, will support muscle growth in response to the demands

anabolic A metabolic process or activity that results in tissue repair or growth. An anabolic hormone or substance is one that stimulates anabolism.

of an appropriate strength training and conditioning program.

How are daily carbohydrate needs calculated for strength/power athletes?

Many strength/power athletes will train intensely three to five times per week; without sufficient dietary carbohydrate intake, this could lead to glycogen depletion and decreased performance. An intake of 5–10 grams of carbohydrates per kilogram of body weight per day has been shown to replenish glycogen stores after daily training sessions.[18] This quantity of carbohydrates should contribute approximately 55–65% of total calorie intake. This percentage can also be used to estimate carbohydrate needs based on total calorie requirements.

As mentioned in Chapter 12 on endurance and ultra-endurance athletes, estimated carbohydrate needs should be compared to total estimated energy requirements to verify that carbohydrate recommendations fall near the range of 55–65% of total calories. Building on the scenarios described in the last section regarding Lyndsi, Jake, and Leo, the following examples demonstrate the importance of fine-tuning carbohydrate recommendations for every athlete:

gaining the performance edge

Carbohydrates are the master fuel for strength/power sports. Consuming adequate amounts of carbohydrates on a daily basis ensures glycogen stores will be sufficient to support high-intensity training and competition. Carbohydrates also act as a support crew for the construction of muscle mass in response to resistance training.

- Lyndsi, the gymnast, requires 216–432 grams of carbohydrates daily based on the 5–10 grams of carbohydrates per kilogram of body weight recommendation (95 lbs ÷ 2.2 = 43.2 kg; 43.2 kg × 5–10 g/kg = 216–432 g). Lyndsi's initial meal plan analysis revealed that she was consuming 66% of her total calories from carbohydrates. Although this percentage sounds appropriate, the absolute value of her carbohydrate intake was only 153 grams, which is only 71% of the low end of her recommended carbohydrate intake range. In addition, Lyndsi's absolute carbohydrate intake is only slightly higher than the RDA for carbohydrates (130 g) for adults and children based on the average minimum amount of glucose utilized by the brain daily.[19] In Lyndsi's revised meal plan, the percentage of calories from carbohydrates decreased to 56%;

however, the absolute value of her intake increased to 290 grams. This number is within the 216–432 recommended range and represents an 89% increase from her previous carbohydrate consumption.

- Jake, the swimmer, requires 375–750 grams of carbohydrates daily based on the 5–10 grams of carbohydrates per kilogram of body weight recommendation (165 lbs ÷ 2.2 = 75 kg; 75 kg × 5–10 g/kg = 375–750 g). Three hundred and seventy-five grams of carbohydrates contribute 1500 calories (375 g carbohydrates × 4 calories/g carbohydrates = 1500 calories). This quantity of carbohydrates represents 51% of 2922 calories (the low end of his recommended calorie range) and 41% of 3654 calories (the high end of his recommended calorie range). Clearly, 375 grams of carbohydrates would not be appropriate for a calorie intake at the low or high end of his recommended range; therefore, it is more appropriate to estimate his carbohydrate needs through a percentage of total calories. For example, 55–65% of Jake's calorie range of 2922–3654 calories equals:

([0.55–0.65] × 2922 calories) /
4 calories per gram of carbohydrates =
401–475 grams of carbohydrates daily

([0.55–0.65] × 3654 calories) /
4 calories per gram of carbohydrates =
502–594 grams of carbohydrates daily

For Jake, estimating an appropriate amount of carbohydrates varies greatly depending on his total calorie intake. In his case, it is best to calculate his carbohydrate needs based on a percentage of total calories. Therefore, a final carbohydrate recommendation for Jake is 401–594 grams of carbohydrates per day. Jake's revised meal plan provides 411 grams of carbohydrates, thus meeting his daily needs.

- Leo, the weight lifter, requires 387–773 grams of carbohydrates daily based on the 5–10 grams of carbohydrates per kilogram of body weight recommendation (170 lbs ÷ 2.2 = 77.3 kg; 77.3 kg × 5–10 g/kg = 387–773 g). Because Leo is attempting to gain weight and thus has higher calorie needs, the estimated carbohydrate intake based on body weight should be checked using the percent total calories method.

By comparing the body weight recommendation range of 387–773 grams of carbohydrate to that of the percentage of total calories range (i.e., 522–682 grams), it is apparent an adjustment is needed for his minimum intake recommendation. In this case, the minimum value of the body weight recommendation range (i.e., 5 grams/kg, or 387 grams) is too low because it accounts for less than 55% of total calories. As a result, adjusting the minimum recommendation to 522 grams is warranted. If you convert the 522 grams of carbohydrate into a gram per kilogram body weight recommendation, it would be 6.8 grams per kilogram of body weight (i.e., 522 grams / 77.3 kg = 6.8 g/kg).

Leo's initial meal plan was providing only 399 grams of carbohydrates per day. The revised meal plan increased his intake 53% to a total of 612 grams of carbohydrates per day.

Keep in mind that these scenarios provide only three examples of individual athlete needs. Most of these cases suggest 55–65% of total calories from carbohydrates; however, this recommendation can be raised or lowered based on the volume of training a strength/power athlete engages in daily. None of these cases recommended carbohydrate intakes at the high end of the range—10 grams of carbohydrates per kilogram of body weight. This does not mean that 10 grams of carbohydrates per kilogram of body weight is not appropriate in some situations. Evaluate each athlete individually, compare estimations to current intake, and then make recommendations based on the athlete's goals and training schedule. Figure 13.2 compares the individual carbohydrate and energy needs of the three athletes discussed here. Each of these athletes has different energy and carbohydrate needs based on his or her body weight, gender, and strength-training program.

Are carbohydrates needed before and during training and competition?

The performance effects of carbohydrate ingestion immediately prior to and during strength/power sports are unclear. The limited research available presents evidence to support a variety of benefits and potential drawbacks. Thus, trade-offs exist, requiring recommendations and nutrition plans to be individualized based on the goals and objectives of the athlete, and a consideration of the specific activity to be performed.

Although engaging in strength/power sports generally does not cause a reduction in blood glu-

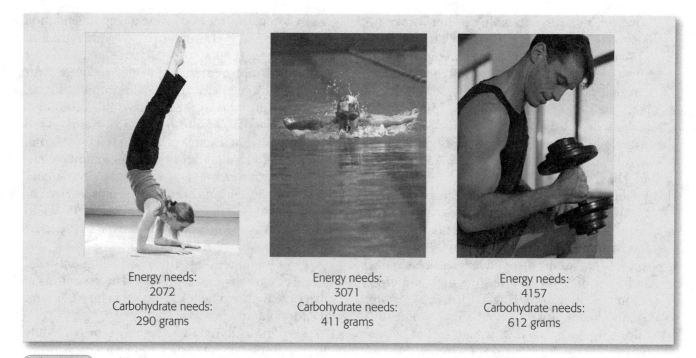

Energy needs:
2072
Carbohydrate needs:
290 grams

Energy needs:
3071
Carbohydrate needs:
411 grams

Energy needs:
4157
Carbohydrate needs:
612 grams

Figure 13.2   Lyndsi, Jake, and Leo have different energy and carbohydrate needs based on their size, sport, and training level.

cose levels during a workout, a considerable glycogenolytic effect has been observed during either intermittent, high-intensity exercise or strength-training-type activities.[8,10,20,21] If depletion of glycogen occurs, then performance suffers as a result of fatigue, and over the long term the athlete can experience muscle loss. Therefore, it appears prudent to consume carbohydrates before and also during strength/power exercise.

A general recommendation for preactivity eating is to consume a carbohydrate-rich meal approximately 2–4 hours prior to the initiation of exercise. The provision of carbohydrates helps to top off the body's glycogen stores prior to training or competition. Many athletes find that the consumption of carbohydrates before a hard training session allows them to complete a tough workout without feeling fatigued prematurely. Therefore, athletes push themselves harder and gain more benefit from the workout. Furthermore, recent research has suggested that the provision of carbohydrates, as well as amino acids, prevents muscle breakdown during intense exercise, potentially leading to a maintenance or enhancement of muscle mass.[17]

Additional benefit has been observed when athletes supplement the preactivity meal with a supply of carbohydrates during the workout or competition, typically in the form of a beverage or liquid supplement. Especially for long training sessions,

consuming carbohydrates periodically during exercise sustains energy levels and work output for longer periods of time.[22,23] In a well-designed study, Haff et al.[22] aimed to determine the performance effects of carbohydrate supplementation on the ability to perform resistance exercise during a second training session on the same day. Subjects performed a glycogen-depleting session of resistance training in the morning (15 sets of various lower body exercises) and then returned to the gym 4 hours later to squat to exhaustion. The carbohydrate-supplemented group outperformed the placebo group by successfully completing a greater number of sets and repetitions. Although higher energy levels and greater strength/power outputs during a training session because of carbohydrate intake sounds like a "no-brainer," not all research findings have yielded similar results.[24,25] In fact, some athletes, coaches, and researchers are suggesting the exact opposite nutrition practice—avoiding carbohydrates before and during training.

This school of thought exists mainly in the world of weight lifting and body building. It is based on the premise that a steady stream of carbohydrates into the bloodstream will prevent the body from tapping into other energy sources, specifically fat stores. Therefore, the recommendation is to avoid eating carbohydrate-rich foods 2–4 hours prior to exercise. In fact, most recommend not consuming any food before a workout. The second half of the recommendation includes the avoidance of carbohydrate beverages, supplements, and food during a workout. Although this practice will cause the body to turn to fats (adipose tissue and intramuscular fats) for energy, it is well known that when glycogen and blood glucose levels begin to run low, the athlete will begin to tire, perception of effort increases, and performance levels can plunge. However, not all athletes experience extreme fatigue, particularly if their diet is adequate at other times of the day when following this practice; therefore, the final recommendation will be based on individual preference and tolerance. If an athlete chooses to avoid consuming food before and during a strength/power workout, a strong emphasis should be placed on consuming the required number of daily calories throughout the rest of the day. Obviously, this carbohydrate avoidance scenario is best implemented with early morning workout sessions to prevent the disruption of regular meal times throughout the day.

The final recommendation should be based on an athlete's preference for carbohydrate consumption, the effects on performance, and the safety of the athlete. Some athletes feel they perform better on an empty stomach whereas others become hungry, distracting them from performing well. In terms of safety, if blood glucose levels run too low, athletes can pass out and injure themselves, especially during an activity such as weight lifting. Athletes should test both methods during practice sessions and determine which recommendation leads to improved performance, increased strength/power, overall safety of the athlete, and a feeling of well-being that they are meeting their goals. At the same time, researchers will continue to examine the effects of macronutrients on strength/power performance and eventually determine specific nutritional guidelines.

Are carbohydrates needed for recovery from strength/power activities?

Similar to endurance sports, strength/power activities can deplete glycogen stores, requiring carbohydrate

consumption after exercise. Complete replenishment of glycogen stores can take as little as 4–6 hours and up to 24–48 hours depending on exogenous carbohydrate availability. It is in the athlete's best interest to consume carbohydrates immediately following exercise as well as throughout the day at regular meals and snacks.

As discussed in Chapter 12, athletes should focus on the timing and quantity of carbohydrates consumed after exercise. A source of carbohydrates should be eaten as soon as possible—ideally within 15–30 minutes—after the cessation of exercise. This will ensure that the carbohydrates are digested and delivered to muscles in the window of time in which the muscles are most receptive to absorbing and storing carbohydrates as glycogen for the next training session. Ideally, athletes should ingest 1.2 grams per kilogram of body weight per hour for 3–4 hours postexercise. Consuming enough carbohydrates is more important than the exact type of carbohydrates. Fruits, vegetables, juices, whole grains, low-fat milk, and dairy products are some of the best choices to supply carbohydrates.

Although the provision of carbohydrates after high-intensity exercise is critical for glycogen replenishment, it has also been suggested that it plays a role in muscle adaptation after intense training. However, carbohydrates cannot act alone in this role; muscle protein synthesis will be much greater when a combination of carbohydrates and protein is consumed immediately after exercise.[26] The quantity and timing of this macronutrient combination for muscle growth and development will be addressed in the upcoming sections on protein needs for strength/power athletes.

Carbohydrates may be important not only for the replenishment of glycogen stores and muscle construction, but also for the attenuation of immunosuppression observed after exercise. Many studies have reported that high-intensity exercise suppresses immune function temporarily after exercise.[27–30] It has been suggested that ingestion of carbohydrates before, during, and/or after exercise may minimize the immune function changes in athletes, leading to less risk of illness.[31–34] Many of the studies related to immunosuppression have been conducted with endurance athletes. However, Chan et al.[31] researched the effects on immune function of carbohydrate consumption before and after resistive exercises. Subjects consumed a low-carbohydrate meal 2 hours prior to the strength-training session. Ten minutes prior to exercise and 10 minutes after exercise, sub-

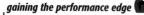
Carbohydrates are the master fuel for strength/power athletes. Each athlete should experiment with different quantities of foods and beverages to determine his or her individual "ideal" plan for before, during, and after exercise.

jects drank either a carbohydrate supplement beverage (one trial) or placebo (second trial). The researchers reported that carbohydrate ingestion minimized the decrease in interleukin-2 and interleukin-5 (an indication of greater immune function as compared to controls) after exercise. More research is needed in this area to verify these results. However, carbohydrate consumption after strength/power exercise is important for glycogen resynthesis and muscle construction regardless of its effect on the immune system. If research does reveal that carbohydrate consumption surrounding high-intensity, short-duration exercise has a positive effect on immune function, it will be a bonus benefit to an already solid nutrition practice.

Are protein needs different for strength/power athletes?

The high intensities that strength/power athletes train at on a daily basis challenge the body and skeletal muscle. This "challenge" creates microscopic tears in muscle tissue, which are the stimuli for subsequent tissue repair and rebuilding. Amino acids, either synthesized by the body or obtained from the digestion and breakdown of dietary protein, are the building blocks for muscle repair and rebuilding. Because of this function, protein has long been a major dietary focus for strength/power athletes. The mantra has typically been "the more protein, the better." Although strength/power athletes do have higher protein needs than their sedentary counterparts, an overdose of protein intake on a daily basis is not ergogenically beneficial.

How are daily protein needs calculated for strength/power athletes?

Strength/power athletes have an increased requirement for dietary protein. Muscle tissue goes through a process of self-repair on a daily basis and, therefore, sufficient amounts of high-quality protein sources need to be consumed at every meal. Dietary proteins are digested and broken down into amino acids, which the body then uses for building blocks for all bodily tissues. Insufficient protein intakes will lead to suboptimal improvements in muscle development,

low energy levels, and poor performance. On the other hand, excessive protein intakes can also lead to adverse effects on performance, body composition, and overall health. Strength/power athletes need to find the right balance between these two extremes. In addition to the total protein intake, the variety of protein sources ingested is also of importance.

How do you determine the "optimal" daily dose of protein for strength/power athletes?

The true "optimal" quantity of daily protein intake for strength/power athletes has been debated over the years. A few articles have reported that active individuals become more efficient at using protein on a daily basis, and therefore protein needs actually decline versus increase in athletes.[26,35] However, a majority of the current research points to protein needs in the other direction, at the higher end of the scale. Some researchers suggest a range of 1.4–1.7 grams of protein daily per kilogram of body weight is appropriate,[36] whereas others recommend a higher upper limit of 2.0 grams of protein per kilogram of body weight.[37] Often magazines, coaches, practitioners, and athletes push the upper limit even higher to levels greater than 2.5–3.0 grams per kilogram of body weight. The bottom line is that strength/power athletes do have increased protein needs; however, there is a limit to the amount of protein that can be used effectively and ingested without adverse effects.

Since the early 1980s, studies have revealed that dietary protein plays an integral role in muscle growth and development. Although all the parameters affecting muscle protein synthesis have not been identified, a few factors such as increased insulin levels and availability of amino acids are obvious. A decline in intracellular amino acid concentration will inhibit protein synthesis. Strength/power exercise has been shown to elicit a decrease in amino acid concentrations.[38,39] Therefore, it seems to follow that the ingestion of protein or amino acids would prevent this decline and in turn stimulate protein synthesis. In fact, studies have shown that the consumption of dietary proteins, which increases endogenous amino acid availability, can stimulate an increase in muscle protein synthesis by 30–100%.[26,40] Muscle growth and development are largely caused by an enhanced protein synthesis, versus a decreased muscle breakdown.[41] Therefore, daily and particularly pre- and postworkout provision of amino acids is of utmost importance in maximizing muscle building.

Because of the essential role of protein and amino acids in the growth and development of muscle tissue, a common misconception is that by increasing protein intake, an athlete can increase muscle mass. As stated in the previous paragraphs, there is no doubt that protein is critical for muscle growth. However, once an athlete has reached the peak of protein assimilation, additional protein will not be used to create even more muscle tissue. Physical training is the strongest stimulus for signaling the muscles to grow and develop. Proper nutrition acts as a support network to the training stimulus; however, it does not necessarily initiate a further stimulus when consumed in quantities that significantly surpass physical requirements. To increase muscle mass, the equation is simple: Train hard and eat well, but do neither in excess.

Similar to carbohydrates and fat, athletic performance and overall health can suffer if too much protein is ingested and macronutrient balance goes astray. Excessive daily protein intake is generally considered to be >2.0 grams of protein per kilogram of body weight. At intakes above this level, protein is either used for fuel or converted and stored as fat. Second, increased protein digestion and breakdown result in greater urea production, thus causing more fluid to be excreted from the body to flush out the toxic urea, potentially leading to dehydration. Third, if calories remain stable and protein intake increases, carbohydrate intake and glycogen replenishment generally suffer, ultimately affecting workouts. Finally, high-protein foods, especially animal products, tend to be high in fat, saturated fat, and cholesterol, all of which can negatively affect cardiovascular health. As with most nutrients, more is not always better.

How do you determine the "optimal" food sources of protein?

In the world of strength/power athletes, "high-quality" and "complete" proteins receive the most attention. Although the quality of a protein is certainly important, true success is achieved with variety. It should be noted that the term *incomplete protein* often is misinterpreted as meaning "inadequate" or "useless" for strength/power athletes. This interpretation is erroneous and misleading. For more information on complete versus incomplete proteins and vegetarian eating, refer to Chapters 5 and 15 of this text. The bottom line is that all sources of protein are valuable for the strength/power athlete. To maximize

> **Training Table 13.4: Tips for Maximizing the Benefits of Dietary Protein for Strength/Power Athletes**
>
> - *Consume enough total calories to meet energy needs.* If calorie intake declines, a higher percentage of ingested protein will be used for energy versus for muscle building and repair.
> - *Consume a level of protein that falls within 1.4–2.0 grams of protein per kilogram of body weight.* This level of protein generally contributes 15–20% of total calories. Athletes should ensure that plenty of carbohydrates and at least minimum amounts of fat are also ingested daily.
> - *Include a protein source in every meal and snack.* By focusing on including a protein source at every meal and snack, protein is digested gradually and continuously throughout the day. This recommendation is especially important for athletes engaging in multiple training sessions daily.
> - *Choose a variety of different protein sources.* Lean meats, poultry, fish, and dairy products are excellent choices because of their amino acid profile and high overall protein content. Vegetarians should consume plenty of soy products, which also contain an ideal amino acid profile and high protein content. Beans, lentils, nuts, seeds, and grains supply protein in smaller amounts and with low levels of one or two amino acids. By consuming a variety of these sources on a daily basis and in larger quantities, strength/power athletes can achieve optimal intakes of protein.
> - *Consume protein supplements in moderation, if necessary.* In general, protein needs can be met through "real" foods consumed throughout the day. Studies have shown that supplemental protein provides no added benefit over whole food sources.[38] However, if an athlete is already eating a well-balanced diet but is still having a hard time obtaining optimal quantities of protein, a supplement can be used in moderation. Protein powders are an appropriate supplement to use because a powder can be added to "real" foods such as milk, yogurt, cereal, and smoothies.

the benefits of dietary protein, consider putting into practice the tips outlined in **Training Table 13.4**.

Do individual amino acids have an ergogenic effect on muscle growth and development?

The ingestion of specific amino acids or groups of amino acids has been purported to enhance muscle strength and development. It has been suggested that amino acids can influence muscle strength and development through the initiation of protein synthesis and/or increase the secretion of various anabolic hormones. The current research provides some insight into the action of various amino acids, but more research is needed to make firm conclusions and subsequent dietary recommendations.

Glutamine is one of the most popular amino acid supplement products on the market because of its touted "anticatabolic" effects in regard to skeletal muscle. It is the most abundant amino acid found in blood plasma and skeletal muscle[42] and accounts for more than 60% of the total intramuscular free amino acid pool.[43] However, glutamine is in high demand by other tissues of the body. For example, glutamine is needed by the cells of the gastrointestinal system to support their continual high protein synthesis rates. Glutamine is also used as a fuel source for cells of the immune system and hair follicles.[43,44] As a result, if glutamine levels are not sufficient to meet the body's total needs, particularly during periods of high stress such as intense training, then glutamine is taken and/or synthesized from amino acids present in skeletal muscle. It appears that glutamine not only prevents muscle **catabolism,** but several studies have reported that glutamine also is critical for protein synthesis within skeletal muscle.[45,46] Although the current research appears promising, the long-term effects of glutamine supplementation on protein synthesis and body composition have yet to be confirmed. As a result, more research is needed before conclusions can be drawn and recommendations made for glutamine supplementation.

catabolism A metabolic process or activity that results in tissue breakdown or destruction.

The branched-chain amino acids, particularly leucine, have been suggested to be positive regulators of muscle protein synthesis.[47] However, the research on the effects of the branched-chain amino acids on exercise performance is still in its infancy. The exact actions of these amino acids before, during, and after exercise and the subsequent requirements and recommendations for intake are yet to be elucidated.

growth hormone A hormone produced by the pituitary gland that results in the growth of many different tissues in the body, including skeletal muscle.

The increased secretion of **growth hormone** is at the center of many amino acid supplement claims; however, study results have shown mixed conclusions. For example, Suminski et al.[48] reported that 1500 mg of arginine and 1500 mg of lysine consumed at rest increased growth hormone levels 60 minutes after ingestion. However, the same quantity of amino acids provided immediately prior to weight lifting did not alter circulating growth hormone levels in males

while exercising. Amino acids and their respective influence on insulin, testosterone, and cortisol have also been highlighted as potential factors in protein metabolism and synthesis. Once again, more research is needed to ascertain the connections and interactions of amino acid ingestion and hormonal responses and the subsequent effects on protein metabolism and muscle protein synthesis.

Is protein needed before and during training sessions and competitions?

The benefits of consuming protein before strength/power sports have recently received more attention in the research. Most of the studies have explored not only the effects of protein, but also the combination effect of carbohydrates and protein on muscle synthesis, catabolism, and performance. The influence of ingesting protein during training or competition on strength/power performance has received minimal attention, and therefore the relationship between these two factors is still under investigation.

Until recently, many of the recommendations related to nutrition and muscle building have focused on the recovery period. Although the 1–4 hours after exercise are still considered a critical time for replenishment, that may not be the only time when the athlete can affect muscle and strength gains. The potential positive impact of consuming a protein–carbohydrate supplement before exercise is a relatively novel concept. The argument for consuming both protein and carbohydrates before strength/power training is based on the anabolic effects of increasing the secretion of insulin and circulating amino acids. By consuming carbohydrates before strength/power exercise, insulin levels will rise and thus decrease the normal exercise-induced catabolism of muscle tissue.[49,50] A supply of exogenous protein results in a greater delivery and increased concentration of intracellular amino acids in the muscle during exercise, enhancing protein synthesis.[39] Although the action of carbohydrates and protein is the same after exercise, the reason that preactivity consumption is preferable to postactivity is related to blood flow. The theory is that when the concentration of nutrients (through the digestion of a preactivity carbohydrate–protein source) and blood flow (caused

gaining the performance edge

Until further research is conducted to elucidate the benefits and drawbacks of consuming individual or groups of amino acids, the best way for athletes to obtain amino acids is from protein-rich, whole foods eaten daily in appropriate amounts.

by exercise) are both increased, the rate of nutrient uptake and utilization as well as protein synthesis is maximized.[39] The positive effects of consuming carbohydrates and protein prior to exercise have been reported with as little as 6 grams of essential amino acids and 35 grams of carbohydrates.[17] Therefore, large volumes of food do not need to be consumed to gain the anabolic benefits.

Strength/power athletes should strongly consider consuming a source of both carbohydrates and protein before a training session to maximize the ability of the body to synthesize new proteins. The benefit of consuming additional protein during strength/power sports still needs to be determined.

Is protein needed for recovery from strength/power activities?

High-intensity exercise and strength training stimulate protein synthesis in muscle tissue. In response to this physical stress, amino acids are released from the free amino acid pools within plasma and cellular spaces of the body.[51,52] To meet the basic metabolic needs of muscle tissue, to repair damage from high-intensity exercise, and to build new muscle tissue, exogenous amino acids are required. Therefore, protein is a critical component of any strength/power athlete's postexercise meal or snack.

Several studies have examined the effects of consuming macronutrients at various intervals after exercise to determine an ideal environment for muscle synthesis and recovery from training. It appears that the provision of amino acids after resistance exercise stimulates greater protein synthesis, producing a net positive effect (more synthesis versus breakdown as compared to fasting after exercise).[53] When a combination of amino acids (6 grams) and carbohydrates (35 grams) is provided, an even greater increase in protein synthesis is observed.[41] This suggested ratio of 6 grams of amino acids to 35 grams of carbohydrates is the same as mentioned previously regarding preactivity protein and carbohydrate ingestion. Therefore, the combination of carbohydrates and protein both before and after high-intensity training is beneficial to protein synthesis.

A study conducted by Chandler[54] and colleagues reported that the combination of carbohydrates and protein was more advantageous than either carbohydrates or protein alone in stimulating anabolic hormone secretion after resistance exercise. Subjects performed a standardized resistance training workout and then consumed an isocaloric amount of one of three supplements (carbohydrates only, 1.5 g/kg;

protein only, 1.38 g/kg; carbohydrates and protein, 1.06 g/kg and 0.41 g/kg, respectively) immediately and 2 hours after the session. Both the carbohydrates and carbohydrate–protein supplements caused an increase in circulating insulin levels. However, only the carbohydrate–protein supplement additionally caused a modest but significant increase in growth hormone levels. The results of this study reveal that the combination of carbohydrate and protein ingestion after strength training can produce a hormonal environment during recovery that may be favorable to muscle growth.

A recent study performed by Borsheim et al.[55] provided more evidence that a combination of protein and carbohydrates after resistance training stimulates muscle protein synthesis to a greater extent than carbohydrates alone. Eight subjects engaged in resistance training on two separate occasions, and consumed either a combination supplement (77.4 g carbohydrates, 17.5 g whey protein, 4.9 g amino acids) or a carbohydrates-only supplement (100 g carbohydrates) 1 hour after the exercise session while net protein balance response was measured. The results revealed the combination beverage not only stimulated protein synthesis at 20–30 minutes after ingestion (as shown in previous studies), but also caused synthesis to peak again at 90 minutes postconsumption. The authors speculate that this second round of enhanced synthesis was caused by the delayed digestion of intact proteins versus rapidly digested amino acids.

Although the optimal balance and ideal quantity of carbohydrates and protein to consume after strength/power activities are yet to be determined, athletes can gain an edge on competitors by consuming a snack or full meal containing both carbohydrates and protein to help recover after training sessions or competitions. So the next question is: When should these macronutrients be ingested?

Similar to consuming carbohydrates immediately after endurance exercise to optimize glycogen replenishment, a combination of protein and carbohydrates should be consumed as soon as possible after strength/power activities. A protein–carbohydrate food or beverage should be consumed immediately following a

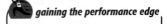
gaining the performance edge

Strength/power athletes should aim for consuming at least 6 grams of amino acids and 35 grams of carbohydrates as soon as possible after training sessions and competitions. The combination of carbohydrates and protein will aid not only muscle protein synthesis, but also glycogen replenishment.

training session or competition, with benefits diminishing 1–3 hours postexercise.[55] This nutrition protocol will stimulate the release of insulin to prevent muscle breakdown while also supplying amino acids needed as building blocks for muscle tissue.

Are fat needs different for strength/power athletes?

Strength/power athletes burn very little fat during the performance of their sport. The bioenergetic demands of the forceful muscle actions performed by strength/power athletes are met by the phosphagen and anaerobic energy systems, neither of which relies on the metabolizing of fats for production of ATP. Does that mean that strength/power athletes do not need to consume fat? No. Essential fatty acids are needed for the general health of all bodily tissues. Fats are also attractive to the strength/power athlete because of their caloric density. A moderate amount of fat should be consumed on a daily basis, with an emphasis placed on unsaturated fats. The timing of fat consumption is also of importance to avoid any potential performance disturbance during training or competition.

How are daily fat needs calculated for strength/power athletes?

For strength/power athletes, the goal is to find the right balance of carbohydrate, protein, and fat intake to supply all essential nutrients and allow athletes to perform at their best. Fat is a controversial topic requiring the consideration of several factors including caloric needs; the athlete's desire to lose, maintain, or gain weight; health history; and ideal sources of fat. All strength/power athletes need fat; however, fat intake recommendations can vary greatly.

A general recommendation cited by Rogozkin[18] suggests a daily fat intake of approximately 2 grams of fat per kilogram of body weight. This quantity of fat may be appropriate for most athletes; however, as always, the calculated estimate should be compared to total calorie needs before a final recommendation is made to the athlete. For general health, a fat intake of 30–35% of total calories is considered an upper limit. A range of 20–25% is more appropriate for strength/power athletes who are trying to lose weight because fat is more calorically dense and it takes less energy to digest, absorb, and assimilate fats than carbohydrates and proteins. What this means is that if excess calories from fatty foods are ingested, then more of the excess will be stored as fat than if the

excess calories had come from proteins or carbohydrates. An athlete who is aiming to gain weight will generally find the 25–30% range sufficient in supplying extra calories as well as decreasing the total volume of food needed to meet total energy needs. General health and specific athletic goals/objectives should be considered when estimating fat needs.

For example, consider two athletes who both weigh 150 pounds: one is a wrestler aiming to lose weight, who consumes about 2500 calories per day, while the other is a shot putter with the goal of increasing muscle mass, who requires 4500 calories per day. Basing their fat needs on 2 grams per kilogram of current body weight, both athletes would require 136 grams of fat per day. Comparing this recommendation to estimated calorie needs, the percentage of total calories from fat would be 49% and 27% for the wrestler and shot putter, respectively. Knowing that the wrestler wants to lose weight, that the fat intake recommendation for overall health is no more than 30–35% of total calories, that fat is calorically dense making it easier to err on the side of overconsumption, and that fats do not increase the metabolic demands for digestion and absorption like proteins and carbohydrates, the 136-gram recommendation is not to the wrestler's advantage. Using the range of 20–25% of total calories from fat to estimate his needs:

(2500 calories × [0.20–0.25]) / 9 calories per gram of fat = 55–69 grams of fat per day

Fifty-five to 69 grams of fat per day will supply the wrestler with a small amount of fat to provide satiety and essential fatty acids, while minimizing the impact on total calorie intake. On the other hand, the 136 grams of fat calculated for the shot putter is appropriate, providing a moderate amount of fat to allow the athlete to meet his increased energy needs while maintaining a healthy diet (see Figure 13.3).

Strength/power athletes should also consider their health history when consuming fats. As mentioned in Chapter 4, saturated and trans fats are the most detrimental to health, whereas monounsaturated and polyunsaturated fats are beneficial to overall health. For those who are at risk for heart disease, high cholesterol, or cancer, special attention should be placed on unsaturated fats. An intake of mainly unsaturated fats is also considered protective for future health problems for all athletes. Strength/power athletes should be guided toward healthy types of fats, especially those who are consuming large quan-

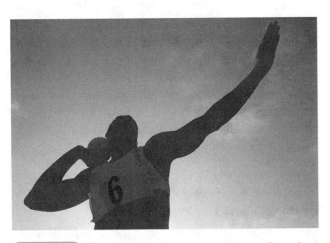

Dietary fat consumed in moderation allows the strength/power athlete to meet increased energy needs while maintaining a healthy diet.

tities of protein, which are often rich sources of saturated fats. Protein sources that are lower in total fat and saturated fat include lean cuts of beef, chicken, turkey, fish, legumes, and soy products.

Are fats needed before and during training sessions and competitions?

Although fats are important to consume on a daily basis, fat intake should be minimized in the hours leading up to, as well as during, an intense training session or competition. Fats take longer to digest, leading to a sense of fullness and potentially gastrointestinal discomfort during exercise. Very small amounts of fat can be included in a preexercise meal consumed several hours prior to the initiation of exercise to provide a feeling of satiety. However, a majority of fat intake should be reserved for after training sessions and competitions, spread evenly throughout the day.

Is fat needed for recovery from strength/power activities?

It is not essential to replace any fat used during strength/power exercise by consuming fat-rich foods immediately following training or a competition. Strength/power sports rely minimally on fat for energy during training sessions and competitions,

gaining the performance edge

Fats are an important component to an overall healthy diet for strength/power athletes. Fat consumption should be kept within the range of 20–35% of total calories, based on total calorie needs and the athlete's goals and objectives. Fats should be obtained from mainly unsaturated sources, while minimizing saturated and trans fat intake. The ingestion of fats before, during, and immediately postexercise should be kept to a minimum. Ingest fats in other meals and snacks spread throughout the day.

and therefore fat "depletion" is not an issue. Even if fat was used during strength/power sports, the body's stores of fat are so great that they will not be depleted in one workout. For athletes aiming to lose weight and become lean, training sessions help to burn calories, leading to a long-term loss of fat mass, and therefore a replacement of fat post-workout would be counterproductive. Instead, the postexercise meal should consist of mainly carbohydrate- and protein-rich foods. However, fats add flavor to foods and create a sense of satiety, and therefore can be included in small amounts in the postexercise meal or snack.

Are vitamin and mineral needs different for strength/power athletes?

The vitamin and mineral needs of strength/power athletes have not been studied extensively. As with all active individuals, nutrient needs may be slightly higher than for sedentary counterparts, but an increased intake of specific vitamins and minerals may or may not be critical for optimal strength/power performance. This section reviews several of the micronutrients that have been suggested to be of importance, including antioxidants, boron, calcium, chromium, iron, magnesium, and zinc. As more research develops, clearer recommendations can be made.

Do strength/power athletes need to supplement with antioxidant vitamins?

The main antioxidants receiving attention in the exercise arena are beta-carotene, vitamin C, vitamin E, and selenium. Antioxidants are touted to combat free radical damage occurring during and after exercise, including strenuous and high-intensity exercise. Most of the current research conducted on the effects of antioxidants and exercise-related free radical damage has focused on endurance athletes. Although strength/power athletes may need more of these nutrients, a specific recommendation cannot be made at this time. The best option is to consume a variety of antioxidant-rich foods such as citrus fruits, dark green and orange vegetables, nuts, seeds, and Brazil nuts.

Should strength/power athletes supplement boron intake?

Boron is a nonessential trace mineral found in foods such as fruits, vegetables, nuts, seeds, and wine. It is readily absorbed by the body, and the average dietary intake is estimated to be between 1 and 2 mg/day. Boron received considerable attention in the world of strength/power sports after a study in 1987 reported elevated testosterone levels in humans after taking boron supplements.[56] Boron supplements quickly appeared in the market, claiming the product could be used as an "anabolic steroid alternative." However, a review of the study reveals that the researchers' conclusions were sorely misinterpreted and taken out of context. Nielsen and colleagues[56] fed a group of postmenopausal women a *boron-deficient* diet, and then once hormone levels had dropped, a boron supplement was provided. After taking a 3-milligram daily dose of boron, serum testosterone and estrogen levels returned to normal levels. Therefore, this study focused on older women who were not athletes, and the supplement was intended to correct a deficiency in the diet. When a study was conducted on young individuals engaged in the sport of body building, a 2.5 mg/day boron supplement had no effect on testosterone levels, lean mass, or strength as compared to the control group.[57] There is no RDA established for boron; however, the estimated daily requirement is thought to be 1 mg/day. A Tolerable Upper Intake Level (UL) has been established at 20 mg/day for adults 19 years or older, and 17 mg/day for adolescents.[58] Low intake of boron, as with all nutrients, can potentially cause adverse effects; however, supplemental boron at levels higher than the 20 mg UL have not been shown to be beneficial and can have negative effects.

Should strength/power athletes be concerned about calcium intake?

Calcium is critical for optimal bone health, muscle development, and nerve transmission in both men and women. Unfortunately, many strength/power athletes are not consuming adequate amounts of daily calcium. This deficiency is often caused by an avoidance of dairy products in the quest for a leaner body. Ironically, recent studies have shown that higher intakes of calcium can actually aid in weight loss and body fat loss.[59] Much of this research has focused on overweight individuals placed on calorie-restricted diets with varied dairy calcium or supplemental calcium intakes. Of potential interest to strength athletes is the growing evidence that high dairy calcium intake aids not only increased weight loss, but also higher body fat losses compared to low dairy or supplemental calcium intakes.[60] In addition, dairy products contain many other essential nutrients for strength/power athletes, including

protein, carbohydrates, vitamin D, and riboflavin. To promote overall health and a strong body, a minimum of three to four servings of calcium-rich foods such as milk, yogurt, calcium-fortified orange juice, green leafy vegetables, soy milk, and other soy-based dairy alternatives should be consumed on a daily basis to meet, but not necessarily to exceed, current recommendations (1000 mg for 19- to 50-year-old men and women).

Is chromium supplementation important for strength/power athletes?

Chromium is an essential mineral involved in the regulation of insulin-mediated metabolism of carbohydrates, fats, and proteins. Some early chromium studies reported positive changes in body composition,[61,62] which have led to a variety of ergogenic claims such as increased muscle mass, decreased fat mass, and enhanced muscular strength. However, most studies reveal no effect on body composition or muscular strength after chromium supplementation.[63–66] Chromium can be easily obtained through the diet in foods such as mushrooms, prunes, nuts, whole grains, brewer's yeast, broccoli, wine, cheese, egg yolks, asparagus, dark chocolate, and some beers.

Should strength/power athletes worry about iron?

"Pumping iron" should not be reserved only for the weight room—it should also happen in the kitchen. Strength/power athletes perform a variety of activities that often involve high-intensity, weight-bearing movements causing hematuria. As mentioned previously, hematuria is the presence of hemoglobin or myoglobin in the urine caused by a breakdown of red blood cells (i.e., hemolysis) or damage to muscle tissue, respectively. Hemolysis has been observed in weight lifters as a result of the mechanical stress of lifting heavy weights. As is the case for hemoglobin, iron is also essential for the formation of myoglobin, which stores oxygen inside muscle cells until it is needed for chemical reactions and muscular contraction.

Sprint swimmers are a unique group of strength/power athletes that have been found to have low iron levels, even though a majority of their training is non-weight-bearing. A study conducted by Brigham and colleagues[67] examined 25 female college swimmers for iron status as well as the effectiveness of iron supplementation during the competitive season. The baseline tests revealed that 17 swimmers had depleted iron stores and 5 swimmers were classified as

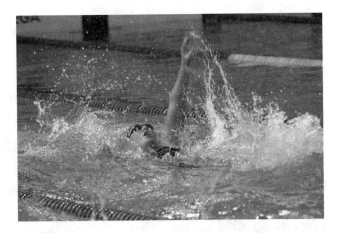

anemic. The experimental group consumed 39 mg of iron per day, which was successful in preventing a further decline in iron status as compared to the control group. However, the authors suggested that a higher dosage might be indicated to increase iron stores to a healthy range. The best line of defense is to prevent an iron deficiency from occurring by ensuring that athletes are consuming plenty of iron-rich foods daily. If anemia is suspected, a physician should be consulted before iron supplements are taken.

Strength/power athletes should focus on sources of heme iron found in foods such as beef, poultry, and fish as well as nonheme iron, which is found primarily in plant foods such as soy products, dried fruits, legumes, whole grains, fortified cereals, and green leafy vegetables. Remember, nonheme iron's bioavailability can be enhanced by eating nonheme foods with either a meat product or a vitamin C source.

Is magnesium supplementation important for strength/power athletes?

Magnesium has become a popular supplement in the area of strength/power sports. Because of its role in muscle contraction and protein synthesis, magnesium supplementation has been touted to increase muscle mass and strength. However, only a few studies have demonstrated an ergogenic effect, and many of the studies have not been well controlled. Therefore, the verdict is still out on whether intake of magnesium above the RDA will provide any benefit. Until the picture becomes clearer, athletes should focus on consuming magnesium-rich foods such as whole grains, green leafy vegetables, legumes, nuts, and seafood.

Why is zinc important for strength/power athletes?

Zinc has a variety of functions in the body, including roles as an antioxidant, a regulator of growth and de-velopment, and a wound healer. Strength/power athletes benefit from all these functions of zinc. Many athletes, especially those on calorie-restricted diets, may not be consuming adequate amounts of zinc and thus it should become a focus of attention. Zinc is found in a variety of foods including beef and other dark meats, fish, eggs, whole grains, wheat germ, legumes, and dairy products. Zinc supplements are generally not necessary when an athlete is consuming enough food.

Is multivitamin/mineral supplementation necessary for strength/power athletes?

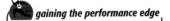

It is a common practice for athletes to take a multivitamin/mineral supplement on a regular basis. Although this may be a good practice for nutrient "insurance," it may not be ergogenic. Several research articles have been published reporting no performance benefit from multivitamin/mineral sup-plementation for athletes participating in strength/power sports.[68,69] If an athlete is looking for insurance, it is best to choose a brand containing no more than 100–200% of the Daily Value for each nutrient to prevent side effects that could be caused by ingesting large doses of vitamins and minerals.

gaining the performance edge

There is little research to support taking specific vitamins or minerals to provide an ergogenic benefit to strength/power athletes, unless an individual is deficient in a nutrient. Athletes should focus on whole foods first, ensuring balance, variety, and moderation of all food groups on a daily basis.

Are fluid needs different for strength/power athletes?

Fluid consumption and hydration are important for all types of athletes. Muscle tissue is composed mainly of water, and therefore when dehydration sets in, muscular function and performance decline. Consuming adequate amounts of fluid before, during, and after strength/power training sessions and competitions will ensure that an athlete feels energetic; has the stamina for long, intense workouts; and recovers well after each session.

What issues are of concern regarding the fluid intake of strength/power athletes?

As mentioned previously, muscle function and performance will decline when athletes are in a dehydrated state. To be well hydrated at the onset of any training session or competitive event, strength/power athletes should follow the daily hydration guidelines stated in Chapter 8 of this book. Remember, fluid losses during exercise are in addition to daily fluid recommendations. Because of the frequency, intensity, and duration of strength/power athletes' training and competition sessions, maintaining euhydration is of utmost importance and should be a dietary focus every day.

One aspect of strength/power sports that often leads to a restriction of daily fluid intake and dehydration is the weight-class system. Sports such as boxing, judo, wrestling, and weight lifting classify athletes based on body weight for competitive events. The goal for these athletes is to maximize their strength/power relative to their body weight. To gain an advantage over a competitor, many athletes will aim for weight reduction immediately prior to a weigh-in for competition so that they can compete in a lower weight category. Competing in a lower body weight category can allow the athlete theoretically to dominate an athlete who legitimately has a lower body weight and possibly also less strength and power. One of the quickest, yet unhealthiest, ways to cut weight quickly is to dehydrate the body through a variety of methods such as rubber suits, steam rooms, and the restriction of fluid intake. The magnitude of weight loss can range from a couple pounds to as high as 9.1 kilograms.[70] Athletes may aim to lose weight on a regular basis, often weekly, during the competitive season. This continuous pattern of weight loss, and then often subsequent weight gain, leads to a pattern of weight cycling, which not only can be detrimental on a daily/weekly basis, but also can have a cumulative effect over the course of an entire season. Some of the negative effects of severe and intentional dehydration include poor thermoregulation; loss of electrolytes, thus increasing the risk for **cardiac arrhythmias**; and extra strain on the kidneys, potentially affecting short-term function. Because of the harmful nature of these practices, many governing bodies have made changes in policies and established strict guidelines to prevent the life-threatening combination of severe dehydration and high-intensity competition.

cardiac arrhythmia A disturbance in the normal rhythmic pattern of heart activity. Severe arrhythmias can lead to sudden death.

The sport of wrestling has recently received attention for its efforts to prevent health-related problems caused by dehydration by changing its policies and procedures related to establishing a minimum weight for all athletes. Currently, both the National Collegiate Athletic Association and the National Federation of State High School Associations have minimum weight standards in place.[71,72] Minimum weight for wrestlers is established through body composition testing to ensure that athletes do not drop to unhealthy weights and body fat levels. In addition to weight and body fat testing, all colleges and many high schools are also measuring hydration through urine specific gravity, requiring a specific gravity of ≤1.020 before assessing a minimum weight. Changes to wrestling policies and procedures are a positive step forward in safeguarding the athletes' health and performance. The established guidelines provide an example to other sports on the importance of enforcing daily hydration for athletes.

Although severe dehydration is mainly a health concern, it should be noted that it can also significantly decrease strength/power performance. The impact on performance for very short duration activities (<30 seconds) is not as profound as for activities requiring more endurance; however, even in short bursts of effort, muscle function has been found to suffer.[73] As the duration of the event increases, the impact of dehydration becomes more evident. **Table 13.3** summarizes the known effects of dehydration on strength/power sports (adapted from Wilmore[74]).

Another unique aspect of weight classification sports is that there typically is a period of time between weighing in and the actual competition. Therefore, in between, food and fluids can be consumed in an attempt to replenish the body for high-intensity efforts and optimal performance. However, can a complete replenishment of the body actually be achieved after such a depletion? Unfortunately, very little research exists to fully explain the physiological responses and performance rebounds with rehydration. Table 13.3 summarizes the current research examining the physiological and performance effects of rapid rehydration after dehydration.

How are fluid needs during strength/power activities determined?

Maintaining euhydration during strength/power sports is similar to endurance and team sports: Athletes need to make accurate estimations of individual sweat rates, practice the consumption of the

gaining the performance edge

Strength/power athletes should make optimal hydration a top nutrition priority on a daily basis. Athletes should be educated on the harmful effects of rapid weight loss caused by dehydration and encouraged to manage weight on a long-term basis using healthy nutrition and exercise practices.

TABLE 13.3	Effects of Rapid and Moderate Rates of Dehydration and Rehydration on Physiological Function and Strength/Power Performance		
Variables		**Dehydration**	**Rehydration**
Cardiovascular			
Blood volume		↓	↓*
Cardiac output		↓	?
Stroke volume		↓	?
Heart rate		↑	?
Metabolic			
Anaerobic power (Wingate test)		↔, ↓	↔, ↓
Anaerobic capacity (Wingate test)		↔, ↓	↔, ↓
Buffer capacity of the blood		↓	?
Muscle/liver glycogen		↓	↓
Blood glucose during exercise		Possible ↓	?
Protein degradation during exercise		Possible ↑	?
Thermoregulation and Fluid Balance			
Electrolytes (muscle and blood)		↓	↔
Core temperature		↑	?
Sweat rate		↓	?
Skin blood flow		↓	?
Strength/Power Performance			
Muscular strength		↔, ↓	↔, ↓
Muscular power		?	↓†
Speed of movement		?	?
Wrestling simulation tests		↓	↔, ↓†

↓, decrease; ↑, increase; ↔, no known change or return to normal values; ?, unknown.

* From Burge et al.[75]

† Oopik et al.[76]

Source: Adapted from Wilmore JH. Weight category sports. In: Maughan RJ, ed. *Nutrition in Sport*. Malden, MA: Blackwell Science; 2000:637–645. Data acquired from reviews written by Fogelholm,[77] Horswill,[78] Keller et al.,[79] and Oppliger et al.[80]

estimated amounts while exercising, and overcome any logistical barriers to fluid availability.

How do you determine individual sweat rates?

Coaches, athletic trainers, and dietitians working to keep athletes well hydrated during training and com-petitions need to be aware of the differences in sweat loss among different sports and treat each athlete individually based on his or her own sweat and fluid replacement needs. Not only do sweat rates need to be determined individually, but athletes also need to discover the impact of various environments on their sweat rates. For example, Grant is a 200-meter sprinter. His training consists of a combination of strength training indoors in an air-conditioned facility and sprint workouts on an outdoor track. His workouts are typically at 4:00 p.m. and therefore the outdoor track can reach temperatures of 80–95 degrees with 70–90% humidity, while the weight room is maintained at 68–72 degrees and 50–60% humidity. Performing two different sweat trials in the two different environments revealed the following:

Weight Room Sweat Trial

1. *Determine body weight lost during exercise:* Grant reported that his body weight before his weight training session was 171 pounds, and 170 pounds afterward. Therefore, he lost 1 pound of water weight during his 1-hour weight-training session indoors (171 – 170 = 1 pound of water weight loss).

2. *Determine the fluid equivalent, in ounces, of the total weight lost during exercise:* Grant lost the equivalent of 16–24 ounces of fluid during his weight training session (1 × 16–24 oz = an additional 16–24 ounces should have been consumed to maintain fluid balance during this weight-training session).

3. *Determine the actual fluid needs of the athlete during a weight room workout:* Grant understands the benefits of euhydration for exercise performance, and therefore brings a bottle to all of his workouts. However, in the weight room he often forgets to drink, consuming only about 8 ounces of fluid in a 1-hour workout. Based on the amount of weight he lost in the weight-training workout, he should be consuming 24–32 ounces of fluid per hour in the weight room (8 oz of fluid consumed + 16–24 oz he should have consumed to establish fluid balance = 24–32 ounces of total fluid needs).

4. *Determine the number of fluid ounces needed per hour of exercise:* Because his sweat trial was performed for a 1-hour workout, Grant knows that he ideally needs to consume 24–32 ounces of fluid per hour to maintain hydration during weight-training workouts indoors in a climate-controlled environment.

Outdoor Track Sweat Trial

1. *Determine body weight lost during exercise:* Grant reported that his body weight before his track workout session was 170.5 pounds, and 168 pounds afterward. Therefore, he lost 2.5 pounds of water weight during his 1-hour outdoor track workout (170.5 – 168 = 2.5 pounds of water weight loss).

2. *Determine the fluid equivalent, in ounces, of the total weight lost during exercise:* Grant lost the equivalent of 40–60 ounces of fluid during his track workout (2.5 × 16–24 oz = an additional 40–60 ounces should have been consumed to maintain fluid balance during this outdoor track workout).

3. *Determine the actual fluid needs of the athlete during an outdoor workout:* Grant brought a bottle to his workout; however, he consumed only a couple of sips equaling about 4 oz. Based on the amount of weight he lost, he should be consuming 44–64 ounces of fluid per hour on the track (4 oz of fluid consumed + 40–60 oz he should have consumed to establish fluid balance = 44–64 ounces of total fluid needs).

4. *Determine the number of fluid ounces needed per hour of exercise:* Because his sweat trial was performed for a 1-hour workout, Grant knows that he ideally needs to consume 44–64 ounces of fluid per hour to maintain hydration during an outdoor track workout in hot, humid temperatures.

Reviewing the two sweat trials, there is a substantial difference between the two trials in different climates: 24–32 oz of fluid are needed in a cool, dry indoor environment, whereas 44–64 oz are required in a hot, humid outdoor setting. Grant should ensure that he is consuming the appropriate amount of fluid for each setting to prevent under- and over-hydration, and to optimize performance.

gaining the performance edge

Each athlete should perform several sweat trials in various indoor and outdoor environments. Sweat rates can vary dramatically, so to promote optimal hydration at all times, individual variations need to be discovered and documented, and appropriate hydration plans need to be implemented.

What should athletes drink and when should they drink it?

Similar to other sports, strength/power athletes should focus on water and sports beverages for fluid replacement during training sessions and competitive events. Water is appropriate for training sessions lasting less than 1 hour, whereas sports beverages are the preferred beverage for any activity lasting longer than 60–90 minutes.

Logistically, it is slightly more challenging for strength/power athletes to actually ingest adequate amounts of fluid during training, but certainly not impossible. Strength/power athletes should take hydration breaks at least every 10–15 minutes during training sessions. Sufficient amounts of water or sports drinks should be consumed at each break to meet individual sweat rate requirements over the course of an hour. Athletes need to take personal responsibility for maintaining hydration by bringing bottles filled with adequate amounts of water and sports beverages to every practice and drinking consistently.

How much fluid should strength/power athletes drink after training sessions and competitive events?

Strength/power athletes can lose modest to copious quantities of fluid while training and competing, which need to be replaced as quickly as possible after exercise. Refer to Chapter 8 for general postexercise hydration guidelines that are appropriate and applicable for strength/power athletes. Athletes should strive to consume optimal (i.e., as determined by sweat trials) amounts of fluids in a timely manner.

What meal-planning/event-planning logistics need to be considered during strength/power events?

The logistics for consuming fuel and fluids during strength/power sports is very manageable, compared to other sports, because of their intermittent nature. However, athletes still need to plan ahead to prepare snacks, water bottles, and recovery foods. The following sections include some ideas for snacks to eat in between efforts at competitive events as well as for quick snacks that provide optimal recovery after high-intensity workouts.

What are high-quality options for snacks between events at meets?

For some strength/power sports such as track and field or swimming meets, an athlete may have several events to compete in over the course of 1 day. These situations usually entail a hard, intense effort, and then a long recovery and wait period before the next event. Athletes need to make sure they are staying fueled and hydrated throughout the day. However, at a meet, their total energy expenditure is relatively small and therefore their nutrition intake in between events should be modest. The goal is to supply enough energy to keep blood glucose and overall energy levels up, while minimizing the risk of gastrointestinal fullness and discomfort. The following small snacks would be appropriate to supply fuel to athletes between events at a meet:

- Whole fruit and juices
- Granola or energy bars
- Half a lunchmeat sandwich (access to a cooler or refrigeration is critical)
- Yogurt and low-fat milk (access to a cooler or refrigeration is critical)
- Bagels or English muffins with jelly or a small amount of peanut butter
- Fig bars
- Sports beverages and water

Athletes should practice consuming snacks during training sessions to ensure that no gastrointestinal distress will occur on competition day. Nothing new should be consumed on the day of a competitive event!

What are high-quality options for snacks after competition?

Similar to training sessions, it is imperative that athletes feed their bodies properly after competitive events to initiate the recovery process. Ideally, athletes should consume a snack within 15–30 minutes of completing their final event at a competitive meet. Often, the athlete is far from home and therefore dependent on packed items or food/fluid that can be purchased on the road. Planning ahead by packing a snack is always the best option. The following are several suggestions of snacks that can be packed, without refrigeration, to be consumed immediately following a competition:

- Peanut butter and jelly sandwiches
- Whole fruit
- Juices and soy milk packaged in aseptic containers (drink boxes)
- Instant breakfast powders that can be mixed with water
- Energy bars containing a combination of carbohydrates and protein
- Homemade dried fruit, dry cereal, and nut mixes

If the athlete relies on fast food or convenience store options, the best choices include:

- Cartons of low-fat milk and yogurt
- 100% juices
- Deli sandwiches
- Grilled meat sandwiches and burgers (skip excessive sauces, mayonnaise, or dips)
- Granola and energy bars

Everyone's appetite is different after hard physical efforts. Athletes need to experiment with a variety of postcompetition snacks to determine what tastes the best, settles well, and can be conveniently packed in a gear bag.

It pays to plan. The nutritional value of food/fluid options on the road is typically not as high quality as snacks packed at home. The benefits of having nutritious, familiar foods and beverages on-hand at all times far outweighs the small amount of time needed to plan ahead.

gaining the performance edge

Strength/power athletes need to take time to plan ahead for day-long meets and competitive events. Nonperishable items should be packed for between events, focusing on carbohydrate sources and fluids. After the day's events are complete, athletes should consume a carbohydrate- and protein-rich snack to begin the recovery process.

Key Points of Chapter

- Strength athletes participate in sports that demand high levels of muscle force production. Power athletes participate in sports requiring the combination of great strength with speed of movement. Despite the difference, strength/power activities can be characterized as short, intense bouts of muscle activity.

- Short, intense bursts of muscle activity require an immediate supply of energy to the muscle. As a result, the primary system relied upon for energy during a strength/power activity is the phosphagen system. As the duration of the activity increases, the anaerobic system begins to contribute to a greater extent.

- The main dietary concern with individuals involved in strength/power sports is the consumption of adequate amounts of total daily calories. Adequate daily caloric intake not only ensures adequate energy for training, competition, and recovery, but also helps the athlete to conserve or build upon his or her current level of muscle mass. Low calorie intake can result in muscle tissue being metabolized to meet the body's energy demands. Loss of muscle tissue is detrimental to strength/power athletes.

- Because many strength/power sports rely on anaerobic metabolism, carbohydrates are the main fuel. However, because of the short duration of the effort, depletion of carbohydrate stores in the muscle is rarely the cause of fatigue in strength/power events. Therefore, carbohydrate-loading prior to competition is not necessary for strength/power sports.

- A daily intake of 5–10 grams of carbohydrates per kilogram of body weight has been shown to replenish and maintain glycogen stores in strength/power athletes. This corresponds to approximately 55–60% of the day's total calorie intake.

- Most research supports carbohydrate consumption 2–4 hours prior to and during strength/power sports; however, some athletes feel they perform better on an empty stomach. Because depletion of energy stores is rarely the cause of fatigue in these sports, the athlete and coach should experiment with various dietary plans and adopt one that is psychologically and physiologically compatible with the athlete.

- Ingestion of carbohydrates as soon as possible after training or sport performance is important to accelerate the replenishment of glycogen stores, provide for muscle tissue growth, and possibly attenuate immunosuppression resulting from intense training or competition.

- Protein intake is essential to accommodate the body's need for muscle repair and tissue building resulting from strength and power training. However, there is a ceiling effect, and excessive protein intake (i.e., >2 g/kg body weight) does not promote more muscle growth than the training in and of itself stimulated. Unused amino acids are converted to fat, not muscle.

- Consuming carbohydrates and protein prior to as well as after strength/power training appears to have a positive synergistic effect in regard to protein synthesis. Consuming at least 6 grams of amino acids with 35 grams of carbohydrates will not only aid in muscle protein synthesis, but will also speed replenishment of energy reserves.

- Fats are not a major energy source during strength/power events, and therefore special dietary consideration prior to, during, and immediately after training or competition is not required. However, fats are critical to a strength/power athlete's balanced diet and should be consumed in moderation (i.e., less than 35% of total daily calories), with the majority of fats being unsaturated.

- Vitamin and mineral supplementation in strength/power athletes has not been shown to speed recovery from training or enhance sport performance above that provided by a balanced diet. A multivitamin/mineral tablet can be taken for nutritional insurance, but the doses provided should not exceed 100–200% of the Daily Value.

- As with any athlete, fluid intake is essential not only for normal physiologic functioning of the body, but also for survival. Because of the differences in environmental conditions in which strength/power sports may occur, performing sweat trials will help assess an athlete's individual fluid needs.

- Rehydrating with water is appropriate for training sessions lasting less than an hour; sports beverages are preferred for activities lasting longer than an hour. A rule of thumb for rehydration is to drink 16–24 ounces of fluid for every pound of weight lost over the course of a training session or competition.

- The logistics for consuming food and fluids during strength/power sports is very manageable because of their intermittent nature. The goal is to supply enough energy to keep blood glucose and overall energy levels up, while minimizing the risk of gastrointestinal fullness and discomfort.

Study Questions

1. What is the difference between strength and power? Which group of competitive weight-lifting athletes relies more on power: power lifters or Olympic lifters? Discuss why.

2. What energy system provides the majority of energy during the performance of a 400-meter sprint? Which macronutrient would be most important to these athletes and why?

3. What energy system provides the majority of energy during the performance of a javelin throw? During recovery between throws, which energy system is most important?

4. How are the daily energy requirements of strength/power athletes different from endurance athletes? Discuss the specific nutritional needs of strength/power athletes and how this might affect their dietary plan.

5. For athletes wishing to gain weight, how many extra calories do they need to consume each week? What problems are associated with gaining weight too fast?

6. How much protein should be consumed and when is it best to ingest protein if maximizing protein synthesis is the goal?

7. How would you rank the three macronutrients in order of importance to the strength/power athlete? Defend your answer.

8. How would you determine the fluid requirements for a particular strength/power athlete? What are current recommendations about the quantity and type of fluid to be used while rehydrating?

9. What are the main nutritional goals for a strength/power athlete on the day of competition?

References

1. Benardot D, Schwarz M, Heller DW. Nutrient intake in young, highly competitive gymnasts. *J Am Dietet Assoc*. 1989;89(3):401–403.

2. Benardot D. Working with young athletes: views of a nutritionist on the sports medicine team. *Int J Sport Nutr*. 1996;6(2):110–120.

3. Kirchner EM, Lewis RD, O'Connor PJ. Bone mineral density and dietary intake of female college gymnasts. *Med Sci Sports Exerc*. 1995;27(4):543–549.

4. Moffatt RJ. Dietary status of elite female high school gymnasts: inadequacy of vitamin and mineral intake. *J Am Dietet Assoc*. 1984;84(1):1361–1363.

5. National Research Council. *Recommended Dietary Allowances*. Washington, DC: National Academy of Sciences; 1989.

6. Forbes GB. Body composition: influence of nutrition, disease, growth and aging. In: Shils ME, Olson JA, Shike M, eds. *Modern Nutrition in Health and Disease*. Philadelphia, PA: Lea and Febiger; 1994:781–801.

7. Kreider RB. Dietary supplements and the promotion of muscle growth with resistance exercise. *Sports Med*. 1999;27:97–110.

8. Tesch PA, Colliander EB, Kaiser P. Muscle metabolism during intense, heavy-resistance exercise. *Eur J Appl Physiol*. 1986;4:362–366.

9. Pascoe DD, Costill DL, Fink WJ, Robergs RA, Zachwieja JJ. Glycogen resynthesis in skeletal muscle following resistance exercise. *Med Sci Sports Exerc*. 1993;25:349–353.

10. Robergs RA, Pearson DR, Costill DL, et al. Muscle glycogenolysis during differing intensities of weight-resistance exercise. *J Appl Physiol*. 1991;70:1700–1706.

11. Balsom PD, Gaitanis GC, Soderlund K, Ekblom B. High-intensity exercise and muscle glycogen availability in humans. *Acta Physiologica Scandinavica*. 1999;165:337–345.

12. Casey A, Short AH, Curtis S, Greenhaff PL. The effect of glycogen availability on power output and the metabolic response to repeated bouts of maximal, isokinetic exercise in man. *Eur J Appl Physiol*. 1996;72:249–255.

13. Maughan RJ, Greenhaff PL, Leiper JB, Ball D, Lambert CP, Gleeson M. Diet composition and the performance of high-intensity exercise. *J Sports Sci*. 1997;15:265–275.

14. Rockwell MS, Rankin JW, Dixon H. Effects of muscle glycogen on performance of repeated sprints and mechanisms of fatigue. *Int J Sports Nutr Exerc Metabol*. 2003;13:1–14.

15. Hirvonen J, Nummela A, Rusko H, Rehunen S, Harkonen M. Fatigue and changes of ATP, creatine phosphate, and lactate during the 400-m sprint. *Can J Sports Sci*. 1992;17(2):141–144.

16. Biolo G, Williams BD, Fleming RY, Wolfe RR. Insulin action on muscle protein kinetics and amino acid transport during recovery after resistance exercise. *Diabetes*. 1999;48:949–957.

17. Tipton KD, Rasmussen BB, Miller SL, et al. Timing of amino acid-carbohydrate ingestion alters anabolic response of muscle to resistance exercise. *Am J Physiol*. 2001;282:E197–E206.

18. Rogozkin VA. Weightlifting and power events. In: Maughan RJ, ed. *Nutrition in Sport*. Malden, MA: Blackwell Science; 2000:621–631.

19. Institute of Medicine. *Dietary Reference Intakes for Energy, Carbohydrate, Fiber, Fat, Fatty Acids, Cholesterol, Protein and Amino Acids (Macronutrients)*. Food and Nutrition Board. Washington, DC: National Academies Press; 2002.

20. Cheetham ME, Boobis LH, Brooks S, Williams C. Human muscle metabolism during sprint running. *J Appl Physiol*. 1986;61:54–60.

21. Spriet LL, Lindinger ML, McKelvie RS, Heigenhauser GJ, Jones NL. Muscle glycogenolysis and H+ concentration during maximal intermittent cycling. *J Appl Physiol*. 1989;66:8–13.

22. Haff GG, Koch AJ, Potteiger JA, et al. Carbohydrate supplementation attenuates muscle glycogen loss during acute bouts of resistance exercise. *Int J Sports Nutr Exerc Metabol*. 2000;10(3):326–339.

23. Lambert CP, Flynn MG, Boone JB, et al. Effects of carbohydrate feeding on multiple-bout resistance exercise. *J Appl Sports Sci Res*. 1991;5:192–197.

24. Conley MS, Stone MH. Carbohydrate ingestion/supplementation or resistance exercise and training. *Sports Med*. 1996;21(1):7–17.

25. Vincent KR, Clarkson PM, Freedson PS. Effect of a pre-exercise liquid, high carbohydrate feeding on resistance exercise performance (abstract). *Med Sci Sports Exerc*. 1993;25:S194.

26. Rennie MJ, Tipton KD. Protein and amino acid metabolism during and after exercise and the effects of nutrition. *Ann Rev Nutr*. 2000;20:457–483.

27. Koch AJ, Potteiger JA, Chan MA, Benedict SF, Frey BB. Minimal influence of carbohydrate ingestion on the immune response following acute resistance exercise. *Int J Sports Nutr Exerc Metabol*. 2001;11:149–161.

28. Kraemer WJ, Clemson A, Triplett NT, Bush JA, Newton RU, Lynch JM. The effects of plasma cortisol elevation on total and differential leukocyte counts in response to heavy-resistance exercise. *Eur J Appl Physiol*. 1996;73:93–97.

29. Nieman DC, Henson DA, Sampson CS, et al. The acute immune response to exhaustive resistance exercise. *Int J Sports Med*. 1995;16:322–328.

30. Potteiger JA, Chan MA, Haff GG, et al. Training status influences T-cell responses following acute resistance exercise in females. *J Strength Cond Res*. 2001;15:185–191.

31. Chan MA, Koch AJ, Benedict SH, Potteiger JA. Influence of carbohydrate ingestion on cytokine responses following acute resistance exercise. *Int J Sports Nutr Exerc Metabol*. 2003;13:454–465.

32. Nehlsen-Cannarella SL, Fagoaga O, Nieman DC, et al. Carbohydrate and the cytokine response to 2.5 h of running. *J Appl Physiol*. 1997;82:1662–1667.

33. Nieman DC, Fagoaga O, Butterworth DE, et al. Carbohydrate affects granulocyte and monocyte trafficking but not function after 2.5 h of running. *Am J Clin Nutr*. 1997;66:153–159.

34. Nieman DC, Nehlsen-Cannarella SL, Fagoaga O, et al. Effects of mode and carbohydrate on the granulocyte and monocyte response to intensive, prolonged exercise. *J Appl Physiol*. 1998;84:1252–1259.

35. Butterfield GE, Calloway DH. Physical activity improves protein utilization in young men. *Br J Nutr*. 1984;51:171–184.

36. Lemon PW. Effect of exercise on protein requirements. *J Sports Sci*. 1991;9:53–70.

37. Rogozkin VA. Principles of athletes' nutrition in the Russian federation. *World Rev Nutr Diet*. 1993;71:154–182.

38. Maughan RJ. The athlete's diet: nutritional goals and dietary strategies. *Proc Nutr Soc*. 2002;61:87–96.

39. Tipton KD, Wolfe RR. Exercise, protein metabolism and muscle growth. *Int J Sports Nutr Exerc Metabol*. 2001;11:109–132.

40. Rasmussen BB, Wolfe RR, Volpi E. Oral and intravenously administered amino acids produce similar effects on muscle protein synthesis in the elderly. *J Nutr Health Aging*. 2002;6:358–362.

41. Rasmussen BB, Phillips SM. Contractile and nutritional regulation of human muscle growth. *Exerc Sport Sci Rev*. 2003;31(3):127–131.

42. Lacey JM, Wilmore DW. Is glutamine a conditionally essential amino acid? *Nutr Rev*. 1990;48:297–309.

43. Rowbottom DG, Keast D, Morton AR. The emerging role of glutamine as an indicator of exercise stress and overtraining. *Sports Med*. 1996;21:80–97.

44. Curthoys NP, Watford M. Regulation of glutaminase activity and glutamine metabolism. *Ann Rev Nutr*. 1995;15:133–159.

45. Rennie MJ, Tadros L, Khogali S, Ahmed A, Taylor PM. Glutamine transport and its metabolic effects. *J Nutr*. 1994;124(8 suppl):1530S–1538S.

46. Rennie MJ. Glutamine metabolism and transport in skeletal muscle and heart and their clinical relevance. *J Nutr*. 1996;126(4 suppl):1142S–1149S.

47. Kimball SR, Jefferson LS. Control of protein synthesis by amino acid availability. *Curr Opinion Clin Nutr Metabol Care*. 2002;5:63–67.

48. Suminski RR, Robertson RJ, Goss FL, et al. Acute effect of amino acid ingestion and resistance exercise on plasma growth hormone concentration in young men. *Int J Sports Nutr*. 1997;7:48–60.

49. Cade JR, Reese RH, Privette RM, Hommen NM, Rogers JL, Fregly MJ. Dietary intervention and training in swimmers. *Eur J Appl Physiol Occup Physiol*. 1992;63:210–215.

50. Carli G, Bonifazi M, Lodi L, Lupo C, Martelli G, Viti A. Changes in exercise-induced hormone response to branched chain amino acid administration. *Eur J Appl Physiol Occup Physiol*. 1992;64:272–277.

51. Poortmans J. Use and usefulness of amino acids and related substances during physical exercise. In: Packer L, Benzi G, Siliprandi N, eds. *Biochemical Aspects of Physical Exercise*. Amsterdam: Elsevier; 1986:285–294.

52. Wagenmakers AJM. Muscle amino acid metabolism at rest and during exercise: role in human physiology and metabolism. In: Holloszy JO, ed. *Exercise and Sport Science Reviews*. Baltimore, MD: Williams & Wilkins; 1998:287–314.

53. Tipton KD, Ferrando AA, Phillips SM, Doyle D, Wolfe RR. Post-exercise net protein synthesis in human muscle from orally administered amino acids. *Am J Physiol*. 1999;276:E628–E634.

54. Chandler RM, Byrne HK, Patterson JG, Ivy JL. Dietary supplements affect the anabolic hormones after weight-training exercise. *J Appl Physiol*. 1994;76:839–845.

55. Rasmussen BB, Tipton KD, Miller SL, Wolf SE, Wolfe RR. An oral essential amino acid-carbohydrate supplement enhances muscle protein anabolism after resistance exercise. *J Appl Physiol*. 2000;88:386–392.

56. Nielsen F, Hunt C, Mullen L, Hunt J. Effect of dietary boron on mineral, estrogen, testosterone metabolism in postmenopausal women. *FASEB*. 1987;1:394.

57. Ferrando AA, Green NR. The effect of boron supplementation on lean body mass, plasma testosterone levels and strength in male body builders. *Int J Sports Nutr*. 1993;3:140.

58. Institute of Medicine. *Dietary Reference Intakes for Vitamin A, Vitamin K, Arsenic, Boron, Chromium, Copper, Iodine, Iron, Manganese, Molybdenum, Nickel, Silicon, Vanadium, and Zinc*. Food and Nutrition Board. Washington, DC: National Academies Press; 2000.

59. Zemel MB. Role of calcium and dairy products in energy partitioning and weight management. *Am J Clin Nutr*. 2004;79(suppl):907S–912S.

60. Zemel MB, Thompson W, Milstead A, Morris K, Campbell P. Calcium and dairy acceleration of weight and fat loss during energy restriction in obese adults. *Obes Res*. 2004;12(4):582–590.

61. Evans GW. The effect of chromium picolinate on insulin controlled parameters in humans. *Int J Biosoc Med Res*. 1989;11:163–180.

62. Hasten KL, Rome EP, Franks BD, Hegsted M. Effects of chromium picolinate on beginning weight training students. *Int J Sports Nutr*. 1992;2:343–350.

63. Campbell WW, Joseph LJO, Anderson RA, Davey SL, Hilton J, Evans WJ. Effects of resistive training and chromium picolinate on body composition and skeletal muscle size in older women. *Int J Sports Nutr Exerc Metabol*. 2002;12(2):125–135.

64. Clancy SP, Clarkson PM, DeCheke ME, et al. Effects of chromium picolinate supplementation on body composition, strength and urinary chromium loss in football players. *Int J Sports Med*. 1994;4:142–153.

65. Hallmark MA, Reynolds TH, DeSouza CA, Dotson RA, Anderson RA, Rogers MA. Effects of chromium and resistive training on muscle strength and body composition. *Med Sci Sports Exerc*. 1996;28:139–144.

66. Trent LK, Thieding-Cancel D. Effects of chromium picolinate on body composition. *J Sports Med Phys Fitness*. 1995;35:273–280.

67. Brigham DE, Beard JL, Krimmel RS, Kenney WL. Changes in iron status during competitive season in female collegiate swimmers. *Nutr*. 1993;9:418–422.

68. Singh A, Moses E, Deuster P. Chronic multivitaminmineral supplementation does not enhance physical performance. *Med Sci Sports Exerc*. 1992;24:726–732.

69. Telford R, Catchpole E, Deakin V, Hahn A, Plank A. The effect of 7–8 months of vitamin/mineral supplementation on athletic performance. *Int J Sports Nutr*. 1992;2:135–153.

70. Steen SN, Brownell KD. Patterns of weight loss and regain in wrestlers: has the tradition changed? *Med Sci Sports Exerc*. 1990;22:762–768.

71. National Collegiate Athletic Association. NCAA Wrestling Rules and Interpretations. Indianapolis, IN: National Collegiate Athletic Association; 2003:WR23–WR34.

72. National Federation of State High School Associations. Wrestling Weight Management Program. Indianapolis, IN: National Federation of State High School Associations; 2001:25–34.

73. Sawka MN, Pandolf KB. Effects of body water loss on physiological function and exercise performance. In: Lamb DR, Gisolfi CV, eds. *Perspectives in Exercise Science and Sports Medicine*. Carmel, IN: Benchmark Press; 1990:1–38.

74. Wilmore JH. Weight category sports. In: Maughan RJ, ed. *Nutrition in Sport*. Malden, MA: Blackwell Science; 2000:637–645.

75. Burge CM, Carey MF, Pyne WR. Rowing performance, fluid balance, and metabolic function following dehydration and rehydration. *Med Sci Sports Exerc*. 1993;25:1358–1364.

76. Oopik V, Paasuke M, Sikku T, et al. Effect of rapid weight loss on metabolism and isokinetic performance capacity: a case study of two well trained wrestlers. *J Sports Med Phys Fitness*. 1996;36:127–131.

77. Fogelholm M. Effects of bodyweight reduction on sports performance. *Sports Med*. 1994;18:249–267.

78. Horswill CA. Physiology and nutrition for wrestling. In: Knuttgen HG, Lamb DR, Murray R, eds. *Physiology and Nutrition for Competitive Sport*. Carmel, IN: Cooper; 1994:131–174.

79. Keller HL, Tolly SE, Freedson PS. Weight loss in adolescent wrestlers. *Pediatr Exerc Sc*. 1994;6:211–224.

80. Oppliger RA, Case HS, Horswill CA, Landry GL, Shelter AC. Weight loss in wrestlers: an American College of Sports Medicine position stand. *Med Sci Sports Exerc*. 1996;28:ix–xii.

Additional Resources

Chesley A, MacDougall JD, Tarnopolsky MA, Atkinson SA, Smith K. Changes in human muscle protein synthesis after resistance exercise. *J Appl Physiol*. 1992;73:1383–1388.

Kleiner SM. *Power Eating*. Champaign, IL: Human Kinetics; 1998.

Phillips SM, Tipton KD, Ferrando AA, Wolfe RR. Resistance training reduces the acute exercise-induced increase in muscle protein turnover. *Am J Physiol*. 1999;276:E118–E124.

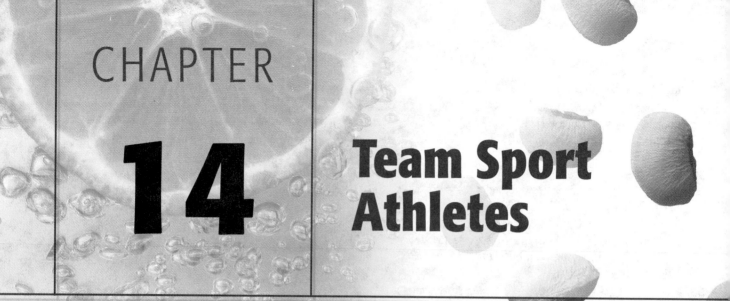

CHAPTER

14

Team Sport Athletes

Key Questions Addressed

- What is different about athletes in team sports?

- What energy systems are utilized during team sports?

- How are energy needs different for team sport athletes?

- Are carbohydrate needs different for team sport athletes?

- Are protein needs different for team sport athletes?

- Are fat needs different for team sport athletes?

- Are vitamin and mineral needs different for team sport athletes?

- What are the fluid recommendations for team sport athletes?

- What are the meal-planning/event-planning logistics that need to be considered during team sport events?

Tomas is a junior in college and is a starting wing on his nationally ranked ice hockey team. He is a hard worker in practice and is highly competitive on the ice. Lately, he has been surprised that he feels fatigued during practices and has even had to come out of the most recent game because he was so out of breath. This concerned both him and his coaches. He describes being very busy in school with studying, exams, and papers. He has plans to go to medical school after graduation and knows he needs excellent grades to get accepted. The team dietitian met with him to determine whether he was meeting the nutrient, fluid, and energy requirements for his busy, active lifestyle.

Questions

- What specific questions should you ask Tomas about his nutrient intake?
- How do you determine his calorie needs?
- How do you determine whether he is meeting his calorie and macronutrient needs?

What is different about athletes in team sports?

For the purposes of this chapter, **team sports** are sports in which two or more athletes work together on a common playing area to defeat an opposing group of competitors. Some commonly identified team sports are football, baseball, ice hockey, soccer, volleyball, and basketball. However, information from this chapter also applies to other less recognized team sports such as rugby, lacrosse, and field hockey. Sports in which individual athletes perform by themselves in an event, and their score is added to that of others to derive a team score, are not considered team sports. Examples of these individual sports are gymnastics, swimming, diving, track and field, tennis, and wrestling. The nutritional practices for these individual athletes participating on a team are discussed in Chapters 12 and 13.

team sports Sports in which two or more athletes work together on a common playing area to defeat an opposing group of competitors. Examples of team sports are football, baseball, hockey, soccer, and basketball.

Team sports have classically been labeled as anaerobic sports because success is often dependent on physical skills that require quick bursts of intense, powerful muscle activity. As discussed in Chapter 2, quick bursts of intense muscle activity are fueled primarily by the adenosine triphosphate/creatine phosphate (phosphagen) and anaerobic energy systems. However, classifying team sport athletes as anaerobic athletes can be very misleading. Sprinting, jumping, throwing, and tackling are indeed anaerobic activities, but it must be remembered that during the less intense moments between anaerobic bursts, the athlete's body is trying to recover. Recovery is an aerobic-energy-requiring process. During recovery the body is attempting to replace the high-energy phosphates (i.e., ATP and CP) used and remove any lactic acid formed during the anaerobic burst of activity. By improving aerobic fitness, an athlete is able to recover more fully between bursts of activity. During a game or practice when the intermittent bursts of activities occur over a 2- or 3-hour time period, the athletes who are not able to recover their ATP and CP levels adequately during the periods of lesser activity begin to run out of energy. Failure to recognize the importance of the aerobic energy system even in team sports traditionally labeled as anaerobic can lead to early-onset fatigue and performance disaster.

What energy systems are utilized during team sports?

Participation in team sports relies upon all three of the body's energy systems; however, the ATP/CP and aerobic systems are the major energy contributors. As depicted by the darker blue area on the left side of region 1 in Figure 14.1, the very high-intensity bursts of muscle activity required to jump, kick, sprint, shoot, and so on are supplied predominantly by the ATP/CP system. The aerobic system comes into play during the lower-intensity activities that occur between the bursts of effort. These between-burst activities are performed at slower, less metabolically demanding (i.e., lower intensity) movement speeds and are depicted by the shaded region 4 in Figure 14.1. The aerobic system not only is supplying most of the energy for the lower-intensity activity itself, but also is helping the athlete to recover. In other words, the aerobic system is working to replenish any ATP and CP that was used in earlier flurries of activity. Failure to completely recharge the muscles' high-energy phosphates (i.e., ATP and CP) between bouts can eventually lead to fatigue

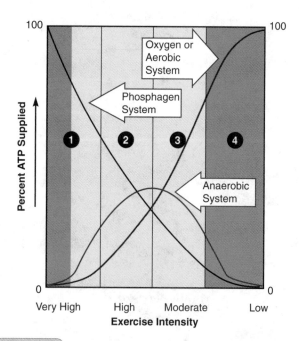

Figure 14.1 Team sport energetics. Participation in team sports relies on all three of the body's energy systems; however, the phosphagen and aerobic systems are the major energy contributors.
Source: Bower RW, Fox EL. *Sport Physiology*. 3rd ed. Dubuque, IA: William C. Brown; 1992. Reprinted with permission of the McGraw-Hill Companies.

and thus decreased sport performance. A realization of the importance of the aerobic system for optimal performance in team sports demonstrates why athletes involved in what have traditionally been considered anaerobic sports need to include endurance training in their conditioning program. Endurance training stresses the aerobic energy system, which adapts and becomes better at producing ATP. This, in turn, enables the team sport athlete to recover more quickly and thus preserves muscle ATP and CP levels over the 2 or more hours it takes to complete many team sport competitions.

How are energy needs different for team sport athletes?

The most significant difference in energy requirements for the category of team sport athletes, versus endurance or strength/power sport athletes, is the huge variation in calorie needs. For an individual athlete, calorie needs can fluctuate greatly on a daily basis because of variations in training and competition schedules. Among team sport athletes, disparities in calorie requirements are caused by several factors such as the nature of the sport, the position played by the athlete, and an individual's body weight. These variations must be considered when calculating energy needs and developing a meal plan for an individual athlete.

Calorie needs can vary greatly among team members within one sport because of variations in their roles, as dictated by their position. For example, soccer players generally expend 3800–3900 calories per day.[1,2] However, actual caloric requirements depend on a player's position on the team. Soccer midfielders and halfbacks run most of the game, chasing the ball and playing both defense and offense. A typical soccer midfielder can run as much as 10 K (6.2 miles) in one game, with a large percentage of the running performed at high intensities.[3] On the other hand, soccer goalies and defensive players play less than half of the field and run less than the forward players, thus using considerably less energy. When calculating energy needs for team sport athletes, the nature of the sport as well as the athlete's position on the team should be considered before making final recommendations.

Some athletes are very heavy, such as football linemen, whereas others weigh significantly less, such as soccer and field hockey players. Larger athletes who require greater mass to perform their sport well may want to increase lean body mass. Football players are getting larger every season. A comparison of NCAA Division I football players from 1987 and 2000 found significant increases in body mass for quarterbacks, running backs, tight ends, offensive linemen, and defensive linemen.[4] The offensive linemen showed the largest increase in body mass (8.8%) when compared to the 1987 study. Larger size means greater calorie needs and higher energy expenditure. It is not unusual for a 300-pound linebacker to have energy needs for weight maintenance of more than 5000 calories per day. In comparison, a 190-pound wide receiver may require only 3500 calories per day for weight maintenance.

Matching energy intake with expenditure can be challenging for competitive athletes. Hassapidou and Manstrantoni studied four groups of female athletes—volleyball players, swimmers, middle distance runners, and ballet dancers—in Greece during one off-season and one competitive season.[5] Researchers found that mean energy intake was lower than mean energy expenditure in all four groups of athletes. Mean energy intake ranged from 1500–2350 calories per day, and mean energy expenditure ranged from 2150–2350 for the athletes in this study. Other studies have shown similar energy intakes and expenditures, with the average intake of female athletes in the range of 1600–2400 calories per day.[6-8] However, in the Hassapidou study, the volleyball players increased energy intake during the competitive season and attained energy balance. The other three teams in the study did not increase intake during the competitive season and were in negative energy balance in both the off- and in-season parts of the study. It is possible that the volleyball team members paid more attention to calorie intake during the competitive season or that their energy expenditure was reduced because they had more competition days and less intense practice. Underreporting of energy intake and energy expenditure could have been inaccurately estimated in all athletes in the study. Although it may be challenging for team athletes to meet energy needs, athletes can achieve energy balance with careful nutrition planning.

How are daily energy needs calculated for team sport athletes?

When calculating energy needs, several things must be considered. An accurate weight should first be obtained because the primary calculation is based on body weight. A good estimate of activity level should be determined based on the sport, amount of daily training, days off, and intensity of training. Age of the athlete is also a determining factor when calculating energy expenditure. The athlete's weight goal and recommended weight must be considered as well. If the athlete's goal is to maintain weight, the calculations do not need to be modified. If the athlete needs or desires weight change, then daily needs should be adjusted.

The calculation equations used to determine energy needs for team sport athletes are the same as for endurance and strength/power athletes. To review the equations, refer to **Table 14.1**.

José's Case Study José is a 22-year-old Triple-A minor league baseball catcher whose long-term goal is to play in the major leagues. During the off-season, he diligently followed an intense training and conditioning program. As a result of his hard efforts, José successfully gained muscle mass, decreased his fat mass, and achieved a body weight of 220 pounds. His current goal is to maintain this weight and body composition throughout the competitive season. Using the equation listed in Table 14.1, José's energy needs are calculated as follows:

1. Calculation for a 22-year-old male: REE = (15.3 × BW in kg) + 679
2. Convert pounds of body weight to kilograms = 220 ÷ 2.2 = 100 kg
3. José's REE = (15.3 × 100) + 679 = 1530 + 679 = 2209 calories
4. Multiply the REE by the activity factor of 1.6–2.4 = 2209 × (1.6–2.4) = 3534–5302 calories per day

The calorie range in the preceding example is quite wide—a difference of 1770 calories. However, as mentioned earlier, it is important to give team sport athletes a large target calorie range to allow for flexibility in daily energy needs. For example, because José is a catcher, he is involved in nearly all defensive plays on the field. The constant crouching, throwing, running between home and first base, and chasing foul balls demand significant energy. Catchers also wear protective gear that adds weight and bulk, causing less efficient movement and thus increasing calorie expenditure. Therefore, José could potentially burn as much as 13 calories per minute during a game.[9] On days when José catches a full game or on hard training days, his energy needs will be on the upper end of his calculated calorie range. On game days when he does not catch or on rest days from training, the lower end of the calorie range would be appropriate. José should be instructed on how to modify his daily intake to match the variances in his training and competition schedule to his daily energy needs, thus allowing him to maintain his current weight.

TABLE 14.1	Resting Energy Expenditure (REE) Equations and Activity Factors	
Gender and Age	Equation (BW in kilograms)	Activity Factor
Males, 10–18 years	REE = (17.5 × BW) + 651	1.6–2.4
Males, 18–30 years	REE = (15.3 × BW) + 679	1.6–2.4
Males, 30–60 years	REE = (11.6 × BW) + 879	1.6–2.4
Females, 10–18 years	REE = (12.2 × BW) + 749	1.6–2.4
Females, 18–30 years	REE = (14.7 × BW) + 496	1.6–2.4
Females, 30–60 years	REE = (8.7 × BW) + 829	1.6–2.4

Source: World Health Organization, Energy and Protein Requirements. Report of a Joint FAO/WHO/UNU Expert Consultation. Technical Report Series 724. Geneva, Switzerland: World Health Organization; 1985:206.

For all team sport athletes, it is important to balance energy needs with recommendations for appropriate macronutrient intake. Many team sport athletes, especially those whose performance may be enhanced by a larger body size, consume excessive amounts of protein. This often is a detriment to their glycogen stores, which need to be replenished daily for optimal sport performance. Team sports require a blending of carbohydrates, protein, and fat because the energy systems utilized during activity are typically a combination of anaerobic and aerobic in nature. **Training Table 14.1** presents examples of sample meal plans for three different calorie levels common for team sport athletes—2500, 4000, and 6000 calories. The lower-calorie meal plan may be appropriate for small, female team sport athletes whereas the higher-calorie meal plan is generally well-suited for larger, heavier male athletes.

Training Table 14.1: Sample Meal Plans for Various Calorie Levels

2500	4000	6000
Breakfast	**Breakfast**	**Breakfast**
Oatmeal, 1 cup	Egg sandwich:	Granola cereal, 1½ cups
Melon chunks, 1 cup	Poached egg, 1	Low-fat milk, 1 cup
Low-fat milk, 1 cup	English muffin, 1 whole	Banana, 1 large
Brown sugar, 1 tbsp	Cheddar cheese, 1 slice	Pineapple juice, 1 cup
Orange juice, 1 cup	Ham, 1 slice	Fruit yogurt, 1 cup
	Blueberry muffin, 1 small	
	Apple juice, 1 cup	
	Low-fat milk, 1 cup	
Lunch	**Lunch**	**Lunch**
Chicken Caesar salad:	Thick crust vegetarian pizza, ½ large	Sandwiches, 2:
Chopped chicken, 4 oz	Orange, 1	Thick whole grain bread, 4 slices
Romaine, leaf lettuce, 2 cups	Cranberry juice, 8 oz	Lite mayo, 2 tbsp
Egg, 1 chopped	Low-fat milk, 1 cup	Turkey, ham, or roast beef, 8 oz
Parmesan cheese, 2 tbsp		American cheese, 2 slices
Tomato, cucumber slices, ½ cup combined		Low-fat milk, 1 cup
Caesar dressing, 1 tbsp		Grape juice, 2 cups
Grapes, large bunch		Fig bars, 4 large
Minestrone soup, 1 cup		
Water		
Dinner	**Dinner**	**Dinner**
Tofu stir-fry with vegetables, 2 cups	Grilled chicken breast, 1 (4–6 oz)	Turkey, 6 oz
Steamed rice, 1½ cups	Baked potato, 1 large, with skin	Mashed potatoes, 2 cups
Sherbet, ½ cup	Green beans, 1 cup	Corn/pea mix, 2 cups
Almond cookie, 1	Carrot/raisin salad, 1 cup	Chocolate pudding with topping, 2 cups
Low-fat milk, 1 cup	Margarine, 1 tsp	Rolls, 2
	Light sour cream, 1 tbsp	Honey, 2 tbsp
	Brownie, 1 small	Margarine, 2 tsp
Snack	**Snack**	**Snack**
Juice, 8 oz	Whole grain crackers, 8–10	Apple juice, 16 oz
Graham crackers, 2 full sheets	Mozzarella cheese sticks, 2	Peanuts, ½ cup
Banana, 1	Sports drink, 16 oz	Raisins, ½ cup
Yogurt, 1 cup	Low-fat milkshake, 12 oz	Soft pretzel, 1 large
	Vanilla wafers, 10–12	Lemonade, 16 oz

How can energy needs during an event be calculated?

Calorie needs during a team sport event are based on the type of event, the length of the event, and the amount of playing time during the event. Single games lasting 1 hour or less, or events lasting 1–2 hours requiring intermittent efforts, generally do not require calories to be consumed while exercising. In these cases, a focus on proper hydration during activity will be all that is needed to keep the athlete in top form. Energy needs for shorter events can usually be met before and after games.

Other events lasting 2–4 hours will require extra calories to be consumed during play to keep performance at its peak. Consuming fluids that contain carbohydrates will provide a small amount of calories, usually sufficient to delay fatigue during games. For example, a starting basketball player might play 35 of the 40 official minutes of a basketball game that might take 2 hours to play. Consuming a sports drink at a rate of 8 ounces every 15 minutes during the game would provide approximately 360 calories in the 2 hours of the game. Although not a large amount of calories, this level of calories, especially from a carbohydrate source, provides readily available energy and decreases the chances of depleting glycogen stores during the game.

Many team sport events have games played throughout a day or weekend, requiring careful nutrition planning for before, during, in between, and after games to ensure adequate fuel. Refer to the team sport event logistics section later in this chapter for examples of how to meet calorie needs during tournament play.

Are carbohydrate needs different for team sport athletes?

As discussed earlier in this chapter, team sport athletes use all three energy systems during activity. The intense bursts of activity usually involved in team sport play depend largely on the anaerobic system for energy, with the aerobic energy system contributing during moderate efforts. Carbohydrates are the main source of fuel for the aerobic system and the only macronutrient that can be metabolized for energy anaerobically. Thus, in the absence of carbohydrates, sport performance deterioration is ensured.

The benefits of carbohydrate ingestion during shorter-duration, high-intensity exercise are beginning to emerge in the literature. Muscle glycogen is the primary substrate used during maximal exercise performed for 30–60 seconds, and repeated bouts of such exercise can substantially reduce glycogen stores in short periods.[10] Davis et al. studied eight trained subjects to determine the effects on fatigue of carbohydrate ingestion using high-carbohydrate drinks during intermittent high-intensity shuttle running.[10] They found that the average run time to fatigue was significantly longer in trials supplemented with carbohydrates when compared to a placebo sports drink. They found a 32% increase

in run time to fatigue during the performance bout. Their research findings are supported by many other studies.[11,12]

Ice hockey provides another example of the importance of adequate daily carbohydrate intake and glycogen storage. For hockey players, maintaining adequate glycogen stores to perform optimally throughout a grueling 8-month season is imperative. A study of Swedish ice hockey players revealed that those who consistently consumed a high-carbohydrate diet versus a mixed diet during a two-game series had higher muscle glycogen concentrations.[13] This increase in glycogen can translate into faster speeds on the ice, a higher number of shifts skated, and better recovery between shifts.

Team sport athletes may not consume the recommended amount of carbohydrates consistently. Those who consume a chronically deficient amount of carbohydrates may experience chronic depletion in muscle glycogen stores. This is especially true with repeated competitions seen in tournament or match play and competitions lasting several days. Because of the profound effect of carbohydrates on performance, one of the main goals of the sports nutrition professional is to ensure that the carbohydrate needs of team sport athletes are met daily, as well as before, during, and after training and competitions.

How are daily carbohydrate needs calculated for team sport athletes?

Team sport athletes vary greatly in their individual training regimens, which influence their daily requirements for carbohydrate intake. Some team members have fairly moderate weekly protocols, whereas other athletes are completing long, intense workouts on a regular basis. Burke et al.[14] reviewed the carbohydrate needs for athletes engaging in training programs that range from moderate to extreme in duration and intensity:

- Moderate duration/low intensity training = 5–7 g/kg body weight/day
- Moderate to heavy endurance training = 7–12 g/kg body weight/day
- Extreme exercise programming (4–6+ hours/day) = 10–12 g/kg body weight/day

For team sports, appropriate carbohydrate recommendations span a majority of the preceding ranges. A general recommendation for carbohydrate intake for team sport athletes is 5–10 g/kg body weight daily. Carbohydrate needs should be calculated on an individual athlete basis, not as a team. Athletes on teams may have very different carbohydrate needs based on position played, amount of training, body weight, need to change body weight, and total calories consumed daily.[15]

Similar to endurance and strength/power athletes, once a carbohydrate gram range is calculated, the recommendation should always be compared to total calorie estimations. Carbohydrates should comprise approximately 55–65% of total calories. It should be noted that for some athletes, carbohydrate recommendations will fall outside of the stated ranges for grams/kilogram of body weight or percentage of total calories. For example, athletes' consumption of carbohydrates based solely on 55–65% of total calories has been shown to fall short of recommendations if total calorie intake is low.[5,6] In these cases, a double-check of carbohydrate needs by calculating a grams/kilogram of body weight recommendation will reveal a shortage in total calories and carbohydrates. Conversely, some football studies have reported that players consume less than half of their calorie intake as carbohydrates, which at face value would indicate a carbohydrate deficiency.[16,17] However, when carbohydrate intake is calculated in grams per kilogram of body weight, it may be discovered that the absolute value of carbohydrate intake is well within the recommended intake range. Bottom line—use both grams per kilogram of body weight and a comparison of carbohydrates to total calorie intake to confirm dietary recommendations. The following examples demonstrate how to calculate carbohydrate needs based on the position played by an athlete on a team.

Cassie and Allison's Case Study Cassie plays goalie and Allison is a midfielder on a semiprofessional soccer team. They are in the beginning of the competitive spring/summer season. Tournaments are played every weekend, with practices nearly every day of the week. Cassie is very tall and muscular. She has played the goalie position all of her life and wants to maintain her weight and muscle mass. Allison is small, trim, and muscular, and wants to maintain her current weight so that she can preserve her exceptional speed and endurance on the field.

The calculation of carbohydrate needs for both players should include calculations based on grams per kilogram as well as percentage of calories. The calculation chart in Table 14.1 is used to determine energy needs.

Calculations of carbohydrate needs for Cassie—163 lbs, 24-year-old female:

1. Calculate carbohydrate needs based on grams per kilogram of body weight.
2. Convert pounds of body weight to kilograms = 163 lbs ÷ 2.2 = 74 kg
3. 74 kg × (6–8 g carbohydrates/kg) = 444–592 g carbohydrates
4. Calculate REE using formula in Table 14.1: REE = (14.7 × 74 kg) + 496 = 1088 + 496 = 1584 calories
5. Multiply REE by activity factors (1.6–2.4) = 1584 × (1.6–2.4) = 2534–3802 calories daily
6. Calculate grams of carbohydrates as a percentage of calorie needs based on the 6–8 grams per kilogram: 6 g/kg = 444 g carbohydrates × 4 calories per gram = 1776 carbohydrate calories ÷ 2534 (low end) and 3802 (high end) = 70% and 47% calories from carbohydrates
   8 g/kg = 592 g carbohydrates × 4 calories per gram = 2368 carbohydrate calories ÷ 2534 and 3802 = 93% and 62% calories from carbohydrates

Calculation of calorie needs for Allison—134 lbs, 25-year-old female:

1. Calculate calorie needs based on grams per kilogram body weight.
2. Convert pounds of body weight into kilograms: 134 lbs ÷ 2.2 = 61 kg
3. 61 kg × (6–8 g carbohydrates/kg) = 366–488 g carbohydrates
4. Calculate REE using the formula in Table 14.1: REE = (14.7 × 61 kg) + 496 = 897 + 496 = 1393 calories
5. Multiply REE by activity factors (1.6–2.4) = 1393 × (1.6–2.4) = 2229–3343 calories daily
6. Calculate grams of carbohydrates as a percentage of calorie needs based on the 6–8 grams per kilogram:
   6 g/kg = 366 g carbohydrates × 4 calories per gram = 1464 carbohydrate calories ÷ 2229 (low end) and 3343 (high end) = 66% and 44% calories from carbohydrates
   8 g/kg = 488 g carbohydrates × 4 calories per gram = 1952 carbohydrate calories ÷ 2229 and 3343 = 88% and 58% calories from carbohydrates

---

The amount of carbohydrates to recommend for these two athletes is determined by the differences in energy cost of their different positions on the team. Allison has high energy costs on the playing field because she is responsible for both offense and defense, and runs a good portion of the playing field with few rests throughout games and practices. Cassie's position is critical to the team on defense, but she has a much lower energy expenditure defending the goal on her end. To achieve the target 55–65% of calories from carbohydrates for team sport athletes, Cassie could consume the mid-point of estimated calorie needs ([2534 + 3802] ÷ 2 = 3168 average calories), and 6 g of carbohydrates per kilogram body weight. This would put her calories from carbohydrates at approximately 56%, meeting her carbohydrate needs for her position (6 × 74 kg = 444 grams of carbohydrates) {[444 × 4] ÷ 3168} × 100 = 56%). Allison's high energy expenditure and need for endurance and carbohydrate usage during her on-field play require more calories from carbohydrates as a percentage of calories. At the high end of Allison's calorie range, she would need to consume 8 grams of carbohydrates per kilogram to obtain 58% of her calories as carbohydrates.

Because carbohydrates are the foundation of soccer players' diet, an intake in the 6–8 g/kg range for these athletes appears appropriate. Most team sport athletes should attempt to consume a minimum of 55–65% of their total calories from carbohydrates. In times of significantly high-intensity or duration training, this percentage may go up. A lower percentage could be appropriate in times where strength training is more of a focus and protein needs are increased. However, carbohydrates are still the primary fuel for the working muscles, and athletes should not decrease carbohydrate intake dramatically (i.e., <50–55%).

Team sport athletes can easily meet their carbohydrate needs by consuming whole grains, fruits, vegetables, and low-fat dairy products throughout the day at meals and snacks. **Training Table 14.2** provides a sample menu that contains approximately 55–65% carbohydrates.

What is the effect of carbohydrate consumption prior to team sport activities?

It is well known that a high-carbohydrate meal prior to team practice or a competitive event helps "top off" glycogen stores and ensures adequate blood glucose levels at practice or game time. As a result, it is recommended that athletes consume approximately 1–4.5 grams of carbohydrates per kilogram of body weight 1–4 hours before a game. The pregame meal can consist of solid and/or liquid sources of carbohydrates (see Figure 14.2). Bagels, cold cereal with skim milk, watery fruits (such as oranges, watermelon, and grapes), and carbohydrate-containing fluids are all good choices.

Many team sport events occur in the late afternoon or evening, which gives athletes the additional

Training Table 14.2: Carbohydrate-Rich Menu

Menu Item (kcal)	Carbohydrates (g)	Calories
Breakfast		
Raisin bran cereal, 1 cup	46	187
1% milk, 1 cup	12	103
Raisins, 1/4 cup	31	130
Grapefruit juice, 1 cup	28	115
Fruited low-fat yogurt, 8 oz	40	210
Subtotal	157	745
	84% of calories	
Lunch		
Black bean soup, 2 cups	40	240
Whole grain bread, 2 slices	24	142
Green salad w/raw vegetables, 2 cups	20	112
Light salad dressing, 2 tbsp	3	138
1% milk, 1 cup	12	103
Peanut butter cookies, 2 small	14	120
Subtotal	113	855
	53% of calories	
Dinner		
Grilled tuna steak, 6 oz	0	240
Rice pilaf, 1 cup	22	115
Broccoli spears, 3 large	15	80
Low-fat frozen yogurt, 1 cup	36	230
1% milk, 1 cup	12	103
Subtotal	85	768
	44% of calories	
Snacks		
Banana, 1 medium	28	109
Fig bars, 2	22	110
Whole grain crackers, 8	20	126
Subtotal	70	345
	81% of calories	
Total	425 g	2713 calories
	63% of total calories	

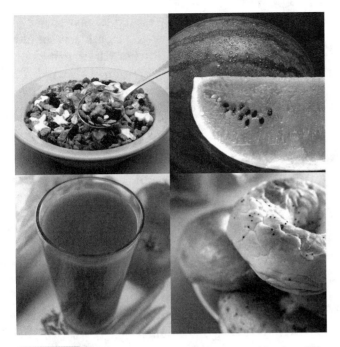

Figure 14.2 Preevent meal options. A variety of foods and beverages that contain mainly carbohydrates, along with a small amount of protein, and that are low in fat are the best preevent meal options.

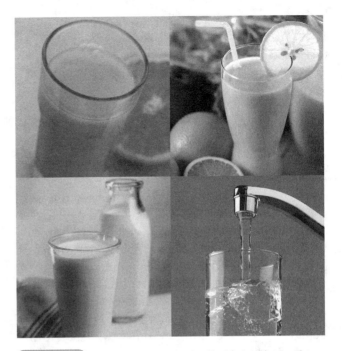

Figure 14.3 Liquid pregame meal options. Liquids may digest more quickly and feel better in the stomach prior to games than solid foods. Athletes with sensitive stomachs and pregame jitters may choose a liquid meal prior to a big game.

opportunity to consume several "game day" meals. In other words, the athletes should not neglect breakfast and lunch just because they know they are going to have a well-balanced pregame meal. They must understand that even the best-planned pregame meal will not erase the effects of prior poor nutritional habits on performance. Game day meals more than 4 hours in advance of competition should consist of easily digestible, familiar foods that are high in carbohydrates (i.e., 55–65% total calories) and also include small amounts of protein and fat for satiety. Athletes should be cautioned to moderate the overall amount of food eaten in a single sitting prior to events to avoid gastrointestinal distress. When combined with a good breakfast and lunch, the odds of the pregame meal fulfilling its mission of topping off energy stores is enhanced.

In team sports there may be several games or matches played on the same day or on multiple days in a row. If an event is an hour or less away, liquid carbohydrates in the form of juices or sports drinks are the best options (see 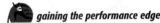 Figure 14.3). Solid carbohydrate foods tend to take longer to digest and could still be in the stomach at game time or during the event, potentially causing gastrointestinal upset. Also, preevent jitters close to game time may prevent

an athlete from consuming solid foods. Liquids tend to be better tolerated and thus provide the nervous athlete with an appropriate dietary option.

Is carbohydrate intake required during team sport activities?

If team sport athletes have followed prudent dietary practices in the days and hours leading up to game time, then rarely are muscle carbohydrate stores exhausted by the end of a game. However, that does not mean that a team athlete's ability to perform isn't affected in the later periods of a game. Liver glycogen stores and blood glucose levels can decrease in later periods of a game, thus negatively affecting performance.[18] Results from studies involving soccer and ice hockey athletes have shown decreased perceptions of effort and an increased capability for maintaining top playing velocities during games when consuming carbohydrates.[19–21] Similar improvements in performance have been shown in studies using activities that simulate team sport activity.[10,11,22] As a result, time-outs and halftime are excel-

> **gaining the performance edge**
>
> Consuming 1–4.5 grams of carbohydrates per kilogram of body weight in solid and/or liquid form 1–4 hours before a game can help top off energy reserves and provide for optimal performance.

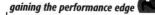
Ingesting carbohydrates during sport competition has been shown to decrease mental fatigue, decrease perceptions of effort, and help maintain playing velocities in team sport athletes.

lent opportunities to supply team sport athletes with carbohydrates in the form of sports drinks or snacks.

Consumption of 1.0–1.1 grams of carbohydrates per minute or approximately 60–70 grams of carbohydrates per hour should be adequate for team sport athletes.[18,23] This is equivalent to ingesting approximately 240 to 280 calories per hour. This level of carbohydrate ingestion is appropriate for sports in which activity levels are consistent and sustained; slightly lower amounts are adequate for team sports in which regular breaks, time-outs, and athlete substitutions occur. Ingesting 60 grams of carbohydrates during competition can be easily achieved if athletes consume a 6–8% carbohydrate sports drink in the amounts recommended for good hydration (i.e., 1 cup approximately every 10–15 minutes).

Is carbohydrate intake needed for recovery from team sport activities?

As is true with any athlete who has been involved in high-intensity activity, the timely consumption of adequate amounts of carbohydrates postevent provides for optimal restoration of glycogen stores.[23,24] Carbohydrate intake should begin as soon as possible after competition or practice to take advantage of muscles' increased ability to take up blood glucose after exercise. Athletes should consume at least 1.2 grams of carbohydrates per kilogram of body weight per hour for 3–4 hours after competition or practice. As much as 2.0 grams per kilogram of body weight may be needed for team athletes who play in highly active sports for most of the game. For example, a 70 kg soccer player should try to consume a minimum of 80–100 grams of carbohydrates after exercise. This can be accomplished by consuming 8 ounces of fruit juice (25 g), one granola bar (25 g), and 1 cup of low-fat fruit yogurt (40 g). Consuming adequate amounts of carbohydrates immediately after exercise is even easier if high-carbohydrate foods and fluids are made available to the athletes before they leave the sport facility or locker room. Fortunately, many high-car-

Ingesting 1.2 grams of carbohydrates per kilogram of body weight per hour for 3 to 4 hours after practice or competition will help speed replenishment of carbohydrate stores.

bohydrate foods are readily available, easy to pack, and relatively inexpensive; therefore, athletes should bring their favorite-tasting carbohydrate drinks or snacks for after practice/competition. This will help ensure that athletes start consuming carbohydrates as soon as possible after activity before outside distractions have the potential to disrupt their dietary recovery practices.

Are protein needs different for team sport athletes?

Protein is rarely used as an energy substrate during team sport activities, particularly if the athlete is meeting energy needs and carbohydrate intake is adequate. In some instances, such as during tournament play and/or long overtime games, the body can use protein for fuel. However, even in these scenarios, the reliance on protein for energy is low. The role of protein for team sport athletes focuses on the provision of daily nutrition. Protein is essential for the repair, construction, and maintenance of muscle mass throughout the season and during off-season training.

How are daily protein needs calculated for team sport athletes?

Calculating protein needs for team sport athletes depends on several factors, including the quantity and methods of training, as well as current body weight and muscle mass goals. Some team sports require more endurance training, whereas others are more focused on strength training. These variations in training, time spent exercising, and the intensity of training will affect protein needs. Protein needs can be determined based on current body weight. Refinement of protein need calculations can be done when change in the athlete's muscle mass is a goal. As with carbohydrates, protein needs based on current body weight should be compared to total calorie recommendations. If protein needs are altered based on training or muscle mass goals, then the percentage of carbohydrates and fat may also need to be adjusted.

Calculating protein needs should be done individually based on the sport and position played. Giving the entire team the same recommended protein intake without calculating the information individually could be a detriment to many players. Differences in playing and practice time, energy expenditure of various positions, and amount of contact in positions all will dictate protein needs.

Abrasions, contusions, and musculoskeletal injuries all may increase protein needs for adequate healing. The athletes on a team who receive the most contact hits during play and training may need slightly higher protein intake.

Strength training during the playing season and in the off-season increases protein needs. Protein needs may increase substantially in the off-season for some team sport athletes if the focus is on muscle mass gains. As strength-training time increases, energy and protein needs will also increase.

Body weight has a significant influence on the amount of protein needed daily. Similar to calculating energy and carbohydrate needs, body weight will significantly alter the overall grams of protein needed by different athletes. If muscle mass gain is a goal, then protein needs may be increased. If weight loss is the goal, protein needs may also be increased to avoid significant losses in muscle mass.

When using body weight to determine protein needs, a range of 1.2–1.6 grams of protein per kilogram of body weight is acceptable for most team sport athletes. Athletes with a goal of increasing muscle mass may require as much as 2.5–3.0 g of protein/kg body weight.[25] This level of protein intake could actually fall within the recommended 15–20% of daily calorie range for large athletes with high energy requirements. If a large football player weighing 110 kilograms consumes 5500 calories per day, at 2.5 g/kg protein intake he would consume 20% of his daily calories as protein.

Scott's Case Study   Scott is an 18-year-old freshman wing on his college hockey team. He is highly competitive and plays the maximum number of minutes possible in each game. He works hard year-round in the weight room and trains for endurance in the off-season. His muscle mass is at the optimal level and his goal is to maintain muscle mass during the long competitive season. The following is a sample calculation of protein needs for Scott, an 18-year-old, male, 210-pound hockey wing:

Calculate protein needs based on grams per kilogram of body weight first:

1. Convert pounds of body weight to kilograms = 210 lbs ÷ 2.2 = 95 kg
2. 95 kg × (1.2–1.6 g protein/kg) = 114–152 g protein/kg

Then, calculate energy needs using the REE calculations listed in Table 14.1:

3. REE = $(17.5 \times 95 \text{ kg}) + 651 = 1663 + 651 = 2314$ calories
4. Multiply REE by activity factors (1.6–2.4) = $2314 \times (1.6{-}2.4) = 3702{-}5554$ calories/day
   Calculate grams of protein as a percentage of calories based on g/kg (1.2–1.6):
5. *Using 1.2 g/kg:* 114 g protein × 4 calories/gram = 456 protein calories ÷ 3702–5554 = 12–8% of calories from protein
   Using 1.6 g/kg: 152 g protein × 4 calories/gram = 608 protein calories ÷ 3702–5554 = 16–11% of calories from protein

---

The preceding calculations show that for Scott to meet his protein needs and achieve an adequate percentage of calories, he must consume the higher end of the grams of protein per kilogram of body weight. This is true for both the low and high end of his estimated calorie needs range. If he consumed only 1.2 g protein/kg, and 3700 calories daily, he would get only 12% of his calories from protein. At the higher end of his calorie needs, only 8% of calories would come from protein. Neither of these levels reaches the 15–20% range recommended for team sports. Because Scott has a high muscle mass, strength-trains year-round, and wants to maintain his muscle mass, protein intake must reach at least 15% daily. This would be achieved if he were to consume the low to middle range of calorie needs and 1.6 grams of protein per kilogram body weight.

Many team sport athletes strive for greater muscle mass and size in attempts to improve performance. These athletes should be encouraged to consume adequate protein daily, but not in excess of needs. To build muscle mass, adequate daily calories are equally as important as adequate protein intake. The extra calories consumed from carbohydrate or fat sources spare ingested protein for muscle repair, building enzymes essential for sport performance, healing, and muscle hypertrophy. The International Olympic Committee (IOC) consensus statement is clear that "a varied diet that meets energy needs will generally provide protein in excess of requirements."[26] **Training Table 14.3** gives a sample day of meals that emphasizes protein without being excessive.

Is protein recommended after exercise for recovery?

There is growing evidence that protein intake after activity does appear to offer some advantages. Protein intake immediately postexercise or postcompetition provides the amino acids for healing of tissues and rebuilding of muscle. Contusions, abrasions, cuts, strains, and sprains are often part of playing team sports, and adequate protein intake is necessary for speeding recuperation. The amount of protein ingested should put the recovering athlete in a state of positive nitrogen balance.

Postgame ingestion of protein, and in particular essential amino acids, has been shown to improve nitrogen balance. Ingestion of essential amino acids appears to stimulate muscle protein synthesis, whereas nonessential amino acids do not have this effect. As little as 6 grams of essential amino acids postexercise can result in dramatic elevations in muscle protein synthesis.[27] Timing of protein intake, along with adequate consumption of carbohydrates and fat, also has an impact on an athlete's state of nitrogen balance. As a result, it is detrimental for athletes to focus just on protein intake after competition, particularly if it is at the expense of adequate carbohydrate and fat intake.[25] It is interesting to note that most athletes already have high protein intakes if they are meeting their energy needs on a regular daily basis, so worrying about adequate protein should not be a concern for most. Timing of protein intake is important; immediately after hard exercise, 6–20 grams of protein consumed in the form of essential amino acids may be beneficial.

> **gaining the performance edge**
>
> Consumption of as little as 6 grams of essential amino acids within 1–2 hours after practice or competition has been shown to increase amino acid use by the body during recovery.

Are fat needs different for team sport athletes?

Fats are a source of energy for any athlete, and as a consequence, the fat needs of team sport athletes are in general not any different from those of other athletes. Even though carbohydrates serve as the primary energy source during the short, intense bursts of movement that are characteristic of many team sport activities, it is important to note that many games can last 1 or more hours. In other words, when considering the energetic demands of team sports, the sports nutrition professional must focus on the energy demands for the entire game, not just that of the short bursts of activity. The reason for this is that the aerobic system is working hard during the rest intervals between bursts to help the athlete recover. During these recovery periods both

Training Table 14.3: Sample High-Protein Menu

Meal Items	Protein (g)	Calories
Breakfast		
Buttermilk pancakes, 3	8	258
Poached eggs, 2	13	156
Grapefruit and orange sections and sliced banana, 1½ cups	2	139
1% milk, 1 cup	8	103
Subtotal	31	656
	19% of calories	
Lunch		
Whole wheat pita, 1 whole	6	170
Chicken breast chunks, 6 oz	54	284
Light mayonnaise, 1 tbsp	0	45
Vegetable juice, 12 oz	2	69
Sprouts, onion, tomato, lettuce, 1½ cup, combined	2	50
1% milk, 1 cup	8	103
Subtotal	72	721
	40% of calories	
Dinner		
Beef and bean burrito with cheese, 1 large	18	470
Chopped tomato and greens, 1 cup	3	60
Light ranch dressing, 1 tbsp	0	45
Soft serve ice cream, ½ cup	3	185
Subtotal	24	760
	13% of calories	
Snacks		
Fresh strawberries, 1 cup	0	120
Graham crackers, 2 full sheets	2	120
Yogurt and fruit smoothie, 2 cups	10	347
Subtotal	12	587
	8% of calories	
Total	139	2724
	20% of total calories	

carbohydrates and fats are used for energy. If adequate fats are available for aerobic metabolism, they can help spare the use of carbohydrates. As a result, it is important for the sports nutrition professional to be able to determine the fat needs of each athlete and recommend intake levels based on the athletes' sport's energy requirement and/or their personal training goals.

How are daily fat needs calculated for team sport athletes?

Fat recommendations for most team sport athletes are the same for the general population. Fat should contribute 20–35% of total calories, providing sufficient amounts of essential fatty acids and aiding in meeting calorie needs. Some studies of team sport athletes report an average fat intake of 30% of total calories,[6,18] whereas others have documented that athletes consume more than 30% of their calories from fat.[1,5,28] Fat intake was reported to provide 37% of total calories in a study of Greek female volleyball players. This same group of athletes consumed 45.9% ± 12.5% of total calories from carbohydrates and 16.0% ± 4.9% of total calories from protein. It appears that the higher percentage of fat intake reduced the percentage of carbohydrates in their diets to well below the minimum 55% for most athletes. Higher fat intake, when consumed at the expense of adequate carbohydrates in the diet, could inhibit optimal sport performance in most team sport athletes.

The level of fat in the diet should provide adequate energy to meet weight goals (maintenance, loss, or gain). For team sports, the macronutrient percentage ranges are 55–65% carbohydrates, 12–20% protein, and 20–35% fat. Team sport athletes may need the middle to high end of the range in fat intake because many of these athletes weigh more and have higher calorie needs. To meet calorie needs, 25–30% fat may be appropriate because fat provides a concentrated source of calories in less volume. The fat consumed should be low in saturated and trans fats and include heart-healthy fat sources that include omega-3 fatty acids. Fat needs can be calculated after calorie, carbohydrate, and protein needs are determined. Total energy intake, carbohydrate intake, and protein intake are more important to team sport athletes, so those values should be calculated first. This does not mean that fat is not important to team sport athletes. It just means emphasis should be placed on the macronutrient intake that fits best for enhanced sport performance.

Joe's Case Study   Joe is a professional football offensive lineman. He does some form of strength or aerobic training almost every day in addition to practice with the team. He complains that he is hungry all the time and feels like he constantly needs to eat to maintain his weight and muscle mass. In fact, he has lost some lean mass recently and wants to regain that lost mass. A sample calculation of Joe's fat needs is listed below. Joe weighs 300 lbs and is 25 years old:

Determine energy needs first using the REE equations listed in Table 14.1:

1. Convert pounds of body weight into kilograms: 300 lbs ÷ 2.2 = 136 kg
2. REE = $(15.3 \times 136 \text{ kg}) + 679 = 2080 + 679 = 2760$ calories
3. Multiply REE by activity factor (1.6–2.4) = $2760 \times (1.6–2.4) = 4416–6624$ calories

Determine carbohydrate needs using 6–7 g/kg body weight:

4. $(6–7 \text{ g}) \times 136 \text{ kg} = 816–952$ grams carbohydrates
5. Calculate the number of calories in 816–952 g = $(816–952 \text{ g}) \times 4$ calories/g = 3264–3808 calories from carbohydrates
6. Determine the percentage of carbohydrates from total calories = $(3264–3808) ÷ 4416 = 74–86\%$ $(3264–3808) ÷ 6624 = 49–57\%$

Determine protein needs based on grams of protein per kilogram of body weight using 1.2–1.6 g/kg:

7. $(1.2–1.6) \times 136 \text{ kg} = 163–218$ g protein
8. Calculate the number of calories in 163–218 g = $163–218 \times 4 = 652–872$ calories from protein
9. Determine the percentage of protein from total calories = $(652–872) ÷ 4416 = 15–20\%$ of total calories from protein $(652–872) ÷ 6624 = 10–13\%$ of total calories from protein

Determine fat needs as a percentage of total calories:

10. Calculate using the highest calorie range = 100 – 57% carbohydrates (7 g/kg) – 13% protein (1.6 g/kg) = 30% of calories left for fat intake
11. Calculate grams of fat per day = $6624 \times .30 = 1987$ calories ÷ 9 calories/g = 221 grams of fat daily

---

In this example, the carbohydrate range was calculated using 6–7 grams of carbohydrates, which is at the lower end of the typical recommendation for athletes of 5–10 g/kg body weight. Because Joe is a lineman and has significant muscle mass and uses short bursts of power for his sport, a lower carbohydrate level, still within the range of recommendations, is appropriate. The 57% of calories determined for carbohydrates is based on the high end of his estimated energy needs. This large amount of calories was chosen for the calculations because Joe has lost muscle mass and needs additional calories to regain that weight. At this high end of the calorie range, the protein calculated at the high end of recommendations (1.6 g/kg) provides only 13% of his intake as protein. This is slightly lower than optimum given his goal of muscle mass gain. If Joe were to consume 1.8 g protein/kg, he would consume 15% of his total calories from protein ({1.8 g/kg × 136 kg} × 4 = 245 × 4 = 980; {980 ÷ 6624} × 100 = 15%).

The calculation of fat needs is based on carbohydrate and protein estimations and therefore was determined last. In this example, fat intake is calculated at 30% of calories, which is within the recommended range. Joe is an athlete who should consume the higher end of fat to meet his goals. He has reported being hungry all the time and has lost weight. Fat is more calorically dense and can help him meet his high-calorie needs for weight gain while providing satiation to curb his hunger. Figure 14.4 shows some healthy sources of dietary fat. If he were to consume more grams of protein to achieve 15% of his total calories, his fat intake would need to decrease slightly as a percentage of total calories.

When calculating energy and macronutrient needs, consideration of both percentage of calories and total grams of each macronutrient is necessary to make sure appropriate levels of all three macronutrients are attained.

Although there is growing evidence that higher fat intake, especially in the form of medium-chain triglycerides, may be helpful for endurance and ultra-endurance athletes, there is no evidence to support the use of high-fat diets by team sport athletes. As noted earlier, fats are an essential part of any athlete's diet; however, too much can have negative effects on performance. A study involving 20 men assessed the effects of high dietary fat intake on high-intensity exercise similar to the bursts of activity encountered in team sports.[29] They found that after 6 weeks on a high-fat diet (i.e., 61% of total calories from fat), peak and mean power output, as determined by an anaerobic power test, significantly decreased compared to that of a control group on a 25% fat diet. In addition, performance on a 45-minute cycling work output test was also reduced compared to the controls. This study indicates that a high-fat diet can lead to decreases in anaerobic exercise performance, which would be deleterious for team sport athletes.

Is fat recommended after exercise for recovery?

The amount of fat stored in adipose tissue, even in lean individuals, is adequate to provide replacement of fats oxidized during most bouts of intermittent-type exercise characteristic of team sport participation. However, there has been growing publicity in athletic circles regarding findings of recent research about the use of intramuscular triglycerides (IMTG) during exercise and how diet affects IMTG replacement during recovery. Burke et al.[14] reviewed research in this area and noted that there is emerging evidence that the consumption of a high-carbohydrate (i.e., ~65% of total calories) / low-fat (i.e., ~20% of total calories) diet during recovery after prolonged exercise may not fully replenish IMTG levels in the muscle. A study investigating the effects of a high-fat (~40% of total calories) versus a low-fat (~24% of total calories) diet on replenishment of IMTG in trained endurance cyclists revealed that the high-fat diet resulted in higher IMTG levels during a 48-hour recovery period.[30,31] Although this might seem to indicate that a higher-fat diet would be beneficial during recovery, it is important to note that the research to date has been done with endurance athletes engaged in continuous prolonged exercise lasting

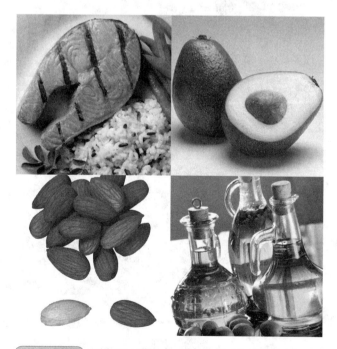

Figure 14.4 Healthful fat sources for athletes with high energy needs. Fat is a rich source of energy and can increase calorie intake in athletes who have high energy needs. Fats should be consumed primarily in the unsaturated form from nutrient-dense food sources.

3 hours or more. The extent to which the team athlete utilizes IMTGs during sport play and the impact depleted IMTGs may have on performance are unknown. What is clear is that carbohydrates are a major fuel source for the team athlete and, as a result, recovery diets for team sport athletes should still focus on replenishment of carbohydrates versus fats.

Are vitamin and mineral needs different for team sport athletes?

Most team sport athletes have higher energy needs than their sedentary counterparts. They may also have slightly increased needs for some vitamins and minerals. However, specific studies documenting increased or different vitamin and mineral needs for team sport athletes are rarely found in the literature. Much research on team sport athletes reports actual intake of energy, macronutrients, vitamins, and minerals and compares this to the appropriate dietary reference intake levels. This section will discuss how team sport athletes may or may not meet dietary intake recommendations for vitamins and minerals, how meeting calorie needs may affect vitamin and mineral intake, and whether a once-daily vitamin and mineral supplement is necessary for team sport athletes.

How does vitamin intake of team sport athletes compare to the dietary intake standards?

Assessing the dietary intake of athletes is accomplished using the typical means of food intake data collection. Self-reported food frequency questionnaires, food recording, interviews, and dietary recalls or combinations of these methods can be used to determine micronutrient intake. Many studies have been completed that assess the dietary intake of athletes and compare that information to recommendations for energy, macronutrient, and micronutrient intakes. Some of this research has focused on one sport; other studies contained data from a variety of sports. The vitamin intake information presented in this section relates to studies that included team sport athletes.

Hinton and colleagues studied 345 NCAA Division I male and female athletes to determine nutrient intake and dietary and weight loss behaviors. They found that the average intakes met or exceeded the Recommended Dietary Allowances (RDAs) for all micronutrients except vitamin E and magnesium.[32] Folate intake was low in a significant proportion of some of the athletes, but average folate intake met the RDA. In this large study of athletes in a variety of sports, it appears that vitamin intakes on average were adequate with only two exceptions. Similar results were found in a study of eight elite male soccer players. Vitamin A intake was 93% of the RDA and the only vitamin found to be deficient.[1] In this study, all of the water-soluble vitamins were well in excess of the RDAs. Beals studied 23 adolescent female volleyball players and found that mean micronutrient intakes met or exceeded the respective Dietary Reference Intakes (DRIs) or RDAs except for folate, calcium, and/or zinc.[33]

Antioxidant vitamins, primarily vitamins A, E, and C, have been promoted aggressively to athletes as a means of improving performance. As noted in two of the preceding studies, vitamin E and vitamin A intakes were reported below recommended levels. However, vitamin C intake was within the recommendations in each of those studies. A majority of studies indicate that vitamin C intake in athletes is adequate at levels of approximately 90–140 mg per day.[34] In attempts to test the theory regarding antioxidant intake and athletic performance, Schroder et al. studied professional basketball players. The athletes were given an antioxidant supplement with 600 mg alpha-tocopherol, 1000 mg vitamin C, and 32 mg beta-carotene, or a placebo, for 32 days during a competitive season. The antioxidant mixture decreased oxidative stress and helped avoid marginal vitamin C status compared to the placebo group.[35] However, improvement in sport performance using any of the antioxidant vitamins in supplemental form is still under investigation. In summary, it appears that male and female athletes in a variety of team sports meet the dietary intake recommendations for most vitamins, except a few. Vitamins A, E, and folate are the exceptions. As a result, sports nutritionists may want to include more foods rich in these vitamins in their athletes' diets.

How does mineral intake of team sport athletes compare to the dietary intake standards?

Much of the concern regarding athletes' mineral intake focuses on iron, calcium, and zinc, especially for female athletes. However, iron intake is of consistent concern in the team sports arena. Mineral losses in sweat, particularly sodium and potassium, can be a concern for athletes in team sports that play in high heat, humidity, and outdoor venues in the sun. Research assessing mineral intake and status in some team sport athletes has been done as a part of intake studies of macro- and micronutrients. This section will focus on iron, sodium, and potassium intake in team sport athletes as it compares to RDAs.

Many studies have documented low iron intakes and poor iron status in female athletes.[36-38] This research often focuses on female athletes in aesthetic sports and in endurance athletes, with less information provided about traditional team sport athletes. Iron depletion and iron deficiency anemia can have deleterious effects on sport performance. Dubnov and Constantini[39] studied the prevalence of iron depletion and anemia in 103 male and female top-level basketball players. They found a high prevalence of iron depletion and anemia in both genders.[39] Fourteen percent of the females and 3% of the males had iron deficiency anemia in this study. Iron intake was not assessed in this study; however, the authors note that to prevent and help treat iron deficiency, athletes should be educated about consuming dietary sources high in iron.

The high incidence of iron depletion in athletes is usually attributed to poor energy intakes; avoidance of meat, fish, and poultry that contain iron in the readily available heme form; vegetarian diets that have poor iron bioavailability; or increased iron losses in sweat, feces, urine, or menstrual blood.[24] Despite the knowledge and abundance of research showing athletes to be at greater risk for iron depletion, the condition appears to persist.

Food sources of dietary iron include meats; fortified breads, cereals, and pastas; and some vegetables. Consuming a vitamin C–rich food with an iron-rich food, especially a nonheme iron food, can enhance the absorption of iron. Team sport athletes can read the labels of foods they commonly consume to determine whether the products are iron-fortified or iron-enriched to increase the iron content of their diets. Female athletes should have their iron status evaluated annually and follow the advice of their medical doctor if supplemental iron is recommended.

Mineral losses through sweat can be high in some sports where high levels of sweat are common. Sports played outside in the summer heat, humidity, and sun are likely to cause high levels of sweating. Athletes should be aware that minerals are lost in sweat, particularly sodium and potassium, and need to be replenished appropriately. Sports drinks with electrolytes help replenish electrolytes during and after exercise. Some energy and sports bars and gels may also contain electrolytes and are often fortified with other vitamins and minerals. When extreme sweat loss occurs, adding salt to food and choosing higher potassium foods such as many fruits, potatoes, and tomatoes can help replace these lost electrolytes.

How does energy consumption affect vitamin and mineral intake?

It is a common principle in nutrition that individuals who meet their energy requirements by consuming a variety of foods will meet their micronutrient needs as well. Indeed, in most cases this is probably true as long as a variety of foods from all the different food groups is eaten regularly. Athletes who have higher energy needs than the general population, however, may have difficulty meeting energy requirements. This may lead to a reduced intake of vitamins and minerals. Athletes at the greatest risk of poor micronutrient status are those who restrict energy intake or use severe weight loss practices, eliminate one or more of the food groups from their diet, or consume high-carbohydrate, low-micronutrient-dense diets.[40]

A study of Greek female volleyball players found energy intake below recommended levels.[41] These athletes also did not meet RDA values for vitamins A, B_1, B_2, B_6, calcium, iron, folic acid, magnesium, and zinc but had sufficient dietary intake of vitamins C, B_3, and B_{12}.[41] Another study of Greek elite female athletes somewhat contradicts this study. Thirty-five female athletes (eight were volleyball players) were assessed for dietary intake and energy balance in the training and competitive seasons.[5] All of the athletes in this study were negative in energy balance during both seasons, yet their intake of all vitamins and minerals except iron were met. The volleyball players in the study were close to meeting their energy needs in the competitive season but not in the training season. It appeared that although the energy intake was low for the athletes, their diets were nutrient-dense. The authors note that this nutrient density in the diets may be related to the high intake of fruits and vegetables consistent with a traditional Mediterranean diet.

In a recent study by Clark et al., female soccer players in the preseason were found to have higher intakes of major vitamins and minerals, except vitamin D and biotin, than in the postseason.[6] However, when energy, vitamin, and mineral intake were assessed immediately postseason, calcium, copper, iron, magnesium, selenium, zinc, vitamin E, vitamin C, and several B-complex vitamins were significantly lower. Daily calorie intake was approximately 2300 preseason and 1800 postseason. The authors noted that both pre- and postseason average energy needs for individual players were met. Preseason energy needs were higher because of increased training demands, and postseason energy needs were significantly lower because training level, time, and intensity had greatly diminished.

This study brings up an interesting question about calorie needs as they relate to vitamin and mineral intake. Is it true that athletes who meet their energy needs will also meet their vitamin and mineral needs as well? Athletes need to make sure to eat a variety of nutrient-dense foods daily to get appropriate amounts of vitamins and minerals in the diet, especially when energy needs/intake are lower. Athletes who may be trying to lose weight may also be at risk for poor vitamin and mineral intake. It becomes more important in times of lowered energy intake to carefully plan a nutrient-dense diet to meet micronutrient as well as macronutrient needs.

In the Hinton study previously discussed, the male athletes did not meet estimated energy requirements but the female athletes did meet the average estimated requirements for their activity level.[32] The majority of females in the study reported that they wanted to decrease their body weight by at least 5 pounds. Approximately 25% of these females reported that they restricted dietary fat or carbohydrates in an attempt to prevent weight gain, yet micronutrient intake was met except for vitamin E and magnesium. When comparing the males to the females in this study, the males had higher total caloric intake than females but did not meet recommended energy requirements. When nutrient intakes were compared between genders, while controlling for energy intake, the diets of the female athletes were more nutrient-dense than those of the male athletes. The male athletes that played football and basketball had lower energy intakes and greater body weights than the other male athletes in the study. This may suggest that it is difficult for these larger athletes with higher energy expenditure to meet caloric needs. Nutrient density appears to have at least as much influence on adequacy of team sport athletes' diets as meeting actual energy requirements.

Are vitamin and mineral supplements recommended for team sport athletes?

Athletes and the general population use a variety of dietary supplements. Many studies report that team sport athletes take vitamin/mineral supplements. Krumbach et al. examined vitamin and mineral supplement use in NCAA Division I athletes and found that 57% of these athletes reported use of vitamin or mineral supplementation.[42] A multivitamin/mineral supplement was most commonly used, and vitamin C, calcium, and iron supplementation was also reported. A study of several different NCAA team athletes found that 18.9% of the athletes regularly used a multivitamin supplement.[43] Herbold et al. studied collegiate female athletes and found that 35.8% of these athletes took a multivitamin with iron supplement regularly, an additional 4.4% took a multivitamin/mineral without iron, and 13.5% took a multivitamin.[44] Twenty-three percent of collegiate freshman football players reported using a vitamin or mineral supplement.[45]

The previous section on team sport athletes' micronutrient intake reported that athletes tend to have adequate vitamin and mineral intake in most cases, especially when energy needs are met. Intake of micronutrients is marginal when less total calories are consumed in some cases, even if energy balance is attained. However, the studies report averages of the study participants; some individual athletes may have vitamin and mineral intakes significantly below recommended levels. Therefore, individual athletes should be assessed for adequate intake, and dietary recommendations should be made for each individual on the team, not a collective recommendation for the whole team. The dietary focus should be on obtaining a nutrient-dense diet with a variety of foods that meet energy demands for exercise.

When eating a variety of foods is difficult, calorie needs are low, or total intake is restricted because an athlete is trying to lose weight, a multivitamin/mineral (MV) supplement may be indicated. The MV should contain close to 100% of the RDA values of all the vitamins and minerals listed on the label. Athletes should choose an MV that is designed for the individual's age and gender. Female athletes may need slightly more calcium, iron, and folate than male athletes, and an MV tailored to females

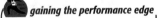
gaining the performance edge

Most team sport athletes who meet their energy needs will meet their vitamin and mineral needs. Athletes with poor appetite, difficult travel schedules where missed meals are common, or those who are trying to lose weight may have a decreased intake of some vitamins and minerals. A once-daily multivitamin/mineral supplement may be indicated for these athletes; however, it should not replace a nutrient-dense nutrition plan.

is likely to provide these additions. It is better to consume a once-daily MV than to consume several single vitamins or minerals in significantly higher than RDA levels. One hundred percent of the RDA is more than enough to provide some "insurance" that the athlete is getting an adequate supply of vitamins and minerals.

Some athletes get very nauseous for a short time after taking an MV supplement. Athletes should be encouraged to take the MV supplement with a full meal to avoid stomach upset. Athletes may choose to omit the MV on a competition day to avoid nausea. Stomach upset is more likely on game day in athletes who tend to get nervous before a game.

Team sport athletes who must make weight or who are overly concerned about weight or appearance should be encouraged to take a daily MV supplement. During times of dieting or when appetite is poor or travel schedules are difficult, the daily MV will help ensure that the major vitamins and minerals are consumed regularly and avoid depletion of vitamin and mineral stores. However, relying on an MV supplement instead of consuming nutrient-dense foods is not recommended. In addition, an MV supplement provides only those nutrients in the supplement. Athletes need to be reminded that vitamins and minerals do not provide energy or macronutrients, and energy needs should be met through adequate caloric intake.

Table 14.2 compares a standard once-daily MV to whole food options as an example of the benefits of obtaining micronutrients from healthful food intake.

TABLE 14.2	Comparison of Whole Foods to Multivitamin/Mineral Supplement				
Vitamin or Mineral	MV Supplement	Raisin Bran Cereal w/Milk	Orange Juice, 1 cup	Nutrients in OJ + Cereal Meal	Meal Compared to MV
Vitamin A	3500 IU	1250 IU	0	1250 IU	1/3 of amount in MV
Vitamin C	60 mg	2 mg	72 mg	74 mg	14 mg more than MV
Vitamin D	400 IU	138 IU	0	138 IU	1/3 of amount in MV
Vitamin E	30 IU	0	0	0	Meal contains no vitamin E; athletes on low-fat diets may need supplemental vitamin E
Folate	400 µg	162 µg	60 µg	222 µg	>1/2 the amount in MV
Vitamin B$_6$	2 mg	0.6 mg	0	0.6 mg	1/4 of the amount in MV
Thiamin	1.5 mg	0.4 mg	0	0.4 mg	1/3 the amount in MV
Niacin	20 mg	5.2 mg	0.4 mg	5.6 mg	1/4 the amount in MV
Calcium	162 mg	327 mg	20 mg	347 mg	>twice the amount in MV
Iron	18 mg	10.8 mg	0	10.8 mg	>1/2 the amount in MV
Zinc	15 mg	3.25 mg	0	3.25 mg	1/5 the amount in MV
Potassium	80 mg	738 mg	450 mg	1188 mg	>10 times the amount in MV; athletes exercising in heat and humidity need to replace potassium with food sources
Sodium	0 mg	484 mg	20 mg	504 mg	MVs typically contain no sodium; athletes exercising in heat and humidity need to replace sodium with food sources
Calories	0	289	110	399	Food provides energy, macronutrients, and fiber plus many more trace elements and phytochemicals that are not found in multivitamin/mineral supplements
Protein	0	12.7 g	2 g	14.7 g	
Carbs	0	58 g	26 g	84 g	
Fat	0	1 g	0 g	1 g	
Fiber	0	7.7 g	0 g	7.7 g	

Note: The 399 calories in this small meal are only a small portion of the total calorie intake that most athletes need in one day. Choosing a variety of other foods to meet calorie needs should complement the nutrients not obtained in the meal, providing a balanced diet with adequate micronutrient intake.

Notice that the MV supplement provides a wide variety of nutrients but no calories, macronutrients, or fiber. The small meal of raisin bran cereal with orange juice provides more potassium, vitamin C, and calcium and nearly two-thirds of the amount of iron found in the supplement. In addition, the meal provides sodium that may be necessary for athletes with high sweat rates, and one-third to one-half of the vitamin A, vitamin D, and folate of the MV. Choosing other nutrient-dense meals throughout the day supplies the rest of the micronutrients not found in the raisin bran and juice meal while providing a variety of other trace elements, healthful phytochemicals, and the energy needed to meet the athlete's energy requirements.

What are the fluid recommendations for team sport athletes?

Despite the intermittent nature of many team sports, maintaining hydration in team sport athletes can be a problem. Many team sports are played outside in the heat and humidity or in warm, humid gymnasiums with poor ventilation. In addition, athletes may wear heavy uniforms, protective equipment, and head gear that prevent heat loss and thus promote heavy sweating. Football gear is by far the worst when it comes to heat dissipation; as a result, these athletes produce as much as 1.5–2 liters of sweat during summer training sessions.[3] Even for ice hockey, which is played in a cool environment, sweat loss can be substantial because of the amount of protective gear that prevents heat dissipation. One study of ice hockey players reported a 3–10 pound weight loss attributed to sweat in one game.[46] Finally, mere observation of a basketball player engaged in practice or a game reveals heavy sweating despite wearing just a jersey and shorts. Clearly, attention must be paid to the maintenance of hydration in team sport athletes.

Why are fluids critical to team sport performance?

In all team sports, preventing dehydration is tantamount to optimal sport performance. As discussed in Chapter 8, athletic performance progressively declines with increasing dehydration. Not only does dehydration negatively affect thermoregulation, but it also compromises cardiovascular function and thus delivery of oxygen and nutrients to the working muscles. Depending upon the metabolic rate; environmental conditions such as heat, sun, and humidity; and clothing worn, exercise can induce significant elevations in body temperatures.[47] As body temperature rises with exercise, especially in warm humid environments, the body increases blood flow to the skin and increases sweat rate. High water and electrolyte losses in sweat can significantly reduce sport performance in athletes. The intermittent, high-intensity outbursts of powerful movements characteristic of team sports require that the athlete be functioning at optimal levels to remain competitive. Failure to maintain hydration decreases sport performance and, even worse, can endanger an athlete's life.

How can dehydration be prevented in team athletes?

Close attention must be paid to the fluid intake of athletes not only during practice or games, but also prior to and after these events. The following sections discuss strategies and considerations regarding hydration in team sport athletes.

What can athletes do prior to practice or competition to prevent dehydration?

Adequate hydration prior to practice or a game is essential, but hyperhydration prior to some sporting events is not necessary or desired. Hyperhydration immediately prior to an event will cause more frequent urination. This can become a bothersome problem in sports such as football or hockey because it is difficult and cumbersome to have to remove clothing and pads to urinate. To minimize this problem, ingesting fluids approximately 2 hours prior to practice/game time allows for adequate hydration and allows time for urine production and elimination before the athlete needs to suit up. The National Athletic Trainers Association (NATA) suggests drinking 17–20 ounces of water or a sports drink 2–3 hours prior to exercise and then an additional 7–10 ounces approximately 10–20 minutes immediately before activity to top off fluid reserves.[48]

What can athletes do during practice or competition to prevent dehydration?

Encouraging fluid intake and having appropriate fluids available at all times will help athletes maintain high levels of hydration. During exercise, the NATA recommends 7–10 ounces of water or sports drink every 10–20 minutes.[48] Flavored drinks may improve fluid consumption in some athletes. Studies have shown that athletes achieve improved fluid balance when drinking flavored beverages, even after expressing a preference for water.[49]

Besides offering a taste advantage over plain water, carbohydrate- and electrolyte-containing drinks also benefit players by increasing blood glucose levels and decreasing utilization of muscle glycogen in addition to helping maintain hydration. Sparing muscle glycogen and maintaining blood glucose levels through ingestion of carbohydrate drinks can help prevent both mental and physical fatigue during events lasting 90 minutes or more. Reilly reported that in soccer the number of goals scored near the end of the game decreases.[50] He surmised that both physical and mental fatigue—in other words, decreased concentration—may be the contributing factors to this phenomenon. Ostojic and Mazic studied professional male soccer players to determine the effects of carbohydrate–electrolyte drinks on soccer performance.[51] Players ingesting the carbohydrate–electrolyte drinks had lower ratings of perceived exertion during the match and completed dribble and precision tests faster than the water-only group after the match.[51] They concluded that drinking a carbohydrate–electrolyte fluid throughout the game helps prevent deterioration in skill performance.

A study of collegiate hockey, rugby, and soccer players found a 22% reduction in muscle glycogen utilization when compared to the control (water-only) group.[28] Similar results were found in a study of soccer and basketball players during practices and shuttle run tests. A 6% carbohydrate and electrolyte solution ingested prepractice and at scheduled intervals four times throughout the practice resulted in a 37% longer run time (i.e., delayed fatigue), faster sprint time at the end of the session, and improved motor skills test performance.[52] The authors concluded that carbohydrate drinks can positively affect sport performance, and their effects are independent of and additive to preventing dehydration.[53] Research certainly seems to indicate that carbohydrate–electrolyte drinks can offer some advantages over water alone for team sport athletes.

During competition, educating athletes on when they can get their fluids can be just as important as what they drink because lack of knowledge may prevent the athlete from ingesting fluids as often as he or she should. Hockey players have many short breaks that allow quick opportunities to replenish fluids. They can consume sports drinks on the bench between shifts and at intermission. Similarly, basketball players have the opportunity to drink during time-outs and during substitutions of players. Breaks between periods and at halftime are opportunities for most team players to replenish substantial fluids and electrolytes. In baseball and softball, quick fluid sips can be taken between the bottom and top of the innings when teams switch offensive and defensive positions. Sports drinks and water should occupy a highly visible position on the bench or near the players. This encourages fluid replacement by acting as a constant reminder to athletes to drink, allows for easy access, and enables trainers to keep track of fluid consumption by athletes.

What can athletes do after practice or competition to prevent dehydration and rehydrate?

Athletes need to work on fully replenishing water losses from previous activity so that they arrive at the next practice/competition well hydrated. As discussed earlier, sweat losses can be very high in team sports, and keeping track of an athlete's success in rehydrating is important. Rehydration should begin as soon as possible after exercise. There is some concern that consuming large volumes of fluid to rehydrate quickly increases plasma volume, thus increasing urine output. Kovacs et al. studied the effects of both high and low rates of fluid intake on postexercise rehydration.[54] They found that higher rates of fluid intake resulted in greater plasma volume increases and thus faster fluid balance restoration when compared to lower rates of intake. The higher rate of rehydration did increase urine output at hours 2 and 3 posthydration, but overall urine output was the same after 6 hours of rehydration in both the high and low rates of hydration.

Some team sports require athletes to compete numerous times in a 24- to 48-hour time span. Tournament play and double headers in baseball are examples. Despite the fact that the athletes are resting and relatively inactive between games, it is imperative that they continue to drink during the short periods of time between competitions. In extreme environmental conditions, it is unlikely that the athletes totally offset sweat loss with fluid intake; as a result, continued rehydration between games is important. Although issues of frequent urination are a concern to athletes, the inconvenience of having to go to the bathroom is more than outweighed by the positive impact of preventing dehydration and its effect on sport performance.

What other special considerations or practices can help prevent dehydration?

Preseason football practice is a special consideration. Twice-a-day practices begin in the late summer and are commonly conducted during times of the day in which the heat and humidity are highest. Encouraging athletes to drink may not be enough to prevent dehydration and the physical dangers associated with it. Athletes need to be educated about the importance of staying hydrated and taught the signs and symptoms of heat illness. In addition, athletic trainers and coaches should be on the lookout for any signs of heat illness in their athletes because the athletes may be too engrossed in learning and practice to drink adequately. Coaches and trainers must adopt practices that help ensure proper hydration. For example, allowing free access to fluids at all times during practice, having good-tasting sports beverages available, and enforcing fluid intake by athletes during mandatory water breaks are excellent practices that can help prevent dehydration.[55]

Another strategy that is effective in preventing dehydration involves having athletes weigh in before practice starts and immediately after practice. Any weight that is lost during practice is the result of water loss and should be replaced prior to the next practice or game. It is recommended that to rehydrate an athlete should consume enough fluid to replace 150% of the body weight lost because of sweat, or approximately 24 ounces of fluid for every pound of body weight lost.[48,54] Over time, this direct monitoring of weight loss during practice and under different environmental conditions will help teach the athlete what his or her typical fluid loss is in varying environmental conditions. Athletes can thus get a better feel for how much fluid they need to ingest to prevent dehydration and thus protect their ability to perform optimally during games.

acclimatization A process in which the body undergoes physiologic adjustments or adaptations to changes in environmental conditions such as altitude, temperature, and humidity. These physiologic changes enable the body to function better in the new climate.

Acclimatization is another practice that must be taken into consideration. Athletes traveling from cooler climates to hotter, more humid environments to compete must be allowed some time to acclimatize to maintain their performance levels. At a minimum, it takes an athlete about 5 days to acclimatize to hot environments, and thus the intensity of practices should be adjusted accordingly. A case study of England's female field hockey team preparing for the 1998 Commonwealth Games in Malaysia describes a 5-day acclimation hydration strategy.[56] They underwent 5 days of low-intensity or high-intensity intermit-

tent cycling in a similar temperature and humidity as the event just prior to leaving for the games. Body mass in the morning and pre- and postexercise, along with urine color measures throughout the day, were recorded. They found a significant reduction in exercising heart rate and core temperature at all time points by days 4 and 5. Urine color decreased from day 1 to day 4, suggesting an improvement in hydration status over these days. As a result, it may be helpful for teams who know they will travel to a more humid or hot environment for a major event to acclimate to these conditions before leaving. Allowing the athletes time to acclimate and get a feel for fluid losses in harsher environments will enable them to adapt their fluid intake levels accordingly.

What are the meal-planning/event-planning logistics that need to be considered during team sport events?

Most team sports are played at scheduled times during the day or evening. Athletes or teams can bring foods and fluids with them to the playing field and often have time to consume these items during breaks in the action. Storage space is available on the sidelines, in the dugout, or in the locker rooms. Back-to-back events, tournament play, traveling, and overnight stays can be challenging for athletes in team sports. These **team sport logistics** need to be considered to obtain proper nutrition for top-notch sport performance.

team sport logistics The planning, implementation, and coordination of details in regard to team practice and competition. For example, nutrition logistics involve dietary considerations prior to, during, and after practice or competition, in addition to issues of food preparation, preservation, and/or when and where to eat while on the road.

Should food be consumed during an event?

Depending on the length of the event, snacks may need to be consumed during an event. Many team sport competitions last between 1 and 3 hours. During the game, players may play only part of the time. Some players only play on offense or defense. Others will get short rest periods during time-outs or substitutions for positions. There usually is a half-time or break between periods when athletes can rehydrate and refuel relatively easily. In most team sports, snacks do not need to be consumed during the event. However, adequate hydration is essential to all athletic endeavors, and sports drinks are recommended as the main fluid for high-intensity competitions.

Although food may not need to be consumed during the event, consumption of food and fluids is essential between events. For example, in a baseball or softball doubleheader, the players will spend as much as 8 hours at the ballpark in a day. They may have pregame warm-ups, play the first game lasting 2–3 hours, get less than an hour break, and then have to play another 2–3 hour game.

Some players will not play both games, or play all of one game. However, every athlete is expected to be ready to play at a moment's notice. There-

fore, proper hydration and fuel for all teammates are essential.

What should athletes consume between games and at tournaments?

Macronutrient intake at all-day or weekend events can be varied based on the timing of events, hours between events, and availability of foods. Athletes should fuel up before an event with a meal several hours prior to the pregame warm-ups. For between-game meals, lower-fat, higher-carbohydrate, moderate protein foods are best. Carbohydrates are more easily digested and absorbed and generally well tolerated immediately prior to events. They are also the primary fuel during activity and need to be consumed after competition to replace muscle glycogen stores. This provides energy for the muscles to use at the next event.

Protein helps athletes by providing satiation, keeping the athlete from becoming hungry during events and while waiting for the next game to start. Protein sources offer more selection and less boredom with eating, often encouraging enhanced nutrition intake during a long day at the event site. Lower-fat foods are necessary during games and tournaments. High-fat foods take longer to digest and may cause stomach upset throughout the day. After the competition is over, a moderate-fat meal can be consumed; however, carbohydrates and protein are still the macronutrients of focus in recovery nutrition. Refer to **Training Table 14.4** for sample meals and snacks that could be used during a 2-day tournament.

Access to food can be a major consideration at ballparks, soccer fields, ice arenas, and gymnasiums. In most cases, a food concession stand will be on-site offering a limited variety of foods. Athletes who do not bring their own food with them or who do not have storage space available may need to choose from concession offerings. This is not ideal because lower-fat, high-carbohydrate, moderate-protein foods generally have limited availability at concession stands.

If the concession stand is the only option, there are some choices that are healthier than others. Athletes should avoid very-high-fat foods such as nachos with cheese sauce, whole fat ice cream, cookies, french fries, onion rings, and other fried foods. Protein sources that might be available are plain hamburgers (no cheese and little mayo), grilled chicken breast sandwiches, deli meat sandwiches, or Italian

Training Table 14.4: Sample Meal Plan for a 2-Day Tournament

Menu Item	Calories	Carbohydrates (g)	Protein (g)	Fat (g)
Breakfast (6:30 am)				
Frosted Mini-Wheats, 1½ cups	285	60	8	1.5
1% milk, 1 cup	105	12	8	2.5
Banana, 1 medium	112	28	0	0
Sports drink, 8 oz	50	14	0	0
Subtotal	552	114	16	4
		83% of calories	12% of calories	6% of calories
First Game (8:30 am)				
Lunch (11:30 am)				
Deli turkey sandwich, no cheese	345	24	29	14
Grapes, 1 cup	62	16	0.5	0
Whole grain crackers, 8	68	10	1	3
Apple juice, 1 cup	117	29	0	0
Subtotal	592	79	30.5	17
		53% of calories	21% of calories	26% of calories
Second Game (3:30 pm)				
Dinner (7:00 pm)				
Spaghetti w/ meat sauce, 3 cups	500	67	34	15
Italian bread w/ butter, 2 slices, 1 tsp	200	30	5	5
Large tossed salad	80	10	4	0
Light French dressing, 2 tbsp	45	7	0	2
1% milk, 1 cup	109	12	8	2.5
Lemon sherbet, 1 cup	100	23	1	1.5
Subtotal	1034	149	52	26
		58% of calories	20% of calories	23% of calories
Snack (10:00 pm)				
Whole grain crackers, 8	175	14	5	10
Peanut butter, 1 tbsp	95	3	3	8
Orange juice, 1 cup	110	28	0	0
Subtotal	380	45	8	18
		47% of calories	9% of calories	43% of calories
Total Day 1	2558	387	106.5	65
		61% of calories	17% of calories	23% of calories
Breakfast (7:00 am)				
Poached eggs, 2	156	1	13	10
Whole grain bagel, 1 small	209	43	8	1.5
Jam, 2 tbsp	108	27	0	0
1% milk, 1 cup	103	12	8	2.5
Cantaloupe chunks, 1 cup	62	15	1.6	0
Subtotal	638	98	30.6	14
		61% of calories	19% of calories	20% of calories
Third Game (11:00 am)				
Lunch/Snack (1:30 pm)				
Soft pretzel, 1 medium, w/mustard	288	33	5	10
Fruited low-fat yogurt, 1 cup	210	40	9	2
Orange, 1 medium	62	15	1	0
Lemonade, 16 oz	200	56	0	0
Subtotal	760	144	15	12
		76% of calories	8% of calories	14% of calories
Finals Game (4:00 pm)				
Dinner on the Road (8:00 pm)				
Grilled chicken sandwich, 1	400	37	25	17
Vanilla milkshake, small	278	45	9	7.5
Side salad	70	13	1	0
Fat-free dressing	35	8	0	0
Subtotal	783	103	35	24.5
		53% of calories	18% of calories	29% of calories
Total Day 2	2181	345	80.6	50.5
		63% of calories	15% of calories	21% of calories

Team sport athletes need adequate fuel during long games or tournament play. Consuming food and fluids at breaks in the action provides essential energy and hydration to continue peak performance during events. Arriving at the competition well fueled and eating for recovery after a long competitive day help athletes stay sharp throughout a several-day tournament.

beef. Carbohydrates available at most concessions include juices, lemonade, soft pretzels, fruit, frozen yogurt, frozen treats such as Popsicles, ices, and smoothies. **Table 14.3** provides a list of healthy food options available at concession stands for between-game snacks or during long tournament play.

Which foods are recommended for athletes while traveling?

In most cases, athletes and their coaches, managers, or parents will be able to transport and store some food and fluids for game time and between games. Packing, storage space, and refrigeration capabilities at the competition site need to be considered. The person in charge of the team's nutrition should call ahead to the event location to determine availability of space and determine whether refrigeration is an option. Some sport facilities have refrigerators in the locker rooms. Others will provide large coolers with ice that teams can use during the events. If neither of these options is available, coolers, ice, and space for storage during transit to the field as well as at the field will need to be planned in advance.

Table 14.4 provides a list of perishable and nonperishable food and beverage items athletes can bring with them for meals and snacks. A variety of both perishable and nonperishable foods and fluids should be available to teammates. Players have different preferences in taste, texture, and type of foods and fluids. Fluids can be brought to the event location already packed in ice, with additional beverages brought at room temperature. As cooled drinks are consumed, room temperature beverages can be added to the cooler. This saves space for the more perishable food items but still allows for cold drinks when athletes need them. Fluids should be consumed cool or cold whenever possible to help keep the athlete cool and to increase palatability, which encourages fluid intake. Having a variety of choices available to meet the individual preferences of each player will encourage consumption of fuel for optimal sport performance.

Overnight stays in hotels, as well as eating on the road, present additional nutrition challenges. Many hotels have small refrigerators where athletes can store fluids and perishable foods. Going to the grocery store nearby and purchasing lean deli meats, whole grain breads, fruits, juices and sports drinks, and cereal and milk can minimize the food budget while ensuring nutritious food options for the team. Athletes may be able to go to the store for themselves, or coaches, trainers, and/or parents can do the shopping for the whole team. A mini-cooler for each athlete or a large cooler for the whole team is essential for any team that plays often on the

TABLE 14.3	Healthier Sports Nutrition Options at Concession Stands	
Sports drinks		Deli sandwiches
Juices		Hamburgers
Lemonades		Cheeseburgers
Smoothies		Grilled chicken sandwiches
Fruit ices		Vegetarian pizza slices
Frozen yogurts		Soft pretzels
Frozen fruit bars		Packaged pretzels

TABLE 14.4	Perishable and Nonperishable Foods and Fluids for Traveling
Perishable—Keep Cold/Serve Cold	**Nonperishable—Do Not Need Refrigeration**
Sports drinks*	Graham crackers
Bottled water*	Vanilla wafers
Low-fat milk	Low-fat whole grain crackers
Yogurt	Animal crackers
Low-fat cheese sticks	Gingersnaps
Deli meats	Granola bars
Hard-boiled eggs	Cereal bars
Bagels	Sports bars
Fruit	Fig or fruit bars
Juices/juice boxes	Pretzels
	Bread sticks
	Canned fruit
	Canned puddings
	Dried fruit
	Dry cereals
	Peanut butter
	Canned tuna, chicken, or salmon

* Nonperishable, but best if served cold.

road. When refrigeration is not available, purchasing nonperishable snacks that can be brought to the playing field and stored in hotel rooms can improve the likelihood that athletes are consuming healthy snacks that meet sports nutrition recommendations for performance.

Lauren's Case Study A competitive club volleyball team has been invited to the national championship tournament. The tournament will be played 500 miles from the team's hometown. They will travel as a group in several vans to the weekend event and stay in a hotel close to the arena. Lauren, the setter on the team, likes to bring food with her because she has very specific food preferences. However, there will be limited space in the vans for all of the players. The hotel does have mini-refrigerators in each room that players will share. She and her roommate plan to share a small cooler with some perishable items, and bring additional nonperishable items in their packs. The following is a list of items Lauren decides to bring.

Nonperishable:

- 3 quarts of her favorite sports drink
- 6 sports bars
- 1 box of whole grain crackers
- 1 bag of dried cherries
- 1 small jar of peanut butter
- Four whole grain bagels
- 1 box of cereal bars
- 4-pack of chocolate pudding cups

Perishable cooler items:

- 2 pints of skim milk
- 6 string cheese sticks
- 4 single-serving yogurt cups

Lauren can consume some of these foods while traveling to the event. Once the team gets to the hotel, she can transfer the perishable items to the hotel mini-refrigerator. Then she and her roommate can fill the cooler with ice at the hotel and use it to transport perishable items to the tournament site. The team can stop at a local grocery or convenience store to purchase additional items as needed throughout the weekend.

By the time events are over and athletes have showered, packed up, and are on their way home or to the next destination, fuel levels are already low. Athletes can have a small snack from the food and fluids they have brought with them to tide them over until the team can stop for a meal. Trainers and coaches should have sports drinks readily available in the locker room for postgame hydration. Carbohydrate intake within 30–60 minutes after exercise or competition increases muscle glycogen replenishment, and fluids with carbohydrates can easily be transported. Full-strength 100% juices after exercise are convenient and contain the carbohydrates and fluids needed postgame.

Restaurants may not be close to the playing field, and when in unfamiliar cities it may be difficult to find a restaurant where teammates want to eat. Coaches and managers should investigate prior to travel which restaurants are close to the competition site or are on the road to the next site and make choices ahead of time. Obtaining travel directions and restaurant menus prior to departure saves time both in deciding where to go and in finding the restaurant.

What restaurant options are recommended for teams that are traveling?

There are many nutrition options in buffet-style, traditional, and fast-food restaurants that can help the athlete meet nutrition needs. Buffets for breakfast, lunch, and dinner offer many selections that are high in carbohydrates, a good source of quality protein, and varied in nutrient composition. Buffets are also excellent for large teams whose individual players may have very different food preferences. More traditional restaurants where players select from the menu can also offer a variety of meal options that help the athlete recover from a long tournament or provide fuel prior to the next competition. Most restaurants offer the option of preparing food with less fat and making substitutions of side dishes. Athletes can make these modifications in the meal choices based on their own individual energy and macronutrient needs.

Fast food can and in many cases has to fit into an athlete's nutrition meal plan. Choosing fast-food restaurants while traveling to and from events can save the team significant time. The time saved may be worth the fewer optimal food choices

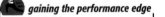

gaining the performance edge

Planning ahead is the key to ensuring team sport athletes will be well nourished on the road. Packing a variety of perishable and nonperishable foods and beverages in coolers and backpacks can keep athletes adequately fueled when restaurant stops are infrequent. Preplanned stops at restaurants where athletes have a variety of choices to meet their personal preferences and nutrition requirements can meet the varied needs of all team members.

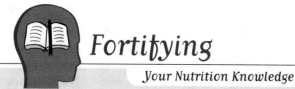

Fortifying

Your Nutrition Knowledge

Planning Nutrition on the Road

- Plan food stops before leaving home. Determine restaurant availability on the road and at the destination. Plan stops according to anticipated budget. Get driving directions from the event location to avoid delays postgame.
- Ask athletes for input on what types of foods and fluids they prefer for snacks and preevent and postevent nutrition.
- Purchase foods and fluids prior to leaving home. Pack a cooler with ice and load it with several food and fluid options based on athletes' preferences and nutrition composition.
- Call ahead to the event location to determine storage space for coolers or refrigeration availability.
- Contact the hotel staff to determine availability of refrigeration in rooms, restaurants on-site, and the menus of the restaurant. Hotel staff can also provide a list of restaurants near the hotel that may be acceptable to the team.
- Pack plenty of bottled water and sports drinks that do not require immediate refrigeration. Pack these in ice in the cooler as athletes consume already-chilled bottles.

available in fast-food establishments. There are, however, many fast-food choices that can benefit the traveling athlete. Emphasis should be placed on consuming carbohydrates and protein while finding lower-fat items on fast-food menus. Grilled meat sandwiches, plain hamburgers or cheeseburgers, salads with low-fat dressing, low-fat or skim milk, yogurt, baked potatoes, chili, and juices are all typically available in fast-food restaurants. Milkshakes can be an excellent option for the athlete with high energy requirements. Many fast-food restaurants use a low-fat milk mix, making shakes a lower-fat, high-calorie, moderateprotein option. Choosing a variety of the preceding food options can make a healthful meal for athletes when chosen in the amounts needed to meet energy and macronutrient needs. **Table 14.5** lists some healthy food options when athletes dine out.

TABLE 14.5   Healthful Food Choices When Dining Out

Carbohydrate Choices	Protein Choices	Lower-Fat Options	Buffet-Style Eating
Low-fat or skim milk	Hamburger	Baked, broiled, roasted, boiled, poached, charbroiled items	Fill one plate first with vegetables, fruit, salads, whole grain breads
Juice	Cheeseburger	Soft flour tortillas or corn tortillas	Broiled, grilled, or steamed meats, fish, chicken
Hot cocoa	Roast beef	Low-fat condiments, salad dressings	Avoid fried foods
Low-fat chocolate milk	Chicken breast	Vinaigrette dressings	Avoid cheesy, creamed foods
Whole grain breads/rolls	Turkey	Steamed instead of fried rice	Baked potato instead of fries
Fruit muffins	Eggs	Salsa, picante sauce instead of sour cream and guacamole	Limit creamy salads, buttery croutons, extra cheese on salads
Pancakes	Chili	Tomato or vegetable juice as appetizers	Put garbanzo, kidney beans on salads
Toast	Meat sauce on pasta	Breads/rolls instead of chips as appetizers	Frozen yogurt or soft-serve ice cream for dessert
Bagels	Fish		Eat until you are full and then stop
Cornbread	Tuna or chicken salad		Avoid the "get your money's worth" mentality
Soups: broth-based, split pea, bean, minestrone, vegetable	Black, pinto, and kidney beans		
Thick-crust vegetable pizza	Lentils		
Salads with corn, beets, carrots, three-bean salad	Tofu, bean curd stir-fry		
Pastas with marinara sauce	Lentil, bean, or pea soup		
Pudding	Low-fat cottage cheese		

The Box Score

Key Points of Chapter

- Teams are made up of athletes whose energy requirements and nutritional needs vary widely. The best dietary plans for team sports are designed around the individual athlete and do not take a "one diet fits the whole team" approach.

- Just as in all sports, the three energy systems work together to provide energy for team sport performance; however, this does not mean that they all contribute equally. The intense, short bursts of activity characteristic of team sport play make team sports more anaerobic in nature, which means that the phosphagen and anaerobic energy systems are the prime contributors during actual sport play. The aerobic system comes into play during the rest intervals between plays when the anaerobic energy stores are being replenished.

- The calorie requirements for team sport athletes vary depending on the sport, the position played by the athlete, and the length of the event. However, the energy requirements for most team sports can usually be met by following healthy dietary practices before and after the game. Consumption of significant amounts of energy during games is generally not necessary for games lasting 1–2 hours.

- The carbohydrate needs of athletes can be determined based on calculated energy requirements (55% to 65% of total calories) or body weight (5 to 10 g/kg of body weight). In most cases, protein and fat intake should range from approximately 15–20% and 20–35%, respectively. It should be realized that carbohydrates are the primary energy fuel for team sports and that their dietary intake should not be decreased at the expense of higher protein or fat diets.

- Pregame meals should consist primarily of carbohydrates and be consumed 3–4 hours prior to competition.

- After practice or a game, carbohydrate levels in the liver and muscle must be restored. The recommendation of consuming 1.2 grams of carbohydrates per kilogram of body weight per hour for 3 to 4 hours after practice or competition helps to ensure that recovery will be optimal.

- During tournaments where multiple games are played over the course of 1–2 days, snacks and small meals should consist primarily of carbohydrates. Athletes should pack food and beverages for the trip if there is room for storage and refrigeration. If packing items is not feasible, then making smart choices at fast-food restaurants and/or the concession stand can serve as the alternative. Educating athletes about making smart nutrition choices when dining out will positively affect their performance in away games.

- Indiscriminant protein supplementation, particularly at the expense of carbohydrate intake, is neither warranted nor recommended. In many instances the athlete's diet supplies enough protein to meet the body's needs.

- The timing of protein intake rather than high-dosage protein supplementation itself may be more important to the athlete. Ingestion of complete protein sources immediately before and after training or practice has been shown to increase cellular uptake and increase protein synthesis, which in turn may speed tissue healing, rebuilding, or adaptation.

- Dietary fat intake for team athletes is no different from a heart-healthy diet. The current recommendation states that 20–35% of total daily calories should come from fats.

- Vitamin and mineral supplementation at high dosages has not been shown to enhance athletic performance. Although intense training can increase the needs for certain micronutrients, the normal diet of most athletes is adequate in supplying the daily micronutrient needs. Although mega-dosing is not recommended, taking a once-a-day multivitamin/mineral tablet as insurance is generally accepted as a prudent dietary practice.

- Preventing dehydration is tantamount to good sport performance. Hydration must be maintained in all-day or weekend tournaments; otherwise, the athletes' performance will deteriorate. A minimum of 3 to 4 liters should be consumed to meet basic needs, with additional water intake occurring prior to, during, and immediately after competition.

- Based on changes in body weight, 2–3 cups of water should be consumed for every pound of body weight lost. Drinking fluids containing carbohydrates within 1–2 hours after practice or games will not only help in rehydration, but also assist in the restoration of muscle glycogen levels.

- Macronutrient intake at all-day or weekend tournaments can be varied based on the timing of events, the number of hours between events, and the availability of foods. In general, foods or snacks eaten before or between games should be composed primarily of carbohydrates because they are more rapidly digested and absorbed. High-fat or high-protein foods or snacks are not recommended because they take longer to digest and may cause stomach upset.

Study Questions

1. Even though team sports tend to be classified as anaerobic sports, why is it important for the athletes to also engage in aerobic conditioning?

2. What information is needed to calculate the daily energy needs for a team sport athlete? What are some of the hurdles encountered by team sport athletes who are trying to meet their energy needs?

3. Which of the macronutrients is the prime source of energy for the interval type of activity encountered in most team sports?

4. What role do proteins play in the diet of team athletes?

5. Once the energy needs of an athlete have been estimated, how are the carbohydrate and protein needs of the athlete determined? In other words, what are the recommended daily intake levels of carbohydrates and proteins for team sport athletes? Provide your answer in a percentage of total calories as well as grams per kilogram of body weight.

6. Should team sport athletes take vitamin and mineral supplements? Defend your answer as to why or why not.

7. Discuss strategies that could help team athletes who practice and compete in hot and humid conditions to stay well hydrated.

8. Discuss strategies that coaches or sports nutrition professionals can employ to increase the chances of athletes adequately hydrating themselves.

9. When a team is on the road, what are some healthy foods to pack for the trip?

10. What are several healthy food choices for athletes when buying food from a concession stand or fast-food restaurant?

References

1. Rico-Sanz J, Frontera WR, Mole PA, Rivera MA, Rivera-Brown A, Meredith CN. Dietary and performance assessment of elite soccer players during a period of intense training. *Int J Sport Nutr*. 1998;8:230–240.

2. Rico-Sanz J. Body composition and nutritional assessments in soccer. *Int J Sport Nutr*. 1998;8:113–123.

3. Wildman R, Miller B. *Sports and Fitness Nutrition*. Belmont, CA: Thompson Wadsworth; 2004.

4. Secora CA, Latin RW, Berg KE, Noble JM. Comparison of physical and performance characteristics of NCAA Division I football players: 1987 and 2000. *J Strength Cond Res*. 2004;18(2):286–291.

5. Hassapidou M, Manstrantoni A. Dietary intakes of elite female athletes in Greece. *J Human Nutr Dietet*. 2001;14:391–396.

6. Clark M, Reed DB, Crouse SF, Armstrong RB. Pre- and post-season dietary intake, body composition, and performance indices of NCAA Division I female soccer players. *Int J Sport Nutr Exerc Metabol*. 2003;13:303–319.

7. Mulligan K, Butterfield G. Discrepancies between energy intake and energy expenditure in physically active women. *Br J Nutr*. 1990;64:23–36.

8. Myerson M, Gutin B, Warren M. Resting metabolic rate and energy balance in amenorrheic and eumenorrheic runners. *Med Sci Sports Exerc*. 1991;23:15–22.

9. Rosenbloom C. *Sports Nutrition—a Guide for the Professional Working with Active People*. 3rd ed. Chicago, IL: American Dietetic Association; 2000.

10. Davis J, Welsh RS, Alderson NA. Effects of carbohydrate and chromium ingestion during intermittent high-intensity exercise to fatigue. *Int J Sport Nutr Exerc Metabol*. 2000;10:476–485.

11. Davis J. Carbohydrate drinks delay fatigue during intermittent, high-intensity cycling in men and women. *Int J Sport Nutr*. 1997;7:261–273.

12. Nicholas C, Williams C, Phillips G, Nowitz A. Influence of ingesting a carbohydrate-electrolyte solution on endurance capacity during intermittent high intensity shuttle running. *J Sports Sci*. 1996;13:283–290.

13. Akermark C, Jacobs I, Rasmusson M, Karlsson J. Diet and muscle glycogen concentration in relation to physical performance in Swedish elite ice hockey players. *Int J Sport Nutr*. 1996;6(3):272–284.

14. Burke L, Kiens B, Ivy JL. Carbohydrates and fat for training and recovery. *J Sports Sci*. 2004;22:15–30.

15. Hawley J, Dennis SC, Noakes TD. Carbohydrate, fluid, and electrolyte requirements of the soccer player: a review. *Int J Sport Nutr*. 1994;3:221–236.

16. Kreider R, Ferreira M, Wilson M, et al. Effects of creatine supplementation on body composition, strength, and sprint performance. *Med Sci Sports Exerc*. 1998; 30(1):73–82.

17. Short S, Short WR. Four-year study of university athletes' dietary intake. *J Am Dietet Assoc*. 1983;82:632–642.

18. Schokman C, Rutishauser IHE, Wallace RJ. Pre- and postgame macronutrient intake of a group of elite Australian football players. *Int J Sport Nutr*. 1999;9:60–69.

19. Leatt PB, Jacobs I. Effects of glucose polymer ingestion on glycogen depletion during a soccer match. *Can J Sports Sci*. 1989;14:112–116.

20. Simard C, Tremblay A, Jobin M. Effects of carbohydrate intake before and during an ice hockey game on blood and muscle energy substrates. *Res Q Exerc Sci*. 1988;59:144–147.

21. Zeederberg L, Lambert EV, Noakes TD, Dennis SC, Hawley JA. The effect of carbohydrate ingestion on the motor skill performance of soccer players. *Int J Sports Nutr*. 1996;6:348–355.

22. Nicholas CW, Tsintzas K, Boobis L, Williams C. Carbohydrate-electrolyte ingestion during intermittent high-intensity running. *Med Sci Sports Exerc*. 1999;31:1280–1286.

23. Shepard RJ. Meeting carbohydrate and fluid needs in soccer. *Can J Sports Sci*. 1990;15:165–171.

24. Hargreaves M. Carbohydrate and lipid requirements of soccer. *J Sports Sci*. 1994;12(suppl):S13–S16.

25. Tipton K, Wolfe RR. Protein and amino acids for athletes. *J Sports Sci*. 2004;22:65–79.

26. International Olympic Committee. IOC consensus statement on sports nutrition 2003. *J Sports Sci*. 2004;22(1):x.

27. Tipton KD. Exercise, protein metabolism, and muscle growth. *Int J Sport Nutr Exerc Metabol*. 2001;11(1):109–132.

28. Nicholas C, Tsintzas K, Boobis L, Williams C. Carbohydrate-electrolyte ingestion during intermittent high-intensity running. *Med Sci Sports Exerc*. 1999;31(9):1280–1286.

29. Fleming J, Sharman MJ, Avery NG, et al. Endurance capacity and high-intensity exercise performance responses to a high-fat diet. *Int J Sport Nutr Exerc Metabol*. 2003;13(4):466–478.

30. Van Loon LJ, Greenhaff PL, Constantin-Teodosiu D, Saris WH, Wagenmakers AJ. The effects of increasing exercise intensity on muscle fuel utilization in humans. *J Physiol*. 2001;536(Pt 1):295–304.

31. Van Loon LJ, Schrauwen-Hinderling VB, Koopman R, et al. Influence of prolonged endurance cycling and recovery diet on intramuscular triglyceride content in trained males. *Am J Physiol Endocrinol Metabol*. 2003;285(4):E804–E811.

32. Hinton PS, Sanford TC, Davidson MM, Yakushko OF, Beck NC. Nutrient intakes and dietary behaviors of male and female collegiate athletes. *Int J Sport Nutr Exerc Metabol*. 2004;14:389–405.

33. Beals KA. Eating behaviors, nutritional status, and menstrual function in elite female adolescent volleyball players. *J Am Dietet Assoc*. 2002;102:1293–1296.

34. Peake JM. Vitamin C: effects of exercise and requirements with training. *Int J Sport Nutr Exerc Metabol*. 2003;13(2):125–151.

35. Schroder H, Navarro E, Tramullas A, Mora J, Galiano D. Nutrition antioxidant status and oxidative stress in professional basketball players: effects of a three compound antioxidative supplement. *Int J Sports Med*. 2000;21(2):146–150.

36. Balaban EP, Cox JV, Snell P, Vaughan RH, Frenkel EP. The frequency of anemia and iron deficiency in the runner. *Med Sci Sports Exerc*. 1989;21:643–648.

37. Haymes EM, Spillman DM. Iron status of women distance runners, sprinters, and control women. *Int J Sports Med*. 1989;10:430–433.

38. Pate PR, Miller BJ, Davis JM, Slentz CA, Klingshirn LA. Iron status of female runners. *Int J Sports Nutr*. 1993;3:222–231.

39. Dubnov G, Constantini NW. Prevalence of iron depletion and anemia in top-level basketball players. *Int J Sport Nutr Exerc Metabol*. 2004;14(1):30–37.

40. American Dietetic Association. Position of the American Dietetic Association, Dietitians of Canada, and the American College of Sports Medicine: nutrition and athletic performance. *J Am Dietet Assoc*. 2000;100:1543–1556.

41. Papadopoulou S, Papadopoulou SD, Gallos GK. Macro- and micro-nutrient intake of adolescent Greek female volleyball players. *Int J Sport Nutr Exerc Metabol*. 2002;12:73–80.

42. Krumbach CJ, Ellis DR, Driskell JA. A report of vitamin and mineral supplement use among university athletes in a Division I institution. *Int J Sport Nutr*. 1999;9(4):415–425.

43. Jacobson B, Sobonya C, Ransone J. Nutrition practices and knowledge of college varsity athletes: a follow-up. *J Strength Cond Res*. 2001;15(1):63–68.

44. Herbold N, Visconti B, Frates S, Bandini L. Traditional and nontraditional supplement use by collegiate female varsity athletes. *Int J Sports Nutr Exerc Metabol*. 2004;14(5):586–593.

45. Jonnalagadda S, Rosenbloom C, Skinner R. Dietary practices, attitudes, and physiological status of collegiate freshman football players. *J Strength Cond Res*. 2001;15(4):507–513.

46. Burns J, Dugan L. Working with professional athletes in the rink: the evolution of a nutrition program for an NHL team. *Int J Sport Nutr*. 1994;4(2):132–134.

47. American College of Sports Medicine. Position stand: exercise and fluid replacement. *Med Sci Sports Exerc*. 2007;39(2):377–390.

48. Casa D, Armstrong LE, Hillman SK, et al. National Athletic Trainers' Association position statement: fluid replacement for athletes. *J Athletic Train*. 2000;35(2):212–224.

49. Minehan M, Riley MD, Burke LM. Effect of flavor and awareness of kilojoule content of drinks on preference and fluid balance in team sports. *Int J Sport Nutr Exerc Metabol*. 2002;12:81–92.

50. Reilly T. Energetics of high-intensity exercise (soccer) with particular reference to fatigue. *J Sports Sci*. 1997;15(3):257–263.

51. Ostojic S, Mazic S. Effects of a carbohydrate-electrolyte drink on specific soccer tests and performance. *J Sports Sci Med*. 2002;1:47–53.

52. Welsh R, Davis JM, Burke JR, Williams HG. Carbohydrates and physical/mental performance during intermittent exercise to fatigue. *Med Sci Sports Exerc*. 2002;34(4):723–731.

53. Murray R. Rehydration strategies—balancing substrate, fluid, and electrolyte provision. *Int J Sport Med*. 1998;19:S133–S135.

54. Kovacs E, Schmahl RM, Senden JMG, Browns F. Effect of high and low rates of fluid intake on post-exercise rehydration. *Int J Sport Nutr Exerc Metabol*. 2002;12:14–23.

55. Coris E, Ramirez AM, Van Durme DJ. Heat illness in athletes. *Sports Med*. 2004;34(1):9–16.

56. Dabinet J, Reid K, James N. Educational strategies used in increasing fluid intake and enhancing hydration status in field hockey players preparing for competition in a hot and humid environment: a case study. *Int J Sport Nutr Exerc Metabol*. 2001;11:334–348.

Additional Resources

Braakhuis A, Meredith K, Cox GR, Hopkins WG, Burke LM. Variability in estimation of self-reported dietary intake data from elite athletes resulting from coding by different sports dietitians. *Int J Sport Nutr Exerc Metabol*. 2003;13:152–165.

Oppliger R, Bartok C. Hydration testing of athletes. *Sports Med*. 2002;32(15):959–971.

Smart L, Bisogni CA. Personal food systems of male college hockey players. *Appetite*. 2001;37:57–70.

CHAPTER

15

Special Populations

Key Questions Addressed

- What is a "special population"?
- What are the special considerations for athletes with diabetes?
- What are the special considerations for athletes who are pregnant?
- What are the special considerations for child and teen athletes?
- What are the special considerations for college athletes?
- What are the special considerations for masters athletes?
- What are the special considerations for vegetarian athletes?

You Are the Nutrition Coach

Ryan is a cross-country athlete running for one of the top collegiate teams in the country. He is a sophomore in college and is living in an apartment with two other runners on the team. He lived in a dorm as a freshman and decided on a more vegetarian style of eating last year because his roommate was vegetarian. There were a variety of vegetarian dishes prepared in the dorm cafeteria that he liked and found convenient after long practices.

Ryan is 5'8" and weighs around 135 pounds. He trains hard daily for 1–2 hours at the track or on the road and lifts weights twice a week with the team. He eats some dairy, mainly yogurt, soy milk, and occasionally eggs. He eats no meat or fish but he does consume some beans, legumes, and frozen veggie burgers. Grocery shopping, meal planning, and vegetarian cooking are all new to Ryan, and therefore he schedules an appointment with the athletic department's sports nutritionist for guidance with eating vegetarian style in his apartment.

Questions

- What nutrients would you be most concerned about being insufficient in Ryan's daily diet?

- What questions should you ask about his typical food intake to help you determine a nutrition plan for Ryan?

- What recommendations, both nutritional and educational, would you give Ryan to help him be successful in sport while practicing a vegetarian diet?

What is a "special population"?

As discussed in earlier chapters, the best dietary plans are designed around the needs of each individual athlete. In a sense, each dietary plan is special. The meal plan must be designed to meet not only the basic metabolic needs of the athlete, but also the unique energetic demands of training, sport participation, and recovery. Although each athlete is certainly "special," the dietary practices followed are basic in regard to nutrition.

The "special populations" discussed in this chapter require nutritional consideration beyond the usual adjustments made to meet individual basic dietary needs. The popularity of sport participation, the advancement of training and conditioning, and the increased sporting opportunities for children and women have expanded the pool of athletes and thus increased the physical diversity of today's athletes. For example, there are athletes who are playing sports with metabolic diseases such as diabetes. The number of older or masters-level athletes is increasing as advances in training and conditioning are keeping athletes in competitive shape later in life; the number of masters-level competitions also is increasing, creating more opportunities for masters athletes to compete. Children are participating in sports at young ages, thus requiring nutritional planning for athletes undergoing growth and development. Title IX has expanded the number of sporting opportunities for women, which in turn has made dealing with the pregnant athlete a growing issue. In the following sections, the nutritional considerations required for these and other special populations are discussed.

What are the special considerations for athletes with diabetes?

According to the American Diabetes Association, there are approximately 23.6 million people with diabetes mellitus (diabetes) in the United States. Of these, approximately three-quarters have been diagnosed and the other one-quarter are unaware they have diabetes. Diabetes is a metabolic disorder that affects carbohydrate availability and utilization by the cells of the body.[1] As described in Chapters 2 and 3 in this text, carbohydrates are one of the main sources of energy for the body, particularly during exercise. As a result, diabetes severely alters normal energy metabolism in the body.

Consumed carbohydrates ultimately appear as glucose in the bloodstream; however, for the blood glucose to be used by cells it must be carried across the cell membranes by special transporter molecules. Activity of the glucose transporters is increased by the hormone insulin, which is produced by the pancreas. In response to rising blood glucose levels after a meal, the pancreas secretes insulin. Insulin activates the cell membrane transporters, thus increasing glucose uptake into the cell (see Figure 15.1), decreasing blood glucose levels back to normal. In diabetes, there is a disruption of insulin release by the pancreas and/or a decreased response of the cells to any insulin that is secreted. In either case, the end result is the inability of cells to uptake glucose.

Because the cells are incapable of uptaking glucose, **hyperglycemia** or high blood glucose results. Despite the fact that blood glucose levels are high, without the increased activity of the cell transporters, the cells of the body are robbed of energy. The body is fooled into thinking the cells are starving for carbohydrates and then, ironically, the liver starts to release its stored glucose into the blood. This makes matters

hyperglycemia An abnormally high blood glucose level; usually a feature of diabetes.

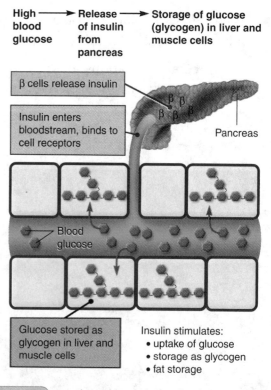

Figure 15.1 Regulating blood glucose levels. In response to high blood glucose levels, the pancreas releases insulin, which increases the uptake of glucose by cells.

worse, raising the glucose levels in the blood even higher. The high blood glucose levels cause sugar to spill into the urine, causing another common symptom of diabetes, frequent urination.

When the body is unable to use glucose as energy, it turns to other sources, namely proteins and fats. As discussed in Chapter 2, in times of energy deficit, proteins can be converted to glucose via gluconeogenesis. The body resorts to breaking down protein from muscle in an attempt to meet its energy demands. The end result is muscle wasting, muscle weakness, and body weight loss, which are three other prominent symptoms of diabetes.

With diabetes, the body also attempts to increase fat utilization, which can also cause problems. When excessive fat is used as an energy source in the absence of glucose, intermediate products of fat metabolism can build up, forming compounds known as **ketone bodies**. The increased production of ketone bodies is known as **ketosis** and can lead to a serious clinical condition named **ketoacidosis**. In ketoacidosis, body fluids, which are normally slightly alkaline, become very acidic, and if left uncorrected can be life threatening and result in coma.

ketone bodies Molecules that are formed from fat metabolic by-products. Ketone bodies are formed when insufficient carbohydrates are available for complete metabolizing of fats.

ketosis A condition that arises from abnormally high levels of ketone bodies in the tissues and body fluids.

ketoacidosis Acidification of the blood caused by a buildup of ketone bodies.

There are many long-term consequences of high blood glucose levels that result from uncontrolled diabetes. The increased blood glucose concentrations can cause damage to many body tissues. Blood vessels in the eyes, kidneys, and heart, along with the cells that make up nerves, are all damaged by high levels of blood glucose. As a result, diabetes can cause blindness, kidney dysfunction, heart disease, and nerve degeneration.[2] Amputations of the lower limbs are a common complication of diabetes because of the nerve and tissue damage caused by diabetes. In fact, statistics from the American Diabetes Association indicate that diabetes is responsible for 60% of all lower extremity amputations and 44% of all new kidney failure cases in adults.

What are the main types of diabetes?

There are two types of diabetes, each requiring different treatment regimens. In **type 1 diabetes**, the pancreas stops

type 1 diabetes A type of diabetes in which the pancreas stops producing insulin. Type 1 diabetics require exogenous insulin injections to help maintain normal blood glucose levels.

producing insulin, and exogenous insulin injections are required. Type 1 diabetes is most often diagnosed in children or young adults and previously was termed "insulin dependent diabetes." In type 1 diabetes, the pancreas fails to produce enough insulin, so the blood glucose has no mechanism to enter the cells. Approximately 5–15% of people with diabetes have type 1 diabetes. The treatment regimen for type 1 diabetes is primarily insulin injections combined with a healthful diet and regular exercise to control blood glucose levels.

In **type 2 diabetes**, the pancreas produces sufficient amounts of insulin—it actually may overproduce insulin—but the body's cells are not responsive. The cells are less responsive to insulin because the number of cell receptors responsible for binding insulin is decreased. If insulin cannot bind to receptors on the cell membrane, then it cannot activate the glucose transporters, and uptake of glucose is affected. Approximately 85–95% of the people with diabetes in the United States have type 2 diabetes. The treatment for type 2 diabetes will depend on the individual's blood glucose levels, amount of endogenous insulin production, and other factors. Some oral medications can enhance insulin sensitivity, helping blood glucose be transported more effectively into the cells for energy. It is interesting to note that exercise can also help in the management of type 2 diabetes. Exercise has been shown to increase the activity level of some of the glucose transporters in the active muscles independent of insulin, thereby increasing the uptake of blood glucose and subsequently lowering blood glucose levels. Exercise also plays a role in weight loss, which in overweight individuals with type 2 diabetes is also effective in treating some of the diabetic symptoms.

type 2 diabetes A type of diabetes in which the pancreas still secretes insulin but the cells are not as responsive to it, resulting in elevated blood glucose levels. Individuals who are obese and over the age of 35 are at increased risk for this disease.

Prediabetes is a condition in which blood glucose levels are elevated but are not high enough to meet the criteria for a diagnosis of diabetes. Most individuals who develop type 2 diabetes have had glucose levels in the prediabetes range for some time prior to their type 2 diabetes diagnosis. The fasting plasma glucose level that typically signifies prediabetes is 100–125 mg/dL.[3] The early identification of prediabetes is essential to the prevention of type

prediabetes A condition where blood glucose levels are elevated but are not high enough to meet the criteria for a diagnosis of diabetes.

TABLE 15.1	Common Symptoms of Diabetes Mellitus
Excessive thirst	Blurred vision
Excessive urination	Unexplained weight loss
Dehydration	Excessive hunger or eating
Dizziness	Poor or slow wound healing
Headache	

2 diabetes and the complications that occur with this disease.

The diagnostic criteria for diabetes mellitus are as follows:[3]

- Diabetes symptoms plus casual plasma glucose concentration ≥ 200 mg/dL (11.1 mmol/L), or
- Fasting plasma glucose ≥ 126 mg/dL (7.0 mmol/L), or
- 2-hour plasma glucose ≥ 200 mg/dL (11.1 mmol/L) during an oral glucose tolerance test.

The diagnostic criteria are the same for type 1 and type 2 diabetes. Physicians can determine which type of diabetes has developed by reviewing the length of onset of symptoms, age at onset, and patient and family history, as well as by performing additional laboratory tests and a physical examination. A list of common symptoms of diabetes is in **Table 15.1**.

What are the considerations related to exercise for athletes with diabetes?

Regular exercise is one of the main recommendations for managing diabetes and blood glucose levels. Regular exercise can decrease insulin resistance and thereby improve blood glucose control. Athletes who are newly diagnosed with diabetes need to consider the effect that exercise training and competition has on their blood glucose levels. More frequent self-monitoring of glucose levels before and after exercise is necessary to avoid complications of low blood glucose levels. As noted earlier, muscular contractions can improve glucose uptake by increasing glucose transporter activity, thereby allowing glucose to enter the cells independent of insulin. This enhanced transport can continue for several hours after exercise and thus can have a prolonged impact on blood glucose levels. Therefore, monitoring of glucose 2–3 hours after exercise may also be necessary because abnormal lows in glucose levels could occur postexercise.

Athletes with type 1 diabetes have to be even more cautious than type 2 diabetic athletes because they have to inject insulin in appropriate amounts and at the proper times to help control their blood glucose. Type 1 diabetic athletes must be very regimented and possess good self-management skills to safely and effectively participate in sports. They must closely monitor the effect of exercise on their blood glucose levels and thus make adjustments in the timing of insulin injections and dosage levels administered. Despite the extra hassle, studies indicate that athletes and active individuals with type 1 diabetes have a decreased risk for cardiovascular disease, which is a major health issue for diabetics. The bottom line is that type 1 diabetic athletes can safely participate in all sports activities as long as they have learned how to control their blood glucose levels, there are no medical complications that would be exacerbated by athletic participation, and they have adopted consistent lifestyle strategies for dealing with their disease.[4]

How can athletes manage their diabetes and excel in sports?

Athletes who manage their diabetes well can excel in their sport and exercise activities. The main objective in managing diabetes is good blood glucose control on a daily basis. Maintaining a fasting glucose level of 70–100 on a regular basis is the primary focus of controlled diabetes.[3] This will prevent the two complications of most concern to diabetic athletes, hyperglycemia and **hypoglycemia**. Preventing hyperglycemia will help keep the athlete from developing some of the chronic diseases defined earlier in this chapter that are related to high circulating glucose levels. Hypoglycemia can be extremely dangerous at any time but is more likely to occur in athletes during and after exercise. To manage diabetes well, athletes need to be very disciplined in the consumption of healthy foods and the timing of food intake and insulin administration relative to exercise. Frequent self-

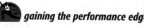

gaining the performance edge

The Diabetes Exercise and Sports Association (DESA) is a nonprofit organization dedicated to encouraging active lifestyles for people with diabetes. It provides education to its members and the public, provides support from other athletes, and promotes education and information exchange to coaches, athletic trainers, teachers, and the public about the positive effects of exercise on people with diabetes (see www.diabetes-exercise.org).

hypoglycemia A condition where blood glucose levels fall below normal.

monitoring of glucose levels prior to, during, and after exercise is a must.

How do athletes self-monitor glucose levels?

Self-monitoring of glucose levels in the blood and urine is essential to any person with diabetes. Self-monitoring on a frequent basis helps individuals determine whether they need to make changes in their diet, exercise program, and/or medications. Athletes should self-monitor more frequently than nonathletes so that they can learn how their sport activity and diet affect their glucose levels. Testing the urine for glucose is one way of self-monitoring. Urine glucose testing consists of placing a small amount of urine on a chemically treated test strip. A change in the color of the test strip indicates a high level of glucose in the urine. Urine tests are less informative to the athlete than blood tests, however, because they only indicate that glucose is spilling over into the urine because blood levels are high. It does not provide the actual blood glucose level.

The monitoring of blood glucose levels is more important to the athlete than urine glucose testing. Athletes can use portable blood glucose testing devices to accurately determine blood glucose levels. Information from this type of self-monitoring is essential to athletes with diabetes because it gives specific information about the actual level of glucose in the blood. The athlete pricks a finger and places a small droplet of blood on a chemically treated test strip. The test strip is inserted into the testing device, which reads the blood glucose level and provides a digital readout of the actual glucose level. This type of monitoring should be done regularly, usually at least once in the morning and several times throughout the day, particularly for individuals who are taking medications for diabetes. Athletes need additional testing prior to exercise, immediately after exercise, and several hours after exercise. Athletes are at risk for hypoglycemia not only during exercise, but also after exercise, when the risk for hypoglycemia may actually be increased. Decisions regarding the safety of initiating exercise and whether to make any adjustments to carbohydrate intake and insulin amounts are based on the preexercise monitoring of blood glucose (see **Table 15.2**).[4]

If the glucose level is greater than 250 mg/dL prior to exercise, the athlete should test the urine for ketones. To test the urine for ketones, a small amount of urine is placed on a chemically treated test strip. These test strips will change color if ketones are present. If ketones are present, exercise should not be ini-

TABLE 15.2	Preexercise Glucose Guidelines
Preexercise Glucose Level	**Recommendation**
<100 mg/dL	Ingest additional carbohydrates prior to initiating exercise: 15–40 g carbohydrates (or more) depending on actual glucose level and athlete's typical response to added carbohydrates.
>250 mg/dL	Test urine for ketones.
>250 mg/dL, with ketones	Do not exercise. Make insulin or medication adjustments and then retest glucose and ketones.
>250 mg/dL, without ketones present	Exercise can be initiated.
>300 mg/dL, without ketones present	Exercise with caution.

tiated until the glucose level is lowered and ketones are not present. A combination of high blood glucose with ketones in the urine can be dangerous and lead to ketoacidosis. Athletes with type 1 diabetes and those with type 2 taking insulin are more prone to this condition and should take additional insulin. It is important that the athlete allow enough time for blood glucose levels to fall before exercise starts. If the athlete's glucose level is greater than 300 mg/dL without ketones present, athletes should exercise with caution. Table 15.2 describes the considerations for these adjustments based on the level of glucose in the blood and ketones in the urine.

When glucose levels are low prior to exercise, then adjustments in insulin dosage and carbohydrate intake must be made, or exercise delayed until blood glucose levels are in a safe range (see Table 15.2). In general, a glucose level of less than 100 indicates that some adjustments should be made in either insulin injections or carbohydrate intake prior to exercise. Consuming a small amount of carbohydrates immediately prior to exercise when blood glucose levels are below 100 will help bring blood glucose up to a level that will be safe to initiate exercise. The amount of carbohydrates to consume at this time varies and depends on the individual athlete. Generally between 15 and 40 grams of carbohydrates will be adequate to bring the blood glucose level up enough to safely initiate exercise.

Monitoring blood glucose levels during exercise, especially exercise lasting greater than 60 minutes, is crucial to the diabetic athlete. It provides the athlete with ongoing information about how the exercise is affecting blood glucose levels and what adjustments need to be made. Any time significant changes in the type, intensity, or duration of exercise are made, close self-monitoring of blood glucose should occur. Once the athlete has a clear picture of how his or her body responds to the change, less frequent monitoring will be necessary. The athlete's physician or a **Certified Diabetes Educator (CDE)** should help with adjusting insulin or medication doses in response to exercise. These professionals can also make suggestions for adjusting preexercise and during-exercise carbohydrate intakes. Athletes may also want to meet with a registered dietitian to devise guidelines for total daily carbohydrate adjustments, as well as formulate specific dietary strategies to better prepare for training and/or competition.

Certified Diabetes Educator (CDE) An allied health professional who has passed a rigorous certification exam documenting his or her advanced knowledge and skills related to dealing with diabetes mellitus.

What are the nutrition recommendations for the athlete with diabetes?

Dietary recommendations for people with diabetes are very similar to healthy recommendations for the general population. The MyPlate food guidance system should serve as the basis for a healthful diet, diabetic or not. Athletes with diabetes should make the various MyPlate selections based on their individual food preferences, cultural food choices, and lifestyle. The basic starting point of a diabetic diet is to consume 45–65% of energy intake as carbohydrates.[5] Carbohydrates consumed in the form of sugars, starch, and fiber should be balanced throughout the day and consumed with a variety of other food groups. Small amounts of sugar or sugar-containing foods are allowed as long as sugar intake does not increase calorie intake above daily needs, thus causing weight gain. Sugary foods should also not replace more nutrient-dense carbohydrates on a regular basis. Protein intake in the range of 15–20%, similar to general athlete recommendations, should be adequate for athletes with diabetes.[5] Total fat intake should be less than 30% of total energy intake with less than 7% of total calories derived from saturated fats.[5] As noted earlier, the athlete may want to consult with a physician, a CDE, and/or a registered dietitian (RD) to help formulate the best diet based on his or her needs and the demands of his or her sport.

Athletes with diabetes should eat at approximately the same time each day and eat a similar amount of food in each meal or snack. There is no need to have a rigid schedule of food intake; however, eating at approximately the same time each day and not varying carbohydrate intake drastically from meal to meal will help maintain blood glucose levels in the recommended range (70–100 mg/dL). If more carbohydrates than usual are eaten, then adjustments in insulin dosage, for diabetics using insulin, can be made. However, determining how much to increase insulin dosage is a learning process and initially requires the athlete to test regularly and often to determine how his or her body responds to higher-than-normal carbohydrate intake. Diabetic athletes requiring insulin also need to learn how to match their carbohydrate intake and insulin dosages to ensure appropriate blood glucose levels are attained at the beginning of exercise. A sample meal plan for a diabetic female basketball player is listed in **Training Table 15.1**.

Diabetic athletes need to be aware of the amount of carbohydrates they are ingesting in a meal or snack. The type of carbohydrate (i.e., simple or complex, high or low glycemic index) is not as important as the total amount consumed. It was once thought that consumption of highly sugared foods caused a higher spike in blood glucose levels than did foods that contain starch or more complex carbohydrates. However, research has shown that in individuals with type 1 or type 2 diabetes, ingestion of either simple (e.g., sucrose) or complex (e.g., starch) carbohydrates does not cause significant differences in glycemic response.[6] Therefore, for diabetic athletes, the key consideration regarding carbohydrate intake during meals is the quantity of carbohydrates being consumed. This gives diabetic athletes freedom to choose various sources of carbohydrates in their diet as long as they pay attention to the amount of carbohydrates being eaten.[6]

Recently, the glycemic index has received considerable attention in both the scientific and popular press. As stated in Chapter 3, for nondiabetic athletes, low glycemic index foods are recommended before exercise, high glycemic snacks/drinks

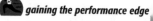
gaining the performance edge

Blood glucose response in diabetic athletes depends on the amount of carbohydrates ingested, not the type. When planning meals and snacks for before, during, or after exercise, carbohydrate content should be the primary consideration.

Training Table 15.1: Sample Meal Plan for a Type 1 Diabetic Athlete

Breakfast	Serving Size
Oatmeal	1 cup
Whole grain toast	2 slices
Peanut butter	2 tbsp
Orange	1 medium
Milk, 1%	1 cup
Total carbohydrates: 81 g	*Total calories: 650*

Lunch	Serving Size
Grilled chicken sandwich:	1
Whole wheat bun	4 oz
Chicken breast	1/2 raw
Tomato	1 tbsp
Light mayo	1 cup
Salad	1 tbsp
Salad dressing, fat-free	1 medium
Apple, raw	1 cup
Milk, 1%	*Total calories: 609*
Total carbohydrates: 80 g	

Dinner	Serving Size
Pork chop, loin, lean	3 oz
Red-skinned potatoes	2 small
Steamed asparagus	1 cup
Margarine	2 tsp
Pineapple chunks, water-packed	1 cup
Water or noncaloric beverage	2 cups
Total carbohydrates: 82 g	*Total calories: 685*

Snack	Serving Size
Pudding, vanilla, sugar-free	1 cup
Sliced strawberries	1/2 cup
Total carbohydrates: 30 g	*Total calories: 161*
Daily total carbohydrates: 273 g **(52% of total calories)**	**Daily total calories: 2105**

during exercise, and moderate-to-high glycemic index foods after exercise. However, this recommendation does not hold true for diabetic athletes. The glycemic index has not been shown to be of much value to people with diabetes; once again, it is the total amount of carbohydrates ingested and the timing of ingestion that are crucial.

What should athletes with diabetes eat during long exercise bouts?

Athletes with type 1 diabetes should have carbohydrates available during and after exercise. During exercise lasting more than 30 minutes, exercisers with type 1 diabetes should consume 15–30 grams of carbohydrates every 30–60 minutes. This can be accomplished by consuming sports drinks, sports gels, diluted juices, sports bars, and/or high-fiber cookies. The following examples all provide the 15–30 grams of carbohydrates appropriate for consumption during exercise:

- 8 oz sports drink, containing 6–8% carbohydrates
- 1 single-serving sports gel
- 1 fig bar
- 8 oz diluted juice, mixed in a 1:1 ratio of juice to water

Another question often asked by endurance diabetic athletes is whether it is appropriate to carbohydrate load. The answer is yes. The modified version of carbohydrate loading, which consists of eating a mixed diet of slightly lower carbohydrates (50% carbohydrates, 30% fat, 20% protein) 4–7 days prior to an event and then increasing carbohydrate intake 3 days prior to the event (up to 60–65% carbohydrates), would be the recommended method of carbohydrate loading. Because this method avoids drastic changes in carbohydrate intake, athletes who self-monitor regularly are better able to adjust their insulin or medication levels to maintain their blood glucose levels while carbohydrate loading. Before trying this method or any other dietary manipulation, however, the athlete should consult with a physician or endocrinologist to ensure good glucose control prior to carbohydrate loading.

How can athletes recognize, treat, and prevent diabetic emergencies during exercise?

Athletes with diabetes can exercise safely if they manage their diabetes well. In type 2 diabetes, with no medications, there should be very little concern of either hypo- or hyperglycemia during exercise. Conversely, any athlete who uses insulin, or type 2 diabetics who take oral medications for their diabetes, may be at risk for experiencing low or high blood glucose levels that could constitute a diabetic emergency. Hyperglycemia can occur as a result of severe insulin deficiency during exercise. This deficiency, when combined with the actions of other hormones that cause the liver to release more glucose into the bloodstream, can cause blood glucose levels to rise precipitously. The signs and symptoms of hyperglycemia are presented in **Table 15.3**.

To be prepared in case of hyperglycemia, the athlete must keep insulin and syringes readily available.

TABLE 15.3	Signs and Symptoms of Hypoglycemia and Hyperglycemia	
Hypoglycemia Signs/ Symptoms	**Hyperglycemia Signs/ Symptoms**	
Sweating	Nervousness	
Pounding heart	Restlessness	
Hunger	Thirst	
Shakiness	Fatigue	
Confusion	Blurred vision	
Lethargy	Muscle cramps	
Incoordination	Nausea	
Slurred or difficult speech	Abdominal pain	
Irritability		
Headache		
Nausea		

The storage and transport of insulin and syringes can be challenging because insulin needs to be kept cool, requiring a refrigerator or portable cooler. Syringes need to be kept secure and in a container to maintain hygiene and to avoid accidental needle sticks to other individuals. Medication adjustments based on high blood glucose levels should be established with the assistance of the athlete's physician.

Hypoglycemia can occur if too much insulin is circulating at the time of exercise. Excess insulin enables cells to uptake more glucose while also causing the liver to release too little glucose into the circulation. This results in too much glucose uptake into the cells and too little left circulating in the blood. The signs and symptoms of hypoglycemia are listed in Table 15.3. Carbohydrate foods should be available during and after exercise in case low blood glucose occurs. Consuming carbohydrates as needed during and immediately after exercise, and continuing intake for several hours after exercise, is the best prevention for hypoglycemia. Carrying a food bag that contains glucose tablets, juice, and regular soda for emergencies is essential for any diabetic athlete. Glucose tablets are particularly helpful to have on-hand because they are small, can be carried in a small pouch on the athlete, and are convenient for times when emergency glucose is needed. The athlete's physician, RD, or CDE can provide guidelines for amounts of carbohydrates to ingest in a hypoglycemic emergency. Sports professionals, friends, parents, and teammates can all help the athlete manage the diabetes. All of these individuals should know the warning signs and symptoms that are typical of low and high blood glucose levels so that they can help recognize and properly address symptoms during training or competition. This is important because in some situations the diabetic athlete may not be aware or recognize the symptoms on his or her own. The athlete's support group (and the athlete) should also know what to do in case of a diabetic emergency. Athletes should keep additional carbohydrate foods on hand before, during, and after exercise to prevent, and treat when necessary, low blood glucose levels. The athlete should inform the coach, athletic trainer, sports nutritionist, and teammates about where he or she keeps the food bag, glucose tablets, insulin, and syringes. In both hypoglycemia and hyperglycemia, calling emergency personnel to the scene may be necessary if self-monitoring and administration of either carbohydrates or insulin do not appear to be effective in alleviating the athlete's symptoms.

What are the special considerations for athletes who are pregnant?

When athletes become pregnant, some may choose to continue training and competing throughout a majority of their pregnancy. For example, Regan Scheiber, an All-American swimmer from Penn State, continued her training postcollege in pursuit of swimming the English Channel. In August 2001, she successfully competed this feat while in her 11th week of pregnancy.[7] This example may be on the extreme end of the spectrum; however, it demonstrates that athletes can continue to train during many months of pregnancy. Many athletes who are pregnant will choose to stay active but decrease their training level and intensity and may not compete, especially in the last two trimesters of pregnancy. Athletes who choose to stay active should be followed closely by their physicians, make modifications to their exercise regimens as medically indicated, and adjust their daily nutrition intake. The growth and development of a baby require adequate energy and proper nutrition. When an individual becomes an athlete, calorie, macronutrient, and micronutrient needs rise. If

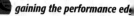

gaining the performance edge

With careful glucose monitoring, regular exercise, and a healthful eating plan, athletes with type 1 or type 2 diabetes should be able to lead an active, competitive life. Regular visits with medical personnel to monitor long-term glucose levels and to make adjustments in treatment regimens will help the athlete with diabetes remain healthy and active.

an athlete becomes pregnant, overall nutrient needs increase again, requiring a renewed focus on a well-balanced and appropriately planned diet.

Although all nutrients are important for the growth of a fetus, several dietary components are of special concern to active mothers. Specifically, pregnant athletes need to ensure the daily consumption of adequate calories, protein, B vitamins (especially folate), vitamin C, vitamin A, magnesium, and iron. The following sections provide the rationale for these increased requirements and suggestions for the development of an individualized nutrition plan for pregnant athletes.

How are an athlete's caloric requirements affected by pregnancy?

In general, athletes will require an additional 300 calories a day as compared to their prepregnancy diet, especially during the second and third trimesters. Because many athletes struggle to meet their own calorie needs, it can be challenging for some to meet the extra caloric demands of pregnancy. However, because training duration, intensity, and frequency often simultaneously, and appropriately, decrease throughout pregnancy, the increase in daily calories required may not be as great. However, special care should be taken to ensure that pregnant athletes are in fact consuming enough calories. Adequate calories from a well-balanced diet will prevent exercise-induced hypoglycemia, which can result in a multitude of problems for both the mother and fetus.

Calorie needs for endurance, strength, and team sport pregnant athletes should be calculated using the equations presented in previous chapters of this text, plus approximately 300 calories. It should be noted that 300 calories is an estimate and may vary among athletes. Similar to nonpregnant athletes involved in heavy training and competition, standard calculation estimates may need to be adjusted based on the individual's response and progression. Recent research has revealed that calorie needs during pregnancy can range from 25 calories per day up to 800 calories per day above prepregnancy values.[8] This is a huge range! If 300 calories a day is used across the board for all pregnant athletes, some women may gain too much weight while others fail to gain enough weight. Therefore, one of the best indicators of adequate calorie consumption is appropriate weight gain throughout pregnancy. In general, athletes should gain 25–35 pounds during the duration of a pregnancy, with variations based on prepregnancy weight (athletes with a BMI < 20 should aim

for a gain of 25–40 pounds), height (shorter athletes should aim for a gain at the low end of the range), and age (teen athletes should aim for the high end of the weight gain range).[9]

The increase in calorie needs during pregnancy can be met by increasing portion size slightly at meals or adding 1–2 small snacks throughout the day. For example, drinking a 12 oz glass of skim milk and eating a 6–8 oz yogurt would provide approximately 300 calories. Many athletes are unaware of the energy value of foods and therefore need assistance in understanding the total quantity of food to consume to obtain 300 calories to prevent under- or overestimation.

The athletes at highest risk for not meeting the energy demands of pregnancy are those in weight-restricted sports, those who were restricting calories with the intention of weight loss before pregnancy, and individuals with disordered eating. These high-risk athletes should work closely with a dietitian to ensure that calorie needs, as well as other macronutrient and micronutrient requirements, are being met. The dietitian should work as a team with the athlete's obstetrician/gynecologist to confirm that the athlete's current consumption level is resulting in the proper growth and development of the baby.

There are several consequences of inadequate calorie consumption. In the first trimester, low energy intake is associated with a higher risk of premature delivery, fetal death, and malformation of the fetal central nervous system. In the second and third trimesters, poor fetal growth and development are the main consequences of inadequate intake. In relation to an athlete's maintenance of fitness, low energy intakes will also lead to fatigue and the inability to recover from even light to moderate workout sessions. If athletes cannot continue to exercise and maintain fitness during pregnancy, making a comeback in their sport after the baby is delivered will be a challenging and potentially lengthy process.

How are an athlete's protein requirements affected by pregnancy?

An athlete's protein needs are increased slightly during pregnancy. Protein is critical for the development of fetal organs and tissues, as well as the maintenance of maternal tissues. In general, an additional 20–25 grams of protein should be consumed daily. The RDA for nonpregnant women is 46 grams/day (based on 0.8 grams of protein per kilogram of body weight), which increases to 71 grams during the second half of pregnancy (requirements in the first

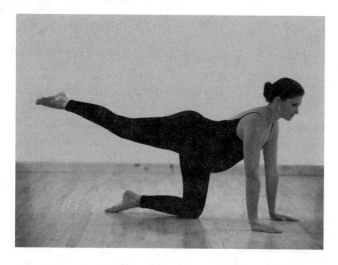

half of pregnancy remain equivalent to nonpregnant women).[10,11] Keep in mind these are baseline requirements, designed mainly for sedentary women. The difference in the baseline requirement is 25 grams; therefore, athletes can use this recommendation to increase their estimated protein needs for their activity level by about 25 grams when pregnant. As with calorie needs, if training duration, intensity, and frequency decline during pregnancy, protein needs may actually stay the same or increase minimally.

An additional 25 grams of protein can easily be obtained through a balanced diet. The consumption of any one of the following would provide 20–25 grams of protein:

- 24 oz skim milk
- 3 oz beef, chicken, or fish
- 1 1/2 cups beans, lentils, or other legumes
- 3 oz nuts

An athlete's success in meeting protein needs is often directly correlated to her energy intake; if calorie intake is low, protein intake is typically low. By increasing total food consumption, from a variety of different food groups, protein needs can be met. Pregnant athletes should not rely on protein supplements to meet daily requirements. Supplements often will provide large quantities of protein, vitamins, and/or minerals that can interfere with the absorption of other nutrients. By focusing on a variety of whole foods, protein needs can be met while also encouraging the athlete to continue meal planning, which will be a critical skill for the whole family once the baby is born.

Inadequate protein intake will affect the mother as well as the baby. Similar to nonpregnant athletes, low protein intake will affect muscle development, immune function, and recovery from exercise. If protein, as well as caloric, intake is low, muscle tissue will be used for energy, altering the body composition of the athlete and affecting her ability to maintain fitness. A lower immune function can endanger the mother's health, thus affecting the health and continued development of the baby. Low protein intakes can also negatively affect the recovery process after exercise sessions, increasing muscle soreness and overall fatigue.

Although protein requirements increase during pregnancy, carbohydrate and fat needs remain proportionately the same. Carbohydrates are still the main source of energy for the mother and fetus. In fact, the respiratory exchange ratio (RER) for active women has been shown to increase during pregnancy, hovering around 1.0.[12–14] This RER value represents a preferential use of carbohydrates versus fats. Therefore, it is important for pregnant athletes to continue eating a moderate to high carbohydrate diet (50–65% of total calories) to provide energy for the growth of the fetus, provide energy for maternal exercise, and prevent ketosis, which can be harmful to the baby.[12] Adequate fiber intake is especially important in preventing constipation and hemorrhoids, which are common during pregnancy. Fat is a good source of concentrated calories and essential fatty acids, and allows for the absorption of fat-soluble vitamins during pregnancy. Overall, a well-balanced diet, with increased calories and protein, will provide the nutrients an athlete needs to produce a healthy baby.

How are an athlete's B vitamin requirements affected by pregnancy?

B vitamins are critical for energy production and tissue development throughout the body of both the mother and the fetus. Thiamin, riboflavin, and niacin needs are slightly increased for athletes and increase again during pregnancy to aid in energy production. Vitamin B_{12} is involved in DNA and red blood cell synthesis, while vitamin B_6 aids in the metabolism of amino acids; daily requirements of both of these nutrients increase slightly during pregnancy. However, the B vitamin deserving the most attention before and during pregnancy is folate.

Folate, or folic acid, plays a role in DNA synthesis, red blood cell production, and the development of the nervous system. Athletes who are thinking about becoming pregnant should begin to monitor their folate intake months before conception to ensure that adequate stores are available at the onset of fertilization. The reason for this focus on meeting folate requirements relates to the development of the fetal nervous system. Adequate intake of folate has been shown to dramatically decrease the risk of neural tube defects in children. The critical stages of neural tube formation occur within the first month after conception—which is typically before a woman knows she is pregnant. If a woman waits to change her eating habits until after she has confirmation of fertilization, she will have missed the window of opportunity to positively affect her baby's health. A focus on folate should occur early and continue throughout pregnancy.

The folate requirements for pregnant women increase from a prepregnancy guideline of 400 micrograms to 600 micrograms during pregnancy.[11,15] Folate can be obtained by consuming a balanced diet containing plenty of fruits, vegetables, and legumes as well as through fortified foods and folic acid supplements. Some of the richest sources of folate are orange juice, strawberries, green leafy vegetables, beans, lentils, and fortified grains. For example, 1 cup of cooked lentils contains about 320 micrograms of folate, which is slightly over half of a pregnant athlete's daily requirement.

Low folate intake will also begin to affect the mother. Active moms need folate for DNA synthesis in relation to red blood cell development. If folate intake is low, megaloblastic anemia can occur, causing the pregnant athlete to feel weak and fatigued. Other signs and symptoms include depression, irritability, and disturbed sleep. A fatigued athlete will not have the energy to keep up with workouts, grocery shop, prepare meals, and continue other healthy behaviors for both the mother and fetus.

How are an athlete's vitamin C requirements affected by pregnancy?

Vitamin C requirements increase minimally during pregnancy. Vitamin C plays a role in collagen formation, hormone synthesis, and proper immune function. Increased vitamin C intake also positively affects the absorption of iron—another nutrient critical for a healthy baby. Vitamin C requirements increase from 75 milligrams to 80–85 milligrams during pregnancy.[11,16] Athlete mothers also benefit from this increase because of the antioxidant functions of vitamin C, aiding in recovery from exercise sessions. Vitamin C is found in foods that conveniently are also good sources of folate: orange juice, strawberries, green leafy vegetables, and some fortified cereals. In general, a strong focus on fruits and vegetables will help an athlete mother achieve her daily vitamin C needs. For example, 1 cup of orange juice contains about 80 milligrams of vitamin C—nearly the entire daily requirement! Therefore, vitamin C supplements are not necessary during pregnancy unless a dietary deficiency exists.

An athlete mother should be aware of the maternal signs of low vitamin C, such as swollen, bleeding gums or fatigue, and work to reverse any deficiencies as soon as possible. Because of its independent and supportive roles (nonheme iron absorption) for both the mother and fetus, a focus on vitamin C should ideally begin before, and continue throughout, pregnancy. Because the increased requirement during pregnancy is small, and vitamin C can easily be obtained through a well-balanced diet, there should be no reason why a pregnant athlete cannot meet her needs.

How are an athlete's vitamin A requirements affected by pregnancy?

Vitamin A requirements increase slightly during pregnancy to assist in cell differentiation and proper immune function. Because vitamin A is a fat-soluble vitamin and therefore can be stored in the body and become toxic, mothers should focus on food sources of vitamin A and avoid supplements.

Vitamin A requirements increase from the prepregnancy level of 700 micrograms (RAE) to 750–770 micrograms (RAE) during pregnancy.[11,17] Similar to vitamin C and folate, vitamin A is most concentrated in fruits and vegetables. Specific foods considered to be excellent sources of vitamin A include spinach, broccoli, tomato juice, carrots, and sweet potatoes.

Beta-carotene, a provitamin form of vitamin A, has also been shown to have antioxidant effects in the body. Active mothers will benefit from adequate vitamin A intake through a stronger immune system, enhanced recovery from exercise, and optimal bone health. However, it should be emphasized that "more" is not necessarily "better" in relation to vitamin A intake; excessive amounts can actually be detrimental to the health of both the mother and fetus. An excessive intake of vitamin A can cause urogenital abnormalities, ear malformations, cleft palate, and neural tube defects in the fetus.[18] By focusing on whole foods, overdoses of vitamin A are generally avoided.

How are an athlete's magnesium requirements affected by pregnancy?

Magnesium has garnered attention recently in the athletic world because of its roles in enzyme and adenosine triphosphate (ATP) production, bone development and maintenance, as well as protein synthesis and muscle contraction. For these same reasons, magnesium requirements increase slightly for women during pregnancy. Once again, there is an overlap of foods that are good sources of magnesium as well as other macro- and micronutrients important during pregnancy.

For women 19–30 and 31–70 years of age, the basic requirement for magnesium is 310 and 320 milligrams per day, respectively. During pregnancy, the requirement increases 40 milligrams a day for all ages.[11,19] Magnesium is generally found in protein-rich foods, providing a two-for-one bonus for pregnant women because protein needs are also increased. The following foods are good to excellent sources of magnesium: whole wheat bread, yogurt, tofu, dried beans, almonds, cashews, peanut butter, and some fish species. Spinach is also an excellent source, providing a four-for-one punch because it is also a good source of folate, vitamin C, and vitamin A. Halibut is an example of a fish that is rich in magnesium—a 6-ounce serving provides about 180 milligrams, which is about 50% of the daily needs for pregnant women of all ages.

If pregnant athletes have low magnesium levels, they may experience several types of symptoms. The first signs are generally loss of appetite, nausea, and weakness. However, these signs are also similar to morning sickness, and therefore symptoms may or may not be caused by low magnesium intake. Morning sickness can indirectly cause low magnesium levels if mothers are chronically vomiting, which can lead to magnesium deficiency over time. Therefore, a consultation with a physician is warranted if morning sickness is severe or continues for an extended period of time. If a true magnesium deficiency develops, the later stages will cause symptoms such as irritability and muscle cramps. Muscle cramps may be experienced more by athletes than sedentary mothers, especially during normal training or exercise sessions. Muscle cramps are another symptom with multiple potential causes, such as dehydration, and therefore mothers should consider all options to ensure that the symptoms are addressed appropriately. If an athlete believes she is low in magnesium, whole foods versus supplements should be the focus. Excessive doses of magnesium can become toxic and lead to respiratory paralysis and death.

How are an athlete's iron requirements affected by pregnancy?

Iron requirements for athletes increase substantially during pregnancy. Iron contributes to the proper development of a baby through energy metabolism, the production of red blood cells, and overall normal growth. Similar to total calories, female athletes generally struggle to meet iron needs before pregnancy; therefore, the increased requirements with pregnancy pose an extra challenge.

Before pregnancy, women should aim for 18 milligrams of iron per day; during pregnancy the goal is boosted up to 27 milligrams per day.[11,17] This quantity of iron can be difficult, but not impossible, for women to actually achieve with consistency on a daily basis. Because of this challenge, iron-deficiency anemia is one of the most common nutrient deficiencies during pregnancy. Iron-rich foods that should be eaten daily include beef, chicken, turkey, fish, legumes, and iron-fortified grains.

As always, the focus should be on iron-rich whole foods first to meet daily needs; however, even with a balanced diet, supplemental iron is often indicated. Iron is typically present in prenatal and pregnancy multivitamins/minerals. Some pregnant athletes may need even more iron than the amount supplied in a standard multivitamin/mineral, requiring an individual iron supplement. However, pregnant athletes should consult with their physician before taking iron supplements because an overdose of iron can be as harmful as a deficiency. High iron intakes can result in diarrhea, constipation, nausea, decreased absorption of other critical nutri-

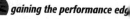

gaining the performance edge

In addition to increased calorie, protein, and certain vitamin and mineral requirements, pregnant athletes should also ensure adequate consumption of fluids, especially during exercise, to aid in thermoregulation. By staying hydrated and cool, the risk for congenital abnormalities resulting from high core body temperature will decrease.[20]

gaining the performance edge

All nutrients are important during pregnancy; however, a special focus should be placed on total calories, protein, folate, vitamin C, vitamin A, magnesium, and iron from whole food sources. These nutrients will ensure the development of a healthy baby while also supporting the mother's quest for maintaining fitness. **Table 15.4** provides an overview of the nutrient requirement changes during pregnancy. The Power-Packed Pregnancy Burritos presented in Training Table 15.2 are a good source of all of the nutrients important during pregnancy.

TABLE 15.4 Differences in Nutrient Needs for Pregnant and Nonpregnant Women

Nutrient	Nonpregnant Recommendation	Pregnant Recommendation
Protein	46 g/day	71 g/day
Folate	400 µg/day	600 µg/day
Vitamin C	14–18 yrs: 75 mg/day	14–18 yrs: 80 mg/day
	19–50 yrs: 75 mg/day	19–50 yrs: 85 mg/day
Vitamin A	14–18 yrs: 700 RAE µg/day	14–18 yrs: 750 RAE µg/day
	19–50 yrs: 700 RAE µg/day	19–50 yrs: 770 RAE µg/day
Magnesium	14–18 yrs: 360 mg/day	14–18 yrs: 400 mg/day
	19–30 yrs: 310 mg/day	19–30 yrs: 350 mg/day
	31–70 yrs: 320 mg/day	31–70 yrs: 360 mg/day
Iron	18 mg/day	27 mg/day

Training Table 15.2: Power-Packed Pregnancy Burritos

2 tbsp olive oil

1 tbsp minced garlic

5 oz frozen spinach ($^1/_2$ box), thawed and drained

2 cups fresh broccoli, chopped

$^1/_2$ medium red onion, diced

1–2 cups canned black beans

1 lb lean sirloin steak, cut into strips, or firm tofu, cut into $^1/_2$-inch squares

1 tbsp chili powder

1 tsp ground cumin

$^1/_2$ tsp garlic salt

8 whole-wheat tortillas

1. Place 1 tbsp of olive oil in a large skillet and add garlic, spinach, broccoli, and onions. Cook 3–5 minutes over medium heat or until tender.

2. If using steak, remove vegetables from the skillet, place in a bowl, and cover with aluminum foil to keep warm. Then place 1 tbsp olive oil and the steak strips in the skillet, cover, and cook 8–10 minutes until cooked through, stirring occasionally. When the steak is done, add the vegetables back to the skillet, add the beans and spices, stir to mix, and cook over low heat for several minutes until warm. Fill one tortilla with $^1/_8$ of the mixture and serve.

3. If using tofu, add the beans, tofu, and spices to the vegetables, stir to mix, and cook over low heat for several minutes until warm. Fill one tortilla with $^1/_8$ of the mixture and serve. Makes 4 servings.

Nutrition Information (per serving):

	Steak	Tofu
Calories	810 kcal	640 kcal
Protein	64 g	28 g
Folate	107 µg (18% RDA)	122 µg (20% RDA)
Vitamin C	45 mg (53–56% RDA)	45 mg (53–56% RDA)
Vitamin A	510 RE (66–68% RDA)	510 RE (66–68% RDA)
Magnesium	70 mg (18–20% RDA)	83 mg (21–24% RDA)
Iron	10 mg (37% RDA)	7 mg (26% RDA)

ents, and for those with hemochromatosis, organ damage or death.

Nonheme iron's bioavailability is enhanced by eating other foods or products containing vitamin C. For example, drinking a glass of orange juice with an iron-fortified cereal will aid in the absorption of the iron in the cereal. Iron absorption can be inhibited by calcium, tannins in tea, phytic acid in grains, or excessive fiber. Therefore, pregnant athletes should consume foods rich in these nutrients in small amounts when consuming a good source of iron (see **Training Table 15.2**).

What are the special considerations for child and teen athletes?

Children are participating in sports at very young ages—from organized peewee football and soccer leagues to a variety of school, club, and other organized sports. Sports provide children and teens with excellent opportunities to build strong muscles and bones as well as confidence and self-esteem. Participation in athletics at a young age can promote health and fitness, establish lifelong healthy activity patterns, and provide for personal development

skills in youngsters. In regard to nutrition, child and teen athletes require adequate daily intake to support a healthy rate of growth and maturation while also meeting the increased energy demands for sport and exercise activities. For the purposes of this chapter, child or teen athletes are defined as those 9–18 years of age.

How does nutrition affect growth and maturation in the child or teen athlete?

Energy needs and caloric intake are of primary importance in supporting growth in children participating in competitive or recreational sports. The growth and maturation process should follow a linear progression with age. Ensuring adequate nutrition to keep growth on the correct progressive track is essential for child and adolescent athletes.

Evaluation of growth is most often accomplished by performing height and weight assessments at regular intervals. This information is compared by age to standardized tables; most U.S. medical facilities use the 2000 Centers for Disease Control and Prevention (CDC) growth charts and Body Mass Index (BMI) charts. The CDC charts are a revised edition of the 1977 National Center for Health Statistics growth charts that were in use prior to the 2000 release of the CDC charts. The newer versions revised the previous 14 charts and consist of 16 charts (8 for boys and 8 for girls) plus two new body mass index-for-age charts for boys and girls ages 2–20 (refer to Appendix E).[21] Figure 15.2 shows a sample weight-for-age chart for boys from 2–20 years of age. The CDC growth charts are used to identify growth patterns as the child ages by comparison to his or her peers, or the "norm." Height, weight, and head circumference measures at regular intervals should be plotted on these charts for each child. This provides a way to determine the trends of growth patterns and aids in health assessment if there is a substantial increase or decrease in the percentiles.

Children past the age of 2 usually maintain their height and weight growth between the same percentiles (such as 50th–75th) during preschool and early childhood years.[22] This consistent height-to-weight growth pattern is often referred to as the **growth channel**. During puberty the growth patterns may not follow as clear of a linear path because of the radical growth spurts that occur at this time. It is cause for investigation if the height or weight of the child falls significantly above or below the growth channel. There is cause for concern of potential nutritional inadequacy or other medical or genetic anomalies if the infant or child is below the 5th percentile or above the 95th percentile on the growth charts.

Growth trends can help determine the nutrition status of a child. Weight in relation to height assesses current nutritional status and growth. This measure is better for assessing current nutrition status than weight-for-age because body weight is dependent on total body size, not age. The height measure at a given age is an indicator of previous nutrition status and growth status. A reduction in the height trend develops more slowly than a reduction in the weight trend and thus can be an indicator of chronic undernutrition. The most important way to assess the child or adolescent athlete's growth is through the trend of growth pattern. This may also reflect the adequacy of energy intake for that athlete's physical activity level.

Growth in adolescence occurs in spurts, with significant growth and leveling off throughout adolescent years. Height growth is linear, with boys growing approximately 8 inches and girls 6 inches during puberty.[23] Significant weight increases in adolescence often occur after the major height growth spurt; however, they can occur throughout the adolescent growth period as well. The main growth spurt in girls occurs approximately 1 year prior to menarche, or the onset of menstruation. Weight gains can be concerning for young athletes. These athletes need to be reassured that height and weight gains are normal and a healthy part of their development.

As mentioned, growth rates are closely related to sexual maturation in adolescence. Development of sex organs, pubic hair, breast tissue (girls), and voice changes (boys) are all signs of sexual growth and maturation. Typical growth spurts begin at approximately 10 1/2 to 11 years of age in girls, with peak in the rate of growth at age 12. For boys, growth spurts typically begin around 12 1/2 to 13 and peak at age 14.[24] Children who are tall prior to sexual maturation have a higher predicted adult height. A shorter child who already possesses sexual maturation characteristics is likely to be a shorter adult as well. Growth of the skeleton is complete when the **epiphyses** (growth plates) at the long ends of the bones close. A poorly nourished athlete who is small of stature at the point of epiphyses closure may not achieve his or her full potential adult height.

Youngsters competing in gymnastics, wrestling, and other sports that emphasize strict weight standards may be at greater risk of growth disorders. Paying close attention to growth trends in child athletes in these types of sports can help prevent growth delays and potential reduction in adult height. Fe-

growth channel The normal height-to-weight growth pattern/ relationship. It is used to assess a child's growth trends and to screen for any potential growth abnormalities.

epiphysis A cartilaginous plate found near the ends of bones that enables bone to grow in length; also known as the growth plate.

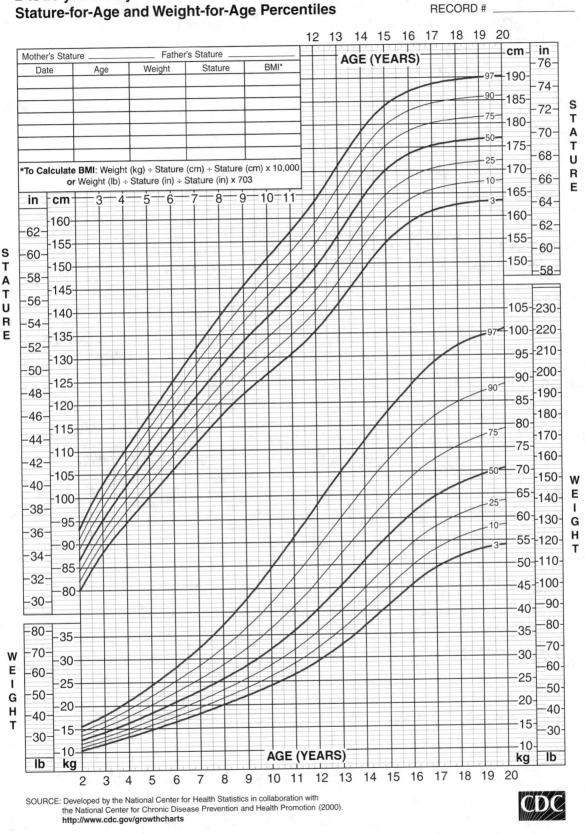

2 to 20 years: Boys
Stature-for-Age and Weight-for-Age Percentiles

NAME _____

RECORD # _____

Mother's Stature _____ Father's Stature _____

Date	Age	Weight	Stature	BMI*

*To Calculate BMI: Weight (kg) ÷ Stature (cm) ÷ Stature (cm) x 10,000
or Weight (lb) ÷ Stature (in) ÷ Stature (in) x 703

AGE (YEARS)

STATURE

WEIGHT

SOURCE: Developed by the National Center for Health Statistics in collaboration with
the National Center for Chronic Disease Prevention and Health Promotion (2000).
http://www.cdc.gov/growthcharts

CDC

Figure 15.2   Boys tend to have a marked increase in stature and weight between the ages of 12^1/$_2$ and 14 years.
Source: Developed by the National Center for Health Statistics in collaboration with the National Center for Chronic Disease Prevention and Health Promotion (2000). Available at: http://www.cdc.gov/growthcharts. Accessed January 22, 2011.

What are the special considerations for child and teen athletes?   **473**

male adolescent gymnasts are consistently found to be shorter of stature, weigh less, and have lower body fat percentages than same-age controls or female athletes participating in less strenuous sports. A study of female gymnasts and swimmers conducted over a 2–3 year interval found that gymnasts had significantly lower growth velocities than swimmers.[25] The gymnasts trained for 22 hours each week compared to 8 hours each week for the swimmers. A different study also found slower growth velocities in adolescent female gymnasts.[26] The girls in this study did not have the typical pubertal growth spurt seen in the inactive controls, and 27% of the gymnasts had less than expected adult heights.

Moderate activity is associated with cardiovascular benefits, positive changes in body composition, and development of bone density. However, excessive physical activity during childhood and adolescence may negatively affect growth and adolescent development.[27] High levels of intense physical activity, as seen in the Theintz study,[25] appear to have effects on growth in some athletes. The nutritional intake of young athletes may also have positive or negative effects on growth. When energy intake matches energy needs, then continued maturation and growth are likely to occur. However, restrictive eating and dieting behaviors in young athletes are likely to negatively affect their growth. Restricting dietary intake to maintain a thin appearance at a time when adequate intake is essential to growth (especially around puberty) can not only restrict growth, but also decrease the nutrients needed for bone mineral accrual. With dietary energy restriction, calcium, vitamin D, iron, and other nutrients necessary for bone density may be limited as well.

For young athletes, the bottom line is to eat enough calories and protein to support growth and enough variety to maintain a wide base of nutrients in the diet. Dietary intake of adequate energy, using the MyPlate food guidance system food groups and serving sizes, will help the young athlete eat adequate energy and nutrients to support all growth functions. Emphasis on complex carbohydrates, adequate protein sources, and moderate fat intake with a variety of foods will provide a complement of nutrients for muscle and bone development. Eating the minimum number of servings per day in each of the food groups, consuming a variety of foods within the food groups, and meeting calorie demands with additional foods from the food groups and some discretionary calories should provide adequate nutrition for growth and development. There is enough flexibility within each food group to allow even the most finicky child to find a choice he or she likes. Calorie needs are based on each individual's hunger and growth. As a child goes through a growth spurt, hunger increases, and he or she should be encouraged to eat more to satisfy hunger. Providing higher-calorie, nutrient-dense meals and snacks during high-growth and high-exercise times will help the child athlete maintain appropriate growth and nutrient intake. Conversely, when growth is slow, hunger and total dietary intake may not be as high.

Establishing a regular meal schedule and providing snacks before practice or after school allow the young athlete to eat when needed to maintain energy levels. The parents or caregivers are responsible for ensuring that a nutrient-rich diet with adequate energy is available for the child. Children can be finicky eaters, and it may be difficult to get them to eat enough nutritious foods during mealtime to meet energy demands. Providing nutrient-dense snacks can help picky eaters consume adequate nutrients even when meal consumption is not optimal. A list of snack options is found in **Table 15.5**. These snacks can be made available in the home; carried with the child for a postschool, prepractice snack; and packed for traveling to sporting events.

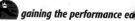

gaining the performance ea

Young athletes need to consume adequate calories to achieve proper height and weight growth. Establishing a regular meal schedule and providing snacks throughout the day will help the child or teen athlete meet dietary needs.

TABLE 15.5	Healthy Snack Options for Young Athletes
Pudding cups	Peanut butter and whole grain crackers
Yogurt	Graham crackers
Smoothies	Whole grain cereal or granola bars
Cheese cubes	Dry cereals
String cheese	Fig bars
Milk/chocolate milk	
Soy milk	
100% fruit juices	
Dried cherries, peaches, apricots, apples	
Raisins	

Are fluid needs for young athletes different from those of adult athletes?

Athletes of any age need proper hydration before, during, and after exercise. Adequate hydration is especially important for child and adolescent athletes for several reasons. Children are less tolerant of heat than adults. Their body surface area is greater as it relates to body weight and absorbs heat from the environment more readily than adults.[28] Children also produce more heat during exercise while sweating less than adults. Because of these factors, special attention should be placed on ensuring that youth and teen athletes are adequately hydrated.

Children may not drink enough fluid even when offered frequently, especially in the heat. To prevent dehydration in young athletes, several strategies can be implemented. Giving each athlete his or her own sports bottle is a way of measuring intake and encouraging adequate hydration. Frequent fluid breaks during practices and competitions along with encouragement from coaches and parents help increase overall fluid consumption. Children should be asked to consume fluids when they are thirsty and until thirst is quenched. Children under the age of 10 may need more reminders to drink adequately than older children. Providing palatable beverages can enhance a child's willingness to drink.[29] Sweet-tasting beverages, such as sports drinks, are often preferred by children; however, as with any athlete, specific flavor preferences will occur. Children should test out a variety of flavors, and parents, coaches, and other sport staff should ensure that these drinks are available and that ample hydration breaks are offered to consume these beverages. Similar to adults, weighing before and after practices and competitions can help determine whether young athletes are consuming adequate amounts of fluids. Athletes who consistently lose 1–2% of body weight during practice should be encouraged to consume more fluids and monitored more carefully by coaches and parents.

gaining the performance edge

Child athletes are at higher risk for dehydration and heat illness during exercise than adults. Offering fluid breaks often, monitoring fluid intake during practice and competitions, and providing flavored beverages during and after practices or competitions will help the young athlete maintain fluid balance.

Do young athletes require higher vitamin and mineral intake?

In general, children who meet energy needs for growth and maturation will consume adequate vitamins and minerals in their daily diets. However, iron and calcium are two minerals that have been identified as being deficient in the diets of children and teens, particularly in young female athletes.[28] Active young female athletes are likely to require more energy and macronutrients to meet the higher demands of sports participation. It is likely that female athletes also have increased needs for calcium and iron, especially during peak growth spurts around puberty and sexual maturation periods. Physical activity and adequate nutrition in younger years allow for optimal bone development during adolescence and adulthood.

The RDA for calcium in males and females aged 9–18 years is 1300 mg/day compared with 1000 mg/day for most adults.[30] The requirement of 1300 mg/day is a rather large amount for children and teens to consume on a daily basis. Children who consume dairy products are likely to meet this level of calcium intake. They should be encouraged to consume at least three servings of dairy daily. Additional calcium intake can be achieved with consumption of calcium-fortified orange juice, many fortified cereals and breads, and fortified soy milk. Adequate calcium in the diet is essential for future bone health because peak bone mass is likely to be achieved in the late 20s or early 30s. Calcium, vitamin D, and magnesium are minerals that are needed regularly in the diet of young people to help achieve peak bone mass. Weight-bearing physical activity in youth also positively affects bone development and achievement of maximal bone mineral density.

Iron requirements are increased during puberty. Iron is essential for the development of muscle and bone for all children, and needs are increased for the active young athlete. The RDA for iron for girls and boys aged 9–13 years is 8 mg/day.[17] For teens aged 14–18, the RDA is 11 mg/day for males and 15 mg/day for females.[17] Females require more iron to account for blood lost during menstruation. The increased need for iron during the 14–18 year age group correlates with the timing of sexual maturation and accelerated growth rates. Increased iron intake supports the increase in body mass, blood volume to maintain the additional mass, and hemoglobin and myoglobin in the cells. Poor iron status was found in nonendurance athletes such as gymnasts, tennis players, and table tennis players, and male gymnasts were found to be particularly prone to nonanemic iron deficiency in a study of elite young athletes aged 12–18 years.[31] Although true anemia is rare in most young athletes, iron deficiency can produce consequences such as fatigue and impaired growth that can significantly affect sport performance.

Teen athletes can meet dietary iron recommendations by consuming a wide variety of foods with iron and consuming adequate calories. Iron-fortified cereals, breads, bagels, granola bars, and sports bars are excellent options that kids typically enjoy eating. A once-daily multivitamin/mineral for teens may help supplement the dietary iron consumed in foods. This can also help with calcium ingestion. The Tolerable Upper Intake Level (UL) for iron for the 14–18 year age group is 45 mg/day. Parents should be careful to instruct their young athletes to take only a once-daily supplement to avoid overconsumption of iron from both the diet and supplements.

What are the special considerations for college athletes?

For many athletes, college presents the first opportunity to live life "on their own." Therefore, athletes are suddenly in charge of food selection, meal planning, and even grocery shopping. Individuals need to learn how to make healthy food choices and balance their intake to meet the increased energy demands from highly competitive practices and competitions. Collegiate athletes also need to navigate the social aspects of college that may involve the use of alcohol, including its deleterious effects on their nutrition status and sport performance.

Are college athletes' energy needs higher than their precollege needs?

Many college athletes participated in three sports and trained year-round in high school. Depending on the level and intensity of training, those multiple-sport high school athletes had extremely high calorie needs and, therefore, becoming a collegiate athlete will not increase calorie demands dramatically. Other collegiate athletes focused on one sport in high school, training and competing seasonally, with long offseasons and preseason training regimens. When these athletes enter college, a change

in training regimens to fewer days off, more competitions, and potentially higher daily activity levels could drastically increase energy needs for the athlete.

Daily walking on campus and busy class schedules may increase baseline energy expenditure. Often, incoming freshmen are not allowed to have cars on campus, so they may have to walk or bike to classes. Some campuses are very large and buildings are spread out over several miles. Practice facilities and playing fields may also be far from residence halls, apartment complexes, and classrooms where college athletes spend most of their time. Getting to and from all of these places is likely to increase energy expenditure and thus energy needs.

Compared to most high school programs, college athletic programs represent a major leap in athleticism and, as a result, incorporate more rigorous strength and conditioning requirements. Although strength and conditioning at the high school level may have been an integral part of some of the more traditional contact sports (e.g., football, wrestling, basketball, hockey), it may not have been as common in other competitive sports (e.g., tennis, swimming, baseball, softball). As a result, the physical demands on the high school athlete transitioning into college may increase substantially, thereby requiring additional calories. Furthermore, increased training usually results in larger muscles, which also increase energy expenditure. As discussed previously, muscle is metabolically active tissue and thus any increases in muscle mass will increase one's total daily energy expenditure.

The physical demands of high-level competition dictate that athletes continue to work on improving—or at a minimum, maintaining—physical conditioning throughout the year. This means that athletes have only brief periods of time off from training. Even in the off-season, most coaches provide their athletes with strength and conditioning programs. The intent is to ensure continued athletic development, even when not under the direct auspices of the sport coach. The physical rigor of being a competitive athlete demands ongoing training, increased energy expenditure, and attention to good nutritional practices.

The combination of higher-intensity training, strength training, daily energy expenditure, and year-round training may equate to high total daily calorie needs for college athletes. Most athletes will find themselves hungry often and will increase caloric intake by eating more at meals and snack times. Many residence hall cafeterias and training tables for athletes offer unlimited buffet-style eating at each meal. College athletes should have the selection and amount of food available to meet additional energy demands in dorm cafeterias. For example, André is a freshman football player at a Division II college. He is 6′3″ tall and weighs 245 lbs. His estimated calorie needs are 4700 per day. He eats in his dorm cafeteria for breakfast and lunch, and with the team at the training table for his evening meal. He is allowed to "carry out" snacks from the training table cafeteria to consume during the day or in the evening. A sample one-day meal plan for André is shown in **Training Table 15.3**.

André is able to meet his calorie needs by increasing calorie- and nutrient-dense beverages (milk, chocolate milk, juices), entrées and side dishes (honey-glazed chicken, baked beans, vegetarian pizza, scrambled eggs), and nutrient- and calorie-dense snacks and desserts (pudding, smoothies, muffins, and crackers). It is important for André to focus on nutrient-rich foods that also have a higher calorie level rather than choosing high-sugar, high-fat, or fried foods and snacks that are high in calories but low in nutrient density.

What are practical tips for the implementation of a college athlete's meal plan?

Most freshman college athletes are choosing for the first time when, how much, where, and what they will eat all day long. This can be a challenge in a college cafeteria environment where huge varieties, and portions, of food are available daily. However, there are many nutritious offerings in a college cafeteria setting. The variety and flexibility of a cafeteria are essential for athletes who have busy practice schedules and demanding academic schedules to juggle. For athletes in apartments, the challenge can be shopping and preparing meals that meet energy and nutrient needs. This needs to be accomplished on an oftentimes limited budget, especially for athletes not on full scholarships.

Making a plan for eating, whether in a cafeteria, at a training table, or in an apartment, is necessary for all athletes' good nutritional health. The plan should include meals and snacks at regular intervals, starting with breakfast, and should focus on a wide variety of foods. Athletes should eat breakfast daily, "breaking the fast" from the overnight sleep. Typical breakfast foods are high in nutrients and provide

Training Table 15.3: Andre's 1-Day Meal Plan

Food Item	Calories
Breakfast	
3 scrambled eggs	188
2 slices whole grain toast	147
2 tsp margarine	67
16 oz orange juice	189
1 cup milk, 1%	105
	Total breakfast: 696
Snack	
1 small blueberry muffin	242
16 oz bottle cranberry juice cocktail	258
	Total snack: 500
Lunch	
2 personal size vegetarian pizzas	1099
	150
Raw vegetables with 2 tbsp Ranch dressing	215
	Total lunch: 1464
12 oz chocolate milk, 1%	
Prepractice Snack	
12 oz low-fat yogurt fruit smoothie	345
	219
1 granola bar	*Total snack: 564*
Dinner	
2 honey-glazed chicken breasts	436
	314
1½ cups baked beans	241
1½ cups cooked corn	159
1 cup butterscotch pudding	125
1 cup milk, 2%	*Total dinner: 1275*
Snack	
Crackers, 12 whole grain	140
2 oz cheese	165
	Total snack: 305
	Daily Calorie Total: 4804

the athlete with the energy needed to start the day. Breakfast can top off glycogen levels and provide the energy needed to get to early eight o'clock classes or team workouts. It can be tempting to sleep in and wake up just in time to rush to early classes without breakfast. A common reason college athletes give for skipping breakfast is the lack of time. However, breakfast does not have to be time-consuming. Many nutritious breakfast items can be kept right in the dorm room or apartment for quick breakfast meals. A few breakfast options include:

- Bagel with 2 tbsp peanut butter or cream cheese
- Yogurt cup and 1 cup juice
- Cold cereal, 1 cup milk, and a banana
- Oatmeal packet, raisins, and 1 cup milk
- Cereal or granola bar and 1 cup milk
- Whole grain toast, 1 cup cottage cheese, 1 cup juice

A refillable cup or mug with a tight-fitting lid and a box of zipper sandwich bags can help athletes make a portable breakfast. Juice and milk can go in the mug, and bagels, dry cereal, and raisins can be placed in the bags for a fast and portable breakfast on the way to class.

Lunch and dinner can also be easy to compile, whether preparing at home or choosing from a cafeteria buffet. Salad or sandwich bars provide a variety of nutrient-dense foods that are rich in carbohydrates and protein. Hot entrées can make the base of the meal; however, they should not be considered the entire meal. Adding a vegetable or salad, soup, milk, or yogurt can round out the meal. For athletes preparing their own meals, the same concepts can be applied. Frozen or prepared entrées can be cooked conveniently, and canned or frozen vegetables, soups, baked beans, and other side dishes can be added for more variety in nutrients and taste. **Table 15.6** lists quick meal ideas that are easy to prepare, relatively inexpensive, and nutrient-dense.

gaining the performance edge

Upon entering college, athletes may be required to plan, purchase, and prepare their own meals and snacks for the first time in their lives. Planning and implementing a healthful sports nutrition diet can be accomplished by using the basic principles of good nutrition combined with adequate intake to meet the demands of training and competition.

For athletes in apartments for the first time, grocery shopping and cooking can be a challenge in terms of time and finances. Athletes should stock the kitchen with a few favorite foods that are easy to prepare when time is limited. Dietitians working with college athletes should be prepared to teach very basic cooking techniques and help athletes plan meals that meet energy and nutrient needs. **Table 15.7** provides a grocery list by food category that may be helpful for college athletes. This list is compiled by food category to help athletes understand the different food groups and to encourage the purchase of a variety of foods.

TABLE 15.6	Quick Preparation Meal and Cooking Ideas

Convenience items such as frozen and canned foods can be part of a healthy sports nutrition diet. A nutritious, well-balanced meal should contain at least three different food groups.

Canned Soups	• Add a can of vegetables, or leftover cooked vegetables to the soup.
	• Serve with whole grain crackers.
	• Add a sandwich and/or fruit.
Hamburgers	• Serve with thick slices of tomato, lettuce, pickle, and onion.
	• Serve with baked frozen fries.
	• Accompany with milk or juice.
Marinated Chicken Breast	• Serve with a microwaved baked potato.
	• Add canned or frozen vegetables.
	• Serve with canned vegetables.
Macaroni and Cheese	• Slice or cube ham and mix into the macaroni and cheese.
	• Add a can of tuna or cooked chicken and heat thoroughly.
Noodles or Rice-in-Sauce packets	• Serve with canned or frozen vegetables.
Any Frozen Entrée	• Serve with a salad or vegetable.
	• Include a roll or bread on the side.
	• Serve fresh fruit for dessert.
Baked Potato	• Melt cheese on top.
	• Top with broccoli or another vegetable (precooked).
	• Cottage cheese mixed with picante or salsa is also a tasty topping.
Pancakes or Waffles	• Top with cut-up fruit or berries.
	• Serve with 1 or 2 eggs.
	• Juice is a healthy beverage choice.
Bean and Cheese Burrito	• Serve with salad or precut raw vegetables.
	• Chop fresh fruit for a side salad.

How does alcohol consumption affect college athletes' nutrition?

Alcohol consumption on college campuses is always a top priority on the list of concerns for academic administrators. Tailgate parties, celebratory occasions, weekend festivities, and other scenarios have led to

TABLE 15.7	Grocery List for Active Individuals

Grocery shopping is the first step to healthful eating. The items athletes purchase at the grocery store will dictate the foods/beverages consumed before, during, and after practices and competitive events, as well as throughout the day. Athletes should develop the habit of making a shopping list to ensure that the kitchen will be stocked until the next shopping trip. Foods should be purchased from all of the food groups to achieve balance, variety, and a wide complement of nutrients. The following is a sample grocery list that includes a wide variety of items.

Fruits	Vegetables	Dairy Products
Bananas	Different-colored veggies	Low-fat yogurt
Berries	Broccoli	Low-fat or skim milk
100% fruit juice	Cauliflower	String cheese
Juice boxes	Carrots	Cheese chunks
Raisins	Dark greens	Cheese slices
Dried fruits	Salad or cabbage mix	Nonfat dry milk powder
Canned fruits (in own juice)	Potatoes	Pudding
Fresh fruits	Sweet potatoes	Cottage cheese
Frozen fruits	Peppers	
	Green and yellow beans	
	Asparagus	

Grains	Proteins
Whole grain cold cereal	Tuna, water-packed
Oatmeal	Fish, frozen or fresh
Whole grain breads	Eggs
Whole grain bagels	Chicken breasts, boneless, skinless
Pasta	Ground beef, 80–95% lean
Brown, wild, or white rice	Lean cuts of pork or beef
Popcorn	Tofu/texturized vegetable protein
Granola bars	Deli or sliced chicken, turkey, roast beef, or ham
Cereal bars	Peanut butter
Graham crackers	Nuts
Whole grain crackers	Starchy beans (black, kidney, pinto, soy)
Frozen foods	Desserts and Snacks
Entrées (variety)	Frozen fruit juice or yogurt bars
Lasagna	Sherbet or frozen yogurt
Veggie burgers	Frozen fruit pieces (berries, grapes, melons)
Flash-frozen chicken breasts	Peanut butter with crackers
Frozen vegetables	Cereal or granola with milk
Stir-fry meals	Yogurt and fruit or granola
Whole grain toaster waffles	Fig bars

a surprisingly high consumption of alcohol by collegiate athletes. This section discusses the incidence of alcohol consumption in college athletes and how excessive alcohol consumption may have negative effects on nutrient intake and athletic performance.

Several studies of college student drinking found that alcohol use is higher in athletes than nonathlete college students.[32–34] Binge drinking episodes have been most commonly researched. Excessive use of alcohol, or a "binge-drinking episode," is considered five or more drinks at a time for men and four or more drinks for women. One study of college athletes stated that 57% of male athletes and 48% of female athletes reported a heavy drinking episode within the past 2 weeks.[33] This is compared to 49% of males and 40% of females who were not athletes in the study. Another study found that almost 81% of varsity athletes had used alcohol in the 12 months prior to the survey.[35] Although not all athletes consume alcohol, when they do, many tend to do so excessively.

Gender differences in alcohol consumption are prevalent in the collegiate athlete population. Male athletes have higher rates of binge-drinking episodes than female athletes. Female athletes typically have the lowest amount of alcohol consumption in both the athlete and nonathlete populations.[34] The National Collegiate Athletic Association (NCAA) has developed programs addressing the issue of alcohol and other drug use in college athletes. Many college and university athletic departments bring NCAA or other sponsored speakers to their schools annually to discuss alcohol issues with their athletes.

Alcohol, namely ethyl alcohol, is an organic compound that holds a unique standing in regard to nutrition. Alcohol is considered to be a food because it provides energy (7 calories/gram) to the body; however, it is not considered a nutrient because of the fact that the body does not need it to survive. It is interesting to note that alcohol is also considered a drug because of its effects on the central nervous system. When ingested, alcohol is very rapidly ab-

sorbed into the bloodstream compared to the rate of other foods. Some absorption of alcohol occurs within the mouth, esophagus, and stomach, with the majority of absorption occurring in the small intestine (see Figure 15.3).

Alcohol, unlike carbohydrates, fats, and proteins, is not stored in the body. Instead, once it is ingested, the body begins to metabolize alcohol in an attempt to quickly eliminate it from the body. As shown in Figure 15.4 , alcohol is converted to acetyl coenzyme A (CoA) and either metabolized further for energy or converted to fat and stored in the body. Increased body fat is not a desirable outcome for most athletes, and thus is a negative aspect associated with alcohol consumption.

ALCOHOL ABSORPTION

Small amounts of alcohol are absorbed in the mouth and esophagus

Alcohol is readily absorbed in the stomach, but food will dilute the alcohol and delay gastric emptying

The primary site of alcohol absorption is the upper small intestine

Figure 15.3 Alcohol absorption. Alcohol easily diffuses into and out of cells, so most alcohol is absorbed unchanged.

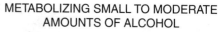

METABOLIZING SMALL TO MODERATE AMOUNTS OF ALCOHOL

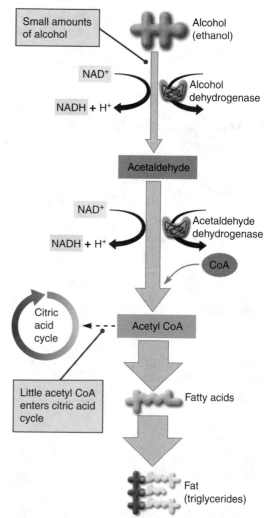

Figure 15.4 Metabolizing alcohol. Alcohol is converted to acetyl CoA and either metabolized further for energy or converted to fat and stored in the body.

Alcoholic beverages can be calorically dense with negligible nutrient content. Alcohol contains 7 calories/gram but virtually no vitamins or minerals. Some alcoholic beverages contain significant calories as a result of the mixers used to make the drinks. Sweet drinks, drinks containing sweet liqueurs, and those with whipped cream or sugar toppings add to the caloric content of the drink without adding nutrients. Alcoholic beverages have been labeled as "empty calories" for good reasons! **Table 15.8** lists the calorie and carbohydrate content of some common alcoholic beverages. Although athletes may be able to consume the additional calories because of their high caloric expenditure, it is better to meet additional calorie needs with nutrient-dense foods.

Some athletes do not consume food before drinking alcohol and/or do not eat anything while they are drinking. Many male and female athletes are conscious of their weight and total caloric intake. In an attempt to "save" calories they practice this abstinence from food strategy before and during drinking. Unfortunately, this strategy makes little sense nutritionally or physiologically. Nutritionally speaking, abstaining from eating nutrient-dense foods while replacing them with nutritionally empty calories from alcohol is not a good idea for many reasons that have already been discussed in this book. Second, absorption of alcohol is much slower if consumed with food. Drinking on an empty stomach leads to rapid absorption of alcohol. Because alcohol affects the central nervous system (i.e., the brain), judgment skills are more quickly affected. As a result, the athlete often ends up drinking more than he or she had intended, thus defeating the purpose of the food abstinence strategy.

Alcohol also has the potential to affect calorie intake because of its effect on appetite. Although alcohol as a drug is a depressant, it appears to stimulate appetite. Appetite is not necessarily physical hunger; it is the desire to eat food. Many individuals who drink alcohol also end up eating either during or after the drinking episode. Hetherington reported that individuals who consumed a preload of alcohol (beer) 30 minutes prior to a test meal consumed more calories than those who consumed a nonalcohol preload.[36] Even when the additional calories from the alcohol preload were taken into account, subjects in the study consumed 30% more at lunch than the nonalcohol preload controls. A common occurrence reported by many college athletes is the "late-night munchies." The foods are consumed after an evening of drinking and are likely calories in excess of the athlete's needs. Typical food choices are less nutritious (pizza, nachos, ice cream, chips) and calorically dense. Athletes who need to maintain weight for optimal sport performance could end up gaining weight if this occurs often. It may not only be the excess calories from the alcoholic beverages, but also the "munchies" that lead to weight gain in some college athletes.

Drinking alcohol after a big game or competitive event is commonplace in college athletics. Athletes who have competed with high intensity have used up their glycogen stores. Postgame nutrition should include nutrient-dense carbohydrates to replenish stores lost during the event. However, athletes who drink alcohol after games or hard practices are less likely to consume adequate amounts of complex carbohydrates from nutrient-dense sources and therefore may not fully replenish glycogen stores. Thus, athletic performance during the next practice or competition will suffer.

A common misconception is that beer is a rich source of carbohydrates because it is made from grains. Actually, one regular domestic beer contains on average 10–12 grams of carbohydrates, a small amount of protein, and zero fat calories; the rest of the calories come from alcohol. Alcohol contains 7 calories per gram. An example of cal-

TABLE 15.8	Calorie and Carbohydrate Content of Alcoholic Beverages	
Beverage	Calories	Carbohydrates (grams)
12 oz regular beer	139	12.6
12 oz light beer	95	4.4
16 oz (1 pint) beer	186	6.8
60 oz pitcher, regular beer	697	63
4 oz wine	77	0.9
1.5 oz shot of liquor	97	0.0
6 oz mixed drink	129	12
7 oz piña colada	526	61
5 oz martini	316	0.5

Sources: Pennington JAT, Douglass JS. *Bowes and Church's Food Values of Portions Commonly Used.* 18th ed. Baltimore, MD: Lippincott, Williams & Wilkins; 2005. Nutrition Analysis Tools and System. 2004. Nutrition Analysis Tool. Available at: http://nat.crgq.com. Accessed August 20, 2004.

culating the alcohol content of one regular beer is shown here:

> Calorie content of a 12 oz beer: 143 total calories
>
> Carbohydrate content: 10.8 g × 4 kcal/g = 43.2 calories from carbohydrates
>
> Protein content: 1.2 × 4 = 4.8 calories from protein
>
> Fat content: 0 calories
>
> Carbohydrate and protein calories combined = 43.2 + 4.8 = 48 calories
>
> Total beer calories = 143 − 48 carbohydrate and protein calories = 95 calories from alcohol
>
> Alcohol calories: 95 ÷ 7 calories/g of alcohol = 13.6 g of alcohol

A beer contains significantly more calories derived from alcohol than from carbohydrates. Beer is not a good source of carbohydrates for the replenishment of glycogen stores after exercise.

An increase in binge drinking is also associated with an increased likelihood of alcohol-related harms. Academic achievement can suffer when social drinking interferes with studying. Missing classes because of a morning hangover can add to the already huge demand on class time for the traveling athlete. Driving while under the influence or riding in a car with a driver under the influence has potential for both injury and legal consequences. Nelson and Wechsler studied college athlete drinking behavior and found that more athletes than nonathletes missed classes, fell behind in school work, forgot where they were/ what they had done, and either drove or rode with another driver while under the influence of alcohol.[33] In summary, the consumption of alcohol by collegiate athletes can be detrimental to overall health, nutrition status, academics, and personal safety, and therefore is not recommended.

What are the special considerations for masters athletes?

Masters athletes are generally defined as athletes over the age of 40 or 50. Nutrition guidelines for sedentary individuals within this age group are different from their younger counterparts.[37] Add regular exercise and high-intensity training into the mix, and those changes in recommendations become even more important because of the extra nutrition demands of physical activity. Masters athletes need to consider the changes to individual nutrient recom-

mendations, the required diet adaptations resulting from chronic disease and medication use, as well as the nutrient needs of their sport.[37]

How do the nutrient needs of masters athletes change?

For apparently healthy masters athletes, total calorie, chromium, iron, calcium, vitamin D, and magnesium needs change. Total calorie, chromium, and iron recommendations decrease, whereas calcium, vitamin D, and magnesium needs increase. By making slight dietary modifications, all of these changes can be easily managed.

How do total calorie requirements change with age?

As athletes age, total calorie needs decrease slightly.[10,11,38] For all aging individuals, several factors contribute to lower energy needs with progressing age, including the loss of calorie-burning muscle mass.[39] Masters athletes are at an advantage over their sedentary counterparts because physical activity helps to maintain muscle mass, keeping their metabolic rate higher; however, some change in calorie needs is inevitable. The result of this decline can be realized when using the resting energy estimation equations presented earlier in this text.

For example, an active 25-year-old man weighing 160 pounds (72.7 kg) will require about 138 fewer calories when he is 50, even if his total weight and activity level remain the same:

> At age 25: REE = $(15.3 \times BW) + 679$ = $(15.3 \times 72.7 \text{ kg}) + 679 = 1791$ calories
>
> Total energy needs = 1791×2 (activity factor) = 3582 calories
>
> At age 50: REE = $(11.6 \times BW) + 879$ = $(11.6 \times 72.7 \text{ kg}) + 879 = 1722$ calories
>
> Total energy needs = 1722×2 (activity factor) = 3444 calories
>
> Difference in total daily energy needs based solely on age = 138 calories

Although this difference may seem to be insignificant, over time it can make a huge impact. If this 50-year-old man continued to eat the same number of calories he required when he was 25, he would gain about 14 pounds in 1 year, even if physical activity remained constant! Eating an extra 138 calories per day for 365 days leads to a calorie excess of 50,370 in 1 year, which is equivalent to 14 pounds of fat mass:

$$138 \text{ extra calories/day} \times 365 \text{ days/year} = 50{,}370$$
$$\text{extra calories in one year}$$

$$50{,}370 \text{ calories} \div 3500 \text{ calories in 1 pound of fat} =$$
$$14 \text{ pounds of fat weight gain per year}$$

Fat mass gain not only can be detrimental to athletic performance, but also is a risk factor for many degenerative diseases such as heart disease and diabetes.

Although masters athletes need to ensure adequate calorie consumption to meet the energy requirements of their sport, they will not need to consume as much as they did earlier in their athletic career. Incongruently, several vitamin and mineral needs increase with age, creating the challenge of eating less but requiring more. As athletes age, it becomes progressively more important to focus on the consumption of nutrient-dense foods while minimizing the intake of "empty" calories.

The proportion of macronutrients should remain relatively constant for masters athletes. Carbohydrates are still the main source of fuel, requiring an intake of 50–65% of total calories. Protein needs remain above the RDA for the sedentary population, with a minimum requirement of 1–1.25 grams of protein per kilogram of body weight.[39] Fat should be kept at a moderate level, ranging from 20–35% of total calories. The key words *balance*, *variety*, and *moderation* still hold true for masters athletes.

How do chromium requirements change with age?

The daily requirements (AI) for chromium decrease from 35 micrograms to 30 micrograms after the age of 50.[17] Chromium plays a role in blood glucose regulation, possibly by maintaining insulin sensitivity and insulin-mediated uptake of glucose into cells. This action has been suggested to be critical in the prevention of diabetes, which in turn promotes overall health. Chromium's role is also recognized in the world of athletics because cells are dependent on insulin to deliver glucose and other nutrients for fuel and repair. Therefore, masters athletes should strive for adequate intakes of chromium, with the goal decreasing slightly after age 50.

However, even if masters athletes were to consume more than 30 micrograms of chromium per day, they would probably not experience any adverse effects. Currently, no upper limit has been set for chromium because toxic effects from food sources are uncommon. Therefore, masters athletes should focus on chromium-rich foods such as mushrooms, dark chocolate, nuts, prunes, whole grains, and wine, and avoid individual chromium supplements. Chromium-containing multivitamin/minerals are safe to continue taking as long as the chromium content does not exceed 85–100% of the Daily Value.

Because the change in the daily recommendation for chromium is small, and there is little risk of overdosing on chromium, this should not be an area of major concern for masters athletes.

How do iron requirements change with age?

As mentioned previously in this chapter, iron is important for a variety of bodily functions related to overall health and athletic performance. Although iron remains a critical nutrient throughout the lifespan, women's needs for iron change after menopause. Postmenopausal women require the same amount of iron as men—8 milligrams a day.[17] This change in recommendations represents a significant decrease from the 18 milligrams women require throughout their childbearing years.[17]

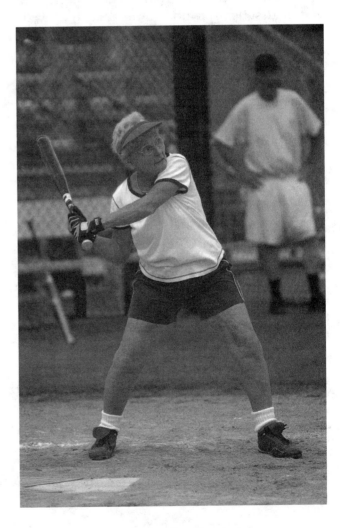

From a practical standpoint, the change in iron requirements creates a major shift in a woman's ability to meet daily requirements. Most female athletes struggle to meet their needs for iron, especially pregnant athletes. Being iron-challenged, younger women are generally urged to eat plenty of iron-rich foods and take iron supplements through a multivitamin/mineral and/or individual iron pill. Once the tables are turned and requirements plunge to only 8 milligrams, postmenopausal women should stop taking supplemental iron and focus solely on iron-rich foods to prevent iron toxicity. Iron-rich foods include beef, poultry, fish, legumes, nuts, and enriched whole grains. The upper limit for iron is 45 milligrams per day, which should not be exceeded through foods and especially supplements. Several multivitamin/mineral manufacturers have developed "senior" or "silver" formulas that contain little to no iron. These specialty formulas are the best choice for postmenopausal women.

Men should continue to aim for 8 milligrams of iron per day. Men are 5–10 times more likely than women to suffer from iron overload and the genetic disorder hemochromatosis. Similar to postmenopausal women, men should focus on whole food sources of iron, keeping intake well below the upper limit of 45 milligrams per day, and avoid iron-containing supplements.

How do calcium and vitamin D requirements change with age?

Calcium requirements increase from 1000 to 1200 milligrams per day for women older than 50 and men older than 70 years.[30] Calcium is important for the maintenance of bone health, nerve function, blood clotting, muscle contraction, and cellular metabolism—all of which are critical for overall health and optimal athletic performance.

Unfortunately, young adults generally do not consume enough calcium, leading to an older population with the same poor habits. Twelve hundred milligrams of calcium can be consumed through foods alone; however, it does require the consumption of four or more calcium-rich servings each day. For example, a glass of skim milk consumed at each meal (providing a total of about 900 milligrams) plus one container of yogurt as a snack (providing another 300–350 milligrams) supplies the daily requirement. Calcium is also found in fortified soy products, green leafy vegetables, legumes, and fortified cereals and juices.

Vitamin D requirements for both men and women increase after age 70 from 600 to 800 IU per day.[30] Vitamin D is unique in that it is found in a very narrow selection of foods. Cow's milk and fortified soy milks are two of the best choices, providing approximately 100 IU per 8 fluid ounces. Some breakfast cereals, orange juices, and even a few yogurts are fortified with vitamin D, although in lower quantities as compared to milk. Canned salmon and sardines, with the bones, can also be a significant source of vitamin D. Most of these foods are also rich sources of calcium, providing a two-for-one deal.

Vitamin D can also be synthesized in the body by spending approximately 15 minutes in direct sunlight each day. However, several factors make sunlight an unreliable source for masters athletes. With age, the body becomes less efficient at synthesizing vitamin D from sunlight. In addition to this impaired function, the application of sunscreen further blocks the body's ability to use sunlight as a precursor to vitamin D. With a stronger emphasis on preventing skin cancer, many masters athletes are wearing, and should be wearing, sunscreen while training and competing outdoors. Thus, sunlight cannot be considered a good source of obtaining a daily dose of vitamin D.

Both calcium and vitamin D are key players in the fight against osteoporosis. These nutrients may also aid in the prevention of cancer and hypertension, as discussed in Chapters 6 and 7. By meeting daily needs, masters athletes can keep their bones strong and decrease their risk for chronic disease.

How do magnesium requirements change with age?

Magnesium is a critical nutrient for enzyme activity and energy production. Magnesium intake is generally suboptimal in the typical American diet, but can be compounded by several factors that may lead to greater magnesium losses or poor absorption. Individuals who have chronic diarrhea or are taking diuretic medications are at higher risk for magnesium deficiency. As athletes age, the incidence of health problems such as high blood pressure increases, often requiring the daily use of medications. Diuretics are a common prescription given to individuals with hypertension. A common side effect of many different medications is diarrhea. Therefore, athletes taking daily diuretic medications, or drugs that cause diarrhea, should ensure an adequate intake of magnesium.

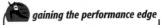
Fortunately, magnesium is found in a large variety of foods, with whole grains, vegetables, and legumes topping the list. The daily requirement for magnesium increases slightly after the age of 31 to 420 milligrams per day for men and 320 milligrams per day for women.[19] These requirements are easily met through whole foods. For example, 1 1/2 cups of black beans contain about 190 milligrams of magnesium, providing 45% and 59% of total daily needs for men and women, respectively. Other specific foods rich in magnesium include cheeses, fish, almonds, spinach, and peanut butter.

If masters athletes fail to meet magnesium needs, loss of appetite, weakness, and muscle cramps can occur. If the deficiency is left untreated, heart rhythm can be disrupted. Fortunately, many of the magnesium-rich foods are also good sources of iron and calcium, providing a three-for-one punch.

How does the presence of chronic disease affect nutrient needs of masters athletes?

The presence of chronic disease generally requires adjustments to daily nutrient intake, regardless of whether the individual is sedentary or an athlete. Increasingly, nutrition is being implicated in the prevention, as well as the treatment, of chronic disease.

The incidence of chronic disease increases with age, so older athletes need to consider not only the nutrient needs of their sport, but also the therapeutic benefits of proper nutrition.

A full explanation of the relationship between nutrition and chronic disease extends beyond the scope of this text. However, there are general nutrition recommendations that should be incorporated into the nutrition plans of masters athletes who have been diagnosed with various conditions. It is important to note that each individual's diagnosis and precipitating factors leading to the disease are different, requiring an individualized approach to each client. **Table 15.9** presents the general recommendations for various chronic diseases; these recommendations should be used as general guidelines and adapted according to the needs of the individual athlete.

In addition to the actual disease state, medications prescribed for the treatment of chronic disease can have their own effects on an athlete's dietary intake. Specific foods and beverages can alter the function, effectiveness, or absorption of various medications. Athletes should consult with their physician, pharmacist, and dietitian to determine whether any dietary modifications are required when starting a new medication. Refer to **Table 15.10** for some common examples of food-drug interactions.

TABLE 15.9	Potential Dietary Modifications Required for Various Chronic Diseases
Disease	**Possible Dietary Modifications**
Atherosclerosis	Decrease total fat, saturated fat, and cholesterol; increase complex carbohydrates, fiber, and antioxidants from fruits, vegetables, and vitamin E–rich foods.
Cancer	Decrease total fat, some meats, alcohol, and salty and cured foods; increase complex carbohydrates, fiber, unsaturated fats, and fruits and vegetables.
Arthritis	Decrease total caloric intake if overweight; increase unsaturated fats, particularly omega-3 fatty acids.
Osteoporosis	Increase calcium, vitamin D, and vitamin K; decrease phosphorus.
Diabetes	Decrease total caloric intake if overweight; decrease total fat and refined sugars; increase fiber and protein; monitor total carbohydrate intake.
Hypertension	Increase calcium, potassium, protein, magnesium, and fiber; decrease sodium, total fat, and saturated fat.
Stroke	Decrease total caloric intake if overweight; decrease total fat and saturated fat; increase complex carbohydrates, fiber, and antioxidants from fruits, vegetables, and vitamin E–rich foods.

TABLE 15.10 Examples of Food–Drug Interactions

Drug	Foods That Interact	Effect of the Food	What to Do
Analgesic			
Acetaminophen (Tylenol)	Alcohol	Increases risk for liver toxicity	Avoid alcohol.
Antibiotics			
Tetracyclines	Dairy products; iron supplements	Decreases drug absorption	Do not take with milk. Take 1 hr before or 2 hr after food or milk.
Amoxicillin, penicillin	Food	Decreases drug absorption	Take 1 hr before or 2 hr after meals.
Zithromax, erythromycin	Food	Decreases drug absorption	Take 1 hr before or 2 hr after meals.
Nitrofurantoin (Macrobid)	Food	Decreases GI distress, slows drug absorption	Take with food or milk.
Anticoagulant			
Warfarin (Coumadin)	Foods rich in vitamin K	Decreases drug effectiveness	Limit foods high in vitamin K: liver, broccoli, spinach, kale, cauliflower, and Brussels sprouts.
Antifungal			
Griseofulvin (Fulvicin)	High-fat meal	Increases drug absorption	Take with high-fat meal.
Antihistamine			
Diphenhydramine (Benadryl), chlorpheniramine (Chlor-Trimeton)	Alcohol	Increases drowsiness	Avoid alcohol.
Antihypertensive			
Felodipine (Plendil), nifedipine	Grapefruit juice	Increases drug absorption	Consult physician or pharmacist before changing diet.
Anti-inflammatory			
Naproxen (Naprosyn)	Food or milk	Decreases GI irritation	Take with food or milk.
Ibuprofen (Motrin)	Alcohol	Increases risk for liver damage or stomach bleeding	Avoid alcohol.
Diuretic			
Spironolactone (Aldactone)	Food	Decreases GI irritation	Take with food.
Psychotherapeutic (MAO inhibitors)			
Tranylcypromine (Parnate)	Foods high in tyramine: aged cheeses, Chianti wine, pickled herring, brewer's yeast, fava beans	Risk for hypertensive crisis	Avoid foods high in tyramine.

Note: Grapefruit juice contains a compound not found in other citrus juices. This compound increases the absorption of some drugs and can enhance their effects. It's best not to take medications with grapefruit juice. Drink it at least 2 hours before or after you take your medication. If you often drink grapefruit juice, talk with your pharmacist or doctor before changing your routine.

Source: Bobroff LB, Lentz A, Turner RE. Food/Drug and Drug/Nutrient Interactions: What You Should Know About Your Medications. Gainesville, FL: University of Florida; March 1999. Publication FCS 8092 in a series of the Department of Family, Youth and Community Sciences, Florida Cooperative Extension Service, Institute of Food and Agricultural Sciences.

What are the special considerations for vegetarian athletes?

Vegetarianism is becoming more popular in both sedentary and active populations (see Figure 15.5). Individuals convert to a plant-based diet for a variety of reasons including long-term health, animal rights, world hunger, finances, and religious beliefs. Many national organizations endorse a vegetarian lifestyle because of a plethora of research revealing a myriad of health benefits such as lower risk of coronary artery disease, hypertension, diabetes, some cancers, and renal disease.[40] However, these health benefits can be realized only when the switch from a carnivorous diet to a vegetarian diet is planned appropriately. The Vegetarian Diet Pyramid has been developed to educate individuals on how to plan a balanced plant-based diet (see Figure 15.6). This section reviews the various types of vegetarianism and the special nutrient needs of these athletes.

The following athletes and coaches follow or have followed a vegetarian diet:

Hank Aaron, Baseball Legend

Danny Garcia, Professional Skateboarder

Billie Jean King, Professional Tennis Player

Tony LaRussa, Professional Baseball Coach

Marv Levy, NFL Coach

Carl Lewis, Track/Field Olympian

Edwin Moses, Olympic Hurdler

Martina Navratilova, Professional Tennis Player

Dave Scott, Ironman World Champion

Bill Walton, NBA Basketball Player

Tyrone Willingham, former Notre Dame Football Coach

Figure 15.5   Past and present vegetarian athletes and coaches.
Source: HappyCow's Famous Vegetarians. Available at: http://www.happycow.net. Accessed January 22, 2011.

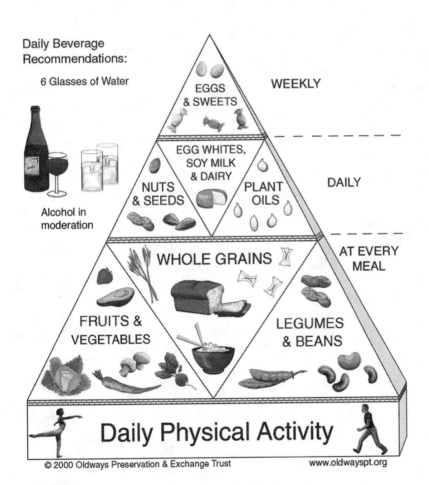

Daily Beverage Recommendations:

6 Glasses of Water

Alcohol in moderation

EGGS & SWEETS — WEEKLY

EGG WHITES, SOY MILK & DAIRY

NUTS & SEEDS

PLANT OILS — DAILY

WHOLE GRAINS — AT EVERY MEAL

FRUITS & VEGETABLES

LEGUMES & BEANS

Daily Physical Activity

© 2000 Oldways Preservation & Exchange Trust   www.oldwayspt.org

Figure 15.6   Vegetarian Diet Pyramid. With careful planning, a diet that lacks animal products can be nutritionally complete.
Source: © 2000 Oldways Preservation & Exchange Trust.

What are the various types of vegetarianism?

Although all vegetarians follow a plant-based diet, the inclusion or exclusion of specific foods can vary greatly based on the type of vegetarianism practiced. Often, individuals who are exploring the idea of becoming a vegetarian begin as a semi-vegetarian, eating dairy, eggs, poultry, and fish but avoiding beef and sometimes pork. The next step is to exclude poultry, thus becoming a pesco-vegetarian (pesco = fish). Lacto-ovo-vegetarians include dairy and eggs but have made the choice to exclude any animal flesh (including fish). Vegetarians can choose to also exclude either dairy or eggs, which is considered lacto-vegetarianism or ovo-vegetarianism. The final progression to what some call "true" vegetarianism is to follow a vegan diet that excludes all animal products including any animal flesh, dairy, eggs, honey (because it is made by bees), and products made with an animal derivative (such as whey or casein from dairy). See **Table 15.11** for a summary of the various types of vegetarian diets. The special nutrition considerations for vegetarians follow the same progression as the dietary practices—the

TABLE
15.11   Types of Vegetarian Diets

Type	Animal Foods Included	Foods Excluded
Semi-vegetarian	Dairy products, eggs, poultry, fish	Red meats (beef, pork)
Pesco-vegetarian	Dairy products, eggs, fish	Beef, pork, poultry
Lacto-ovo-vegetarian	Dairy products, eggs	Beef, pork, poultry, fish
Lacto-vegetarian	Dairy products	Beef, pork, poultry, fish, eggs
Ovo-vegetarian	Eggs	Beef, pork, poultry, fish, dairy products
Vegan	None	All animal products and animal derivatives

greater the exclusion of foods from the diet, the more special considerations exist.

It should be noted that these special considerations are mainly focused on helping individuals discover the wide variety of protein foods and dairy alternatives available. Vegetarianism is often erroneously viewed as being insufficient for supporting the training and competitive demands of athletics. The reality is that vegetarianism is just a different pathway to the same destination. An analogy can be made to coaching techniques: Two football coaches may have very different training/conditioning practices based on what they view as the best way to prepare for a winning season; likewise, a carnivore and a vegetarian will have very different dietary practices based on their beliefs, both with the intention of supporting overall health, training, and competition. Therefore, athletes should consider vegetarianism as a healthy alternative to mainstream eating. The major mistake that athletes make when converting to a vegetarian diet is the exclusion of foods from the protein foods and/or dairy group without introducing plant-based substitutions. Simply cutting out the meat and dairy choices in the MyPlate food guidance system causes the pyramid to collapse and crumble because of poor planning and the exclusion of many nutrients. Instead, vegetarians advocate finding alternatives that are equivalent to the foods found in the MyPlate food groups, thus creating a well-balanced, appropriately planned diet.

The protein foods and dairy/milk alternative groups are rich in protein, iron, zinc, calcium, vitamin D, and vitamin B_{12}. Therefore, vegetarians need to substitute plant-based foods that are rich sources of these nutrients.

Which vegetarian foods are rich in protein?

Protein is critical for tissue growth and repair, the formation of hormones and enzymes, and proper immune function in athletes. Protein can be found in a variety of meat and dairy alternative foods. Beans, nuts, seeds, and soy products fit into the protein foods group, providing not only protein, but also iron, zinc, magnesium, and calcium. Semi-, lacto-, and ovo-vegetarians are the least likely to experience a challenge in meeting protein needs; vegans can meet protein needs with a little extra meal planning and creativity, particularly when traveling. Overall, vegetarians can meet their protein needs, positively affecting athletic performance in a similar fashion to carnivores.[41]

As mentioned in Chapter 5 of this text, vegetarians should aim to consume a variety of meat alternative sources each day to meet essential amino acid requirements. Soy protein is the only plant protein that contains high amounts of all essential amino acids, making soy foods convenient and complete. Nuts, seeds, legumes, and grains provide all the essential amino acids; however, they may contain low levels of one or more of these amino acids, thus requiring a combination of protein sources throughout the day. Figure 15.7 presents the various combinations of plant proteins that provide complementary essential amino acids. These combinations do not need to occur within one meal; a variety of plant proteins can be consumed throughout the day to provide all essential amino acids.

A heavy emphasis should be placed on soy products because soy is considered a complete protein. Also, from a practical standpoint, soy can be found in many forms, allowing for creative and varied meal planning. See **Table 15.12** for a description of commonly used soy products and associated meal-planning ideas. Figure 15.8 lists various online soy resources.

The greatest challenge for vegetarians, especially vegans, is finding protein sources while traveling and when dining out. Ideally, athletes should seek

gaining the performance edge

Athletes seeking information about becoming vegetarian will find the following Web sites helpful: Vegetarian Resource Group, www.vrg.org; Vegetarian Times, www.vegetariantimes.com; Vegetarian Recipes, www.vegweb.com; and Vegetarian Societies and Organizations in North America, www.greenpeople.org/vegetarian.htm.

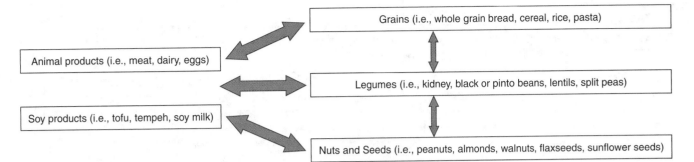

Figure 15.7 Complementary proteins for vegetarians. Because animal and soy products contain high levels of all essential amino acids, they can be consumed with any grain, legume, or nut/seed. Grains are complemented by legumes, and legumes are complemented by nuts/seeds. Grains are not a complementary match to nuts/seeds, but the two make a tasty combination in recipes.

TABLE 15.12	Incorporating Soy into a Vegetarian Diet	
Soy Product	**Description**	**Meal Planning Ideas and Uses for Cooking**
Edamame	Green soybeans; beans are harvested early and are therefore more sweet than mature soybeans.	Edamame can be boiled and lightly salted for a snack or side dish. Edamame are also perfect in pasta dishes, stir-fries, and cold summer salads.
Soy breakfast links/patties and soy dogs	Often called meat analogs, these products are meat alternatives made from soy.	The soy links/patties are perfect for breakfast or Sunday brunch. The soy hot dogs are a favorite among kids and work great on the grill.
Soy cheese and cream cheese	These cheeses are made with soy milk instead of cow's milk. Some cheeses include whey or casein and therefore may not be appropriate for vegans.	Cheddar, mozzarella, and Monterey jack–type soy cheeses can be used in sandwiches and omelets and on pizza. Soy cream cheese is delicious on bagels or muffins and can also be used in recipes.
Soy crumbles	Soy crumbles are the vegetarian version of ground beef. They are typically found in the freezer section of a grocery store.	Use soy crumbles in any recipe that calls for ground beef, such as sloppy joes, chili, lasagna, or tacos.
Soy flour	Ground, roasted soybeans produce soy flour.	Soy flour can take the place of one-quarter of the all-purpose flour in a recipe.
Soy milk	Soy milk is an alternative for cow's milk made from whole soybeans. Soy milk comes in low-fat and nonfat versions as well as vanilla and chocolate flavors.	Soy milk can be consumed by the glass, on cereal, and in smoothies, as well as in any recipe calling for milk. Many coffeehouses carry soy milk to make delicious soy lattes and mochas.
Soy nuts	Roasted whole soybeans. They often are found in trail mix with other nuts and dried fruits.	Soy nuts are perfect for a midday snack or on top of salads.
Soy yogurt	Made from soy milk instead of cow's milk.	Soy yogurt can be served at breakfast in a parfait, at lunch with a sandwich, or as a snack with dried fruits, nuts, or granola.
Soybeans	Mature beans, found in yellow, brown, and black varieties.	Whole, cooked soybeans can be used in any dish calling for beans, such as chili, soups, stews, and burritos.
Tempeh	Whole soybeans, often mixed with a grain, are fermented into a soybean cake with a nutty flavor.	Tempeh's firm texture makes it perfect for marinating and grilling. Tempeh also works well in soups, stews, casseroles, or cubed for BBQ sandwiches.
Texturized soy protein (TSP)	Made from soy flour or soy protein concentrate, it typically is found in a dehydrated form and used as a meat extender.	TSP is generally inexpensive and can be stored for long periods of time because it is dehydrated. When rehydrated, TSP can be used in recipes similar to soy crumbles.

(continued)

TABLE 15.12 Incorporating Soy into a Vegetarian Diet *(Continued)*

Soy Product	Description	Meal Planning Ideas and Uses for Cooking
Tofu	Made in a similar fashion as cottage cheese, tofu is formed by mixing soy milk with a coagulant. Tofu comes in silken, soft, firm, and extra-firm varieties.	Silken tofu is used as a replacement for sour cream in recipes such as vegetable dip or as a replacement for cream cheese in recipes. Firm and extra-firm tofu are best for stir-fries, soups, stews, chili, burritos, casseroles, grilling, etc.
Veggie burgers	Burgers made from soy protein and/or tofu as well as other ingredients such as vegetables.	Veggie burgers can be warmed in the microwave, in a skillet, or on the backyard grill for a quick lunch.

Online Soy Resources

National Organizations	Web Sites
Soy Protein Partners	www.soybean.org
Soyfoods Association of America	www.soyfoods.org
U.S. Soyfoods Directory	www.soyfoods.com

State Organizations	Web Sites
Illinois Center for Soy Foods	www.nsrl.illinois.edu/nutrition.html
Iowa Soyfoods Council	www.iasoybeans.com
Missouri Soybean Council	www.mosoy.org
Nebraska Soybean Board	www.soycooking.com
Ohio Soybean Council	www.soyohio.org

Figure 15.8 Many organizations provide information, recipes, and research briefs on the benefits of soy.

out vegetarian restaurants in their area, on the road, and at their final travel destination (see Figure 15.9). Vegetarian restaurants will provide a large variety of protein sources, along with whole grains, fruits, and vegetables. Unfortunately, vegetarian restaurants are not found on every street corner, and therefore athletes need to improvise at other types of dining establishments. The following is a listing of common restaurants and the vegetarian protein sources typically found on the menu:

- *American:* Mainly steakhouses, these restaurants will typically have fish and pasta dishes with cheese on the menu.
- *Casual dining:* Mainly "chain" restaurants, veggie burgers are now commonly found in the burger section of the menu.
- *Chinese:* Chicken and fish can typically be substituted in any dish for beef. Tofu is found in the vegetable section of the menu.

- *Greek:* Fish dishes, lentil soup, and hummus (made from chickpeas) are traditional Greek foods.
- *Italian:* For semi-vegetarians, many dishes will be served with chicken. For lacto-vegetarians, dishes with pasta, vegetables, and cheese are easy to find. Vegans will most likely need to eat a protein source before heading to the restaurant because legumes, nuts, and soy products are hard to find in these restaurants.
- *Mexican:* Bean burritos can be made at any Mexican restaurant. Refried beans are typically served with main entrées. If available, ask for whole beans in dishes and as a side instead of refried beans, which are often prepared with lard or oil.
- *Pizzeria:* Chicken and shrimp can be found on the menu in gourmet pizzerias. Lacto-vegetarians can easily order a vegetable supreme pizza. Similar to Italian restaurants, vegans will typically

Vegetarian Dining Resources

The following resources can be provided to vegetarian athletes to locate vegetarian restaurants across the country:

- Vegetarian Journal's Guide to Natural Foods Restaurants in the U.S. & Canada, Third Edition, www.vrg.org, 1998
- Online Guide to Vegetarian Restaurants Around the World, www.vegdining.com
- Online Vegetarian Restaurants Guide, www.vegetarian-restaurants.net
- Vegetarian Travel Sites, www.happycow.net

Figure 15.9 Athletes who are vegetarian and travel throughout the United States and abroad can obtain vegetarian restaurant information and locations online.

need to eat more protein at breakfast, lunch, and as snacks if a pizzeria is the restaurant of choice for the evening.

- *Thai:* Similar to Chinese restaurants, chicken, fish, and tofu are commonly included in main entrée options, catering to all types of vegetarians.

The protein needs of athletes can be met by plant protein sources. More attention to protein substitutions is necessary as an athlete progresses from a semi-vegetarian to a vegan. However, the food industry has made it very easy to substitute nearly any animal product with a soy/vegetable product. Because of the American meat-focused society, it can take some time to adjust to a plant protein–based diet, but after some education and experimentation with foods, athletes can discover the health, performance, and taste benefits of being vegetarian.

Which vegetarian foods are rich in iron?

Athletes need iron for the synthesis of red blood cells and enzymes, as well as for proper immune and brain function. Iron is concentrated mainly in foods within the meat and protein foods group. As mentioned in Chapter 7 of this text, there are two forms of iron found in foods: heme (animal sources) and nonheme (plant sources). Nonheme iron is not absorbed as readily as heme iron, therefore justifying a special focus on iron for vegetarians.[42] Vegetarians can beat the iron challenge by consuming sufficient quantities of iron-rich foods, and possibly supplements, each day and pairing those foods with a source of vitamin C.

The main issue with iron in vegetarian diets is not necessarily the total quantity of iron obtained from plant foods, but the bioavailability of the iron ingested. Several studies have shown that vegetarian diets contain as much, if not more, total iron as compared to carnivorous diets.[40,43,44] However, because of the chemical form of iron (nonheme) and other constituents that may enhance or inhibit iron absorption, less iron from food may be absorbed into the bloodstream for use by the body. To compensate for the lower bioavailability of iron from plant sources, the RDA for iron intake for vegetarians is increased nearly 80% above the recommendation for individuals consuming a carnivorous diet. Male vegetarians should aim for 14 milligrams per day while female vegetarians (of childbearing age) should consume 33 milligrams per day.[17]

Iron is found in calcium-processed tofu, legumes, nuts, seeds, and iron-fortified cereals. For example,

1 cup of fortified corn flakes provides 9–10 milligrams of iron, supplying 68% and 29% of the daily requirement for men and women, respectively. Blackstrap molasses is also a good source of iron, and can be consumed as a spoonful dose or mixed with hot cereals. Semi-vegetarians can easily meet iron needs through several servings of chicken, fish, and plant foods each day.

Consuming a source of vitamin C at every meal will help vegetarians absorb the nonheme iron from foods. For example, a glass of orange juice will aid in the absorption of iron from a bowl of fortified corn flakes. Green peppers and tomatoes, which are packed with vitamin C, are a tasty match to tofu in burritos or spaghetti sauce. Every vegetarian meal should include a source of iron (iron-rich foods typically also contain a solid dose of protein) and fruits/vegetables, which are excellent sources of vitamin C.

If vegetarian athletes fail to meet their iron needs, low serum ferritin levels and iron-deficiency anemia can ensue.[45-47] Symptoms include fatigue, decreased tolerance of cold, and decreased physical stamina, which all obviously impair athletic performance. By making wise food selections, iron needs can generally be met and iron-deficiency anemia avoided. In fact, studies have shown that even though iron stores may be low, vegetarians are no more likely to develop iron-deficiency anemia than nonvegetarians.[48] However, for insurance, vegetarian athletes should be followed by a physician to monitor for low iron stores and iron-deficiency anemia.

Which vegetarian foods are rich in zinc?

Zinc is critical to the health, performance, and well-being of an athlete in many ways. Zinc is required for gene expression, cell growth and development, immune function, hormone production, protein and fat metabolism, and proper vision. The content and absorption of zinc from plant products are slightly lower than from animal products (mainly because of phytic acid, an inhibitor of zinc absorption), so vegetarians need to ensure their well-balanced diet includes plenty of rich sources of zinc.[42]

For the general population, daily zinc requirements for men and women have been set at 11 milligrams and 8 milligrams, respectively.[17] However, vegetarians may require up to 50% more zinc daily because of the lower availability of zinc from plant sources.[17] Vegetarian sources of zinc include whole grains, fortified cereals, legumes, nuts, seeds, and dairy products. For example, 1 cup of fortified bran flakes provides 4–5 milligrams of zinc, supplying about 40% and 55% of the daily requirement for men and women, respectively. These foods are often high in iron as well, providing the convenience of obtaining two critical nutrients in one food.

Zinc deficiency can cause a variety of problems, including an increased risk of infections, loss of appetite, diarrhea, and decreased thyroid hormone synthesis. Infections can take athletes out of training and competition for several days to weeks while healing and recuperating. Loss of appetite and diarrhea can cause failure to fuel the body properly, poor recovery, and malabsorption of nutrients. Decreased thyroid hormone synthesis can cause fatigue, weakness, and diminished capacity for high-intensity training. Athletes should focus on food sources of zinc because high doses via supplementation can cause decreased absorption of other nutrients, vomiting, and cramping.

Which vegetarian foods are rich in calcium and vitamin D?

Calcium and vitamin D are often thought of as being synonymous only with dairy products, so these two nutrients are often cited to be of special concern to vegetarians, especially vegans. However, because of the food industry and calcium-rich plant foods, calcium and vitamin D needs can easily be met on a vegetarian diet.

There has been an explosion of dairy/alternative products produced by the food industry, giving vegetarians many choices for calcium- and vitamin D–rich foods. Most common dairy products, such as milk, yogurt, and cheese, can be found in a "veggie" form, typically made from soy or grains. Most of these alternatives are fortified with calcium and vitamin D, providing equivalent amounts as compared to dairy products. Some varieties are not fortified, however, so vegetarians should read food labels to choose dairy alternatives that contain added calcium and vitamin D. Calcium is also found in dark green leafy vegetables, calcium-fortified cereals, legumes, and some nuts (e.g., almonds). The calcium availability from green leafy vegetables, legumes, and nuts is lower than from dairy products and other fortified

foods, and therefore should not be considered the sole source of calcium in the diet.[49] Calcium-fortified orange juice is widely available in supermarkets, with a few newer varieties fortified with vitamin D as well. In addition to fortified dairy/alternatives and orange juice, vitamin D is found in eggs and fortified cereals. Athletes aged 19–50 years require 1000 mg of calcium and 600 IU of vitamin D each day.

The largest problem related to calcium and vitamin D deficiency in vegetarian athletes is the long-term effect on bone health. Osteoporosis has been linked to low intake of these nutrients, as well as other dietary, lifestyle, and genetic factors. By maintaining adequate intakes of these nutrients, athletes can prevent bone-related athletic injuries and osteoporosis later in life.

Which vegetarian foods are rich in vitamin B_{12}?

Vitamin B_{12} is produced by microorganisms, bacteria, fungi, and algae; animals and plants cannot produce this nutrient. Animal foods are a rich source of vitamin B_{12} because animals can absorb the vitamin B_{12} produced by bacteria in the intestinal tract. Because plant foods do not have an "intestinal tract" with vitamin B_{12}–producing bacteria, plant foods do not contain any vitamin B_{12}. Semi-, pesco-, lacto-, and ovo-vegetarians generally, but not always, consume plenty of vitamin B_{12}. Vegans can fall short in this category because their diets are devoid of any animal products, potentially causing vitamin B_{12} deficiency and associated ramifications.[50] However, vegans and other vegetarians can consume more than adequate amounts of vitamin B_{12} through the wide range of fortified foods and multivitamin/mineral supplementation.

Athletes need vitamin B_{12} for metabolizing folate, which prevents megaloblastic anemia, and for maintaining the myelin sheath surrounding all nerves, allowing for proper functioning of the nervous system. Symptoms of vitamin B_{12} deficiency can include decreased sensation, loss of bowel and bladder control, depression, and general weakness. Long-term vitamin B_{12} deficiency can lead to irreversible nerve damage. Therefore, vitamin B_{12} is of great importance to athletes and deserves special attention, especially for vegans.

The daily requirement of vitamin B_{12} for both men and women is 2.4 micrograms per day. For vegetarians eating fish and dairy, a full daily dose of vitamin B_{12} can be obtained by eating 3 ounces of salmon, or 1 cup of yogurt plus 1 cup of milk. For vegans, 2 cups of fortified soy milk or 1½ cups of fortified cereal will provide 100% of the daily requirements. Therefore, it is not difficult to consume adequate amounts of vitamin B_{12}; it just requires an awareness of wise food choices.

Most multivitamin/mineral supplements will also supply 100% of the daily value for vitamin B_{12}.

Many sport-specific supplements also contain significant quantities of vitamin B_{12}. As always, vegetarian athletes should focus on whole foods first, and then use vitamin/mineral and sport supplements as extra insurance. A sample meal that contains a variety of nutrients essential to a healthful vegetarian diet is shown in **Training Table 15.4**.

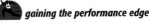

gaining the performance edge

Vegetarianism can be a healthy alternative to mainstream eating for athletes. By following a well-balanced diet and focusing on nutrient-dense protein foods and dairy/alternatives, vegetarians can consume all required nutrients in adequate amounts, leading to optimal health and athletic performance.

Training Table 15.4: Example of Vegetarian Dinner Meal

This dinner can be prepared and on the table in less than an hour, with leftovers ready for the rest of the week. The veggie burgers and greens should be served with an 8–12 oz glass of fortified soy milk to create a well-balanced meal, representing four different food groups. The entire dinner provides a significant source of protein, iron, zinc, calcium, vitamin D, and vitamin B_{12}.

Homemade Veggie Burgers

1¼ cups water
½ cup lentils, rinsed and drained
1 15 oz can of kidney, black, or garbanzo beans, drained and rinsed
⅓ cup wheat germ
¼ cup finely chopped pecans or walnuts
¼ cup chili sauce
½ tsp ground cumin
¼ tsp garlic salt
2 tsp dried parsley
Cooking spray
4 whole-wheat hamburger buns
Lettuce, tomato, cucumber, and avocado slices (optional)

1. In a small saucepan, combine the water and lentils and bring to a boil over high heat. Reduce the heat to low-medium, cover, and cook for 20–25 minutes, or until tender. After cooling for 25–30 minutes, drain the lentils if all the water has not been absorbed.

2. Place lentils and beans in a food processor and process until smooth.

3. Place the lentil/bean mixture in a medium bowl. Add the wheat germ and next five ingredients; mix to combine.

4. Form 4 patties with the mixture. Grill the burgers in a shallow frying pan coated with cooking spray for 5 minutes on each side. Burgers that will not be eaten at the meal can be stored (uncooked) in an airtight container for several days and cooked when desired.

5. Place each burger on a bun with your choice of toppings.

Good-for-You Greens

1 lb kale, washed and chopped coarsely
2 tbsp olive oil
½ lb mushrooms, washed and sliced
¼ tsp salt
¼ tsp ground black pepper
½ tsp dried oregano or basil

1. Place about ¼-inch of water in the bottom of a Dutch oven or other large pot. Place all the kale in the pot, cover, and cook over medium-high heat for 5–8 minutes or until slightly tender. Drain the water, but keep the kale in the pot.

2. Add the olive oil and mushrooms to the pot, sautéing the kale and mushrooms over medium heat. Add the spices.

3. Cook the kale and mushrooms about 5 minutes or until mushrooms are soft. Serve immediately with Homemade Veggie Burgers and a glass of fortified soy milk.

Makes 4 servings.

Nutrition information for entire meal, consisting of one Homemade Veggie Burger, one serving of Good-for-You Greens, and 12 oz fortified soy milk:

Calories: 800 kcal

Protein: 39 g

Iron: 12 mg (86% men, 36% women RDA)

Zinc: 5 mg (45% men, 63% women RDA)

Calcium: 705 mg (71% AI)

Vitamin D: 150 IU (25% RDA)

Vitamin B_{12}: 1.2 µg (50% RDA)

Source: Adapted from Rosensweig L and the food editors of Prevention magazine. *New Vegetarian Cuisine.* Emmaus, PA: Rodale Press; 1994.

The Box Score

Key Points of Chapter

- Special populations are those groups of athletes who find themselves in unique situations, physiological or otherwise, that impose nutritional demands beyond those of their sport alone.

- Diabetes is a metabolic disorder affecting the body's ability to regulate blood glucose levels. Athletes with diabetes must learn to regulate their blood glucose levels through the consumption of healthy food choices, the regular monitoring of blood glucose, and the coordinated timing of food intake, physical activity, and administration of medications.

- Diabetic athletes should consume diets similar in composition to the healthy nutrition recommendations for the general population with the exception of a special focus on the total quantity and timing of carbohydrate consumption. Athletes with diabetes should follow a consistent meal pattern in regard to time of meals, caloric content, and number of carbohydrates in each meal.

- Athletes with type 1 diabetes should check their blood glucose level prior to exercise and adjust food or insulin accordingly. During exercise lasting longer than 30 minutes, 15–30 grams of carbohydrates in simple form should be consumed every 30–60 minutes. Sports drinks, gels, and/or bars are excellent sources of carbohydrates for the diabetic athlete.

- Pregnancy demands that the female athlete consider not only her own nutrient requirements, but also those necessary to support the normal growth and development of a fetus. Pregnant athletes need to ensure the daily consumption of adequate calories (approximately 300 extra calories/day), protein (20–25 grams extra/day), B vitamins, vitamins A and C as well as magnesium and iron.

- Young athletes must follow a nutrition plan that meets the needs of their sport and at the same time allows for normal growth and maturation of body tissues. Parents and dietitians can follow the growth trends of a young athlete to help determine nutrition status over time.

- Child athletes are at a higher risk for dehydration and heat illness. As a result, monitoring fluid intake during practice and competitions and encouraging fluid intake will help maintain their fluid balance.

- Iron and calcium are two minerals that have been identified as being deficient in the diet of young athletes, particularly female athletes. Consumption of dairy products and/or calcium and iron-fortified foods along with a once-daily multivitamin/mineral supplement will help ensure that the vitamin and mineral needs of young athletes are being met.

- College athletes find themselves in the unique situation of being on their own for the first time in their lives and must learn how to take responsibility for their own nutritional practices. Poor eating and drinking habits, along with the added demands of college life, can spell disaster for a college athlete. Dietitians must do more than provide a meal plan to college athletes. They must also educate them about grocery shopping, meal planning, food preparation, and other healthy dietary practices to help ensure their overall health and athletic success.

- The number of masters athletes over the age of 40 is growing. Masters athletes need to consider their individual nutrient requirements, the needs of their sport, and any other special considerations resulting from chronic diseases or medication use. The rule of thumb is that masters athletes need to work on getting "more for less" from their diet via consumption of nutrient-dense foods and decreasing "unnecessary calories."

- Vegetarianism is being practiced by a growing number of athletes. It can be a healthy alternative to a traditional diet as long as substitutions are made. Depending on the type of vegetarian diet being followed, food choices may vary greatly. If planned appropriately, vegetarians and vegans can obtain the nutrition they need from whole foods and fortified products. One multivitamin/mineral per day can provide extra insurance that all micronutrient needs are being met.

Study Questions

1. What is the difference between type 1 and type 2 diabetes? Which type is most prevalent in athletes?

2. What nutritional habits should diabetic athletes adopt to enhance their ability not only to perform, but also to cope with their disease?

3. What are some of the nutritional concerns associated with the pregnant athlete? How many extra calories should a pregnant athlete consume daily?

4. What is a growth channel, and how might a nutrition expert use it?

5. Which sports tend to increase the chances of dehydration in young athletes? What recommendations should be given to young athletes to prevent dehydration?

6. Discuss the various factors that contribute to college athletes being considered as a "special population" in regard to nutrition.

7. What impact does alcohol have on one's diet and overall energy consumption?

8. Discuss how the nutrient needs of the young athlete differ from those of the masters athlete.

9. What is meant by "complementing proteins"? Which special population needs to be concerned most with complementing protein sources? Give two examples of food sources providing complementing proteins.

10. What are the different types of vegetarianism? What nutritional considerations must be taken into account when dealing with vegetarian athletes?

11. What suggestions for protein source alternatives would you give a vegetarian athlete who dines out frequently at nonvegetarian restaurants?

References

1. Barnes DE. *Action Plan for Diabetes*. Champaign, IL: Human Kinetics; 2004.

2. Anderson J, Geil PB. Nutritional management of diabetes mellitus. In: Shils ME, Olson JA, and Shike M, eds. *Modern Nutrition in Health and Disease*. Philadelphia, PA: Lippincott, Williams & Wilkins; 1999:1259–1286.

3. American Diabetes Association. Diagnosis and classification of diabetes mellitus. *Diabetes Care*. 2007;30:S42–S47.

4. American Diabetes Association. Physical activity/exercise and diabetes. *Diabetes Care*. 2004;27(suppl 1):S58–S62.

5. American Diabetes Association. Nutrition recommendations and interventions for diabetes. *Diabetes Care*. 2007;30:S48–S65.

6. Franz MJ, Bantle JP, Beebe CA, et al. Nutrition principles and recommendations in diabetes. *Diabetes Care*. 2004;27(suppl 1):S36–S46.

7. Pivarnik JM, Perkins CD, Moyerbrailean T. Athletes and pregnancy. *Clin Obstet Gynecol*. 2003;46(2):403–414.

8. Pitkin RM. Energy in pregnancy. *Am J Clin Nutr*. 1999;69(4):583.

9. Institute of Medicine. *Nutrition During Pregnancy*. Washington, DC: National Academies Press; 1990.

10. Institute of Medicine. *Dietary Reference Intakes for Energy, Carbohydrate, Fiber, Fat, Fatty Acids, Cholesterol, Protein, and Amino Acids*. Food and Nutrition Board. Washington, DC: National Academies Press; 2002.

11. Trumbo P, Schlicker S, Yates AA, Poos M. Dietary reference intakes for energy, carbohydrate, fiber, fat, fatty acids, cholesterol, protein and amino acids. *J Am Dietet Assoc*. 2002;102(11):1621–1630.

12. Artal R. Exercise and pregnancy. *Clin Sports Med*. 1992;11(2):363–377.

13. Artal R, Masaki DI, Khodiguian N, Romem Y, Rutherford SE, Wiswell RA. Exercise prescription in pregnancy: weight-bearing versus non-weight bearing exercise. *Am J Obstet Gynecol*. 1989;161:1464–1469.

14. Clapp JF III, Wesley M, Sleamaker RH. Thermoregulatory and metabolic responses prior to and during pregnancy. *Med Sci Sports Exerc*. 1987;19(2):124–130.

15. Institute of Medicine. *Dietary Reference Intakes for Thiamin, Riboflavin, Niacin, Vitamin B_6, Folate, Vitamin B_{12}, Pantothenic Acid, Biotin, and Choline*. Food and Nutrition Board. Washington, DC: National Academies Press; 1998.

16. Institute of Medicine. *Dietary Reference Intakes for Vitamin C, Vitamin E, Selenium and Carotenoids*. Food and Nutrition Board. Washington, DC: National Academies Press; 2000.

17. Institute of Medicine. *Dietary Reference Intakes for Vitamin A, Vitamin K, Arsenic, Coron, Chromium, Copper, Iodine, Iron, Manganese, Molybdenum, Nickel, Silicon, Vanadium and Zinc*. Food and Nutrition Board. Washington, DC: National Academies Press; 2001.

18. Bernhardt IB, Dorsey DJ. Hypervitaminosis A and congenital renal abnormalities in a human infant. *Obstet Gynecol*. 1974;43:750–755.

19. Institute of Medicine. *Dietary Reference Intakes for Calcium, Phosphorus, Magnesium, Vitamin D, and Flouride*. Food and Nutrition Board. Washington, DC: National Academies Press; 1997.

20. Wiggins DL, Wiggins ME. The female athlete. *Clin Sports Med*. 1997;16(4):593–612.

21. Centers for Disease Control, National Center for Health Statistics. CDC Growth Charts: United States. 2001. Available at: www.cdc.gov/nchs/about/major/nhanes/growthcharts/background.htm. Accessed March 13, 2005.

22. Berning JR, Steen SN. *Nutrition for Sport and Exercise*. 2nd ed. Gaithersburg, MD: Aspen Publishers; 1998.

23. Insel P, Turner RE, Ross D. *Nutrition, 2002 Update*. Sudbury, MA: Jones and Bartlett Publishers; 2002.

24. Insel P, Turner RE, Ross D. *Nutrition*. 2nd ed. Sudbury, MA: Jones and Bartlett Publishers; 2004.

25. Theintz GE, Howald H, Weiss U, Sizonenko PC. Evidence for a reduction of growth potential in adolescent female gymnasts. *J Pediatr*. 1993;122:306–313.

26. Lindholm C, Hagenfeldt K, Ringertz BM. Pubertal development in elite juvenile gymnasts: effects of physical training. *Acta Obstet Gynecol Scand*. 1994;73:269–273.

27. Rogol AD, Clark PA, Roemmich JN. Growth and pubertal development in children and adolescents: effects of diet and physical activity. *Am J Clin Nutr*. 2000;72(suppl):521s–528s.

28. Petrie HJ, Stover EA, Horswill CA. Nutritional concerns for the child and adolescent competitor. *Nutr*. 2004;20:620–631.

29. Bar-Or O. Children's responses to exercise in hot climates: implications for performance and health. *Gatorade Sports Sci Exchange*. 1994;7(2):1–5.

30. Institute of Medicine. *Dietary Reference Intakes for Calcium and Vitamin D*. Food and Nutrition Board. Washington, DC: National Academies Press; 2010.

31. Constantini NW, Eliakim A, Zigel L, Yaaron M, Falk B. Iron status of highly active adolescents: evidence of depleted iron stores in gymnasts. *Int J Sports Nutr Exerc Metabol*. 2000;10:62–70.

32. Leichliter JS, Meilman PW, Presley CA, Cashin JR. Alcohol use and related consequences among students with varying levels of involvement in college athletics. *J Am Coll Health*. 1998;46(1):257–262.

33. Nelson TF, Wechsler H. Alcohol and college athletes. *Med Sci Sports Exerc*. 2001;33(1):43–47.

34. Wilson GS, Pritchard ME, Schaffer J. Athletic status and drinking behavior in college students: the influence of gender and coping styles. *J Am Coll Health*. 2004;52(6):269–273.

35. Green GA, Uryasz FD, Petr TA, Bray CD. NCAA study of substance use and abuse habits of college student athletes. *Clin J Sport Med*. 2001;11:51–56.

36. Hetherington MM, Cameron F, Wallis DJ, Pirie LM. Stimulation of appetite by alcohol. *Physiol Behav*. 2001;74:283–289.

37. American Dietetic Association. Position of the American Dietetic Association: nutrition, aging and the continuum of care. *J Am Dietet Assoc*. 2000;100(5):580–595.

38. McGandy RB, Barrows CH, Spanias A, Meredith A, Stone JL, Norris AH. Nutrient intake and energy expenditure in men of different ages. *J Gerontol*. 1966;21:581–587.

39. Evans WJ. Exercise, nutrition and aging. *Clin Geriatr Med*. 1995;11(4):725–734.

40. American Dietetic Association. Position of the American Dietetic Association: vegetarian diets. *J Am Dietet Assoc*. 1997;97:1317–1321.

41. Haub MD, Wells AM, Tarnopolsky MA, Campbell WW. Effect of protein source on resistive-training-induced changes in

body composition and muscle size in older men. *Am J Clin Nutr*. 2002;76:511–517.

42. Hunt J. Bioavailability of iron, zinc and other trace minerals from vegetarian diets. *Am J Clin Nutr*. 2003;78(suppl):633S–639S.

43. Calkins BM, Whittaker DJ, Nair PP, Rider AA, Turjman N. Diet, nutrition intake, and metabolism in populations at high and low risk for colon cancer. *Am J Clin Nutr*. 1984;40(suppl):896–905.

44. Craig WJ. Iron status of vegetarians. *Am J Clin Nutr*. 1994;59(suppl):1233S–1237S.

45. Alexander D, Ball MJ, Mann J. Nutrient intake and haematological status of vegetarians and age-sex matched omnivores. *Eur J Clin Nutr*. 1994;48:538–546.

46. Anderson BM, Gibson RS, Sabry JH. The iron and zinc status of long-term vegetarian women. *Am J Clin Nutr*. 1981;34:1042–1048.

47. Hua NW, Stoohs RA, Facchini FS. Low iron status and enhanced insulin sensitivity in lacto-ovo vegetarians. *Br J Nutr*. 2001;86:515–519.

48. National Research Council, Food and Nutrition Board. *Diet and Health: Implications for Reducing Chronic Disease Risk*. Washington, DC: National Academies Press; 1989.

49. Weaver CM, Proulx WR, Heaney R. Choices for achieving adequate dietary calcium with a vegetarian diet. *Am J Clin Nutr*. 1999;70(suppl):543S–548S.

50. Herrmann W, Schorr H, Obeid R, Geisel J. Vitamin B_{12} status, particularly holotranscobalamin II and methylmalonic acid concentrations and hyperhomocysteinemia in vegetarians. *Am J Clin Nutr*. 2003;78:131–136.

Additional Resources

American College of Sports Medicine. *ACSM's Guidelines for Exercise Testing and Prescription*. 7th ed. Philadelphia, PA: Lippincott, Williams & Wilkins; 2006.

Colberg SR. *The Diabetic Athlete: Prescriptions for Exercise and Sports*. Champaign, IL: Human Kinetics; 2001.

Hammill PVV, Drizd TA, Johnson CL, Reed RB, Roche AF, Moore WM. Physical growth: National Center for Health Statistics percentiles. *Am J Clin Nutr*. 1979;32:607–629.

Key Questions Addressed

- Why should you consider becoming a registered dietitian?

- What are the steps to becoming a registered dietitian?

- Is continuing education required once the RD credential is obtained?

- What is the Board Certified as a Specialist in Sports Dietetics credential?

- Is licensure necessary for registered dietitians?

- How can students and professionals obtain practical experience in the field of sports nutrition?

- What are the potential job markets in sports nutrition?

- What are some of the daily responsibilities of a sports dietitian?

You Are the Nutrition Coach

Caroline will finish her dietetic internship and master's in nutrition in one month. She has been in competitive sports all of her life and is interested in pursuing a career in sports nutrition. She completed a 2-week rotation in a sports medicine clinic during her internship and did nutrition assessment and counseling with a variety of athletes in the clinic. Her master's thesis research included pre- and post-body composition assessments of middle-aged women in a 12-week strength-training program. During her job search, she finds there are a lot of jobs in hospitals and clinics, and one job open for a sports dietitian at the university close to her home.

Questions

- What education and experience does Caroline need to land the university sports dietitian job?

- How could her master's thesis help her compete with other dietitians applying for the university job?

- What can Caroline do to help her be more competitive for a similar sports dietitian job that might come up in the future?

Why should you consider becoming a registered dietitian?

A **registered dietitian (RD)** is a health care professional trained to provide food and nutrition information to the public. Approximately 70,000 registered dietitians work in the United States in a variety of settings, including hospitals, public health organizations, universities, research facilities, food service venues, corporations, consulting practices, fitness and wellness centers, and nonprofit businesses. The registered dietitian credential is the only one recognized nationally in the nutrition field. Therefore, RDs are the experts in the nutrition profession providing the link between dietary advice and optimal health. Regardless of the professional setting, becoming an RD is essential for working in the nutrition field because most, if not all, positions require the credential for employment.

gaining the performance edge

The educational background and professional recognition of becoming a registered dietitian are critical for succeeding in a sports nutrition career.

Sports nutrition is a relatively new specialty area for registered dietitians. The field of sports nutrition is growing exponentially because of the recognition that proper nutrition is paramount for optimal performance. The explosion of dietary supplements marketed to athletes has also created a need for these knowledgeable professionals who can help individuals decipher fact from fiction. Sports dietitians, who are also registered dietitians, provide the unique expertise in planning a practical, individualized meal plan for training and competition and educating athletes on the science behind nutrition recommendations for sport, while also determining the pros and cons of incorporating supplements for improving athletic performance.

The definitions and differences between a *dietitian* and a *nutritionist* warrant explanation. A dietitian is an individual who has successfully completed the requirements for the nationally recognized RD credential. A **nutritionist** may or may not have the same background as a dietitian. Anyone can claim to be a nutritionist without proving background, degrees, or certifications. In the job

market, including the area of sports nutrition, employers look for individuals who are RDs. Likewise, athletes are seeking out credentialed registered dietitians versus self-proclaimed nutritionists for nutrition guidance.

What are the steps to becoming a registered dietitian?

There are three main requirements to becoming a registered dietitian. The first requirement is to obtain a 4-year degree at an accredited college or university. The undergraduate coursework must meet the **Didactic Program in Dietetics (DPD)** requirements set by the **Commission on Accreditation for Dietetics Education (CADE)** within the **American Dietetic Association (ADA)**. Students can receive a 4-year degree in a variety of nutrition practice areas, but the core DPD requirements must be met as the first step in becoming an RD.

The second requirement for obtaining the RD credential is to complete a required amount of post-baccalaureate experience in nutrition. This is completed in one of two ways: either a 6–12 month dietetic internship at an accredited facility or acceptance into a coordinated undergraduate program. On either pathway, at least 900 hours of experience and practice supervised by registered dietitians are required.

After the internship or coordinated program is completed, the individual is then eligible to take the national board exam for dietitians. Successfully passing this exam is the third and final step in becoming a registered dietitian. All of these steps must be completed in the order described before the RD credential can be awarded. Each step is explained in greater detail in the following sections.

What are the curriculum requirements for an undergraduate degree in dietetics?

Students who are striving to become registered dietitians must complete specific coursework at an accredited 4-year educational institution. The required curriculum must meet the CADE standards set by the American Dietetic Association. To maintain accreditation, the college or university must be accredited by a body for higher education; integrate the DPD administratively and fiscally into the college structure; provide the required didactic instruction, which culminates in a baccalaureate degree; and designate a director who is credentialed as a registered dietitian and has earned at least a master's degree. The various accredited institutions provide similar coursework; however, they may have different departmental or major names. A majority of universities use the term *Dietetics* as the major name, and it can be housed in the College of Health and Applied Sciences, Consumer and Family Sciences, or Agriculture. Completion of the program culminates in a 4-year bachelor of science degree.

The curriculum is designed to teach students the science and practical application of food and nutrition for long-term health. The curriculum is demanding and provides a challenging academic experience starting in the first year of college. Students should be interested in and prepared for coursework involving several levels of chemistry, including biochemistry, microbiology, beginning and advanced medical nutrition, food sciences, communication, business management, food service, and research. Didactic program curricula are based on the foundation knowledge, skills, and competency statements for dietitians. There are eight foundations that are required to maintain CADE accreditation to ensure students' competency in the field. The foundations are in the following areas:

- Communication
- Physical and biological sciences
- Social sciences
- Research
- Food
- Nutrition
- Management
- Health care systems[1]

In addition to the core requirements, curriculum variations are allowed, including recommended electives, which are typically based on the direction of the individual university and the faculty advisors for the dietetics program. One of the fast-growing additions to the dietetics core curriculum is a course in sports nutrition. Several universities have even created a major or minor in sports nutrition. The sports nutrition courses are often open to exercise science, athletic training, and physical therapy students as well. The dietetic undergraduate student who is in-terested in becoming a sports dietitian would also benefit from taking electives in the exercise sciences. Classes in exercise physiology, kinesiology, sports management, and sports psychology will help prepare students for a sports nutrition career.

Do individuals need a graduate degree to be a sports dietitian?

Graduate degrees are not yet required to obtain the RD credential. However, because sports nutrition is a specialty area that requires significant knowledge of general nutrition, plus exercise physiology, body composition, and eating disorders, a graduate degree is helpful. In addition, many jobs in sports nutrition will require a master's degree for employment. Therefore, to be competitive in the sports nutrition job market, a master's degree is likely a necessity. Graduate degrees can be obtained in several areas, including advanced human nutrition, sports nutrition, exercise science, kinesiology, sports management, athletic training, and sports medicine. Any of these graduate programs provide a perfect complement to undergraduate studies for registered dietitians who work with recreational through elite athletes.

What do the dietetic internships entail and how does the experience relate to becoming a dietitian?

As mentioned previously, students have two main options for completing the second phase of becoming a registered dietitian: complete an accredited dietetic internship after undergraduate work or apply for a coordinated program that combines undergraduate work and the internship. There are approximately 260 accredited internship programs and 55 coordinated programs available in the United States. As shown by the numbers, most students complete their postbaccalaureate experience through an accredited dietetic internship. A third internship option that is gaining popularity is the distance internship option. Approximately 10 sites in the United States offer this option in which interns go to the sponsor site for some of the internship experience but also gain their practice-hour experiences in their home geographic region with approved registered dietitian preceptors. As with the undergraduate DPD and coordinated programs, internships must also maintain CADE accreditation through the ADA.

If a student chooses the popular route, after completing undergraduate work, the student applies for a dietetic internship. The application process works on a computer matching system, requiring students and internship sites to rank their preferences on sites and applicants, respectively. The computer system matches preferences on both ends and then notifies students of their placement. Dietetic internships are competitive, and some students who complete the 4-year DPD and gain a BS in Dietetics do not get into an internship program. There are not enough internship spaces available for the number of graduating students each year. Maintaining high grades throughout the entire 4-year undergraduate program, gaining volunteer or work experience in nutrition or food science, excelling in other academic areas, and leadership in extracurricular activities will help students during the internship matching process.

Dietetic internship sites must meet the requirements established by the CADE,[1] including:

- The internship must be housed in a college or university, health care facility, federal or state agency, business, or corporation. In addition, only individuals who have a 4-year BS and have completed all of the DPD requirements can be admitted.
- Interns must complete at least 900 hours of supervised practice experience, which must be completed within 2 years of starting the experience.

The sponsoring organization must designate a director who has at least a master's degree and is credentialed as a registered dietitian. Preceptors working with the interns must also be registered dietitians.

Coordinated programs in dietetics require only one application process. This pathway offers undergraduate coursework and internship practicum hours intermixed throughout the program. There are limited spaces available in the coordinated programs as well, and therefore students need to shine academically coming out of high school. Some students prefer this pathway because of the streamlined nature of the experience and guaranteed internship hours.

There is a long list of competencies that individuals are required to master before completing the dietetic internship or coordinated program. The competencies are designed to ensure that all entry-level dietitians will possess core knowledge, skills, and abilities in a variety of nutrition-related areas prior to employment in the field. The competencies presented in broad categories include individual/group education and counseling, regulations, food service, program and material development, interpreting medical/scientific data and applying them in clinical settings, medical nutrition therapy, advanced nutrition support, and competency in working with diverse cultures. Only after students have successfully met the core competency standards can graduation occur, making them eligible to take the RD examination.

Dietetic internships and coordinated programs can also offer an emphasis area in addition to the core competencies. Sites are required to develop their own set of competencies to establish an emphasis area for their program. These areas include advanced nutrition therapy, community nutrition, sports nutrition, food service management, business, and research. Emphasis areas are considered a "bonus"; therefore, time spent in the specialty area is in addition to time allotted to mastering core competencies.

Dietetic internships and coordinated programs are standardized and regulated to provide each potential registered dietitian with similar background knowledge, skills, and abilities. The training is rigorous and demanding; however, because the RD credential is the only one recognized in the field, the profession demands a high level of knowledge, skill, and analytical ability from each dietitian. This process helps ensure that the profession maintains its high level of credibility in the health care, food science, education, and research fields.

How is the board exam taken, and what topic areas are covered?

After successfully completing a dietetic internship or coordinated program, each individual is then eligible to take the RD board exam. This is a standardized test taken on a computer at various sites across the nation. The exam tests the student's knowledge and practical application of all of the core competency areas from the DPD and internship, including clinical nutrition, food service management, and community nutrition. Scoring of the exam occurs immediately following the test. Successful scores are sent to the ADA Commission on Dietetic Registration. Shortly thereafter, the commission issues a registration card that allows the dietitian to use the RD credential.

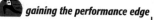
gaining the performance edge

The process of becoming a registered dietitian includes obtaining an undergraduate degree in dietetics from an accredited university, successfully completing postbaccalaureate work through a dietetic internship or coordinated program, and passing the RD board exam. The RD credential is essential for individuals interested in the field of sports nutrition.

Is continuing education required once the RD credential is obtained?

All registered dietitians must obtain continuing education credits to update their knowledge and skills in their area of practice. The continuing education process for RDs includes developing a professional development portfolio plan following guidelines set by the Commission on Dietetic Registration (CDR) of the ADA. This plan guides the registered dietitian in selection of continuing education activities that will enhance, update, and provide new knowledge in the primary practice area in which they work. Registration renewal occurs every 5 years, requiring 75 hours of continuing education. Completion of these hours can be obtained through various means including, but not limited to, the following:

- Attending continuing education seminars and conferences
- Completion of dietetics-related academic coursework
- Conducting research
- Attaining CDR-approved certification such as the Certified Specialist in Sports Dietetics (CSSD)
- Participating in journal clubs and study groups

Requiring continuing education for RDs encourages and ensures that each dietitian will regularly maintain a high level of knowledge in the area in which he or she works. The portfolio system allows each dietitian to choose one or several areas of nutrition for professional development based on his or her current career path.

What is the Board Certified as a Specialist in Sports Dietetics credential?

Specialty board certification for registered dietitians is offered by the Commission on Dietetic Registration in the areas of sports dietetics, pediatric nutrition, renal nutrition, oncology nutrition, and gerontological nutrition. The Board Certified as a Specialist in Sports Dietetics credential (CSSD) was first offered as a specialty certification in 2006. Certification is granted in recognition of the applicant's documented practice experience in sports nutrition and successful completion of a computerized examination. Sports dietetics practitioners are defined as registered dietitians who are experienced in applying evidence-based nutrition knowledge in exercise and sports. They assess, educate, and counsel athletes and active individuals. They design, implement,

and manage safe and effective nutrition strategies that enhance lifelong health, fitness, and optimal performance.[2]

To be eligible for the CSSD, applicants must:

- Be a registered dietitian for a minimum of 2 years.
- Document a minimum of 1500 hours of practice directly in the sports nutrition area within the past 5 years.
- Submit an application and a $250 application fee.[2]

Once the application is reviewed and accepted, the applicant can select a test site in his or her geographical area, then schedule and take the computerized examination. If a passing exam grade is achieved, the applicant can use the credential RD, CSSD for the 5-year certification period. At the end of the 5-year period, specialists can apply for recertification by successfully submitting the application, application fee, and achieving a passing grade on the CSSD examination.

Is licensure necessary for registered dietitians?

Forty-six states have laws regulating dietitians and/or nutritionists through registration, certification, or licensure. Certification and registration are much less strict than licensure; they limit the use of some titles for dietetic practice and/or may require a state examination but do not limit the practice of nutrition for nonregistered or uncertified persons. Licensure is the strictest of the state regulations, and 35 states and Puerto Rico currently have licensure laws.[3] Licensure laws regulate both the definition of titles that can be used and the scope of practice for the profession. The licensure process was initiated in many states to ensure that only qualified professionals, with proof of adequate education and experience, provide nutrition services or advice to individuals seeking nutrition care. Nonlicensed professionals are subject to prosecution for practicing without a license. The licensure process is similar to other allied health care professionals such as pharmacists, physical therapists, athletic trainers, and nursing professionals. Consumers, especially athletes, should inquire about the RD and CSSD credentials and licensure before choosing a dietitian to provide them with nutrition education.

In states where licensure is required, dietitians can obtain a license if they are a registered dietitian in good standing with the ADA. Licensure requires proof of dietetic registration and a fee. Some differences in the licensing laws and fees occur from state to state. The license usually indicates who is allowed to practice as a dietitian in the state. This includes allowing only licensed dietitians to use the name "dietitian" and most often means the title "nutritionist" is not a recognized dietetic professional. **Licensed Dietitian (LD)** and **Licensed Dietitian Nutritionist (LDN)** are two common examples of how the licensure laws distinguish the titles of licensed nutrition professionals. Continuing education is also required to maintain licensure, which is renewed on an annual or bi-annual basis. The continuing education that dietitians maintain for their dietetic registration usually can also be used for the licensure continuing education requirement.

Licensed Dietitian (LD) or Licensed Dietitian Nutritionist (LDN) Dietitian who has obtained a state license to practice dietetics following the state-regulated practice guidelines.

What if you are not an RD and don't have a license—can you still give nutrition advice to athletes?

There are many times when an athletic program does not have a dietitian available to provide all of the sports nutrition education. Sports professionals other than dietitians can provide some nutrition education; however, there are limitations. It is important for non-RDs to understand these limitations and recognize when a referral to an RD is appropriate.

The non-RD professionals that athletes typically obtain nutrition information from include athletic trainers, strength and conditioning coaches, team coaches, and physicians. Non-RD sports professionals can do a great job of imparting nutrition information because they often have an excellent rapport with the athlete, which encourages good communication of nutrition needs, practical applications, and goals for improving athletic performance. However, these nonlicensed individuals need to be careful not to break licensure laws by providing specific nutrition counseling or medical nutrition therapy. Medical nutrition therapy, individualized nutrition assessment, and development of nutritional plans are functions that registered dietitians and CSSDs are specifically trained (and in 35 states licensed) to do. As discussed in Chapter 10, non-RD sports professionals can provide athletes with general nutrition information that is considered "public domain." Examples of public domain information include the MyPlate food guidance system, dietary guidelines, hydration recommendations, and precautions for

training/competing in the heat. This information is easily accessible from large government, business, and educational or professional organizations.

It is important that nonlicensed nondietitians have a good working knowledge of nutrition before conveying advice to athletes. Several nondietetic undergraduate programs, such as athletic training, require at least one course in nutrition. Any non-RD who is interested in providing some nutrition guidance to athletes is encouraged to take additional nutrition courses in college as well as attend continuing education seminars. These professional development opportunities will help non-RDs understand the science behind recommendations as well as methods for communicating the practical application of concepts in the sport setting.

When athletes need more information and counseling beyond the public domain information, a referral should be made to an RD. Referrals should be made at minimum when:

- An athlete presents with an eating disorder.
- An athlete has a medical condition such as diabetes, high cholesterol, hypertension, and others that require nutrition education and treatment.
- Medical information such as laboratory data, medical history, and consultation with medical providers is needed to accurately educate the athlete.
- Nutrition assessment and a nutritional care plan need to be developed.
- The athlete needs specific nutrition information that the professional does not have the knowledge and expertise to provide.

The sports professional and RD will then work together as a team to ensure that the nutrition plan matches the athlete's training regimen and addresses health or performance concerns.[4] One of the most important aspects of a team approach is the delivery of a consistent message from all sports professionals working with the athlete to ensure consistency and to increase the likelihood of success.

How can students and professionals obtain practical experience in the field of sports nutrition?

For any student or sports professional who is interested in pursuing a career in sports nutrition, practical experience is of the utmost importance. Sports nutrition is a specialty area and therefore requires a solid educational background as well as practical experience in a "real-world" setting. Even registered dietitians cannot be an "expert" in sports nutrition without the experience of applying nutrition knowledge specifically to athletes. Practical experience can be obtained in a variety of ways including, but not limited to, the following:

- *Teaching/graduate assistantships*. Both undergraduate and graduate students can pursue opportunities on campus for assistantship positions. These assignments may involve teaching a sports nutrition course, counseling student athletes in a campus wellness center, or working with a specific athletic team.
- *Research*. Professors in nutrition and exercise science departments are usually looking for eager students to assist with gathering and analyzing data for research projects. Students should inquire about current projects as well as potential upcoming data collection related specifically to sports nutrition and athletic performance.
- *Hospitals*. Many local hospitals have a sports medicine department that employs sports physicians, athletic trainers, physical therapists, and possibly also a sports dietitian. These sports medicine or performance departments are a great way to observe a wide variety of professionals working as a team to assist athletes. These centers often can provide the opportunity to work with athletes in endurance, strength/power, and team sports, ensuring a well-balanced experience.
- *Health clubs*. Depending on the size and extent of a health club or fitness center, a dietitian may be on staff and work with a variety of recreational athletes. Many people who are fitness enthusiasts are also interested in working on their nutrition to enhance their workouts. For most sports dietitians, a majority of their clients are recreational athletes (versus elite or professional), so experience working with this population will be valuable regardless of your final career path.
- *Internships*. Many businesses and nonprofit organizations will offer short-term internship programs for students and/or professionals in the areas of nutrition, exercise physiology, or other sport sciences. Typically 12–16 weeks in length, these part-time or full-time positions allow an individual to have the experience of what happens on a daily basis in the world of sports nutrition. Often these positions will provide a wide range of opportunities and responsibilities, giving an individual a well-rounded experience.
- *Volunteer work*. One of the best ways to get experience and to network is to volunteer within a professional organization. Working on a committee, assisting at regional or national conferences, writing book reviews, or giving student presentations on campus are excellent opportunities for gaining sports nutrition/science knowledge while also learning the art of organization, planning, and facilitating.

Students should begin seeking opportunities for practical experience in their sophomore and junior years in college. Dietetic and other sports science students should continue to search for positions throughout college, aiming for variety, to allow for an educated decision on a final career path.

What are the potential job markets in sports nutrition?

Once an individual has acquired the necessary educational background and practical experience, the next step is to look for a permanent position in the field of sports nutrition. Dietitians and other sports professionals can be involved in counseling fitness enthusiasts, as well as recreational, elite, or professional athletes through a variety of venues. A full-time position performing only sports nutrition duties is becoming more common; however, professionals should be prepared to bring other skills to the table in order to be qualified for an existing position or to create a new job in an established facility. The following are a sampling of the most likely places to find a career in sports nutrition:

- *Clinical settings*. Mainly associated with a hospital, these positions may be incorporated into an outpatient dietitian position or as part of a sports medicine clinic. In the outpatient setting, athletes are typically referred to a dietitian for a non-sports-related medical issue. In a sports medicine clinic, athletes are generally counseled on sports injury treatment/prevention or techniques for improving overall performance. A sports medicine clinic is one of the most likely places to find a full-time sports nutrition position.
- *Sport performance companies*. These relatively new companies or programs with sports medicine facilities provide team and individual coaching to improve speed, agility, power, and overall sport performance.

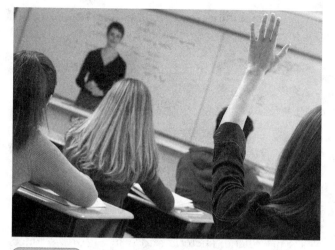

Figure 16.1 Nutrition education in action. Sports dietitians provide education to athletes in many different settings, including on the field, in the athletic training room, in the classroom, or in private consultation offices.

- *Fitness/wellness facilities.* There are many fitness centers, park districts, and wellness centers in private companies that hire sports dietitians. Opportunities to teach group nutrition classes and provide one-on-one sports nutrition counseling, wellness education, and clinical nutrition management are abundant in these settings.

- *College sport teams.* Many athletic departments now hire a full-time or part-time sports dietitian to provide nutrition assessment and education for a specific team or all teams in the athletic department.

- *Academics* (see Figure 16.1). Universities provide a wealth of opportunities to be involved in sports nutrition. One option is to teach a sports nutrition class for undergraduate or graduate students in a dietetics or exercise science department. Several universities and colleges have a unique pairing of the health center and recreation center, which lends itself perfectly to therapeutic and preventive nutrition education, including sports nutrition. Many professors are now concentrating their research in the area of sports nutrition, providing another possibility for a full-time position on a university campus.

- *Professional teams.* Working with a professional sporting team can be one of the most challenging jobs to obtain because so few positions actually exist. Although there are some exceptions, most of the dietitians who work with professional teams do so on a part-time, consultant basis. These positions are generally filled by sports dietitians who have worked in the field for many years and have extensive experience counseling athletes.

- *Corporations/food industry.* Companies who either produce or market sports nutrition products often prefer to hire a dietitian over a general research or sales professional to have the experts working on their products. These jobs can include research, development, marketing, and sales responsibilities.

- *Private consulting.* Currently one of the most popular avenues for sports dietitians, a private consulting business allows an individual to "create" his or her own position. As mentioned previously, sports nutrition is a relatively new field, and therefore permanent positions are not abundant. Often, the best option for a dietitian is to open a private practice that can cater to local and regional athletes. Dietitians should be prepared to include other areas of nutrition and wellness in their business plan because sports nutrition will typically not generate enough revenue to completely sustain a business, at least not initially.

There are several ways to keep abreast of job openings and opportunities in sports nutrition. Networking with sports dietitians and viewing job postings at professional conferences are a couple of targeted ways to find a job. Often, superior performance during an internship or other practical experience in a professional setting can lead to a permanent position. Several Web sites are also helpful in the search for a job in sports nutrition:

- www.eatright.org: American Dietetic Association, CareerLink
- www.acsm.org: American College of Sports Medicine
- www.jobsindietetics.com: Jobs in Dietetics newsletter
- www.hpcareer.net: Health promotion career finder
- www.nsca-lift.org: National Strength and Conditioning Association
- www.higheredjobs.com

What are some of the daily responsibilities of a sports dietitian?

Two of the authors of this book, Lisa Burgoon and Heather Fink, are practicing sports dietitians. To give others a peek into their history, experiences, and daily roles and responsibilities, Lisa and Heather share their stories on how they became sports dietitians, what's involved in their current jobs, and advice to those pursuing a career in sports nutrition.

Lisa Burgoon, MS, RD, CSSD, LDN

How did I become a sports dietitian?

I grew up in a sports-minded and active family. My siblings and I started competing on the local swim team at age 5, and we continued swimming through high school. Our summers were filled with outdoor swim meets, and leisure time was spent at the pool racing our friends. I played T-ball and softball from a youngster through high school as well. My parents are avid golfers and our family vacations often included hiking, biking, and fun outdoor activities. This active lifestyle from a very young age instilled an interest in human physiology and how the body can be pushed to perform better.

I enrolled in the Dietetics program at Michigan State University and found the nutrition classes interesting and challenging. The class that really sparked my interest in sports nutrition was an exercise physiology course. I was fascinated with the human physiology behind exercise and movement.

After completing my bachelor of science degree from Michigan State, I was accepted into the dietetic internship program at the Hines Veterans Administration Medical Center near Chicago, Illinois. This internship was an intense 9 months of clinical, educational, and food management work and included an elective project that interns completed as a group. My group designed the first-ever wellness program at the medical center. Adding the wellness aspect to my nutrition and exercise science interest helped me narrow the focus of my eventual career path as a registered dietitian.

My first job after the internship was at the Veterans Administration Medical Center in Denver, Colorado. I was primarily in charge of the dietary needs of patients on the medical and surgical floors. I loved the work and learned an incredible amount about medical nutrition therapy in my first few years within the center. That experience and knowledge have helped me over the years in my consultations with athletes and other clients seeking to improve their nutrition habits.

Although I enjoyed the work at the hospital, I knew I wanted to further my education and learn more in the exercise science area. Chapman University, in California, opened a branch of their college in Denver. They offered a unique master's degree in sports medicine, with an affiliation with Metro State University, also in Denver. I worked full time

and took evening classes for nearly 5 years before completing my master's degree in sports medicine. The program was unique, allowing me to take sports nutrition, advanced exercise physiology, athletic training, kinesiology, and research courses that truly hooked me on sports nutrition as a career. When I had time, I conducted seminars on sports nutrition with local high school teams and with several medical residency programs at the many hospitals in downtown Denver.

Shortly after completing my thesis, I interviewed for and was offered a position at the University of Illinois at Urbana-Champaign as the dietitian at the McKinley Student Health Center. I worked in that position for 5 years, learning a lot about eating disorders, weight management, and working with some athletes on campus. Heather Fink was one of the graduate assistants who worked with me and the sports dietitian at the SportWell Center. After that dietitian left, I moved into the sports nutrition position and worked as the SportWell coordinator/ sports dietitian.

After 8 years as coordinator of the SportWell Center, and after completing the first edition of this text, I decided to change the direction of my career. I began teaching at the University of Illinois in the Department of Food Science and Human Nutrition and became Board Certified as a Specialist in Sports Dietetics. I taught an upper-level dietetics capstone course in nutrition assessment and therapy and created the first sports nutrition course on our campus. In addition, I served as a coordinator on a USDA Higher Education Challenge Grant in student leadership development in the College of Agricultural, Consumer, and Environmental Sciences.

My career continues to evolve in higher education. I teach an introductory level leadership theory course, and facilitate leadership development programs for students on campus. I continue to teach the sports nutrition course at least once per year in either a blended or fully online format. I am also revising a curriculum in sports nutrition for athletic trainers to gain continuing education hours.

What are my daily roles and responsibilities as a sports dietitian?

My job responsibilities are quite different as an instructor of sports nutrition and dietetics when compared to being a practicing sports dietitian. While at SportWell, I completed individual assessment of clients, provided group and one-on-one counseling to athletes in the Division of Intercollegiate Athletics, and educated hundreds of recreational and NCAA athletes each year on sports and general nutrition topics. Now I teach juniors, seniors, and graduate students about sports nutrition and general wellness, and I give them practical information that they will be able to use with their own clients after they obtain their degrees, certifications, and first jobs. Teaching at the college level has been a great experience in which I am able to integrate my practical experiences working with athletes with the academic side of teaching. I have the added pleasure of working with students in many majors including dietetics, human nutrition, exercise physiology, food industry, and athletic training.

My teaching philosophy includes providing experiential learning in the classroom. I draw on my 20-plus years as a practicing dietitian to provide real-life examples, cases, and interactive discussions and assignments to help students learn. During the school semester I spend at least one-half of my workweek creating or revising course material, developing classroom activities, teaching, grading, and maintaining close contact with my students. I have maintained the practical aspects and skills of one-on-one and group education for athletes through providing some private consulting.

What are my three key pieces of advice for individuals pursuing a career in sports nutrition?

1. *Gain individual consultation experience.* You will need excellent communication skills when working with athletes in individual or group settings. You can gain these skills during your internship, while in a clinical or outpatient setting, or in any job where you meet individually with clients. Learn the language of athletes and how the various sports are played. This will help you communicate with athletes on their level and you will gain credibility by knowing (and caring about) their sport.

2. *Join professional organizations.* There are many state and national organizations that will help you stay current with sports nutrition information and provide excellent networking opportunities. The American Dietetic Association, American College of Sports Medicine, **Sports, Cardiovascular and Wellness Nutritionists (SCAN)**, and other dietetic practice groups all have national and regional confer-

Sports, Cardiovascular and Wellness Nutritionists (SCAN) Dietetic practice group of nutrition professionals with expertise and skills in promoting the role of nutrition in physical performance, cardiovascular health, wellness, and disordered eating.

ences annually. Attend these conferences to update your knowledge. Seek out mentors in these organizations as well. Many mentors not only help you improve your skills as a sports dietitian, but also may be able to help you obtain a job in sports nutrition.

3. *Maintain focus in education and experiences.* It will take some effort to obtain a sports nutrition job in a somewhat limited job market. The better qualified candidate will get that job. Focus your education on sports nutrition, exercise science, and other aspects of the sports environment. A master's degree in nutrition with an emphasis on exercise science will be highly desirable to potential employers. Get paid work experience with a sport team or in a clinic (even on a part-time basis) so that you gain practical hours in the sports nutrition arena.

Heather Hedrick Fink, MS, RD, CSSD

How did I become a sports dietitian?

My passion and enthusiasm for food and nutrition began in junior high. I had an excellent home economics teacher who sparked my interest in proper nutrition and cooking. I continued to register for food and nutrition courses throughout high school, finding my interest deepening with each class. In my senior year of high school, there was no question in my mind of what my major would be in college—I was determined to be a dietitian.

I graduated from the University of Illinois in Urbana/Champaign with a bachelor of science degree in dietetics. While in my undergraduate program, I began to discover another area of interest that was a perfect match to dietetics—exercise physiology. I took one class in my undergraduate work in the exercise science department, but continued to focus mainly on obtaining the RD credential. After graduating, I spent a year at the University of Wisconsin, Madison, Hospital and Clinics successfully completing my dietetics internship. Several months into the internship I realized that clinical nutrition was not my passion. It was then that I decided to go back to school for a graduate degree in exercise science. I returned to the University of Illinois after receiving an offer for an assistantship that would combine several experiences: performing individual nutrition consultations (after I passed the RD exam) in the student health center, working within the nutrition department as a teaching assistant for a communication and sports nutrition course, and conducting a variety of programs and services through the student recreation center in a facility called SportWell. My duties within SportWell consisted of facilitating a weight management class, performing body composition measurements on students and faculty, presenting peer review sessions around campus on body image and healthy eating, and working with athletes. The assistantship gave me an ideal opportunity to begin practicing as a dietitian, while also working on my master of science degree in a different academic area. Not only did I get hands-on experience working as a dietitian, I had two incredible dietitian mentors to learn from, one of whom was Lisa Burgoon.

During my graduate work but outside my assistantship, I had one of the most valuable experiences of my education. I volunteered to be the dietitian for the 70+ Team who competed in the Race Across America (RAAM). I compiled the nutrition plans for all four riders and accompanied the men on their journey across the United States, preparing food, monitoring hydration status, and ensuring that they were fueled at all times. Although I was not paid, this position gave me another opportunity for hands-on, practical experience in sports nutrition.

During my last semester in graduate school, I attended the SCAN professional conference. While networking at the conference, I learned of a full-time dietitian position at the National Institute for Fitness and Sport in Indianapolis. I applied, interviewed, and was hired within 2 weeks of the conference. My educational background and the practical, hands-on experience I had gained during my graduate assistantship and volunteer opportunities made my résumé well-balanced and my qualifications a perfect match for the job. Most recently, I have advanced my career by obtaining the Certified Specialist in Sports Dietetics credential. This new designation has helped me to gain more credibility, visibility, and marketability in the local community and nationwide.

What are my daily roles and responsibilities as a sports dietitian?

The National Institute for Fitness and Sport (NIFS) is a nonprofit organization located in downtown Indianapolis, Indiana. NIFS's mission is to enhance human health, physical fitness, and athletic performance through research, education, and service for people of all ages and abilities. I am the Assistant Director of Educational Services, a job with a plethora of roles and responsibilities.

Specific to the area of sports nutrition, I educate individuals and groups in a variety of ways. I conduct one-on-one nutrition consultations with ath-

letes, ranging from the fitness enthusiast to the elite athlete. Most of my nutrition clients are triathletes, duathletes, swimmers, and runners because I also train and compete in these sports. I provide group presentations on sports nutrition and dietary supplements to athletes, parents, athletic trainers, and coaches at local high schools, universities, medical centers, and club teams. I coordinate and facilitate a half-marathon training program for runners and walkers in which I disseminate daily training nutrition information. I write informational articles for publications such as the NIFS newsletter, the National Federation of State High School Association's publications, as well as other local magazines/newsletters on a variety of sports nutrition topics. I am routinely interviewed regarding sports nutrition topics by local television stations and newspapers as well as national magazines and periodicals. Fueling individuals for fitness and performance is an exciting and fulfilling aspect of my job.

In addition to sports nutrition, I have many other responsibilities at NIFS. I present wellness seminars to corporations, schools, churches, and other groups related to nutrition, fitness, and wellness. I coordinate our team-building program, helping groups to come together to work as a cohesive team. We employ undergraduate and graduate students within our full-time internship program, which I coordinate throughout the year. I plan and facilitate educational workshops for professional organizations, sports teams, and individuals in the community. Educational Services also acts as an in-house resource to all the other departments within NIFS, providing advice, consultations, and written education materials.

My position within NIFS is a unique combination of nutrition, fitness, and wellness. Each day is different, providing new challenges and adventures. I thoroughly enjoy all of my opportunities to work with athletes on sports nutrition, and treasure the variety and balance of my other roles and responsibilities.

What are my three key pieces of advice for individuals pursuing a career in sports nutrition?

1. *Gain practical experience.* Anyone interested in sports nutrition needs to seek out opportunities to put knowledge into practice. Volunteering, finding part-time jobs, writing articles, performing book reviews, helping conduct research, or taking advantage of any other means of getting hands-on experience will be vital to future success.

2. *Keep current.* Our knowledge of sports nutrition is always changing and expanding. Join professional organizations, read peer-reviewed journals, attend conferences, and take courses in sports nutrition to keep your knowledge up-to-date.

3. *Be active in athletics.* Athletes relate best to other athletes. If you are truly interested in sports nutrition, get involved in a sport and be active. A dietitian who not only talks the talk, but also walks the walk, will be highly respected and regarded in the athletic community.

The Box Score

Key Points of Chapter

- To become a registered dietitian, individuals must meet specific requirements in undergraduate college courses and obtain a minimum of a bachelor's degree at an accredited college or university.

- Registered dietitians have to obtain a minimum of 900 hours of supervised experience after obtaining a bachelor's degree before they can take the registration exam for dietitians.

- In some states, registered dietitians must be licensed, in addition to being registered. Laws in states that require licensure are developed to protect the public from harm that could potentially be done by individuals who say they are "nutritionists." These individuals typically have not had the same education, training, or supervision as registered and licensed dietitians.

- Non-nutrition-credentialed professionals should check licensure laws in their state to be sure they are not providing nutrition services outside of the law. Much public domain information is available for all professionals to educate athletes, in order to help them with performance nutrition.

- The Board Certified as a Specialist in Sports Dietetics (CSSD) credential is a certification offered by the Commission on Dietetic Registration of the American Dietetic Association. Individuals with this credential are recognized as knowledgeable and experienced in working with athletes and nutrition for performance enhancement.

- Obtaining the RD credential is the first step to becoming a sports dietitian. Additional work and volunteer experience in the sports nutrition arena, as well as possible graduate studies in the exercise science field, will prepare dietitians for a job in sports nutrition.

Study Questions

1. What, if any, are the differences between a sports nutritionist and a dietitian?

2. In what job settings can registered dietitians be found?

3. What are the three required steps that must be completed in order to become a registered dietitian?

4. What academic coursework should students be prepared to take when pursuing a BS degree in dietetics?

5. Discuss the various ways in which a registered dietitian may obtain continuing education credits.

6. Discuss some of the various ways that students interested in sports nutrition can get field experience.

7. What are some of the daily roles and responsibilities of a registered dietitian involved in sports nutrition?

8. What nutrition information can an individual who is not a licensed or registered dietitian provide to athletes? What are the legal and ethical issues surrounding noncredentialed nutrition assessment and therapy?

9. Explain the qualification requirements for the CSSD credential. Why is this credential important in the sports nutrition field?

References

1. Commission on Accreditation of Dietetics Education. 2002 Eligibility Requirements and Accreditation Standards. Chicago, IL: American Dietetics Association; 2002:1–25.

2. American Dietetic Association, Commission on Dietetic Registration. Sports Dietetics Application Booklet. Available at: www.cdrnet.org/PDFs/SportsDieteticsApplicationBooklet3=20=07.pdf. Accessed July 25, 2007.

3. American Dietetic Association. Advocacy and the Profession, Licensure, and Certification. Available at: www.eatright.org/ada/files/licensure_laws1.pdf. Accessed June 25, 2005.

4. Driskell JA, Wolinsky I. *Nutritional Assessment of Athletes.* Boca Raton, FL: CRC Press; 2002.

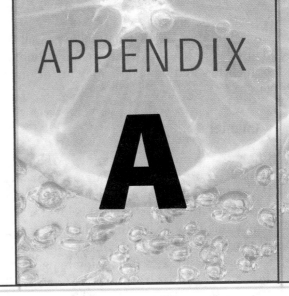

You Are the Nutrition Coach— Answers

APPENDIX A

Chapter 1

Jennifer has several top priorities—the first consists of her athletic goals/objectives and the second relates to her cholesterol levels. As mentioned in this chapter, the stated athletic goals/objectives are often the main reason why an athlete seeks advice regarding nutrition. If these objectives are not addressed, the athlete will leave the appointment frustrated and disappointed, and may disregard other topics that were discussed (although they may be valid issues). Second, because high cholesterol levels put an individual at high risk for heart disease, it is important to discover how successful she has been at lowering her blood cholesterol levels to an appropriate and healthy range.

As Jennifer struggles with maintaining her weight, she may be cutting out nutrients her body needs to maintain energy levels and to recover quickly from exercise. A quick assessment of her overall calorie intake and a review of the types of foods she is consuming should help reveal whether she is missing out on valuable nutrients needed for health and exercise performance. To address her concerns regarding her constant hunger, she may need to eat more often or choose foods that provide satiation for longer periods of time. Often, when individuals start a weight loss plan, they decrease intakes of fat and protein. Both protein and fat provide satiety, and if they are decreased too drastically, hunger can result. She should be encouraged to include a variety of foods, balance the food choices within all of the food groups, and eat all foods in moderation. This pattern of eating will aid in weight maintenance, curb her hunger, provide adequate calories to sustain daily energy levels, and decrease her recovery time.

Chapter 2

Kay is making a bad decision. Although it is true that fats are a more energy-dense macronutrient than proteins or carbohydrates, that does not mean that they are the fuel of choice for all activities. Intense sprint events lasting up to 3 minutes in length rely very heavily on the anaerobic energy system, with strong support from both the phosphagen and aerobic energy systems. As a result, Kay's decision to switch to a high-fat, high-protein, low-carbohydrate diet is not an appropriate one for the following reasons:

- Fats cannot be metabolized for energy anaerobically.
- If not closely monitored, high-fat diets can result in excess calories and increased body fat.
- Proteins rarely are used for energy in short running events.
- Proteins cannot be metabolized for energy anaerobically.
- Excess protein intake can lead to increased body fat.
- Carbohydrates are the only macronutrient that can be metabolized anaerobically.
- Low-carbohydrate diets do not restore muscle carbohydrate stores between training sessions.
- Low-carbohydrate diets combined with training can significantly reduce or deplete muscle carbohydrate stores, which are the sole source of energy for anaerobic metabolism.

Kay should be advised to follow a well-balanced daily diet consisting of adequate amounts of carbohydrates and moderate amounts of protein and fat.

Chapter 3

It appears that consuming a low-carbohydrate diet could be causing Meggan's fatigue. In an attempt to lose weight, Meggan mistakenly lowered her total carbohydrate intake to a level below the minimum requirements for health and endurance performance. Instead, she should focus on slightly lowering her total calorie intake while maintaining the percentage of total calories from carbohydrates at 60–65%. Carbohydrates are the main fuel for her sport; therefore, if Meggan's glycogen stores are low at the onset of a soccer session, she will fatigue quickly.

Second, as an alternative to a sports beverage, Meggan chose to drink juice during practice. Juices typically have a carbohydrate concentration of 10–14%, which is well above the recommended range of 6–8%. Highly concentrated fluids consumed during exercise delay gastric emptying, thus affecting the absorption of fluids and carbohydrates into the bloodstream; they can also cause gastrointestinal cramping, diarrhea, and nausea. Meggan should experiment with various flavors and brands of sports drinks, supplying 6–8% carbohydrates, to discover one that tastes appealing and digests well. Meggan's endurance and performance will be positively affected by consuming an appropriate amount of fluids and carbohydrates during her soccer practices and competitions.

Chapter 4

Because of the extremely cold water temperature of the English Channel, it would behoove Shelley to gain a small amount of fat weight to protect and insulate her body during the swim. However, to prevent a decline in her marathon performance, Shelley should gain a small amount of weight gradually over the upcoming year. To gain weight, Shelley will need to consume more calories than she expends daily. To gain weight gradually and in a healthy way, she should increase her calories by only about 100–200 calories a day through the consumption of nutrient-dense foods. Shelley should be deterred from eating candy bars, chips, and sodas to obtain her extra calories. Calorie-dense and nutrient-dense foods that are rich in unsaturated fats such as nuts, seeds, olives,

and avocados, as well as other low-fat foods such as fruit juices, thick breads, and low-fat milk/yogurt shakes are excellent choices.

As with all sports, a small amount of fat can be included in her preswim meal for flavor and satiety. Minimal amounts of fat should be consumed during the channel swim to prevent gastrointestinal distress; however, if practiced and tolerated during training, a small amount of fat can be consumed to prevent flavor fatigue from the sweet foods and beverages traditionally consumed while swimming. Fat should also be kept to a minimum after the swim to leave plenty of room in the postswim meal for carbohydrates and proteins.

Chapter 5

Based on what Jamar has revealed about his diet, it appears that he could be consuming excessive amounts of protein. To confirm this suspicion, a calculation of his daily protein needs and an estimation of his current protein intake should be determined.

For athletes with the goal of gaining weight, 1.6 to 2.0 grams of protein per kilogram of body weight daily are recommended. Jamar weighs 175 pounds, which is approximately 80 kilograms; therefore, his protein requirements range from approximately 128–160 grams of protein per day. Based on his diet recall, Jamar is consuming approximately 160 grams of protein just from his snacks and protein supplements. When additionally accounting for his protein intake at breakfast, lunch, and dinner, the suspicion that he is overconsuming protein is confirmed.

It should be explained to Jamar that consuming protein above daily requirements does not directly cause an increase in muscle mass; challenging the muscles through an appropriately planned training regimen coupled with consuming calories slightly above his daily needs from a balance of carbohydrates, proteins, and fats will ultimately lead to muscle mass gains. Jamar should also understand that protein not used by the body is converted to fat, which can be detrimental to his sport performance because increasing body fat can negatively affect his speed and quickness.

A meal plan should be developed for Jamar that provides adequate calories to support his current training regimen plus additional calories for gradual weight gain. The plan should focus on whole food sources of protein versus supplements, because whole foods will provide a variety of nutrients for a lower cost than supplements.

Chapter 6

The first step is to determine Roger's typical daily intake. Because his energy intake is below recommended levels for his high activity level, he needs to eat more to meet his energy requirements. Performing a quick diet history that includes questions about the frequency of fruit, vegetable, and grain intake is beneficial to help determine why vitamins A and C and folate are low. Asking about his daily routine, how he plans for meals and snacks, and if he carries food with him on campus will help establish his typical food intake and the best time during the day to add some nutrition breaks.

Roger should eat three to five meals and/or snacks daily. This will increase his energy intake, providing fuel for practices and adequate recovery nutrition. Because of his low intake of vitamins A and C and folate, Roger should strive for a minimum of five daily combined servings of fruits and vegetables, which will supply vitamins A and C, as well as folate. At least three servings of low-fat dairy products should be included in Roger's daily diet, especially milk and yogurt, which are vitamin A–fortified.

The following tools will help Roger to implement the preceding recommendations:

- A shopping list to stock his apartment with a variety of foods including fresh, frozen, or canned fruits and vegetables
- Suggestions for including more dairy products in his meals and snacks, such as yogurt parfaits, milk/yogurt smoothies, and creamy soups made with milk
- Advice on how to choose wisely at the training table meals that are provided to him at dinner by the team
- A list of local eateries with examples of entrées and side options that include a variety of foods, as well as general information about dining out healthfully to help him plan balanced meals when the team plays on the road

Chapter 7

The magnesium content of the sports beverage she is using could have caused the nausea, intestinal cramping, and diarrhea. In one 8 oz serving of the beverage, the magnesium content, as well as the other macro- and micronutrients, are present in appropriate amounts. However, considering that she consumed 100 oz of the beverage during the bike portion of the race, she actually drank 12.5 servings of the product within a couple of hours (100 oz ÷ 8 oz/serving = 12.5 servings). When multiplying all of the nutrients present in the beverage by 12.5, it becomes apparent that the magnesium content exceeds the daily upper limit of magnesium (12.5 servings × 30 mg of magnesium = 375 mg consumed during the race; the UL for magnesium is 350 mg). All of the other nutrients remain within reasonable limits in the quantities she consumed during the race. Side effects of high doses of magnesium include nausea and diarrhea.

In the future, Anne should consider using a different sports beverage with lower quantities of magnesium. The most important factors to consider when evaluating a sports beverage include the carbohydrate, sodium, and potassium content of the product. Other minerals included in the beverage formula should be in small amounts that will not exceed the daily upper limit when consumed in the quantities required to maintain proper hydration during long-duration activities.

Chapter 8

The athletes' complaints of fatigue, lethargy, and lightheadedness can stem from several things, including dehydration. The following suggestions would help the athletes make sure they are on the right track with their hydration protocol:

- Each athlete should perform a sweat test to ensure he is consuming enough fluid per hour during long practices.
- After determining their individual sweat rates, the athletes should bring their own water bottle to practice, knowing the total volume of the bottle. Therefore, the athletes can drink according to their sweat losses by measuring their intake by the number of water bottles consumed during practice.
- The athletes should take full advantage of the fluid breaks during practices. Based on the number of breaks per hour, athletes can calculate how much fluid should be consumed at each break to match their sweat losses.
- Challenging the beliefs of the coach regarding water versus sports beverages is not an easy task, and must be approached with respect and tact. A few options for discussing this topic with the coach include asking the coach for a more thorough explanation of when he or she will and will not permit the consumption of sports beverages

and why; inquiring about the athletic department's guidelines or rules regarding the provision of sports beverages for athletes; and asking for the opportunity to provide a sports beverage on a short-term basis to determine whether it will improve or hinder the team's performance.

Chapter 9

Jason should first focus on taking time to plan and prepare a healthful breakfast and lunch as well as several snacks. Eating regularly throughout the day will enable him to comfortably consume the total calories, carbohydrates, protein, and fat required to help him gain muscle mass, strength, and power. Through thoughtful snacking, he can also optimize the timing of his protein intake. Snacking will enable him to take advantage of the increases in protein assimilation that research has shown can be caused by protein intake prior to and after training.

Boron, ornithine, and arginine supplementation, as well as supplemental chromium picolinate, have not been shown to deliver on their claims as ergogenic aids for increasing muscle mass, strength, or power. Likewise, mega-dose vitamin and mineral supplements have not been shown to have an ergogenic effect. He would be better served to save some money by purchasing only a basic once-daily multivitamin/mineral tablet as a nutrition insurance policy.

Protein supplementation may not be needed, depending on his current protein intake. For athletes, protein intake of up to 2 g/kg of body weight has been shown to provide benefits above that provided by the RDA recommendation. Protein consumption above 2 g/kg of body weight will provide little additional benefit and possibly increase fat mass, which is not desirable for an athlete wanting to increase speed. Jason should focus on foods first, and then include moderate amounts of protein supplements if indicated.

Chapter 10

It would be helpful if Jennifer brought a 3-day food record to the initial consultation. This information can be used to understand Jennifer's usual dietary patterns and assess her basic nutrient intake. Jennifer should also be asked to complete a basic questionnaire that includes at least her demographic details, contact information, medical history, current med-

ications, and questions about dietary supplement use.

Assessing readiness to change can be determined by asking a few questions about past nutrition experiences and expectations of dietary changes needed to meet her current goals. Simply asking Jennifer, on a scale of 1 to 10, how likely she is to increase her calorie intake will help the dietitian determine Jennifer's level of motivation and readiness to make the effort needed to change dietary habits. With some experience working with athletes, it becomes fairly clear which individuals are ready for change and which ones are not. An athlete who is engaged in the conversation, asks questions about how to make changes, and is able to detail how the recommended changes will be implemented is one who is ready for behavior changes. It is important to assess readiness for change and gear the education provided to Jennifer according to her level of readiness.

Follow-up appointments should be scheduled approximately every 2–4 weeks for the first 2 months. This will allow enough time for Jennifer to make dietary changes to increase caloric intake that will help facilitate weight gain. Follow-up appointments should include a weight check. Body composition assessments could be conducted once every 3–4 months as a way of monitoring progress toward increasing muscle mass. Jennifer should be encouraged to keep food records each week and bring them to each appointment. The dietitian can review these to determine any needed changes in food intake. Follow-up appointments can conclude when an appropriate weight is reached and maintenance of that weight has occurred for several weeks.

Chapter 11

Accurate measures of height, weight, and body composition are important first steps in assessing Ian's weight. Of these measurements, body composition is the most important because it provides information on Ian's fat mass and lean mass. If Ian's body composition falls within the healthy range for teenage gymnasts, he may be encouraged to maintain his current weight. If his level of body fat is above the recommended ranges, Ian could attempt weight loss.

Assuming that Ian may benefit from some weight loss, a healthful eating plan should be developed. Resting metabolic rate and total energy expenditure should be calculated based on his body weight, level of activity, and duration and intensity of exercise. A low-fat, high-fiber eating plan that contains adequate carbohydrates and protein is recommended for any athlete performing high-intensity exercise daily. Protein is essential for maintenance of muscle mass, and carbohydrates will help replenish glycogen stores needed for daily exercise. A low-fat diet is recommended because fat is more calorically dense than carbohydrates or protein, thus providing an easy way to cut calories from the daily diet. Sample meal plans should be provided to help Ian translate nutrition recommendations into actual food selections.

Because Ian participates in a sport that places athletes at higher risk for disordered eating, an additional concern is that Ian could develop disordered eating patterns. He reports he wants to lose weight to improve sport performance. However, if the weight loss diet is taken too far, he could potentially develop an obsession about food intake and body weight. Ian should be monitored for his food intake and his feelings about his body, weight loss program, and sport performance. The coach, parents, and sports nutrition professional working with Ian on his weight loss plan need to be aware of the warning signs of eating disorders with athletes and watch for these signs in Ian.

Chapter 12

To determine Adam's daily calorie needs, use the energy estimation calculations presented in Table 12.1:

> For a 14-year-old male, REE = (17.5 × BW) + 651
>
> Adam's REE = (17.5 × 63.6 kg) + 651 = 1764 × activity factor (1.6–2.4)
>
> Adam's daily calorie needs = 2822–4234 calories per day

Adam does not need to increase his intake of ice cream, candy bars, and other "junk" foods to meet his calorie needs. It would be better for Adam's health and swimming performance to consume calorie- and nutrient-dense foods. Desserts and snack foods will certainly add calories, but very little nutrition.

Suggestions for calorie- and nutrient-dense foods from each food group include:

- Grains: Thick-cut, dense breads; hot whole grain cereals; granolas

- Fruits: Dried fruits, juices
- Vegetables: Avocados; olives; starchy vegetables such as potatoes, corn, peas, and squash
- Milk/alternatives: Fruited yogurts, cottage cheese, instant breakfast mixes added to low-fat milk
- Meat and beans/alternatives: Mixed nuts, seeds, nut butters

Adam was losing about 1 pound per week, which means his intake was deficient by approximately 500 calories per day. The first step is to determine how many calories Adam is currently eating. After establishing a baseline, compare his current intake to the recommendations calculated above (2822–4234 calories per day). Adam should strive to consume 500 extra calories a day from his baseline, aiming for a total intake within the calculated recommendations, to keep his weight stable.

Chapter 13

Robert is having trouble controlling his body weight because he is consuming more calories than he is expending. His information indicates that he has a sedentary office job, and his weight training and mile walks do not burn that many calories. Using Table 13.1 to estimate his total daily calories and using a low activity factor (i.e., 1.6 or 1.7), his total daily calories should be closer to the 2950 to 3150 range.

The most glaring concerns about his diet are its high-protein (i.e., 250 grams per day), high-fat, and low-carbohydrate content. His protein consumption is the equivalent of 3 grams per kilogram of body weight (250 grams / 82 kilograms = 3 grams/kilograms). This is well above the recommended 1.4 to 2.0 grams per kilogram of body weight for strength athletes. It is important to note that excess protein converts to fat in the body, and this could certainly be contributing to his body fat changes. Given that his caloric intake from protein is 1000 calories (250 grams × 4 kilocalories per gram = 1000 calories), or about 30% of his total calories, carbohydrate consumption is low; thus the fat composition of his diet is approximately 40%. Forty percent is higher than the recommended fat intake of 30–35% or less of total calories. Finally, low-carbohydrate intake is detrimental to strength/power athletes. Strength and power athletes rely on the phosphagen and anaerobic energy systems during training and competition. It is important for athletes to understand that carbohydrates are the only energy nutrient that can be metabolized anaerobically. As a result, carbohydrates should predominate fats and proteins in Robert's diet, not the reverse.

Chapter 14

Many factors could be at play with Tomas's fatigue in the game. He is a busy college student trying to make great grades to get accepted into medical school. He is on a nationally ranked hockey team and has added the pressure of maintaining a high caliber of competitiveness.

Some questions that should be asked of Tomas to determine whether his nutrition is a factor in his fatigue include:

- Have you changed your diet recently? Are you following any particular diet?
- Have you lost or gained weight recently?
- How many times per day do you eat?
- What is an example of 1 day's worth of meals and snacks?
- How much fluid on average do you consume daily? Has this amount changed recently?

To determine Tomas's calorie needs, use the energy calculations listed in Table 14.1:

Tomas is 20 years old and weighs 185 lbs
(185 lbs = 84 kg)

REE = (15.3 × BW) + 679

Tomas's REE = (15.3 × 84 kg) + 679 =
1964 = activity factor (1.6–2.4)

Tomas's daily calorie needs = 3142–4714

The answers to the preceding questions will help determine whether Tomas is meeting his daily calorie needs. If he has changed his diet recently, the nutrition coach must determine whether the amount of calories and/or types of nutrients have decreased. The 1-day dietary recall, along with interview questions to determine specific types of foods consumed, will provide this information. His fatigue could simply be related to negative energy balance. He may not be eating meals at regular times, could be skipping meals to study, or might not be preparing enough food to eat at his meals and snacks. Adequate fluid intake can be determined from an inquiry of his daily fluid choices as well as from the dietary recall. Many athletes can become severely fatigued if they are not meeting fluid requirements. Once the answers to these questions are compared to Tomas's

daily energy and fluid needs for his sport, the nutrition coach can help him modify his diet to prevent future fatigue.

Chapter 15

Ryan may be obtaining adequate levels of all nutrients if he is consuming a varied diet supplying sufficient daily calories. Because he is not well versed in planning and preparing vegetarian meals, he needs to ensure the inclusion of protein, calcium, and iron-rich foods. Protein can easily be consumed in adequate amounts without the consumption of animal products; however, it does take some planning. At least two servings of yogurt and calcium-fortified soy milk will help him meet both protein and calcium needs. Two to three servings from nonmeat protein sources such as dried beans, peas, lentils, veggie burgers, tofu, and other soy products will also contribute to his protein intake. Good sources of iron-rich nonmeat foods include fortified cereals and breads, spinach, broccoli, legumes, and some dried fruits.

The nutrition professional should ask several questions about Ryan's intake to help understand his regular eating patterns. A 24-hour recall or dietary assessment will provide information about his current intake and where he may be deficient in nutrients or energy. Asking how often he grocery shops, what he purchases, and inquiring about his food preparation knowledge is important for the development of an example grocery list and/or meal plan.

Education on how to improve nutrition intake can be provided to Ryan based on current dietary intake and information he gives about his shopping and cooking abilities. It is helpful to provide a grocery list of staple items to purchase that are high in protein, calcium, and iron as well as nutrient-dense. Suggestions for quick, easy vegetarian meals and cooking techniques will encourage Ryan to eat a greater variety of whole foods.

Chapter 16

Caroline has completed her undergraduate degree in dietetics, which provides assurance that she has a good balance of knowledge in a variety of nutrition therapy and education areas. As soon as she completes her internship she is eligible to take the Registered Dietitian exam. In most cases, the university sports dietitian job will require the RD credential and they will look for a dietitian with an advanced degree. Because Caroline will be finished with her master's degree in nutrition at the same time as her internship, she is likely to meet the minimum education requirements for the job. She may, however, lack experience when compared to other potential candidates. She did gain experience in the 2-week sports medicine rotation, but other dietitians applying for the job may have much more experience.

One thing that potentially sets Caroline apart from the other candidates is her research thesis related to body composition and physical activity. This shows that she has worked for the better part of 2 years on a research project that looks at two major parts of athletics—body composition and strength training. She can use this thesis as a topic of discussion in her application and cover letter and in an interview for the sports dietitian job. It is quite likely that her competitors for the position will not have this type of research experience.

If she is not offered the university sports dietitian job immediately following her internship, Caroline can do several things to help her compete for the next similar job opening. She should try to find a job where she will be able to work with athletes in some capacity on a regular basis. This could happen in a hospital dietitian position that has a rehabilitation or sports medicine clinic. She might even go back to the sports medicine clinic where she did her 2-week rotation and ask if they need a part-time RD to perform sports nutrition consulting. She needs to get the practical hours working with athletes and active people so that she will be eligible to obtain the board certification as a Specialist in Sports Dietetics (CSSD) credential. Completing the 1500 hours necessary in consultation with athletes and maintaining the RD credential for a minimum of 2 years will allow Caroline to take the CSSD exam. Once certified, she will have excellent credibility and the credential to show potential employers that she is knowledgeable and experienced in providing nutrition education and therapy to athletes.

APPENDIX B

The Gastrointestinal Tract

Mouth

In the mouth, food is broken up by chewing with the teeth and tongue. Saliva lubricates food and makes swallowing easier. Salivary amylase begins the digestion of starch. The mouth warms or cools the food so that it is closer to body temperature. When the food bolus (a fairly liquid ball of food) is ready, swallowing is consciously initiated.

Tongue

The tongue is a mobile mass of muscle that helps teeth tear food into pieces by forcing it against the bony palate. The tongue contains receptors for sweet, salty, sour, and bitter tastes. Umami, a fifth taste elicited by monosodium glutamate, is a meaty, savory sensation. Flavor is a complex combination of taste, smells (the nose has about 6 million olfactory receptor cells), physical sensations (e.g., spicy foods), and food texture.

Salivary glands

The three pairs of salivary glands produce saliva. The water in saliva helps dissolve food particles, facilitating taste sensations. The mucus in saliva lubricates food for swallowing and transport. Digestive enzymes in saliva begin breaking down foodstuffs. Salivary amylase begins the chemical breakdown of starches into simple sugars. Lingual lipase initiates the breakdown of fat. The mineral sodium and the enzyme lysozyme in the saliva act as disinfectants, destroying bacteria and other microorganisms in food.

Epiglottis

The epiglottis is a flap of tissue that acts as a valve during swallowing. It closes the entrance to the larynx and prevents food from entering the respiratory passages.

Trachea

This tube allow air to pass to and from the lungs.

Esophagus

The esophagus is the tube that connects the mouth to the stomach. Wavelike muscle action (peristalsis) moves food through the esophagus to the stomach. The upper one-third of the muscles of the esophagus are under voluntary control, the middle third are a mixture of voluntarily controlled muscle and automatically controlled smooth muscle, while the lower third is smooth muscle alone.

Inferior esophageal sphincter

The inferior esophageal sphincter is a muscular valve at the lower end of the esophagus. This control valve relaxes to allow food to pass into the stomach. When contracted, it prevents backflow (reflux) of stomach contents into the esophagus. A malfunction can cause painful esophageal reflux (heartburn), which can be so severe that it is mistaken for a heart attack.

Stomach

The upper baglike portion of the stomach acts as a hopper to receive and hold the food prior to deliv-

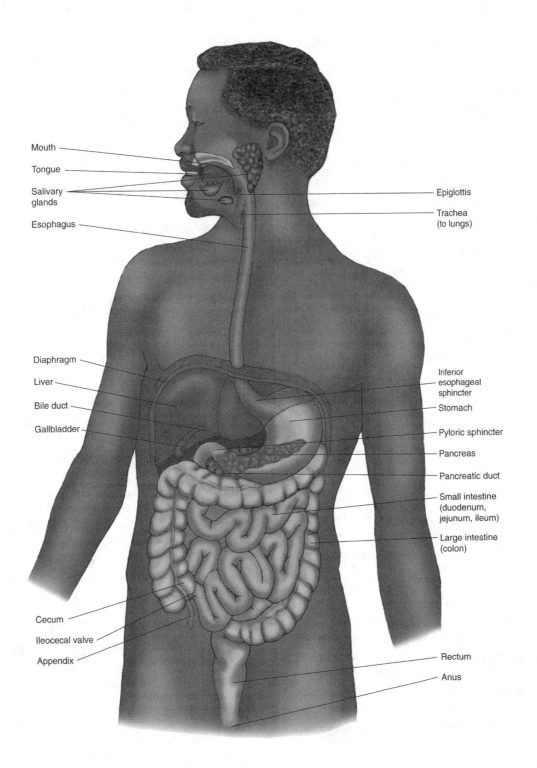

Mouth

Tongue

Salivary
glands

Esophagus

Epiglottis

Trachea
(to lungs)

Diaphragm

Liver

Bile duct

Gallbladder

Inferior
esophageal
sphincter

Stomach

Pyloric sphincter

Pancreas

Pancreatic duct

Small intestine
(duodenum,
jejunum, ileum)

Large intestine
(colon)

Cecum

Ileocecal valve

Appendix

Rectum

Anus

ery to the lower two-thirds. Three layers of smooth muscle surround this lower portion of the stomach. Muscular contractions churn the food, so the solids can ferment and mix with acids, fluid, and protein-splitting enzymes. The result is a sticky semi-liquid, called chyme, that is gradually released into the duodenum (the first part of the small intestine). Stomach acid halts the digestion of starch, but the stomach also produces gastric lipase, an enzyme that begins the digestion of fat.

Pyloric sphincter

The pyloric sphincter is a muscular valve that controls passage of chyme from the stomach to the small intestine. When contracted, it prevents backflow from the small intestine into the stomach.

Liver

The liver is the body's chemical factory and detoxification center. It has many functions in controlling metabolism and deactivating hormones, drugs, and toxins. It also produces bile—a mixture of bile salts, phospholipids, cholesterol, pigments, proteins, and inorganic ions such as sodium. The detergent-like action of bile emulsifies fat, facilitating fat digestion.

Gallbladder

The gallbladder stores and concentrates bile. The arrival of fatty food in the duodenum stimulates the release of the duodenal hormone CCK, which signals the gallbladder to contract. The bile is then released into the duodenum, where it aids fat digestion.

Bile duct

The bile duct carries bile from the gallbladder to the duodenum.

Pancreas

The pancreas is a complex gland that produces a pancreatic juice, rich in bicarbonate and enzymes. The pancreatic juice is released into the duodenum, where it does its work. Pancreatic amylase breaks down starch into maltose. Lipase splits fats into monoglycerides, fatty acids, and glycerol. The pancreatic proenzyme trypsinogen is converted to the enzyme trypsin. Trypsin splits polypeptides and proteins into amino acids. Bicarbonate produced by the pancreas neutralizes the acid chyme that enters the small intestine. In addition, the pancreas produces insulin and glucagon—hormones that have important roles in regulating carbohydrate metabolism and blood glucose.

Pancreatic duct

The pancreatic duct carries pancreatic juice from the pancreas to the duodenum.

Small intestine

The small intestine is a tube approximately 10 feet long that is divided into three parts: the duodenum (the first 10 to 12 inches), the jejunum (about 4 feet), and the ileum (about 5 feet). Whereas the duodenum is mainly responsible for breaking down food, the jejunum and ileum primarily deal with the absorption of food. The duodenum secretes mucus, enzymes, and hormones to aid digestion. Most digestion and absorption occur in the small intestine. Intestinal cells secrete disaccharidases and peptidases to help complete carbohydrate and protein digestion. The intestinal lining is highly folded to increase its surface area and is richly supplied with circulatory vessels that carry absorbed nutrients away in the blood and lymph. Undigested material is passed on to the large intestine.

Ileocecal valve (sphincter)

The ileocecal valve is the sphincter at the lower end of the small intestine. When open, it permits food residue to move from the small intestine to the large intestine. When closed, it prevents backflow from the large intestine.

Large intestine

The large intestine is made up of the appendix, cecum, colon, rectum, and anus. The colon is about 2.5 inches in diameter and about 4 feet long. In the large intestine, bacteria break down dietary fiber and other undigested carbohydrates, releasing acids, and gas. The large intestine absorbs water and minerals while dehydrating and processing the remaining undigested material into solid feces. The colon walls secrete a viscous mucus to help lubricate and mold the feces. This mucus also helps protect the colon wall from mechanical damage.

Appendix

The appendix is a fingerlike appendage attached to the cecum, the first part of the colon. The appendix has no known function.

Cecum

The cecum is the pouch-like beginning of the large intestine. The small intestine's ileum empties into the cecum.

Rectum

The rectum stores waste prior to elimination.

Anus

The anal sphincter holds the rectum closed. Either voluntary or involuntary control may open it to allow elimination.

Major Metabolic Pathways

- Glycolysis
- Beta Oxidation Pathway
- Citric Acid Cycle
- Electron Transport Chain
- Urea Cycle

Glycolysis

Glycolysis is the first step in metabolizing glucose and other monosaccharides for energy. Unlike the reaction that converts blood glucose to glucose 6-phosphate, the reaction that converts glucose from glycogen to glucose 6-phosphate does not require ATP. Thus the glycolysis of glucose from glycogen directly yields 3 ATP as compared to the 2 ATP from blood glucose. Additional ATP is produced from glycolytic NADH in the electron transport chain.

The reactions that convert fructose to fructose 6-phosphate require ATP, so fructose produces the same amount of ATP as blood glucose. The same is true for galactose, which enters at glucose 6-phosphate.

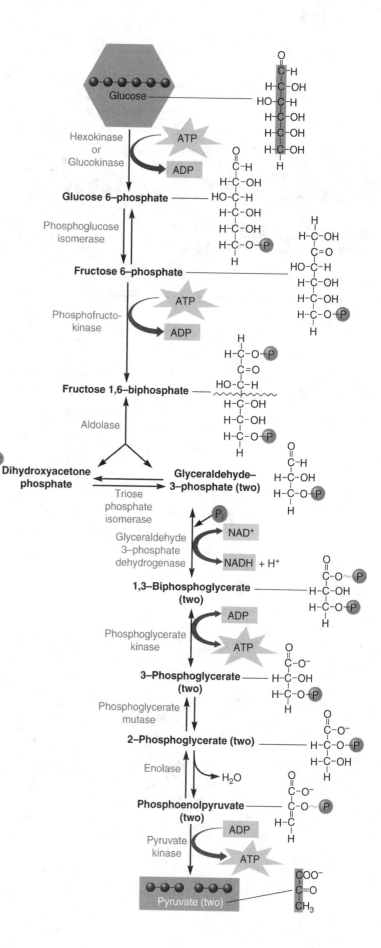

Beta Oxidation Pathway

Beta-oxidation reactions repeatedly clip the two-carbon end off a fatty acid until it is degraded entirely. Beta-oxidation of 18-carbon stearic acid produces 9 acetyl CoA, 8 FADH$_2$, and 8 NADH.

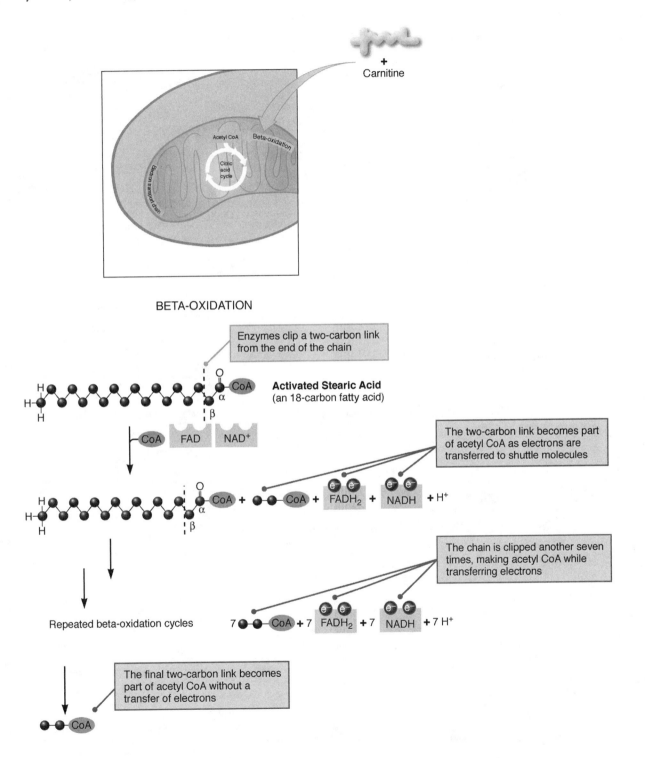

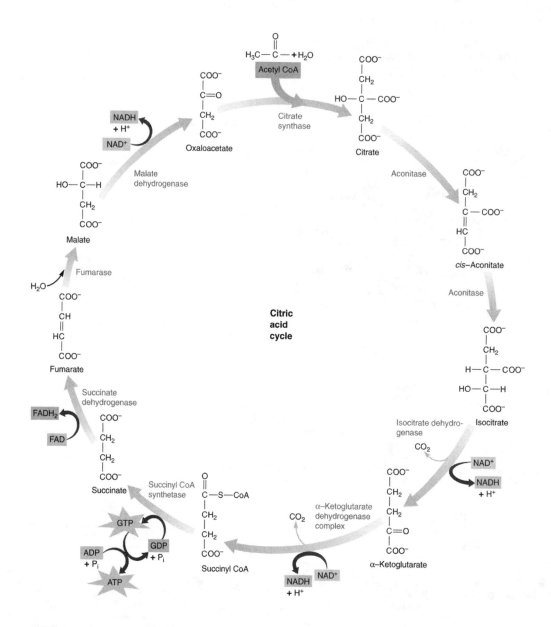

Electron Transport Chain

(site of oxidative phosphorylation)

1. NADH: A pair of electrons from NADH enters the chain at complex I (NADH-Q reductase). The flow of electrons from NADH to ubiquinone leads to the pumping of 4 H^+ from the matrix to the intermembrane space. The flow of electrons from ubiquinone to cytochrome c through complex III (cytochrome reductase) pumps another 2 H^+ into the intermembrane space. As complex IV (cytochrome oxidase) catalyzes the transfer of electrons from cytochrome c to O_2, it pumps another 4 H^+. (Complex IV actually uses 4 electrons to produce 2 H_2O from a single O_2.) The transit of the NADH electron pair through the electron transport chain pumps a total of 10 H^+ into the intermembrane space. Each 3 H^+ returning to the matrix through the ATP synthase produces 1 ATP. Another H^+ is consumed in transporting ATP from the matrix to the cytosol. Thus the two electrons from NADH produce about 2.5 ATP (10 pumped / 4 = 2.5).

2. $FADH_2$: A pair of electrons from $FADH_2$ enter the chain at complex II (succinate-Q), which is the nonpumping complex. The flow of electrons from $FADH_2$ to ubiquinone does not pump any protons to the intermembrane space. The flow of electrons through complexes III and IV is the same as for NADH. Thus the transit of the two $FADH_2$ electrons through the electron transport chain pumps a total of 6 H^+ into the intermembrane space and produces about 1.5 ATP (6 / 4 = 1.5).

3. Cytosolic NADH: Glycolysis forms NADH in the cytosol, but the outer mitochondrial membrane is impervious to NADH. How can NADH deliver its electrons to the electron transport chain? NADH transfers its pair of electrons to special carriers that can cross the mitochondrial membrane. One carrier, glycerol 3-phosphate, shuttles the electrons to the matrix and delivers them to FAD, thereby forming $FADH_2$. This $FADH_2$ delivers the electrons to the chain where they form 1.5 ATP.

    In the heart and liver, malate shuttles the electrons from cytosolic NADH to the matrix. Malate crosses the mitochondrial membrane and delivers the electrons to NAD^+, thereby forming NADH inside the mitochondrion. This NADH delivers the electron pair to the chain where they form 2.5 ATP.

    Depending on the carrier, cytosolic NADH may produce 1.5 or 2.5 ATP.

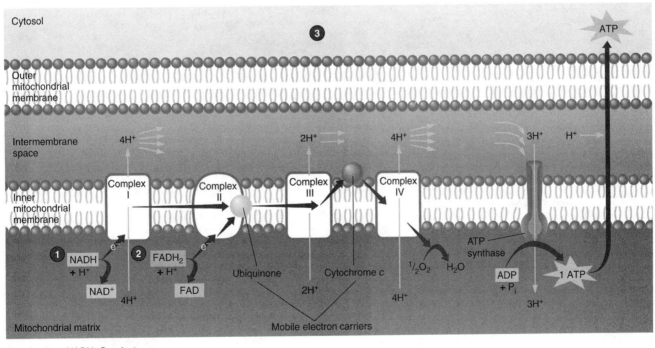

Complex I   NADH–Q reductase
Complex II   Succinate–Q reductase
Complex III   Cytochrome reductase
Complex IV   Cytochrome oxidase

Complexes I, III, and IV are proton (H^+) pumps. Complex II does not pump protons.
The three proton pumps are linked by the mobile electron carriers ubiquinone and cytochrome c.

Urea Cycle

Some NH_4^+ from the breakdown of amino acids is used for biosynthesis of nitrogen compounds. Excess NH_4^+ is converted to urea and excreted.

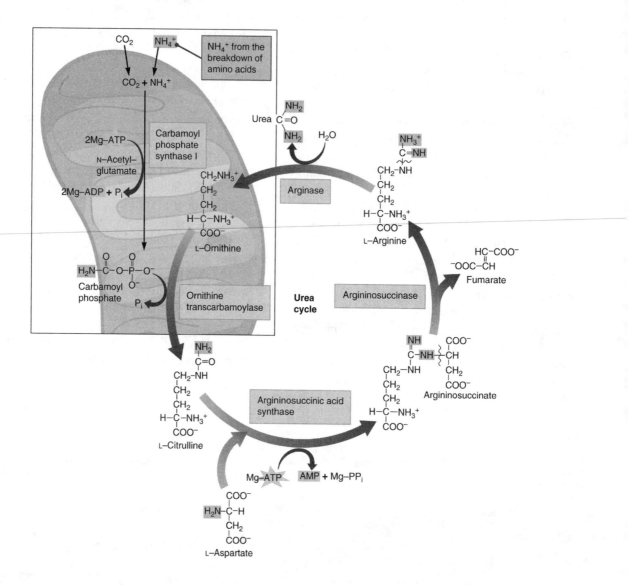

APPENDIX D

Calculations and Conversions

Energy from food

Total energy intake = sum of energy from macronutrients

grams carbohydrate × 4 kcal/g
grams protein × 4 kcal/g
grams fat × 9 kcal/g
grams alcohol × 7 kcal/g

Example

Carbohydrate	275 g × 4 kcal/g = 1100 kcal
Protein	64 g × 4 kcal/g = 256 kcal
Fat	60 g × 9 kcal/g = 540 kcal
Alcohol	15 g × 7 kcal/g = 105 kcal
Total Energy	2001 kcal

Calculating the percentage of calories for each

Carbohydrate	(1100 kcal / 2001 kcal) × 100 = 54.97% (55%)
Protein	(256 kcal / 2001 kcal) × 100 = 12.79% (13%)
Fat	(540 kcal / 2001 kcal) × 100 = 26.99% (27%)
Alcohol	(105 kcal / 2001 kcal) × 100 = 5.25% (5%)

1 kilocalorie = 4.184 kilojoules
1 kilojoule = 0.239 kilocalories

Body mass index (BMI)

U.S. formula

BMI = [weight in pounds / (height in inches)^2] × 703

Example

A 154-pound man is 5′8″ (68 inches) tall

BMI = [154 / (68 in × 68 in)] × 703
BMI = (154 / 4624) × 703
BMI = 23.41

Metric formula

BMI = weight in kilograms / [height in meters]^2 or BMI = [weight in kilograms / (height in cm)^2] × 10,000

Example

A 70-kg man is 1.75 meters tall

BMI = 70 kg / (1.75 m × 1.75 m)
BMI = 70 / 3.0625
BMI = 22.86

Metric prefixes

giga-	G	1,000,000,000
mega-	M	1,000,000
kilo-	k	1000
hecto-	h	100
deka-	da	10
deci-	d	0.1
centi-	c	0.01
milli-	m	0.001
micro-	μ	0.000001
nano-	n	0.000000001

Length: metric and U.S. equivalents

1 centimeter	0.3937 inch
1 decimeter	3.937 inches

1 foot	0.3048 meter
1 inch	2.54 centimeters
1 meter	39.37 inches
	1.094 yards
1 micron	0.001 millimeter
	0.00003937 inch
1 millimeter	0.03937 inch
1 yard	0.9144 meter

Food measurement conversions: U.S. to metric

Capacity

1/5 teaspoon	1 milliliter
1 teaspoon	5 milliliters
1 tablespoon	15 milliliters
1 fluid ounce	30 milliliters
1/5 cup	47 milliliters
1 cup	237 milliliters
2 cups (1 pint)	473 milliliters
4 cups (1 quart)	0.95 liter
4 quarts (1 gallon)	3.8 liters

Weight

1 ounce	28 grams
1 pound	454 grams

Food measurement conversions: metric to U.S.

Capacity

1 milliliter	1/5 teaspoon
5 milliliters	1 teaspoon
15 milliliters	1 tablespoon
100 milliliters	3.4 fluid oz
240 milliliters	1 cup
1 liter	34 fluid oz
	4.2 cups
	2.1 pints
	1.06 quarts
	0.26 gallon

Weight

1 gram	0.035 ounce
100 grams	3.5 ounces
500 grams	1.10 pounds
1 kilogram	2.205 pounds
	35 ounces

Conversion factors

To change	To	Multiply by
centimeters	inches	0.3937
centimeters	feet	0.03281
cubic feet	cubic meters	0.0283
cubic meters	cubic feet	35.3145
cubic meters	cubic yards	1.3079
cubic yards	cubic meters	0.7646
feet	meters	0.3048
gallons (U.S.)	liters	3.7853
grams	ounces (avdp)	0.0353
grams	pounds	0.002205
inches	millimeters	25.4000
inches	centimeters	2.5400
inches	meters	0.0254
kilograms	pounds	2.2046
liters	gallons (U.S.)	0.2642
liters	pints (dry)	1.8162
liters	pints (liquid)	2.1134
liters	quarts (dry)	0.9081
liters	quarts (liquid)	1.0567
meters	feet	3.2808
meters	yards	1.0936
millimeters	inches	0.0394
ounces (avdp)	grams	28.3495
ounces	pounds	0.0625
pints (dry)	liters	0.5506
pints (liquid)	liters	0.4732
pounds	kilograms	0.4536
pounds	ounces	16
quarts (dry)	liters	1.1012
quarts (liquid)	liters	0.9463

Growth and Body Mass Index Charts

A complete set of growth charts is available at www.cdc.gov/growthcharts. There are three sets, each with a different set of percentiles. Each set includes the following charts for girls and boys:

- Weight-for-age percentiles: birth to 36 months
- Length-for-age percentiles: birth to 36 months
- Weight-for-length percentiles: birth to 36 months

- Head circumference-for-age percentiles: birth to 36 months
- Weight-for-age percentiles: 2 to 20 years
- Stature-for-age percentiles: 2 to 20 years
- Weight-for-stature percentiles
- Body mass index-for-age percentiles: 2 to 20 years

2 to 20 years: Girls
Stature-for-Age and Weight-for-Age Percentiles

NAME _____

RECORD # _____

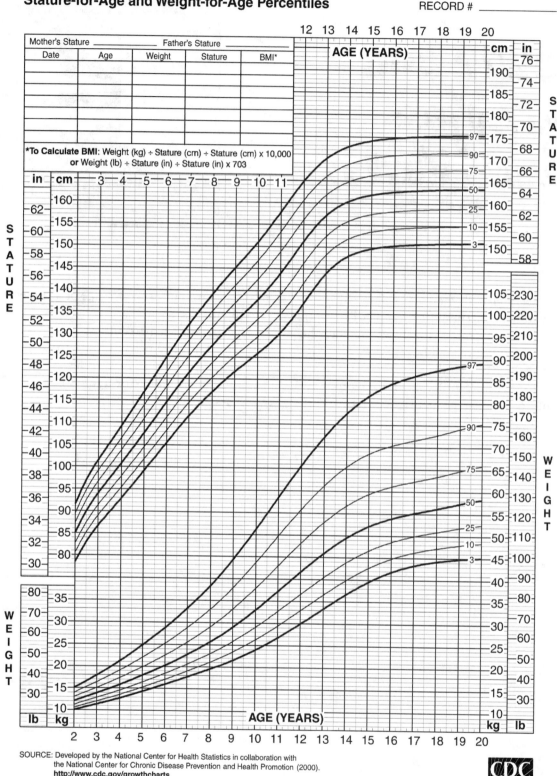

Mother's Stature _____		Father's Stature _____		
Date	Age	Weight	Stature	BMI*

*To Calculate BMI: Weight (kg) ÷ Stature (cm) ÷ Stature (cm) x 10,000
or Weight (lb) ÷ Stature (in) ÷ Stature (in) x 703

AGE (YEARS)

SOURCE: Developed by the National Center for Health Statistics in collaboration with
the National Center for Chronic Disease Prevention and Health Promotion (2000).
http://www.cdc.gov/growthcharts

CDC

2 to 20 years: Boys
Stature-for-Age and Weight-for-Age Percentiles

NAME _____

RECORD # _____

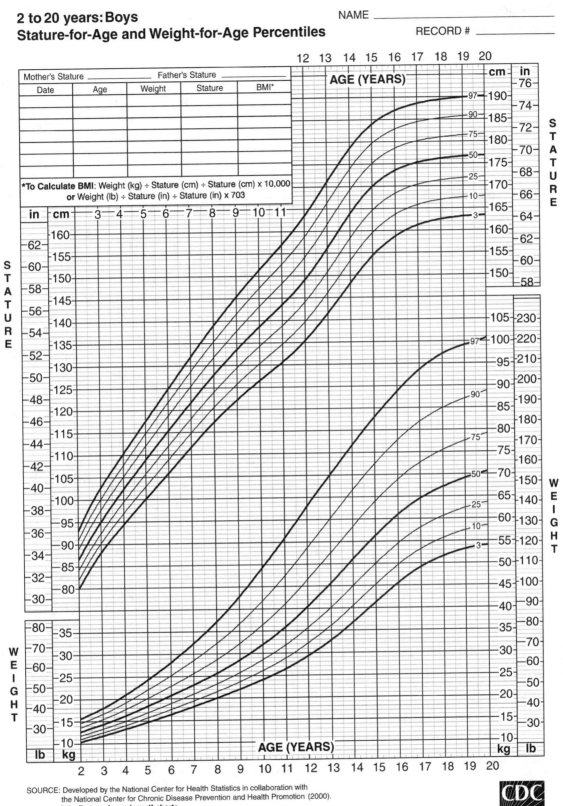

Mother's Stature		Father's Stature		
Date	Age	Weight	Stature	BMI*

*To Calculate BMI: Weight (kg) ÷ Stature (cm) ÷ Stature (cm) x 10,000
or Weight (lb) ÷ Stature (in) ÷ Stature (in) x 703

AGE (YEARS)

STATURE

WEIGHT

CDC

2 to 20 years: Girls
Body mass index-for-age percentiles

NAME _____

RECORD # _____

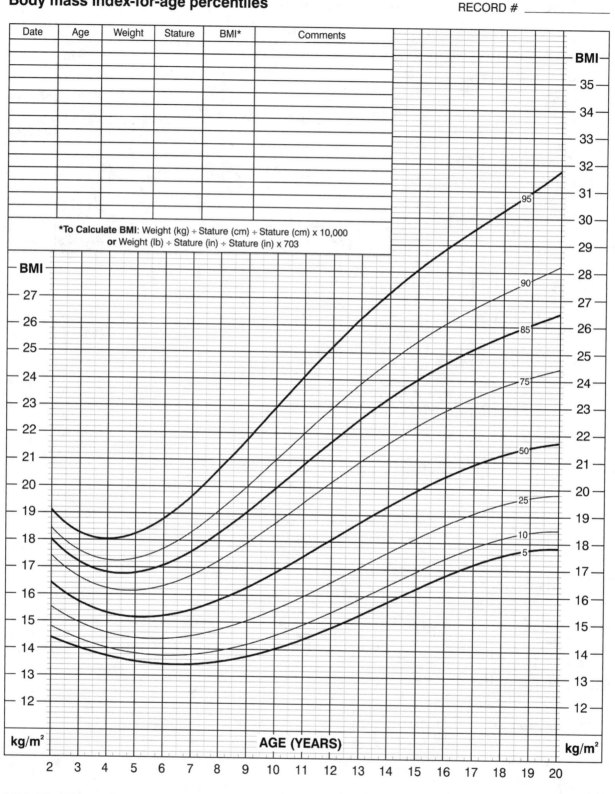

*To Calculate BMI: Weight (kg) ÷ Stature (cm) ÷ Stature (cm) x 10,000
or Weight (lb) ÷ Stature (in) ÷ Stature (in) x 703

Published May 30, 2000 (modified 10/16/00).
SOURCE: Developed by the National Center for Health Statistics in collaboration with
the National Center for Chronic Disease Prevention and Health Promotion (2000).
http://www.cdc.gov/growthcharts

SAFER · HEALTHIER · PEOPLE™

2 to 20 years: Boys
Body mass index-for-age percentiles

NAME _____

RECORD # _____

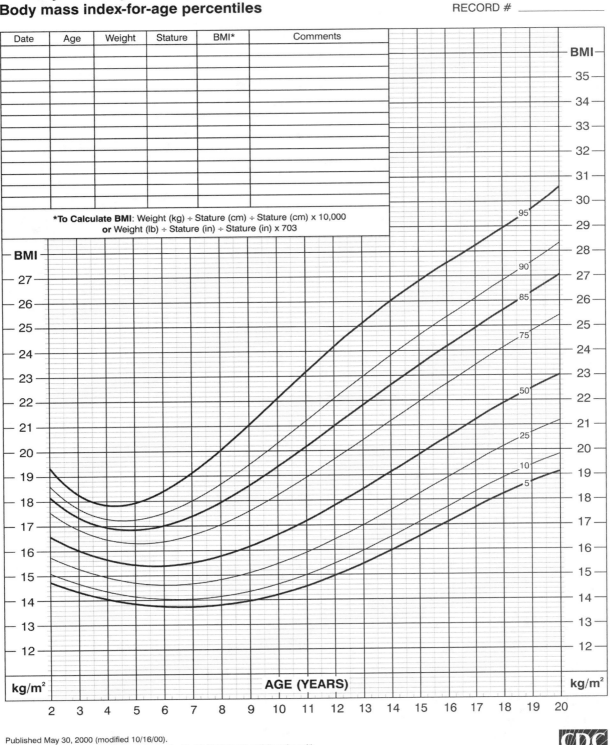

Date	Age	Weight	Stature	BMI*	Comments

*To Calculate BMI: Weight (kg) ÷ Stature (cm) ÷ Stature (cm) x 10,000
or Weight (lb) ÷ Stature (in) ÷ Stature (in) x 703

AGE (YEARS)

Published May 30, 2000 (modified 10/16/00).
SOURCE: Developed by the National Center for Health Statistics in collaboration with
the National Center for Chronic Disease Prevention and Health Promotion (2000).
http://www.cdc.gov/growthcharts

SAFER · HEALTHIER · PEOPLE™

Glossary

acceptable daily intake (ADI) The FDA-established safety limit for food additives and artificial sweeteners. The ADI is set at approximately 100 times below the level required for toxic or adverse effects.

acclimatization A process in which the body undergoes physiologic adjustments or adaptations to changes in environmental conditions such as altitude, temperature, and humidity. These physiologic changes enable the body to function better in the new climate.

active transport An energy-requiring means of cellular absorption in which substances are carried across membranes by protein molecules. Active transport is not dependent on concentration gradients.

adenosine diphosphate (ADP) A chemical compound that contains two phosphate groups attached to an adenosine molecule. ADP, when phosphorylated, becomes ATP.

adenosine monophosphate (AMP) A chemical compound that contains a single phosphate group attached to an adenosine molecule.

adenosine triphosphate (ATP) The molecule that serves as the body's direct source of energy for cellular work.

Adequate Intake (AI) A reference intake for nutrients that is used instead of the Recommended Dietary Allowance. When insufficient scientific evidence is available to calculate an Estimated Average Requirement (EAR), then an AI is used. Similar to the EAR and the Recommended Dietary Allowance (RDA), the AI values are based on intake data of healthy individuals.

adipocyte A single fat cell.

aerobic power The rate of aerobic ATP production. It is usually represented by the fastest pace or rate of physical activity an athlete can sustain and is an indicator of cardiorespiratory fitness.

aerobic system The energy system that relies upon the presence of oxygen to make ATP. Of the three energy systems, it is the slowest at producing ATP but has an almost unending capacity to make ATP.

air displacement plethysmography A technique that measures the volume of air displaced by an object or body. In body composition assessment, air displacement plethysmography is used to determine the volume of the body so that the density of the body can be determined.

amenorrhea The absence or abnormal cessation of menstruation; defined as less than four cycles per year.

American Dietetic Association (ADA) Organization of over 70,000 dietetic practitioners that oversees dietetic accreditation and provides timely and accurate nutrition information to the public.

amino acid A molecule that serves as the basic building block for proteins. Amino acids are composed of atoms of carbon (C), hydrogen (H), oxygen (O), and nitrogen (N).

amino acid pool The collection of amino acids found in body fluids and tissues that is available for protein synthesis.

amylase A digestive enzyme that breaks down carbohydrates into simple sugars.

anabolic A metabolic process or activity that results in tissue repair or growth. An anabolic hormone or substance is one that stimulates anabolism.

anabolic agent A substance that enhances the body's ability to build tissue. In regard to sports, anabolic agents are typically those that lead to an increase in muscle mass by promoting protein synthesis.

anabolic pathway A metabolic pathway that requires energy and results in the formation of more complex molecules.

anaerobic A term used to describe a condition in which oxygen is not present.

anaerobic system (also known as anaerobic glycolysis) The energy system that has the capability to generate ATP in the absence of oxygen. The anaerobic system results in the formation of ATP and lactic acid.

anorexia athletica (AA) A subclinical condition in which individuals practice inappropriate eating behaviors and weight control methods to prevent weight gain and/or fat increases. Anorexia athletica does not meet the criteria for a clinically defined eating disorder, but the behaviors exhibited are on a continuum that could lead to the more severe clinically recognized eating disorders.

anorexia nervosa A clinical condition manifested by extreme fear of becoming obese, a distorted body image, and avoidance of food. Anorexia nervosa can be life-threatening and requires medical and psychiatric treatments.

anticatabolic A nutritional compound that slows the breakdown processes in the body (catabolism), thus tilting the metabolic balance toward increased tissue building (anabolism).

antioxidants Compounds that protect the body from highly reactive molecules known as free radicals.

appetite A psychological or emotional desire for food.

atherosclerosis The progressive narrowing of the lumens of arteries caused by fatty deposits on their interior walls. Over time, these fatty plaques can block blood supply to vital tissues, causing poor delivery of oxygen; complete blockage results in cell death.

ATP pool   The muscle cell's inventory of readily available ATP.

basal metabolic rate (BMR)   The minimum amount of energy required to sustain life in the waking state. BMR is usually measured in the laboratory under very rigorous conditions.

beta cells   Specialized cells within the pancreas that secrete the hormone insulin.

beta-oxidation   The first metabolic pathway of fat metabolism, which cleaves off two carbon molecules each time a fatty acid chain cycles through it.

bioelectrical impedance analysis (BIA)   A body composition assessment technique that measures the resistance to flow of an insensible electric current through the body; percent body fat is then calculated from these impedance measurements.

bioenergetics   The study of energy transfer within a biological system.

body mass index (BMI)   An indicator of nutritional status that is derived from height and weight measurements. Body mass index has also been used to provide a rough estimate of body composition even though the index does not account for the weight contributions from fat and muscle.

bone mineral mass (BMM)   The weight of the mineral content of bone.

bonking   A condition in which the endurance athlete experiences extreme fatigue and an inability to maintain the current level of activity. It is also known as "hitting the wall" and results when the body has depleted muscle and liver glycogen levels.

branched-chain amino acids (BCAA)   A group of amino acids whose carbon-side chain, unlike other amino acids, is branched. The branched-chain amino acids include leucine, isoleucine, and valine.

brush border disaccharidases   Digestive enzymes produced by cells of the intestinal wall that break disaccharides into simple sugars.

bulimia nervosa   A clinical condition characterized by repeated and uncontrolled food bingeing in which a large number of calories are consumed in a short period of time, followed by purging methods such as forced vomiting or use of laxatives or diuretics.

calcitriol   The active form of vitamin D in the body. It plays a vital role in calcium regulation and bone growth.

carbohydrate loading   A high-carbohydrate dietary plan commonly used by endurance athletes that is designed to engorge muscle cells with glycogen.

cardiac arrhythmia   A disturbance in the normal rhythmic pattern of heart activity. Severe arrhythmias can lead to sudden death.

cardiorespiratory endurance   The ability of the cardiovascular and respiratory systems to deliver blood and oxygen to working muscles, which in turn enables the working muscles to perform continuous exercise. It is an indicator of a person's aerobic or cardiovascular fitness.

carnitine   A compound that transports fatty acids from the cytosol into the mitochondria, where they undergo beta-oxidation.

carotenoids   A class of colorful phytochemicals that give plants and their fruit the deep colors of orange, red, and yellow. There are hundreds of different carotenoids; however, the ones most identified as vital to health include alpha- and beta-carotene, lycopene, lutein, zeaxanthin, and cryptoxanthin.

catabolic pathway   A metabolic pathway that degrades complex compounds into simpler ones and in the process gives off energy.

catabolism   A metabolic process or activity that results in tissue breakdown or destruction.

cell membrane   The membrane that makes up the outer boundary of a cell and separates the internal contents of the cell from the external substances.

Certified Diabetes Educator (CDE)   An allied health professional who has passed a rigorous certification exam documenting his or her advanced knowledge and skills related to dealing with diabetes mellitus.

chemical energy   Energy that is released as the bonds holding chemicals together are broken. In the human body the foods ingested provide chemical energy to make ATP, which is the ultimate source of chemical energy in the body.

cholecystokinin (CCK)   A hormone produced by cells of the small intestine that stimulates the release of bile salts and pancreatic enzymes.

chylomicron   A droplet made of resynthesized triglycerides wrapped in lipoproteins that is produced inside the intestinal cells. Chylomicrons are released from the intestinal cells and then pass into the lymphatic system.

CINAHL   The acronym used for the Cumulative Index to Nursing & Allied Health, which is a reference database that provides authoritative coverage of the literature related to nursing and allied health.

cis   A type of molecular configuration in which the atoms surrounding a double bond are arranged on the same side of the molecule. Most naturally occurring unsaturated fatty acids exist in the cis configuration.

citric acid cycle   One of the major metabolic pathways of the aerobic energy system. It is also known as the Krebs cycle or the tricarboxylic acid cycle. Its main role is to strip hydrogens off compounds passing through it.

coenzymes   An organic molecule, usually a B vitamin, that attaches to an enzyme and activates or increases its ability to catalyze metabolic reactions.

collagen   A fibrous protein found in connective tissues of the body such as tendons, ligaments, cartilage, bones, and teeth.

Commission on Accreditation for Dietetics Education (CADE)   Agency of the American Dietetic Association that oversees educational programs preparing students for careers in dietetics.

complementing proteins   A group of two or more incomplete protein foods that when eaten together provide the full complement of essential amino acids.

complete protein   A protein source that supplies the body with all of the essential amino acids in high amounts.

complex carbohydrate   A carbohydrate composed of two or more linked simple sugar molecules.

condensation   A chemical process that results in the formation of water molecules. Condensation occurs when peptide bonds are formed between amino acids.

conditionally essential amino acid   An amino acid that under normal conditions is not considered an essential amino acid, but because of unusual circumstances (e.g., severe illness) becomes essential because the body loses its ability to make it.

creatine kinase   The enzyme that catalyzes the reaction transferring phosphate from creatine phosphate to adenosine diphosphate to make ATP.

creatine monohydrate   A dietary supplement that can help improve an athlete's anaerobic strength and power by increasing levels of creatine phosphate in muscles.

creatine phosphate (CP)   A high-energy phosphate stored inside muscle cells.

crossover point   The point on an increasing continuum of exercise intensity where fats and carbohydrates each contribute 50% of the needed energy and beyond which carbohydrates become the predominant energy source.

cytoplasm   The interior of the cell. It includes the fluid and organelles that are enclosed within the cell membrane.

cytosol   The watery or fluid part of the cytoplasm.

deamination   The metabolic pathway that is responsible for removing the nitrogen or amine group from the carbon structure of amino acids.

defecation   The physical process of excreting feces from the rectum.

dehydration   A condition resulting from a negative water balance (i.e., water loss exceeds water intake).

denaturation   A process by which proteins lose their three-dimensional shape and as a consequence their enzymatic activity.

deoxyribonucleic acid (DNA)   The molecular compound that makes up the genetic material found within the nuclei of cells.

diabetes   A medical disease that is characterized by high blood glucose levels. Diabetes results when either the beta cells of the pancreas do not produce enough insulin or the body's tissues do not respond normally to insulin when it is produced.

Didactic Program in Dietetics   Core academic course requirements to obtain a 4-year degree in dietetics.

diet history   The most comprehensive form of dietary intake data collection. It involves an interview process that reviews recorded dietary intake, eating behaviors, recent and long-term habits of food consumption, and exercise patterns. A skilled and trained interviewer is needed to take the diet history.

dietary fiber   A complex carbohydrate obtained from plant sources that is not digestible by humans. Although dietary fiber provides no energy for cellular activity, it does help maintain a healthy digestive system, lower blood cholesterol levels, and regulate blood glucose levels.

Dietary Reference Intakes (DRI)   A newer way to quantify nutrient needs and excesses for healthy individuals. The DRI expands on the older Recommended Dietary Allowance (RDA) and takes into consideration other dietary quantities such as Estimated Average Requirement (EAR), Adequate Intake (AI), and Tolerable Upper Intake Level (UL).

dietary supplement   A product (other than tobacco) that is not intended to be used as a food or a sole item of a meal or diet. To be considered a dietary supplement, the product must contain one or more of the following dietary ingredients: vitamin, mineral, herb or other botanical, amino acid, dietary substance to supplement the diet by increasing the total dietary intake or concentrate, metabolite, constituent, extract, or combination of any of these ingredients.

Dietary Supplement Health and Education Act (DSHEA)   A legislative act passed in 1994 to help regulate the dietary supplement industry. DSHEA broadened the regulatory definition of dietary supplements and altered the federal government's oversight of supplement products.

digestion   The process of breaking down ingested foods into their basic units in preparation for absorption by the cells of the gastrointestinal tract.

diglyceride   A lipid that is composed of a glycerol molecule with two attached fatty acids.

dipeptide   A simple protein consisting of two amino acids linked via peptide bonds.

disaccharide   A simple carbohydrate that consists of two linked sugar molecules.

doping   The practice of enhancing performance through the use of foreign substances or other artificial means.

dual-energy X-ray absorptiometry (DEXA)   A method of body composition assessment that involves scanning the body using radiography technology to distinguish between fat and lean body tissue.

Eating Disorder–Not Otherwise Specified (EDNOS) An eating disorder that does not meet all the criteria needed for it to be diagnosed as either bulimia nervosa or anorexia nervosa but that meets enough of the diagnostic criteria to be labeled as a true eating disorder.

eicosanoids A group of localized, hormone-like substances produced from long-chain fatty acids.

electrolytes Positively or negatively charged ions found throughout the body. The body uses the electrolytes to establish ionically charged gradients across membranes in excitable tissues such as muscle and nerves so that they can generate electrical activity. The most well-known electrolytes are sodium (Na+), potassium (K+), and chloride (Cl–).

electron transport chain (ETC) The final metabolic pathway of the aerobic energy system. It is responsible for transferring hydrogens from one chemical to another and in the process making ATP and water.

emulsifier A substance that breaks lipids into very small globules so that they are more manageable in watery fluids.

endocytosis A means of cellular absorption in which substances are encircled by the cell membrane and internalized into the cell.

endurance athlete An athlete who participates in sports involving continuous activity (30 minutes to 4 hours, as defined in this chapter) involving large muscle groups.

energy balance A state in which energy intake is equal to energy expenditure.

energy continuum A continuum of activity levels spanning from lowest to maximum, with all points in between requiring slightly increasing rates of energy production.

energy nutrients Carbohydrates, proteins, and fats serve as the body's source of energy and are considered the energy nutrients.

enrichment The addition of vitamins and minerals to refined/processed products to increase their nutritional value.

enzymes A group of complex proteins whose function is to catalyze biochemical reactions in the body.

epiphysis A cartilaginous plate found near the ends of bones that enables bone to grow in length; also known as the growth plate.

ergogenic aid Anything that enhances a person's ability to perform work, or in the case of athletics, to perform better in sport.

esophagus The segment of the digestive system that connects the oral cavity to the stomach.

essential A nutrition descriptor referring to nutrients that must be obtained from the diet.

essential amino acid An amino acid that must be obtained from the diet because the body is unable to make it on its own.

essential body fat Fats found within the body that are essential to the normal structure and function of the body.

essential fatty acids Fatty acids that must be obtained from the diet. Linoleic acid and linolenic acid are considered essential fatty acids.

Estimated Average Requirement (EAR) The estimated daily intake level of a vitamin or mineral needed to meet the requirements, as defined by a specified indicator of adequacy, of half of the healthy individuals within a given life stage or gender group.

euhydration A state of fluid balance in which water loss has been replaced by adequate water intake.

eumenorrhea A term used to describe normal menstruation consisting of at least 10 menstrual cycles per year.

extracellular A term used to describe structures, fluids, or other substances found outside of the cell.

extracellular water Body water that is found outside of cells that make up the various tissues of the body. Examples of extracellular water are saliva, blood plasma, lymph, and any other watery fluids found in the body.

facilitated diffusion A means of cellular absorption in which protein carrier molecules are required to move substances across membranes driven only by differences in concentration gradient.

fat loading The dietary practice of eating a diet high in fats (i.e., >60% of total daily calories) 3 to 5 days prior to competition.

fat mass (FM) The portion of body composition that is fat. Fat mass includes both fat stored in the fat cells and essential body fat.

fat substitutes Artificial fats derived from carbohydrates, proteins, or fats that provide foods with the same texture and taste functions of fat but with fewer calories.

fat-free mass (FFM) The weight of all body substances except fat. Fat-free mass is primarily made up of organ weight and the skeletal muscles, including minerals, protein, and water.

fatigue A physical condition marked by the point in time at which the work output or performance cannot be maintained.

fat-soluble vitamins A group of vitamins that do not dissolve easily in water and require dietary fat for intestinal absorption and transport in the bloodstream. The fat-soluble vitamins are A, D, E, and K.

Federal Trade Commission (FTC) A government agency whose mission is to ensure truth in advertising on supplement labels, in print advertising, and in commercials, thereby preventing unfair competition and protecting consumers from unfair or deceptive practices in the marketplace.

female athlete triad A group of three interrelated conditions, typically diagnosed in young female athletes—disordered eating, menstrual irregularities, and osteopenia/osteoporosis.

flavin adenine dinucleotide (FAD) One of two electron carriers that is responsible for shuttling hydrogens from one metabolic step or pathway to another.

fluorosis A condition resulting from the overconsumption of fluoride that can lead to pitting and discoloration of the teeth and/or bone and joint problems.

Food and Drug Administration (FDA) The governing body responsible for ensuring the safety of foods sold in the United States. This includes oversight of the proper labeling of foods.

food frequency questionnaire A nutritional analysis survey tool that asks an athlete or client to record how often common foods are eaten on a daily, weekly, monthly, or even yearly basis.

food record The most common method for collecting food intake data. It requires the direct recording of all food and beverage intake over a 1-, 3-, or 7-day period. Documentation of intake should occur at the time of consumption or as soon as possible afterward to obtain the most accurate information.

fortification The process of adding vitamins or minerals to foods or beverages that did not originally contain them.

free fatty acids Compounds composed of long hydrogen-carbon chains that have a carboxyl group on one end and a methyl group at the other. Free fatty acids can be formed when a fatty acid is cleaved off of a triglyceride molecule.

free radicals Highly reactive molecules, usually containing oxygen, that have unpaired electrons in their outer shell. Because of their highly reactive nature, free radicals have been implicated as culprits in diseases ranging from cancer to cardiovascular disease.

fructose A simple sugar known for its sweet taste that is commonly found in fruits.

functional fiber Isolated, nondigestible carbohydrates that have beneficial physiological effects in humans.

galactose A simple sugar found in milk.

gastric lipase A fat-digesting enzyme secreted by cells of the stomach.

gastrointestinal tract (GI tract) The regions of the digestive system that include the stomach, small intestine, and large intestine.

gene A specific sequence of DNA found within cell nuclei that contains information on how to make enzymes or other proteins.

Generally Recognized as Safe (GRAS) Substances that have not been conclusively proven to be safe but are generally accepted by experts as being safe for human consumption and therefore can be added to foods by manufacturers.

gluconeogenesis The formation of glucose from noncarbohydrate sources such as proteins.

glucose One of the most commonly occurring simple sugars in nature. It is the carbohydrate that humans rely upon for cellular energy.

glucose transporters (GluT) Specialized membrane carrier proteins that are responsible for the active transport of glucose into muscle cells.

glycemic index (GI) An index for classifying carbohydrate foods based on how quickly they are digested and absorbed into the bloodstream. The more quickly blood glucose rises after ingestion, the higher the glycemic index.

glycemic load A way of assessing the overall glycemic effect of a diet based on both the glycemic index and the number of carbohydrates provided per serving for each food ingested.

glycerol A three-carbon molecule that makes up the backbone of mono-, di-, and triglycerides.

glycogen The storage form of carbohydrates in animal cells. Glycogen consists of intricately branched chains of linked glucose molecules.

glycolysis A metabolic pathway that is responsible for the breakdown of glucose. It is unique in that it can function with or without the presence of oxygen.

goiter A clinical condition resulting from iodine deficiency. Goiter causes enlargement of the thyroid gland and results in an observable enlargement of the lower neck.

good manufacturing practices (GMP) A set of quality control measures adopted by the United States Pharmacopeia that establishes guidelines for personnel, facilities design and cleanliness, equipment, testing, storage, production and process controls, yield, packaging, and shipping of products.

growth channel The normal height-to-weight growth pattern/relationship. It is used to assess a child's growth trends and to screen for any potential growth abnormalities.

growth hormone A hormone produced by the pituitary gland that results in the growth of many different tissues in the body, including skeletal muscle.

health claim A description placed on a food label that describes potential health benefits of a food or nutrient.

health history questionnaire A survey that includes a variety of questions about current health, past medical history, and other daily health and wellness topics. The information collected in the health history questionnaire about chronic diseases, current or past injuries, surgeries, and regular medications helps nutrition professionals make a thorough assessment of the athlete's needs and subsequently develop a sound nutritional program.

hematuria   The presence of hemoglobin or myoglobin in the urine. Hematuria is an indicator of hemolysis.

hemochromatosis   A clinical condition associated with the accumulation of iron in the body's tissues, particularly the liver, which can result in liver failure or cancer.

hemolysis   The breakdown of red blood cells in the body. This, in turn, results in the release of hemoglobin into body fluids.

high-quality protein   Source of protein that contains a full complement of all the essential amino acids, has extra amino acids that are available for nonessential amino acid synthesis, and has good digestibility.

hormone releaser   A substance or substances that stimulate an increased quantity and/or frequency of release of hormones within the body.

hunger   A physical cue such as gurgling or growling of the stomach that prompts an individual to eat.

hydrogenation   A chemical process in which hydrogen atoms are added to unsaturated fatty acids. Hydrogenation of fatty acids leads to the formation of trans fatty acids, which are a growing health concern in regard to cardiovascular disease.

hydrolysis   A chemical process that requires utilization of water to break the chemical bond between elements or molecules. Hydrolysis is required to break peptide bonds between amino acids.

hydrolyzed protein   A source of protein that is usually in supplement form and contains proteins that have undergone a predigestion process, breaking the more complex proteins into smaller di- and tripeptide complexes.

hydrophobic   Term used to describe molecules or compounds that are water-insoluble. Lipids are hydrophobic substances.

hyperaminoacidemia   A condition describing abnormally high levels of amino acids in the blood.

hypercalcemia   A clinical condition in which blood calcium levels are above normal.

hyperglycemia   An abnormally high blood glucose level; usually a feature of diabetes.

hyperhydration   A condition resulting from a positive water balance (i.e., water intake exceeds water loss).

hyperkeratosis   A clinical condition resulting from the overproduction of the skin protein known as keratin. Overproduction of keratin plugs skin follicles, thickens the skin surface, and causes skin to become bumpy and scaly. Vitamin A deficiency is related to hyperkeratosis.

hypoglycemia   A condition in which blood glucose levels fall below normal.

hyponatremia   Low blood sodium levels resulting from sodium deficiency and/or the intake of large volumes of water.

immediate energy system   The energy system composed of the high-energy phosphates ATP and creatine phosphate; as a result it is also known as the phosphagen system. Of the three energy systems, it is capable of producing ATP at the fastest rate.

inadvertent doping   A situation resulting from an athlete ingesting a dietary supplement that unbeknownst to him or her can result in a positive test for a banned substance.

incomplete protein   Sources of proteins that do not contain the full complement of essential amino acids.

inorganic   A descriptor given to a compound that does not contain carbon atoms in its molecular structure.

insensible perspiration   Loss of water from the body via seepage through tissues and then eventual evaporation into the air. It is labeled as insensible because, unlike sweating, the water loss via seepage through the skin or respiratory passageways occurs relatively slowly and thus goes unnoticed.

insoluble fiber   A type of nondigestible plant carbohydrate that does not dissolve in water. Insoluble fiber sources are primarily whole grain products, nuts, seeds, and some vegetables.

insulin   A hormone secreted by specialized cells within the pancreas that lowers blood glucose levels after snacking or meals.

international units (IU)   An outdated system used to measure vitamin activity.

intracellular   A term used to describe structures, fluids, or other substances found inside the cell.

intracellular water   Body water that is found inside the cells. Approximately 66% of the total amount of water in the body is located inside the cells.

iron deficiency anemia   A clinical condition commonly resulting from poor iron intake that affects the red blood cells and their ability to transport oxygen.

isomer   Compounds like unsaturated fats that may have the exact same molecular makeup as another compound but exist in a different geometric shape.

ketoacidosis   Acidification of the blood caused by a buildup of ketone bodies.

ketone bodies   Molecules that are formed from fat metabolic by-products. Ketone bodies are formed when insufficient carbohydrates are available for complete metabolizing of fats.

ketosis   A condition that arises from abnormally high levels of ketone bodies in the tissues and body fluids.

kilocalories (kcals)   The unit of measure for energy. It is the amount of heat energy required to raise the temperature of 1 liter of water 1 degree centigrade.

lactase   A digestive enzyme that breaks lactose into the simple sugars galactose and glucose.

lactose The disaccharide found in milk that is composed of the simple sugars glucose and galactose.

large intestine The terminal portion of the gastrointestinal tract that receives undigested, partially digested, and unabsorbed contents from the small intestine. It is in the large intestine that the formation of feces occurs. The large intestine consists of the colon, rectum, and anal canal.

lean body mass (LBM) The portion of a body's makeup that consists of fat-free mass plus the essential fats that comprise those tissues.

Licensed Dietitian (LD) or Licensed Dietitian Nutritionist (LDN) Dietitian who has obtained a state license to practice dietetics following the state-regulated practice guidelines.

limiting amino acid The essential amino acid that is in short supply is an incomplete protein source.

lingual lipase An enzyme for fat digestion that is secreted by cells located at the base of the tongue.

lipid peroxidation A chemical reaction in which unstable, highly reactive lipid molecules containing excess oxygen are formed.

lipids A class of organic compounds that is insoluble in water and greasy to the touch. Lipids are commonly referred to as fats and exist in the body primarily as triglycerides.

lipophilic Substances that are fat-soluble.

lipoprotein lipase A specialized enzyme that breaks down triglycerides into glycerol and free fatty acids.

lipoproteins Substances that transport lipids in the lymph and blood. These substances consist of a central core of triglycerides surrounded by a shell composed of proteins, phospholipids, and cholesterol. Various types of lipoproteins exist in the body and differ based on size, composition, and density.

macronutrients These include carbohydrates, proteins, and fats and are classified as such because they have caloric value and the body has a large daily need for them.

major minerals The minerals required by the body in amounts greater than 100 milligrams per day. The major minerals include calcium, phosphorus, magnesium, sodium, chloride, potassium, and sulfur.

maltase A digestive enzyme that breaks down maltose into two glucose molecules.

maltose A disaccharide made up of two linked molecules of glucose.

mastication The process of chewing.

medium-chain triglycerides (MCT) A glycerol molecule with three medium-chain fatty acids attached.

Medline The U.S. National Library of Medicine's premier bibliographic database that provides information from the following fields: medicine, nursing, dentistry, veterinary medicine, allied health, and preclinical sciences.

messenger ribonucleic acid (mRNA) A type of nucleic acid that carries the genetic instructions for protein synthesis from the cell nucleus to the ribosomes located in the cell cytoplasm.

metabolic factory The cellular enzymes, organelles, and metabolic pathways responsible for the production of energy within the cells.

metabolic pathways Sequentially organized metabolic reactions that are catalyzed by enzymes and result in the formation or breakdown of chemicals within the body.

metabolism The sum total of all the energy required to power cellular processes and activities.

micelles Tiny bubbles made up of monoglycerides and long-chain fatty acids that are wrapped in bile salts. Micelles help transport digested fats to the intestinal wall for absorption.

micronutrients Vitamins and minerals are classified as micronutrients because the body's daily requirements for these nutrients are small.

mitochrondrion A specialized cellular organelle responsible for the aerobic production of ATP within the cell.

monoglyceride A lipid composed of a glycerol molecule with one attached fatty acid.

monosaccharide A single sugar molecule. Monosaccharides are the building blocks for more complex carbohydrates.

monounsaturated fatty acid A fatty acid whose hydrocarbon chain contains one double bond.

muscle dysmorphia A type of distorted body image in which individuals have an intense and excessive preoccupation and/or dissatisfaction with body size and muscularity. Muscle dysmorphia is most prevalent in male body builders and weight lifters.

muscular endurance The ability of a muscle or group of muscles to repeatedly develop or maintain force without fatiguing.

negative energy balance A state in which the total calories consumed are fewer than the total calories expended. A negative energy balance will result in weight loss.

nicotinamide adenine dinucleotide (NAD) One of two electron carriers that is responsible for shuttling hydrogens from one metabolic step or pathway to another.

nitrogen balance A way of monitoring nitrogen status in the body. When dietary input of nitrogen (i.e., protein gain) equals the output of nitrogen (i.e., protein loss) then nitrogen balance has been achieved.

nonessential A nutrient descriptor referring to nutrients that can be made within the body.

nonessential amino acid A type of amino acid that can be made by the body from other amino acids or compounds and thus does not need to be supplied by diet.

nonessential body fat Fat found in adipose tissue. Nonessential body fat is also called "storage fat."

nonessential fatty acid   A fatty acid that can be made by the body and thus does not have to be consumed in the diet.

nutrient content claims   Nutrition-related claims on food labels that highlight certain characteristics of the food.

nutritionist   Individual who may or may not have the same background as a registered and/or licensed dietitian.

oligomenorrhea   A condition in which the female menstrual period is irregular, with cycles occurring only four to six times per year.

oligopeptide   A protein molecule made up of 4 to 10 amino acids that are linked via peptide bonds.

oligosaccharide   A complex carbohydrate made up of 3 to 10 linked simple sugars.

oral cavity   Another name for the mouth, which makes up the first segment of the gastrointestinal tract.

organelles   Specialized structures found inside cells that perform specific functions. For example, the mitochondria are organelles responsible for the aerobic production of energy for the cell.

osmolality   An indicator of the concentration of dissolved particles per kilogram of solvent (mOsm/kg). Osmolality affects the movement of water across membranes when the concentrations on either side of the membrane are different. A beverage with a high osmolality tends to draw water to it rather than be absorbed.

osmolarity   Similar to osmolality, it is an indicator of the concentration of dissolved particles per liter of a solvent (mOsm/L). The higher the osmolarity, the greater the tendency to attract water rather than be absorbed.

osteoporosis   A clinical condition that can result from inadequate calcium intake and is characterized by a significant decrease in bone mass. The result is weak bones that can be easily fractured.

outcome-oriented goal   The final outcome or end result that an athlete would like to achieve as a result of changing dietary habits. For example, a slightly overfat athlete may have an outcome-oriented goal of losing 3 pounds of body fat in 6 weeks. Outcome-oriented goals help guide the athlete and dietician to develop a nutrition plan, revise the plan as needed, and continue behavior change toward meeting the desired end result.

pancreatic amylase   An enzyme secreted by the pancreas into the duodenum that assists in the digestion of starches.

pancreatic lipase   A digestive enzyme secreted by the pancreas into the duodenum that breaks down triglycerides.

passive diffusion   A means of cellular absorption in which the movement of molecules through permeable cell membranes is driven only by differences in concentration gradient.

peptidases   A group of protein-digesting enzymes that are released from cells of the small intestine. Peptidases work on breaking the chemical bonds of short-chain proteins (i.e., three or fewer amino acids), thereby yielding single amino acids.

peptide bond   A type of chemical bond that links the amine group of one amino acid to the acid group of another amino acid when forming a protein.

percent body fat (PBF)   The amount of fat mass found on the body expressed as a percentage of total body weight.

phosphagen system   The energy system composed of the high-energy phosphates ATP and creatine phosphate. It is also known as the immediate energy system. Of the three energy systems, it is capable of producing ATP at the fastest rate.

phosphocreatine   A high-energy phosphate stored inside muscle cells. It is also known as creatine phosphate.

phospholipid   A type of lipid that consists of a glycerol backbone, two fatty acids, and a phosphate group. Phospholipids are derived from both plant and animal sources and are both water and fat soluble. Phospholipids constitute the cell membranes of tissues throughout the body.

photosynthesis   An energy-requiring process in which plants capture light energy from the sun and use the energy to combine carbon dioxide and water to form carbohydrates.

phytochemicals   A large class of biologically active plant chemicals that have been found to play a role in the maintenance of human health.

polyols   A class of food sweeteners that are found naturally in some plants but are not easily digested and thus yield fewer calories. Polyols, also known as sugar alcohols, include xylitol, sorbitol, and mannitol and often are added to sweeten products such as mints, candy, and gum.

polypeptide   A protein molecule made up of more than 10 amino acids that are linked via peptide bonds.

polysaccharide   A complex carbohydrate composed of 11 or more linked simple sugars. Starches and glycogen are examples of polysaccharides.

polyunsaturated fatty acid   A fatty acid whose hydrocarbon chain contains two or more double bonds.

positive energy balance   A state in which the total calories consumed are greater than the total daily calories expended. A positive energy balance will result in weight gain.

power   The ability of a muscle or group of muscles to generate force at high movement speeds. In other words, the more work performed per unit of time, the greater the power output of the muscle. Power is also known as speed-strength.

prediabetes   A condition in which blood glucose levels are elevated but are not high enough to meet the criteria for a diagnosis of diabetes.

process-oriented goal   An achievement based on following or complying with procedures designed to cause a specific outcome. Process-oriented goals are focused on the steps required to reach the desired outcome and not so much on the final outcome itself. For example, an athlete wishing to lose weight may formulate a process-oriented goal of training 30 minutes longer 4 days of the week. The end result is to lose weight, but the goal is to meet the additional exercise requirements.

prohormone   A molecule or substance that can be readily converted to a biologically active hormone.

proteases   A class of protein-digesting enzymes that break the chemical bonds holding amino acids together.

pyruvate   The end product of glycolysis.

reactive oxidative species (ROS)   Free radical molecules that contain oxygen in their molecular formula and that are formed during aerobic metabolism. Commonly occurring reactive oxidative species in the human include superoxidases, hydroxyl radicals, and peroxyl radicals.

Recommended Dietary Allowance (RDA)   The average daily dietary intake level that is sufficient to meet the nutrient requirements of the overwhelming majority (i.e., 98%) of a healthy population.

registered dietitian (RD)   Individual trained to provide food and nutrition information to the public and who has successfully passed the national registration examination for registered dietitians.

resting metabolic rate (RMR)   The minimum amount of energy required to meet the energy demands of the body while at rest. RMR is typically measured instead of BMR because it is only slightly higher than BMR and is determined under less rigorous conditions.

retinoids   A class of compounds that have chemical structures similar to vitamin A. Retinol, retinal, and retinoic acid are three active forms of vitamin A that belong to the retinoid family of compounds.

retinol activity equivalent (RAE)   A unit of measure of the vitamin A content in foods. One RAE equals 1 microgram of retinol.

ribosomes   Cellular organelles that are responsible for protein synthesis.

salivary glands   Glands of the mouth that produce and secrete saliva.

satiation   The feeling of fullness that accompanies food intake and signals the time to end a meal.

satiety   The feeling of fullness that maintains after a meal and helps determine intervals between meals.

saturated fatty acid   A fatty acid in which all hydrogen-binding sites are filled and thus no double bonds exist in its hydrocarbon chain.

secretin   A hormone released from the duodenum that stimulates the release of bicarbonate from the pancreas.

simple carbohydrate   A form of carbohydrate that exists as a monosaccharide or disaccharide.

simple sugars   Another name for simple carbohydrates. These are sugars that exist as single sugar molecules (i.e., monosaccharides) or two linked simple sugar molecules (i.e., disaccharides).

skinfold calipers   An instrument used to measure the thickness of skinfolds in millimeters.

small intestine   The portion of the gastrointestinal system where the bulk of digestion and absorption occurs. The small intestine is divided into three segments: duodenum, jejunum, and ileum.

social physique anxiety   A feeling of personal uneasiness or nervousness about how other people view or perceive the athlete's body shape or fatness level.

sodium bicarbonate   A chemical compound found in the blood that helps maintain the body's normal acid-base balance. Sodium bicarbonate is considered the blood's most potent chemical buffer.

soluble fiber   A type of indigestible plant carbohydrate that dissolves in water. Soluble fiber has been shown to help lower blood cholesterol levels in some individuals. Sources of soluble fiber are oats, barley, legumes, and some fruits and vegetables.

speed-strength   This term is synonymous with power.

SportDiscus   A reference database of citations, books, conference proceedings, dissertations, reports, monographs, journals, magazines, and newsletters covering information in the following areas: sports medicine, exercise physiology, biomechanics, psychology, training techniques, coaching, physical education, physical fitness, active living, recreation, history, facilities, and equipment.

sports anemia   A condition caused by the combination of intense training and poor protein intake; it results in reduced levels of hemoglobin in the blood.

Sports, Cardiovascular and Wellness Nutritionists (SCAN)   Dietetic practice group of nutrition professionals with expertise and skills in promoting the role of nutrition in physical performance, cardiovascular health, wellness, and disordered eating.

sports nutrition   A specialty area of study and practice within the field of nutrition.

starch   The major plant storage form of carbohydrates. Starch is composed of long chains of linked glucose molecules.

steady state exercise   Any level or intensity of physical activity in which the energy demand for ATP is met by the aerobic production of ATP.

steatorrhea An abnormal condition in which large amounts of fat are found in the feces.

sterols A category of lipids that possess carbon rings in their structure rather than carbon chains. Cholesterol is the most commonly known sterol.

stomach The distensible, pouch-like portion of the gastrointestinal system that receives foods from the esophagus. It has muscular walls that mechanically churn foods and assist in the digestive process. Ingested foods pass from the stomach into the duodenum.

strength The ability of a muscle or group of muscles to generate force. Strength is purely a measure of how much weight can be successfully lifted by an athlete. Strength is highly dependent on the amount of muscle tissue an athlete possesses.

sucrase A digestive enzyme that breaks down sucrose into glucose and fructose molecules.

sucrose A commonly consumed disaccharide also known as table sugar. It is composed of linked glucose and fructose molecules.

sweat glands Specialized glands located in the deep layer of the skin responsible for the production of sweat and its delivery to the surface of the skin for the purpose of evaporative cooling.

tapering A scheduled decrease in the volume and intensity of training 6 or more days prior to competition. The purpose is to allow for recovery from training and replenishment of glycogen stores in the liver and muscle.

team sport logistics The planning, implementation, and coordination of details in regard to team practice and competition. For example, nutrition logistics involve dietary considerations prior to, during, and after practice or competition, in addition to issues of food preparation, preservation, and/or when and where to eat while on the road.

team sports Sports in which two or more athletes work together on a common playing area to defeat an opposing group of competitors. Examples of team sports are football, baseball, hockey, soccer, and basketball.

thermic effect of activity (TEA) The amount of energy required to meet the energy demands of any physical activity.

thermic effect of food (TEF) The increase in energy expenditure associated with food consumption.

Tolerable Upper Intake Level (UL) The highest level of daily nutrient intake that poses no adverse health effects for almost all individuals in the general population.

total fiber The sum of dietary and functional fiber.

trace minerals Minerals required by the body in quantities less than 100 milligrams per day. The trace minerals include iron, zinc, chromium, fluoride, copper, manganese, iodine, molybdenum, and selenium.

trans A type of molecular configuration in which the atoms surrounding a double bond are arranged on opposite sides of the molecule. Trans fatty acids are not common in nature but are formed during the process of hydrogenation.

transcription The process of copying genetic information from a specific DNA sequence through the formation of messenger RNA.

transfer ribonucleic acid (tRNA) A type of ribonucleic acid that is responsible for delivering specific amino acids to the ribosome during production of protein.

translation The process in which proteins are produced by ribosomes as they read the genetic instructions found on messenger RNA.

Transtheoretical Model A conceptual model of how humans go about changing their behaviors. It involves six stages, each of which represents a different mind-set toward change. Knowing which change stage an athlete or client is in can be helpful in developing strategies for altering their health or nutrition behaviors.

triacylglycerols A category of lipids more commonly referred to as triglycerides (see triglyceride).

triglyceride A lipid that is composed of a glycerol molecule with three attached fatty acids.

tripeptide A protein molecule made up of three amino acids linked via peptide bonds.

24-hour dietary recall A method of collecting food intake information that requires the athlete to remember all foods and beverages consumed within the past day (i.e., 24 hours). Although not the most accurate way of collecting food intake information, it can provide an idea of an athlete's nutritional intake in the first consultation session if other types of food records are not available.

type 1 diabetes A type of diabetes in which the pancreas stops producing insulin. Type 1 diabetics require exogenous insulin injections to help maintain normal blood glucose levels.

type 2 diabetes A type of diabetes in which the pancreas still secretes insulin but the cells are not as responsive to it, resulting in elevated blood glucose levels. Individuals who are obese and over the age of 35 are at increased risk for this disease.

ultra-endurance athlete A subgroup of endurance athletes who engage in extremely long bouts of continuous activity lasting more than 4 hours. Ironman triathletes and ultra-marathoners are examples of this group of endurance athletes.

underwater weighing The gold standard of body composition determination that involves weighing a person while he or she is totally immersed in water.

United States Anti-Doping Agency (USADA) A national-level, nongovernmental organization that serves as an extension of the World Anti-Doping Agency. Its mission is to educate athletes about doping, reinforce the ideal of fair play, and sanction those who cheat.

United States Pharmacopeia (USP) A not-for-profit organization that establishes and verifies standards for the quality, purity, manufacturing practices, and ingredients in supplement products.

unsaturated fatty acid A fatty acid whose hydrocarbon chain contains one or more double bonds.

villi Small rod-shaped projections that cover the walls of the small intestine.

waist circumference A measure of abdominal girth taken at the narrowest part of the waist as viewed from the front.

waist-to-hip ratio A comparison of waist girth to hip girth that gives an indication of fat deposition patterns in the body.

water balance Term used to describe the body's state of hydration. If water intake equals water loss, then water balance has been achieved. If water loss exceeds water intake, then negative water balance results. The converse is positive water balance.

water intoxication A condition resulting from the excessive intake of water. The end result can be a clinical condition known as hyponatremia.

water-soluble vitamins A class of vitamins that dissolve in water and are easily transported in the blood. The water-soluble vitamins are the B vitamins, vitamin C, and choline.

weight cutting The practice of losing weight, usually in preparation for a competitive event in hopes of making a lower weight class and thus improving performance.

World Anti-Doping Agency (WADA) An international, nongovernmental organization whose mission is to foster a doping-free culture in sports. WADA was established in 1999 and is headquartered in Montreal, Canada.

Index

Fats, dietary, 98–127. *See also* Lipids
  absorption of, 34–36, 36*f*
  assimilation into body, 36–37, 37*f*
  breakdown, aerobic, 53, 54*f*
  calories from, 298–299
    athlete's goal for, 115
    in food, 113–115, 113*t*, 115*t*
    Percent Daily Value and, 114, 115*t*
  competitive performance and, 118–120, 120*f*
  definition of, 3, 100
  as energy source, 3
  food sources, 105*t*, 111–113, 111*t*, 112*t*
    healthful, at restaurants, 453*t*
    high, 448
    high-protein diets and, 140
  functions of, 3, 100
    as carriers, 102
    enhancement of sensory qualities of food, 102
  glycemic index and, 78
  health claims for, 16
  intake
    after exercise, 123, 123*t*
    during endurance activity, 378–379
    enhancement of sensory qualities of food, 102
    before exercise, 120–122, 122*t*
    overconsumption of, 109–110
    prior to exercise, recommendations for, 121–122
    recommendations for, 109–110
    for recovery from endurance activities, 379
    satiety level and, 102
    for team sport athletes, 448
    too high, 110–111
    too low, 110
  malabsorption, 35
  needs/requirements
    calculation, for endurance athlete, 378
    for endurance athletes, 376–378
    for master athletes, 483
    preexercise, 415
    for strength/power athletes, 414–415, 415*f*
    for team sport athletes, 438–441
    during training and competition, for strength/power athletes, 415
  Nutrition Coach scenario, 99, 512
  in oil group, 113, 113*t*
  percentage of calories from, on Nutrition Facts panel, 12–13
  RDA, 109
  saturated, on Nutrition Facts panel, 13
  storage, *vs.* carbohydrate storage, 101, 101*t*
  total, on Nutrition Facts panel, 13
  training effects, 118–120, 120*f*
  transport of, 35–36, 36*f*, 37*f*
  triglycerides (*See* Triglycerides)

  utilization during exercise, 119
  in weight loss diet, 335
Fat-soluble vitamins
  absorption of, 42, 102
  definition of, 156
  for endurance athletes, 377
  vitamin A (*See* Vitamin A)
  vitamin D (*See* Vitamin D)
  vitamin E (*See* Vitamin E)
  vitamin K (*See* Vitamin K)
Fat substitutes, 108–109, 108*t*
Fatty acids
  classification of, 34, 35*f*
  essential, 106
  hydrogenation of, 103
  increasing, preexercise, 120
  nonessential, 106
  production, 40*f*
  saturation level, 103, 104*f*
  structure, 102–103, 102*f*, 103*f*
FDA. *See* Food and Drug Administration
Federal Trade Commission (FTC), 265
Felodipine (Plendil), 486*t*
Female athletes
  eating disorders and, 346–347, 346*f*
  iron-deficiency anemia, 442
  iron requirements, age-related changes in, 484
  pregnant (*See* Pregnant athletes)
  sports at risk for eating disorder development, 343
  supplements and, 263
Female Athlete Screening Tool (FAST), 346
Female athlete triad, 195, 346–347, 346*f*
Ferritin, 205
FFM (fat-free mass), 321, 322
FFQ (food frequency questionnaire), 289, 291–292, 292*f*
Fiber, dietary
  bloat/flatulence and, 66–67
  cancer and, health claims for, 16
  colon cancer and, 69
  as complex carbohydrate, 65–66
  content, on Nutrition Facts panel, 14
  coronary heart disease risk and, 16
  definition of, 66
  functional, definition of, 66
  glycemic index and, 78
  health and, 69–71
  insoluble, 66
  intake, recommendations for, 66
  soluble, 16, 66
  total, definition of, 66
Fit Day, 295*t*
Fitness/wellness facilities, sports nutrition jobs in, 506
Flavin adenine dinucleotide (FAD), 52
Flavonoids, 183
Fluid. *See also* Water
  daily intake, 234
    for endurance athletes, 382

  recommendations for, 232–233, 232*t*
  intake during exercise
    amount of, 237
    for endurance athletes, 382–387
    gastric emptying and, 238–239
    guidelines for, 246, 249
    intestinal absorption and, 238–239
    Nutrition Coach scenario, 61, 512
    osmolality of fluid and, 242–243, 244*t*
    ounces needed per hour of exercise, 238
    session length and, 249
    temperature of fluid and, 243, 244*t*
    timing during session, 249
    during training/competitive events, 448
    types of fluids for, 240
  losses, 233
    beverages and, 233
    high-protein diets and, 234
    medications and, 234
  needs/requirements
    assessment of, 232–233, 232*t*
    calculation, for endurance athletes, 382
    daily and exercise-specific, 250*t*
    determination of, 238
    for endurance exercise recovery, 386
    for strength/power athletes, 417–420
  Nutrition Coach scenario, 223, 513–514
  preexercise intake, 87
  recommendations, for team sport athletes, 445–448
  for recovery, 249–251, 250*t*
    amount of fluid for, 249
    guidelines, 251
    types of fluid for, 249–250
  replacement, 237
Fluid balance, proteins and, 134–135
Fluid equivalents, determination of, 238
Fluid replacement beverages
  carbohydrate, 240, 374–375
  electrolytes in, 241–242, 244*t*
  protein in, 243, 244*t*
  taste of, 241, 244*t*
Fluoride
  deficiency, 211
  DRIs, 193*t*
  food sources, 211, 211*f*
  functions of, 211
  importance for athletes, 211
  RDA/AI, 211
  supplements, 211
  toxicity, 211–212, 212*f*
Fluorosis, 211–212, 212*f*
FM (fat mass), 320
Folate (folic acid)
  deficiency
    anemia of, 206*t*

Protein (Cont.)
  timing of, 151
  total energy intake and, 137
  for weight gain, 137–138, 352
  for weight loss, 137–138
  metabolism, carbohydrate intake and, 53–54, 55f
  needs/requirements
    age and, 139
    based on body weight, 136–137, 136t
    calculation, for endurance athlete, 378
    changes during pregnancy, 471t
    of endurance athletes, 370–375, 371t, 372t, 374f
    for master athletes, 483
    of pregnant athletes, 467–468
    for recovery from endurance activities, 374–375
    for strength/power athletes, 410–414, 411t
    for team sports athletes, 436–438, 438t
  nitrogen balance and, 135–136
  Nutrition Coach scenario, 129, 512
  optimal daily dose, for strength/power athletes, 410–411, 411t
  quality of, in supplements, 143–145, 143t, 144t
  during recovery
    for endurance athletes, 374–375
    for strength/power athletes, 413–414
    for team sport athletes, 438
  structure of, 130, 130f, 131–132, 132f
  supplements, 142–146, 411t
    cost of, 145, 145t
    performance enhancement and, 145
    powder/bars, 271t, 276t
    quality of protein in, 143, 143t, 144t
    risks from, 146
    Supplement Facts list, 144, 144t
  synthesis of, 41–42, 41f
  tissue content, water and, 224
  transport of, 39–42, 39f–41f
  types of, for preexercise, 147
  utilization
    intensity/duration of exercise and, 138
    training state/fitness level and, 138
  in weight loss diet for athletes, 334–335
Protein foods group
  carbohydrate-rich, 76, 76t
  fat content, 112, 112f
  protein content, 142, 142t
Provitamin A carotenoids, 175
Puberty, iron requirements during, 475
Public domain information, on nutrition, 285–286

PubMed, 278t
Pyloric sphincter, 520
Pyridoxal. See Vitamin B_6
Pyridoxamine. See Vitamin B_6
Pyridoxine. See Vitamin B_6
Pyruvate
  conversion to acetyl CoA, 52, 52f
  definition of, 52
  for endurance athletes, 275t

Race Across America, diet for Team 70+, 73
Radiation, for heat transfer, 225
RAE (retinol activity equivalent), 172, 173f
RAND report, on ephedrine alkaloids, 261, 262
Rapport, establishing for nutritional consultation, 299–300
RDAs. See Recommended Dietary Allowances
RDIs (reference daily intakes), 14t
RDs. See Registered dietitians
Reactive oxidative species (ROS), 180
Recipes
  badminton beans and rice, 141t
  baseball barbecue sandwiches, 112t
  berry soy smoothie, 185t
  black-eyed peas with Chinese greens, 167
  cross-country chicken parmesan, 142t
  goalie guacamole, 111t
  good-for-you greens, 493t
  handball hummus, 76t
  homemade veggie burger, 493t
  nutty black bean salad, 178
  poolside parfait, 196
  power-packed pregnancy burritos, 471
  roasted broccoli and cauliflower, 169
  salmon pepper salad, 185t
  soccer smoothie, 74t
  summertime salad, 203
  sunshine broccoli salad, 185t
  sweet potato fries, 214
  teriyaki tofu stir-fry, 199
  volleyball veggie dip, 112t
Recommended Dietary Allowances (RDAs)
  carbohydrates, 71
  definition of, 4, 5t
  in Dietary Reference Intake, 5, 296
  protein, 136
  of vitamins/minerals, 299
Recovery
  alcohol and, 481
  carbohydrates intake for, 90–92, 90f, 92t
    for strength/power athletes, 409–410
    for team sports athletes, 436
  from endurance sports
    carbohydrate intake during, 369–370

  fat intake and, 379
  fluids needs for, 386
  protein needs for, 374–375
  fat intake, 123, 123t
    for strength/power athletes, 415
    for team sport athletes, 440–441
  fluid intake, guidelines for, 251
  hydration status and, 249–251
  products for, 250–251
  protein intake, 374–375, 438
  supplements for, 250–251
Rectal temperature, dehydration and, 228, 228f
Rectum, 27, 520
Red blood cell count, 205
"Reduced," as nutrient content claims, 18
REE. See Resting energy expenditure
Reference daily intakes (RDI), 14t
Refined grain foods, 7
Registered dietitians (RDs)
  board certified as specialist in sport dietetics credential, 503
  board examination, 500, 502
  continuing education for, 502
  definition of, 500
  educational requirements, 500
  functions of, 285
  internship/experience for, 500
  internships, 501–502
  licensure, 286, 503–504
  referrals to, 504
  in sports nutrition, 501, 506–510
  undergraduate degree curriculum requirements, 500–501
  vs. nutritionist, 500
Rehydration, in strength/power sports, 418, 419t
Renfrew Centers and Foundation, 350t
RER (respiratory exchange ratio), 468
Research, in gaining practical sports nutrition experience, 505
Resistance training
  athletes (See Strength/power athletes)
  protein needs, during recovery, 413–414
  protein utilization and, 138
  for weight gain, 351–352
Respiratory exchange ratio (RER), 468
Restaurants
  meal options, for team sports athletes, 451–452, 453t
  vegetarian protein sources in, 490–491, 490f
Resting energy expenditure (REE)
  calculation, 298f, 330t
    for endurance athletes, 361, 361t
    for strength/power athletes, 400t, 499
    for team sport athletes, 429
  interpretation of, 297
Resting metabolic rate (RMR)
  definition of, 43

Photo Credits

Tolerable Upper Intake Levels (UL[1])

Life stage group	Vitamin A[2] (µg/d)	Vitamin D (µg/d)	Vitamin E[3,4] (mg/d)	Niacin[4] (mg/d)	Vitamin B$_6$ (mg/d)	Folate[4] (µg/d)	Vitamin C (mg/d)	Choline (g/d)	Calcium (g/d)	Phosphorus (g/d)	Magnesium[5] (mg/d)	Sodium (g/d)
Infants												
0-6 mo	600	25	ND[7]	ND	ND	ND	ND	ND	ND	ND	ND	ND
7-12 mo	600	25	ND	ND	ND	ND	ND	ND	ND	ND	ND	ND
Children												
1-3 y	600	50	200	10	30	300	400	1.0	2.5	3	65	1.5
4-8 y	900	50	300	15	40	400	650	1.0	2.5	3	110	1.9
Males, females												
9-13 y	1,700	50	600	20	60	600	1,200	2.0	2.5	4	350	2.2
14-18 y	2,800	50	800	30	80	800	1,800	3.0	2.5	4	350	2.3
19-70 y	3,000	50	1,000	35	100	1,000	2,000	3.5	2.5	4	350	2.3
>70 y	3,000	50	1,000	35	100	1,000	2,000	3.5	2.5	3	350	2.3
Pregnancy												
≤18 y	2,800	50	800	30	80	800	1,800	3.0	2.5	3.5	350	2.3
19-50 y	3,000	50	1,000	35	100	1,000	2,000	3.5	2.5	3.5	350	2.3
Lactation												
≤18 y	2,800	50	800	30	80	800	1,800	3.0	2.5	4	350	2.3
19-50 y	3,000	50	1,000	35	100	1,000	2,000	3.5	2.5	4	350	2.3

Life stage group	Iron (mg/d)	Zinc (mg/d)	Selenium (µg/d)	Iodine (µg/d)	Copper (µg/d)	Manganese (mg/d)	Fluoride (mg/d)	Molybdenum (µg/d)	Boron (mg/d)	Nickel (mg/d)	Vanadium[6] (mg/d)	Chloride (g/d)
Infants												
0-6 mo	40	4	45	ND	ND	ND	0.7	ND	ND	ND	ND	ND
7-12 mo	40	5	60	ND	ND	ND	0.9	ND	ND	ND	ND	ND
Children												
1-3 y	40	7	90	200	1,000	2	1.3	300	3	0.2	ND	2.3
4-8 y	40	12	150	300	3,000	3	2.2	600	6	0.3	ND	2.9
Males, females												
9-13 y	40	23	280	600	5,000	6	10	1,100	11	0.6	ND	3.4
14-18 y	45	34	400	900	8,000	9	10	1,700	17	1.0	ND	3.6
19-70 y	45	40	400	1,100	10,000	11	10	2,000	20	1.0	1.8	3.6
>70 y	45	40	400	1,100	10,000	11	10	2,000	20	1.0	1.8	3.6
Pregnancy												
≤18 y	45	34	400	900	8,000	9	10	1,700	17	1.0	ND	3.6
19-50 y	45	40	400	1,100	10,000	11	10	2,000	20	1.0	ND	3.6
Lactation												
≤18 y	45	34	400	900	8,000	9	10	1,700	17	1.0	ND	3.6
19-50 y	45	40	400	1,100	10,000	11	10	2,000	20	1.0	ND	3.6

[1]UL = The maximum level of daily nutrient intake that is likely to pose no risk of adverse effects. Unless otherwise specified, the UL represents total intake from food, water, and supplements. Due to lack of suitable data, ULs could not be established for vitamin K, thiamin, riboflavin, vitamin B$_{12}$, pantothenic acid, biotin, or carotenoids. In the absence of ULs, extra caution may be warranted in consuming levels above recommended intakes.

[2]As preformed vitamin A (retinol) only.

[3]As α-tocopherol; applies to any form of supplemental α-tocopherol.

[4]The ULs for vitamin E, niacin, and folate apply to synthetic forms obtained from supplements, fortified foods, or a combination of the two.

[5]The ULs for magnesium represent intake from a pharmacological agent only and do not include intake from food and water.

[6]Although vanadium in food has not been shown to cause adverse effects in humans, there is no justification for adding vanadium to food and vanadium supplements should be used with caution. The UL is based on adverse effects in laboratory animals and these data could be used to set a UL for adults but not children or adolescents.

[7]ND = Not determinable due to lack of data on adverse effects in this age group and concern with regard to lack of ability to handle excess amounts. Source of intake should be from food only to prevent high levels of intake.

Sources: Data compiled from *Dietary Reference Intakes for Calcium, Phosphorus, Magnesium, Vitamin D, and Fluoride.* Washington, DC: National Academies Press; 1997. *Dietary Reference Intakes for Thiamin, Riboflavin, Niacin, Vitamin B$_6$, Folate, Vitamin B$_{12}$, Pantothenic Acid, Biotin, and Choline.* Washington, DC: National Academies Press; 1998. *Dietary Reference Intakes for Vitamin C, Vitamin E, Selenium, and Carotenoids.* Washington, DC: National Academies Press; 2000. Institute of Medicine, Food and Nutrition Board. *Dietary Reference Intakes for Vitamin A, Vitamin K, Arsenic, Boron, Chromium, Copper, Iron, Manganese, Molybdenum, Nickel, Silicon, Vanadium, and Zinc.* Washington, DC: National Academies Press, 2000. *Dietary Reference Intakes for Water, Potassium, Sodium, Chloride, and Sulfate.* Washington, DC: National Academies Press; 2005. These reports may be accessed via http://nap.edu.

Daily Values for Food Labels

The Daily Values are standard values developed by the Food and Drug Administration (FDA) for use on food labels.

Nutrient	Amount
Protein[1]	50 g
Thiamin	1.5 mg
Riboflavin	1.7 mg
Niacin	20 mg
Pantothenic Acid	10 mg
Biotin	300 μg
Vitamin B₆	2 mg
Folate	400 μg
Vitamin B₁₂	6 μg
Vitamin C	60 mg
Vitamin A[2]	5,000 IU
Vitamin D[2]	400 IU
Vitamin E[2]	30 IU
Vitamin K	80 μg
Chloride	3,400 mg
Calcium	1,000 mg
Phosphorus	1,000 mg
Magnesium	400 mg
Iron	18 mg
Zinc	15 mg
Selenium	70 μg
Iodine	150 μg
Copper	2 mg
Manganese	2 mg
Chromium	120 μg
Molybdenum	75 μg

The Daily Values for protein vary for different groups of people: pregnant women, 60 g; nursing mothers, 65 g; infants under 1 year, 14 g; children 1 to 4 years, 16 g.

The Daily Values for fat-soluble vitamins are expressed in International Units (IU), an old system of measurement.

Food Component	Amount	Calculation Factors
Fat	65 g	30% of kcalories
Saturated fat	20 g	10% of kcalories
Cholesterol	300 mg	Same regardless of kcalories
Carbohydrate (total)	300 g	60% of kcalories
Fiber	25 g	11.5 g per 1000 kcalories
Protein	50 g	10% of kcalorine
Sodium	2,400 mg	Same regardless of kcalories
Potassium	3,500 mg	Same regardless of kcalories

NOTE: Daily Values were established for adults and children over 4 years old. The values for energy-yielding nutrients are based on 2,000 kcalories a day.

Dietary Reference Intakes (DRI) for Carbohydrates, Fiber, Fat, Fatty Acids, and Protein

Life stage group	Carbohydrate (g/d)	Fiber (g/d)	Fat (g/d)	Linoleic Acid (g/d)	α-Linolenic Acid (g/d)	Protein[1] (g/d)
Infants						
0-6 mo	60*	ND[2]	31*	4.4*	0.5*	9.1*
7-12 mo	95*	ND	30*	4.6*	0.5*	11
Children						
1-3 y	130	19*	ND	7*	0.7*	13
4-8 y	130	25*	ND	10*	0.9*	19
Males						
9-13 y	130	31*	ND	12*	1.2*	34
14-18 y	130	38*	ND	16*	1.6*	52
19-30 y	130	38*	ND	17*	1.6*	56
31-50 y	130	38*	ND	17*	1.6*	56
51-70 y	130	30*	ND	14*	1.6*	56
> 70 y	130	30*	ND	14*	1.6*	56
Females						
9-13 y	130	26*	ND	10*	1.0*	34
14-18 y	130	26*	ND	11*	1.1*	46
19-30 y	130	25*	ND	12*	1.1*	46
31-50 y	130	25*	ND	12*	1.1*	46
51-70 y	130	21*	ND	11*	1.1*	46
> 70 y	130	21*	ND	11*	1.1*	46
Pregnancy						
≤ 18 y	175	28*	ND	13*	1.4*	71
19-30 y	175	28*	ND	13*	1.4*	71
31-50 y	175	28*	ND	13*	1.4*	71
Lactation						
≤ 18 y	210	29*	ND	13*	1.3*	71
19-30 y	210	29*	ND	13*	1.3*	71
31-50 y	210	29*	ND	13*	1.3*	71

This table presents Recommended Dietary Allowances (RDA) and Adequate Intakes (AI).
An asterisk (*) indicates AI. RDAs and AIs may both be used as goals for individual intake.

[1]Based on 1.52 g/kg/day for infants 0-6 mo, 1.2 g/kg/day for infants 7-12 mo, 1.05 g/kg/day for 1-3 y, 0.95 g/kg/day for 4-13 y, 0.85 g/kg/day for 14-18 y, 0.8 g/kg/day for adults, and 1.3 g/kg/day for pregnant women (using pre-pregnancy weight) and lactating women.
[2]ND = Not determinable due to lack of data on adverse effects in this age group and concern with regard to lack of ability to handle excess amounts. Source of intake should be from food only to prevent high levels of intake.

Source: Data compiled from *Dietary Reference Intakes for Energy, Carbohydrate, Fiber, Fat, Fatty Acids, Cholesterol, Protein, and Amino Acids.* Food and Nutrition Board. Washington, DC: National Academies Press; 2005. This report may be accessed via http://nap.edu.